Praise for
The Motherly Guide to Becoming Mama

"During a time of renewed awareness of the need to improve maternal health and wellness, *The Motherly Guide to Becoming Mama* provides a resounding response. Mothers around the world deserve the guidance that this book offers: unconditional support and access to expert-backed, non-judgmental information. This book is the first of its kind to support the whole woman through the whole journey—from getting pregnant, to birth, postpartum, and beyond. The maternal wellness revolution has arrived."

CHRISTY TURLINGTON BURNS
FOUNDER, EVERY MOTHER COUNTS

"Motherly is leading the conversation about how pregnancy, birth, and postpartum transforms a woman's world—and *The Motherly Guide to Becoming Mama* is their greatest contribution yet. Women deserve all the support as their bodies, minds, and lives transform, and this book delivers it with so much heart."

KATRINA SCOTT
COFOUNDER, TONE IT UP

"*The Motherly Guide to Becoming Mama* is like having an entire birth team on your nightstand. So many of us are in our bodies, completely body illiterate and unaware of its complexity until we find ourselves trying to conceive and/or be pregnant. *Becoming Mama* gave me so much insight into all (and I do mean all) the layers of pregnancy. But more than that, it offers grace, empowerment, and support for however and wherever you find yourself on the becoming mama journey."

ANTHONIA AKITUNDE
FOUNDER AND EDITOR-IN-CHIEF, MATER MEA

"THE essential guide to pregnancy and birth is finally here. *The Motherly Guide to Becoming Mama* is the only book you need to get you through this adventure. It's woman-centered, warm, and informative . . . it's the book I wish I would've had, and the one I'm so excited for you to have."

NATALIE GORDON
FOUNDER AND CEO, BABYLIST

"This epic book is a cross between an encyclopedia and a wise aunt. In this thorough and comprehensive resource, the Motherly team offers equal doses of wisdom, love, and cold hard facts so that each new mother can develop the confidence that she desperately needs on her pregnancy and motherhood journey. A soulful and dependable guide for all women."

KIMBERLY ANN JOHNSON
AUTHOR OF *THE FOURTH TRIMESTER*

The Motherly Guide to

Becoming Mama

The Motherly Guide to
Becoming Mama

Redefining the Pregnancy, Birth, and Postpartum Journey

JILL KOZIOL *and* LIZ TENETY, FOUNDERS *of* MOTHERLY
with DIANA SPALDING, MSN, CNM

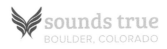

sounds true
BOULDER, COLORADO

Sounds True
Boulder, CO 80306

This book is not intended as a substitute for the medical
recommendations of health-care providers and mental health
professionals. Rather, it is intended to offer information to help the
reader collaborate with health-care providers and mental health
professionals in a mutual quest for optimal well-being. We advise readers
to carefully review and understand the ideas presented and to seek
the advice of a qualified professional before attempting to use them.

Published 2020

Cover design by Rachael Murray and Anne Hill
Book design by Karen Polaski
Cover and interior illustrations © 2020 Stepha Lawson

Printed in South Korea

Library of Congress Cataloging-in-Publication Data
Names: Spalding, Diana (Certified midwife), author. |
        Koziol, Jill, author. | Tenety, Liz, author.
Title: The motherly guide to becoming mama : redefining
        the pregnancy, birth, and postpartum journey / by
        Diana Spalding, Jill Koziol, and Liz Tenety.
Description: Boulder, CO : Sounds True, 2020. | Includes
        bibliographical references and index.
Identifiers: LCCN 2019012251 (print) | LCCN 2019015526 (ebook) |
        ISBN 9781683643555 (pbk.) | ISBN 9781683644286 (ebook)
Subjects: LCSH: Pregnancy—Popular works. | Childbirth—
        Popular works. | Prenatal care—Popular works.
Classification: LCC RG525 .S6464 2020 (print) | LCC
        RG525 (ebook) | DDC 618.2—dc23
LC record available at https://lccn.loc.gov/2019012251
LC ebook record available at https://lccn.loc.gov/2019015526

10 9 8 7 6 5 4 3 2 1

To the generations of
mothers whose strength,
sacrifice, tenacity, and
tenderness gave birth to
a better world for women
and children. We carry
your life's work within us.

Contents

Dear Mama

Pregnancy is about more than simply growing a baby. It's about becoming a mama.

These 9 months are also the season of your own metamorphosis because when a child is born, a mother is born, too. And that has been the most powerful revelation of our lives as women.

Motherhood changes you long before your baby is born. The changes begin with the decision to focus on your health, to start saving up for your first home, to accept a work promotion, or to connect more deeply with your partner—all with the goal of someday, somehow welcoming a little one into your life.

In each small moment on that journey—meeting with your medical provider, starting your prenatal vitamins, taking your first pregnancy test—you begin to transform into this new being: a mother.

Perhaps motherhood for you started with an unplanned pregnancy. Or perhaps motherhood has been a long-fought journey, full of incredible waiting, pain, or loss. Maybe your pregnancy experience is just like you anticipated. Or maybe it's nothing like you'd ever envisioned.

In many ways, pregnancy epitomizes the highs and lows of motherhood: the dreams and the despair, the magic and the ambiguity, the strength and the sacrifice, even the absurdity and the beauty. The discomfort of pregnancy, which can make it hard to sleep, is a bellwether of sleepless nights to come. The joy of a positive pregnancy test becomes a peek into the ecstasy of seeing your baby's face for the first time. The marks that pregnancy leaves on your body are a reminder of the permanent shift in your identity.

Motherhood will also mold you in unexpected, amazing ways, but becoming a mama doesn't mean leaving the woman you are behind. It means you have an opportunity to nurture, not lose, your true sense of self. You'll discover superpowers you never knew you had. You'll endure greater challenges than you've ever known. And you'll experience an indescribable love that will change your life.

We created *The Motherly Guide to Becoming Mama* to coach and inspire you through this season of transformation. It is the pregnancy book we wish we'd had when we first became mothers. It is the one pregnancy book focused on you—the pregnancy book women deserve.

This book won't bog you down with demands or give you more to be worried about or tell you what to do. (We promise!) Because the truth is, we don't know quite how your story will unfold. It's impossible to know exactly what to expect during *your* pregnancy; after all, you are your own amazing woman with unique dreams, experiences, and needs. Instead, we asked Diana Spalding, a certified nurse-midwife, pediatric nurse, Motherly's

Digital Education Editor, and mother of three (we *know*, we're impressed, too!) to write this book, drawing on her deep experience walking alongside women like you to help you feel confident during this time of massive change, to remind you of your strength, to give you the courage to face difficult choices, and to help you define—and redefine along the way—what becoming a mama means to you.

At Motherly, we want to be with you along this journey. We're so proud of the supportive, nonjudgmental community of women we've built together and are thrilled to bring their wisdom to your pregnancy. Every woman, every baby, every pregnancy is different, but mama, we know this is true: *You were made for this moment.*

You are powerful. You are capable. You are becoming a mama.

You've got this.

xo,

Jill + Liz

Founders of Motherly

Welcome, and
How to Use This Book

My heart is bursting for you.

Maybe you are already pregnant. Maybe this is your first baby, or maybe it's your fourth. Or perhaps you are not pregnant yet but have decided that it is time to start preparing for what comes next.

Whatever the reasons that inspired you to pick up this guide, you are on the verge of something tremendous. This is the start.

You are on your journey to *becoming mama*. And *becoming mama* is everything.

It is thrilling, blissful, scary, exhausting, empowering, confusing, and awe-inspiring—all in a single moment.

And it is a whole-self journey. This is not just something that happens in your uterus.

Becoming mama involves your whole body and mind, emotions, lifestyle, career, relationships, home, bank account, schedule, spirituality, worldview, and your heart. Oh, your heart. You will always be you, but you will never be the same.

And I am so deeply honored to begin this adventure with you.

My path to midwifery started when I was a little girl. I am the daughter of a midwife and have been surrounded by birth my entire life. I didn't play "normal" games as a child. Instead of tea parties with my dolls, I pretended to deliver their babies. The very first word I learned in Spanish was *empuja*—push. I read baby name books and made notes in the margins.

I've been obsessed with pregnancy and birth for a very long time.

In college, I studied anthropology. My fascination for the ways culture, health, and medicine influence each other led me to Central America, where I conducted public health research focusing on parasitic diseases.

Inspired to become a nurse, I moved to New York City for nursing school, and as it turned out, to fall in love with the guy who would become my husband and father of my kids. I spent 5 years working as a registered nurse on a pediatric hematology-oncology unit in the Bronx, learning just how strong children and their parents can truly be.

I then started midwifery school, which for me was a master's degree in nursing (more on the different paths to midwifery on page 91). I was trained and guided by wonderful midwives and was then hired to work with them.

Midwifery is not my job; it is my life. Being with women as they grow and give birth to their children is more of an honor than I can describe. I get invested in women's stories.

I still cry at every birth. Bearing witness as a woman crosses the threshold into motherhood fills me with joy, reverence, and hope that everything really will be okay.

Through it all, my most profound teachers have always been the women I have had the honor of working with. I learned very quickly that it was never going to be my job to tell women what they *needed*. My role is to provide information, evidence, and compassion and then to hold space for a woman as she finds her way to motherhood.

My way to motherhood started on a warm spring day—after 32 hours of labor—when we welcomed our daughter into our lives. Three years later, our middle guy joined us, and then in an unexpected plot twist, our youngest, another boy, came into the world a short 15 months later. And since we are all about birth stories here, I will share that they were all born vaginally in hospitals with midwives and with epidurals.

I am the founder of a motherhood wellness center called Gathered Birth in the suburbs of Philadelphia.

And now, in what still seems like a surreal dream, I get to work with Motherly and give birth to this book.

The Motherly Guide to Becoming Mama was inspired by what we saw as an overwhelming need to provide evidence-based, nonjudgmental nurturing to women when they need it most.

As I said, my job is not to tell you what matters: It is to listen to you and then walk alongside you accordingly. Therefore, to create this book, we started with you. We spoke to thousands of women in the Motherly community in order to understand what you needed this guide to be.

Here is what you told us: You are fiercely dedicated to your baby (who already exists or who will one day exist). You want to know everything about them, from the ways they develop through pregnancy and beyond, to how to create the best possible start in life for them.

You are also committed to staying true to yourself, to self-nurturing, and to thriving in the way that fills your soul.

And you do not believe that these two things are mutually exclusive.

You are part of a generation of women who believe that the love we have for our children and our own well-being can be woven together into a tapestry that radiates balance and love. Yet weaving that tapestry is hard.

Our lives often do not leave room for optimal self-care. Careers and relationships take work, sometimes sapping us of the energy we need to focus back on ourselves. We are often lacking the foundation of a strong and nearby village when we need support. Systemic racism, misogyny, and heteronormative expectations can leave us without a voice to stand up and say, "This is what I need," and to be heard. And the constant swirling of judgment, conflicting messages, and "shoulds" is exhausting and depleting.

But you have decided, despite the difficulties and the obstacles, that this is not the experience you want. You have decided that you will bring your baby into this world differently, and in doing so, become part of the radical movement of strong women making this world better for each other and for each other's babies.

You are redefining the pregnancy, birth, and postpartum journey. And Motherly is with you.

HOW THIS BOOK IS ORGANIZED

In part I of this guide, "Getting Pregnant," you will find chapters on preparing for pregnancy, conception through the many ways people grow their families, infertility struggles, and miscarriage—because loss can be a part of our stories, and you should not have to go through it alone. Lastly, I've guided you through how to decide where to give birth and who you'd like your care provider to be during your pregnancy and birth. I know it feels early, but these decisions can impact your prenatal care from the beginning, so it's important to start thinking about it now. That said, it is often possible to make changes during the course of your pregnancy, so return to these pages if you find that you'd like to switch birthing places or providers.

Part II, "Pregnancy Month by Month," guides you through each month of pregnancy. In these chapters, you'll find prompts to "pause and reflect" (because *oh, my goodness*, you are having a baby, and this is huge) and ways to bond with your growing baby.

You'll also see a list of symptoms that you may be feeling each month—but maybe not! Each woman experiences pregnancy differently. I've created a "Symptom Checker," which you'll find on page 429, that you can turn to at any time to learn more about what you're feeling and what you can do about it (remembering, of course, that your provider is always your point person for all things medical and symptom-related).

You'll read about what might happen at each month's prenatal appointment(s). Because pregnancy is a holistic adventure, each of the month-by-month chapters will give you information from a renowned team of experts. (Seriously, they are amazing. Check them out on page 535.) They'll share how to nourish and move your body for the specific time of pregnancy you are in, how to build strong relationships with your partner (if applicable) and village, and how to deal with potential changes at work as well as providing you with unique ways to consider finances, life plans, baby gear, and so much more.

And, I know you will be excited to start thinking ahead to birth and beyond, so starting in a few months you'll find cues to read ahead so you can envision and plan!

Part III, "Giving Birth," breaks the labor process into four distinct stages. Then, once you know what to anticipate during your labor, you'll find a chapter on coping techniques to help you rock your experience like the amazingly strong woman you are. I've also included full chapters on potential interventions and Cesarean birth. Giving birth is a story that will unfold as it moves forward; if your story involves interventions, you deserve to feel prepared and confident so that you can experience your birth with empowerment. Finally, with all this information to support you, you'll be guided through how to make your birth plan.

You also told us that you needed much more postpartum support: what to anticipate with your own healing after pregnancy and birth and how to care for this new little human being. So, it is my honor to guide you through this as well in part IV, "The Fourth Trimester."

Now this part is big: When we asked, you told us you felt very strongly that you did not want to spend every day worrying about all the possible complications, but you did want to have access to that info should it come up for you. We've got you!

Possible complications, details on most of the testing, and the "scary stuff" are in a separate section called "Tests and Complications," on page 451 (a few live within the main text). This way, you can choose how and when to see this information. From reading it all, to reading none of it, to just focusing on the things that apply to you, you are in charge here.

Where applicable, I've included notes for your partner (whether this is a significant other, friend, or family member) to help them through this monumental time as well. And speaking of your village, the Motherly community had a lot to share with you about this journey, so you will find quotes from them throughout the book, too.

Of course, there is a ton of info on birth throughout this book—and all the beautiful ways that birth happens. I am so excited for you already, but I'll be patient. We'll get there soon enough, and I'll give you prompts throughout about what sections to read ahead to become a total birth boss.

While this book focuses on pregnancy, we want to take a moment to reflect on all the amazing ways that women become mothers—adoption, gestational carriers, and fostering. We are all in this together, the rich variety of our stories enhancing the beauty of the experience of motherhood. In addition, within these pages you'll often find the word *woman*, but I want to take a moment to acknowledge and celebrate all people who are on the conception and pregnancy journey, regardless of their gender identity. We welcome you to our community.

Throughout the creation of this book, we worked hard to be sure that every mama could see herself within this guide—to have all women represented, and all concerns voiced. Yet despite our efforts, we acknowledge that we are far from perfect and will be on a lifelong quest to learn more and grow. We are so grateful for the opportunity to serve our diverse community, and to paraphrase Maya Angelou, we will always strive to do better as soon as we know better.

Mama, this is *your* journey. Whether you feel scared or confident (or a mix of both), know that you are not alone. Your journey to becoming mama starts now.

You've got this.

xo,

Diana

PART I

Getting Pregnant

Jill and Liz here, co-founders of Motherly. We are honored to walk this journey with you as guides, sharing our experiences and inviting you to define what motherhood looks like for you. Just as motherhood looks and feels different for each of us, your story is your own to shape. And, while you may not have a child in your arms just yet, in so many ways, your motherhood story has already begun.

Whether you've been trying to get pregnant for some time or find yourself unexpectedly expecting (or anything in between), you have already begun the massive transformation that occurs when you begin taking the first steps on the motherhood path.

This momentous adventure can seem daunting. There are so many steps, so many things to consider, so many potential worries. But here is the thing: Becoming doesn't happen overnight, it is a journey. Mama is a role you will continue to grow into—forever. We have six children between us and continue to learn and grow as women and mothers, every single day.

We invite you to reflect on what this powerful moment means to you.

If you are thrilled, that's awesome—though prepare to steel yourself for the tough patches. If you are ambivalent, scared, or any of the thousands of other complex emotions that can—and will—present for you, that's okay too. *Becoming mama* is not a simple, straight trajectory. It is layered and deep and winding and ever-changing—just like you.

We have had unexpected pregnancies that took time to fully embrace. We have had losses that we thought would break us, and subsequent newfound strength that remains with us every day. And we have had sobbed tears of joy as we gazed at our children and told them, "I never wanted anything more than you."

So how can you become the mama you want to be, starting today? The first, and most profound, step of becoming mama is learning how to mother yourself. To treat yourself during this time with grace and understanding. To honor the incredible changes that this new life brings into your world and take some time to reflect on what you need to feel whole and supported on this journey. And to stand strong and proud of the mama you're becoming.

And so today, as you wonder whether this is the month you'll finally get pregnant or you're busy scheduling those first trimester doctor's appointments, remember that these early steps are the beginning of your motherhood story, and that this story is yours to write.

You deserve it—you are becoming mama. You've got this.

xo,

Jill + Liz

Deciding to Have a Baby and Preparing to Get Pregnant

I am crossing a threshold that will forever change the way I exist in this world.

We all come to pregnancy in different ways. For some, it arrives as a surprise. Others make a plan for when they will start trying to conceive. And others use fertility treatments, which can require an extensive amount of planning (not to mention money, time, and emotional resources).

The decision to have a child is without a doubt one of the most consequential of your whole life. There is the obvious stuff: the changes your body will go through and the ways your social, professional, and financial life will shift. You will evolve profoundly.

But then there are the changes you don't expect:

- How surreal it feels to get a positive pregnancy test.
- How odd and wonderful it is the first (and one-hundredth) time you feel your baby flutter inside your womb.
- How in awe of yourself you are when you give birth to your baby—*however* you give birth to your baby.
- How soft the fuzz on a newborn baby's back is.
- How you can alternate between feeling scared, conflicted, and confident, all in the course of one afternoon.

Motherhood is one thousand things all at once. It's beautiful, chaotic, messy, confusing, intuitive, scary, energizing, and exhausting, all in the same instant.

It is the hardest thing you will ever do. And mama, it's breathtaking.

You are at the core of this entire experience, which means that you will carry everything: the baby, of course, but also the symptoms that come with growing that baby, the joys, the possible heartbreaks, the worries. It's all you, mama.

So, it's essential that you remember two things: you are a phenom, and you will not do this alone.

At your highest highs and your lowest lows, there is a village of professionals and peers to traverse this path with you. Simply the decision to become a mother—whatever that means for *you*—means that you have joined the circle of generations upon generations of women who have embarked on this adventure (and those who will). And of course, you've got an entire village of women at #TeamMotherly rooting for you every step of the way. Come hang out with us at mother.ly/becomingmama and follow us on Instagram @motherly for even more support, information, and inspiration. We've got you. Welcome.

Before your baby becomes your number one focus, it is time to focus on yourself. After all, you are your baby's mother. Doesn't your baby's mother deserve the best? (Your baby would certainly think so.)

xo,

Diana

TTC: "TRYING TO CONCEIVE" OR "TRYING TO BE CALM"?

Throughout these pages, you will find reminders about how important the various aspects of your health are as you make your way on this journey. That importance starts now.

Psst: Already pregnant? You can still use the materials in this chapter to take tremendous steps toward improving your health that will positively impact your pregnancy and baby.

This period of trying to conceive (TTC) has the potential to be stressful. In fact, studies have been done to examine how anxiety-provoking it can be. The answer: very.

Women may struggle with the unpredictability and uncertainty involved. And there are so many personal factors that may contribute to how you are feeling these days—past experiences, resources, your health, finances, relationships, feelings about impending medical tests and treatments—and of course, what your conception journey will look like.

It's a lot! That's why it is vital to tend to your emotional well-being as much as possible.

Actively supporting your mental health will look different for everyone. Maybe you will add a meditation practice into your routine. Perhaps you find that you are at your happiest when you can swim or take long walks several times per week. You might also consider starting to talk to a therapist if you are not currently. (For the record, I believe that *everyone* would benefit from regular mental health care. We get routine physicals, pap smears, and prenatal checkups. Why should our emotional health be any different?)

Now, never in the history of calming down has anyone calmed down by being told to calm down. However, it is possible that high levels of stress can make it more difficult to

get pregnant. So taking time to nurture yourself is key.

Even more essential is that throughout this journey, you will continue to be a person—a very important one. Yes, becoming a mother is huge, and something we'll talk about a lot, but it does not mean that you stop having human needs (even though you *will* be a new kind of superhero). You deserve to go through this process feeling strong and healthy. Checking in with yourself and being honest about your mental and emotional well-being is essential. Be gentle with yourself and get help when you need it.

pause AND REFLECT

Mindfulness is the act of bringing your attention to the current moment, recognizing what you are experiencing—physically, emotionally, and externally—and allowing those feelings to be, without judgment.

It is incredibly hard to do. Our fast-paced lives and busy brains are constantly pulling our focus elsewhere. My mind, for example, seems to excel at going through my to-do list and all the things I have not done yet, instead of settling into the present moment.

Know that mindfulness is deeply personal and will look different for everyone. Some people prefer to sit quietly, while others may find that uncomfortable or upsetting, so they may choose to be more active and try walking, painting, or something else that feels right. As you encounter mindfulness guides in this book, please adapt them to your level of comfort.

Mindfulness is indeed a lifelong practice in which there is always room for improvement. But it's worth it. Researchers are finding more and more benefits when people can incorporate mindfulness into their lives—stress reduction, less anxiety and depression, and overall improved mental well-being. Um, yes, please!

Throughout the book, I'll share guided opportunities to reflect or meditate. I invite you to return to those pages as often as you like, and include your partner and village in them too, if you wish to. Tons of resources and apps also await you online to guide your journey to mindfulness.

Take some time this month to set up a meditation nook in your home—any place that you can go to that feels peaceful and safe. It might be your bed, a lawn chair in your backyard, or a pillow on the floor of your living room. You can keep it simple or decorate with a few meaningful and beautiful items. The point is to create a space that you love being in, that you can return to throughout your pregnancy (and beyond) to recenter and reground.

How to Practice

When you have a few moments of calm in your day (even just 3 to 5 minutes will do), find a journal and retreat to your nook. Close your eyes and focus on your breath. Every time you inhale, see if you can visualize a soft, warm light entering your body with your breath and filling you with its gentle presence. Allow the light to illuminate your emotions and sensations. As you exhale, allow your awareness to come into your body in this present moment—emotional, physical, and environmental.

- What does your body feel like? Is there a place that feels discomfort or pain?
- What other sensations are with you? What can you hear, smell, taste, see, and feel?
- What thoughts are arising? Do you feel those thoughts anywhere in your body?

Now let the adventure you are about to embark on emerge into your consciousness. You are becoming mama.

- How does that make you feel?
- What changes does it provoke in your body, thoughts, and feelings?

Try not to fight what comes up; just observe it without judgment.

Your body is incredibly intuitive and wise, and you can learn from what surfaces during this practice.

Take a few moments to journal about what you learn and return to this exercise throughout your pregnancy to see what stays constant and what changes.

PREPARING TO BE PREGNANT

The moment you decide that you want to have a baby, an internal switch flicks on, and suddenly it seems like it is the *only* thing you want. So, if you are feeling excited to get this show on the road, that is completely normal. (I am excited for you to be pregnant, too!)

However, if you have the opportunity to wait just a bit before you start trying, so you can focus on your health first—about 2 to 3 months, to be specific—it is *possible* that your journey will be easier. In fact, research has found that when women can focus on their own well-being before trying to conceive, they tend to get pregnant faster and have healthier pregnancies and babies. Ultimately, you know yourself and your situation better than anyone else. Ask for professional guidance and listen to that inner voice. She knows what she's talking about.

Following are ways you can get baby-ready.

Schedule a Preconception Health Visit

A preconception visit is an overall wellness checkup that is usually scheduled with a women's health-care provider. If you currently see someone you love, you can schedule with them. You could also start to think about who you might like to care for you during your pregnancy and schedule the visit with them. For information about choosing a birth attendant, jump to page 89.

The goal of this visit is to help you reach a state of optimal health before pregnancy. That is going to look different for everyone, and your provider can help you personalize the best plan for you.

The appointment itself will likely involve a thorough conversation about your health history—any chronic illnesses or health issues you have, medications you take, past pregnancies, and current concerns. You may also discuss your family's medical and pregnancy history if you know it. And if you have a partner or known sperm donor with whom you plan to make this baby, you will likely talk about any relevant health concerns with them as well.

There will also be a physical exam, which may include a pelvic exam.

Psst: Dislike pelvic exams? Me, too! Check out "What Else Will Happen at This Month's Prenatal Visit?" on page 102 for some tips.

This visit is also a great time to make sure that any vaccinations you choose to receive are up-to-date. There are some vaccines that you cannot get when you are pregnant, so if you need one, now is the time. Some vaccines may require a period of time before you can safely get pregnant, so be sure to ask your provider. Of note, the Centers for Disease Control (CDC) recommends that pregnant women receive the flu shot.

PLANNING FOR HEALTH-CARE COVERAGE

This is a great time to check in with your insurance company. Ask them about what you are (and are not) covered for in terms of conception and prenatal care, so you can plan accordingly. For example, some health insurance companies cover some of the costs associated with assisted reproductive technologies, and some do not.

If you do not have health insurance, you may be eligible for coverage under the Affordable Care Act of 2010.

Your male partner or sperm donor may also benefit from a preconception health visit because his health contributes to fertility, too!

Visit Your Dentist

Scientists are finding more and more connections between oral hygiene and overall health, and pregnancy is one of the most important times to focus on those pearly whites.

Here are just a few of the ways that a healthy mouth can benefit your future baby:

- Decreased risk of preterm birth
- Possible decreased risk of preeclampsia
- Healthier birth weight of baby
- Improved dental health for your child, such as fewer cavities

A healthy mouth can also decrease your lifetime risk of developing diabetes, heart disease, and cancer.

So plan a visit to your dentist before you get pregnant, and continue to see them throughout your pregnancy. Almost all dental procedures are considered safe during pregnancy (especially when you consider the potential risks of an unhealthy mouth). Just be sure to let your dentist know that you are pregnant.

Stop Taking Birth Control . . . Maybe

The effects of hormonal birth control on a woman's future fertility have long been questioned.

The findings from a 2018 review of 14,884 women found that, in general, previous use of hormonal contraception does not (by itself) seem to make it harder to get pregnant. Translation: If you have been using the pill, an IUD, a patch, a ring, an injection, or an implantable device, chances are you will be fine!

There is a potential delay in conceiving, though, while the hormones fully leave your body. So, you could consider stopping the hormonal method of birth control now in preparation for trying to conceive in a few months. If you plan to have sex with a man between now and then, you could use a condom instead. Just be careful. Condoms tend to be less effective than hormonal methods, so if you absolutely cannot get pregnant right now (for example, if you are taking a medication that would be dangerous to take while pregnant), you might want to keep using your existing birth control method until you are ready.

Start Taking Prenatal Vitamins

Prenatal vitamins are designed specifically to meet the needs of pregnant women and their growing babies. Though getting nutrients through food is ideal, the American College of Obstetricians and Gynecologists (ACOG) recommends prenatal vitamins to ensure that you are getting what you need. While vitamins benefit you and your baby throughout your pregnancy, they work best when started before you become pregnant.

Prenatal Nutrition Guidelines

Requirements per day:

- Calcium: 1,000 mg
- DHA: at least 200 mg
- Fiber: 25 grams
- Folic acid: 600 micrograms
- Iron: 27 mg
- Vitamin A: 770 micrograms
- Vitamin B6: 1.9 mg
- Vitamin B12: 2.6 micrograms
- Vitamin C: 85 micrograms
- Vitamin D: 600 international units

Of note, some women find that prenatal vitamins make them nauseous. If this is the case, experiment with when you take the vitamin: Some women have better luck taking them with food or just before bed. They may also make you constipated from the iron (more on this soon).

In recent years, there has been some concern raised about the potential inclusion of lead in prenatal vitamins. According to ob-gyn Dr. Sarah Bjorkman:

> As it turns out, all prenatal vitamins have a small amount of lead in them. However, these levels are well below previously established safe and tolerable exposure doses. Knowing this has allowed me to have informed conversations with my

patients where I still stress the importance of prenatal vitamins and their role in preventing birth defects (specifically open neural tube defects), while also directing them to the vitamins with the lowest concentrations of lead when possible. These can be found on the FDA website.

Following are some of the essential components of prenatal vitamins.

Folate and Folic Acid   Folate, also known as vitamin B9, is an essential nutrient that our bodies can synthesize from leafy vegetables. However, many of us do not consume sufficient levels of it naturally, so vitamins are recommended. Folic acid is the synthetic form of B9, which is virtually interchangeable with folate in the body.

Registered Dietician Nutritionist Crystal Karges, who guides the "Nourish" sections of this book (and who wrote the delicious recipes throughout the book), says that folate and folic acid offer protective benefits against neural tube defects such as spina bifida and anencephaly, lowering the risk as much as 70 percent. Getting enough of this vitamin in the earliest days and weeks of pregnancy is key.

"Because most common neural tube defects can occur within the first few weeks of pregnancy, it is ideal to start getting more of this nutrient at least 1 month before you start trying for baby, with a goal of 600 micrograms of folic acid per day," she advises.

Calcium   ACOG also recommends getting 1,000 milligrams of calcium per day while you're pregnant and breastfeeding. The increase in calcium will protect you from

losing bone density because your growing bundle is now sharing your calcium for their own bone growth. Calcium intake can include supplements as well as four daily servings of dairy products or foods that are rich in calcium such as nuts and seeds, sardines and salmon, beans and lentils, and leafy greens.

Iron   Iron enhances how blood carries oxygen, and it also helps to guard against anemia, which occurs from the reduction in the concentration of red blood cells and hemoglobin (oxygen-carrying protein) in your blood. Blood volume increases by 40 to 45 percent during pregnancy. It's as if your blood has been diluted, so anemia is actually quite common! In fact, 40 to 50 percent of women develop it during pregnancy. To avoid anemia, ACOG recommends 27 milligrams of iron per day for pregnant and breastfeeding women.

Be aware that the high levels of iron in prenatal vitamins—along with the digestion-slowing effects of a hormone called progesterone (more on this later)—can cause some constipation. Make sure you are drinking at least ten 8-ounce glasses of water per day and eating at least 25 grams per day of dietary fiber from fruits, vegetables, and whole grains to help prevent constipation.

There is a caveat to be aware of: Iron comes in different forms, and there is some concern that iron pills may not be the best option, as they usually contain iron that is not well absorbed by your body (but still cause some unpleasant side effects). So, if you are diagnosed with anemia, talk to your provider about all your iron options. Increasing iron-rich foods is often the best way to start: white beans, liver, and dark chocolate are some great foods to start with. (Yes, I said *chocolate*!) Iron supplements also come in liquid form, which is often better tolerated than the pills.

One last recommendation about iron. Vitamin C helps iron get absorbed into the bloodstream, while calcium inhibits its bio-availability. Translation: When you take your iron (either pill or food), take it with something high in vitamin C (like orange juice) and avoid calcium-rich foods like dairy for about an hour before and after. Generally speaking, our diets are varied enough that you don't need to worry about this too much, but if you really need to give your iron a boost, this could help.

DHA   DHA, an acronym for docosahexaenoic acid, is an omega-3 fatty acid. Research is showing that people in developed countries are increasingly deficient in omega-3 due to the prevalence of vegetable oils in our diets. Since our bodies don't naturally produce it, getting more of it in the form of supplements or food is important, especially during pregnancy and breastfeeding.

Research has also shown that DHA supplementation during pregnancy can boost your baby's immune system and decrease their risk for allergies. And continued supplementation during childhood is correlated with higher level reading and spelling skills.

The recommended daily amount is at least two servings of fish or shellfish (8 to 12 ounces), but due to the presence of heavy metals in some seafood, you may also want to opt for 200 milligrams of a supplement.

A note for women with a plant-based diet: It is absolutely possible to get all the nutrients you need during pregnancy as a vegetarian or vegan; it might just be a little harder. Speak with your provider about your specific concerns or meet with a nutritionist if you are able to.

Quit Smoking
A nonjudgmental note for smokers: An estimated 7.2 percent of pregnant women smoke cigarettes, so you are certainly not alone. "Just quitting" is nowhere near most people's experience of leaving cigarettes behind. It is a complex issue with tons of emotional and physical factors to consider. In short, it's really hard.

But cigarette smoking can harm fertility. Substances in cigarettes can make it harder for the fertilized embryo to implant into the uterine lining; thus, getting pregnant may be harder, and your risk of miscarriage may increase.

Cigarettes can lead to serious pregnancy complications for you and your baby, such as low birth weight, hypertension, placental abruption, preterm birth, and stillbirth. And children who were exposed to cigarettes in the womb have a higher risk of breathing problems, ear infections, future obesity, sudden infant death syndrome (SIDS), and behavioral problems.

When you quit smoking, your body instantly starts to mend the damage—within

20 minutes! And the longer you go without smoking, the more dramatic those benefits are. One year from now, when you will possibly be holding your baby in your arms, your lungs will be significantly healthier and ready to keep up with the demands of taking care of your new little person. How awesome are you?

You don't have to quit alone: It's also a good idea for your partner to quit so that when the baby arrives, they can have a smoke-free home. Lastly, research indicates that when conception is proving challenging, it may be helpful for the man (partner or sperm donor) to quit smoking cigarettes to improve the chances of getting pregnant.

Consider Leaving the Wine Behind

Alcohol's potential effect on fertility is controversial: Some studies have said it's just fine to continue drinking, while others have found the opposite. A 2017 review of nineteen studies involving more than ninety-eight thousand women found that alcohol intake decreased the chances of getting pregnant by an average of 13 percent each cycle. Light drinking (less than one glass of wine per day) results in an 11 percent decrease, while drinking more than one drink a day can decrease your fertility by 23 percent.

Also of note, despite the possible impact of alcohol on fertility, it does not appear that light to moderate prepregnancy alcohol consumption increases the risk of miscarriage or stillbirth.

Once you are pregnant, most medical authorities recommend not drinking at all since it can lead to miscarriage or fetal developmental problems, known as fetal alcohol syndrome (see page 460). Alcohol crosses into the placenta, which means that when you drink, your baby is getting some alcohol in their system.

Ultimately, you have to make the decision here that feels right for you, and you can always speak with your provider to help you make those choices.

Cut Back on Caffeine

You may also be wondering if you can continue to drink coffee and other caffeinated drinks. The jury is out on this one. While some studies have found that caffeine does not impact fertility, others find that it does—for women and men.

When we asked Crystal Karges for her take on caffeine, she recommended limiting your intake to about 200 milligrams per day, which is about one 12-ounce cup of coffee.

"Since caffeine is a stimulant that can cross the placental barrier during pregnancy, there is also a risk that it can reach your growing baby, who won't be able to metabolize it as efficiently as you can," Karges says. "While you don't have to cut caffeine cold turkey, you may consider slowly tapering off to support optimal functioning before baby."

Evaluate Your Drug, Medication, and Supplement Use

Prescription and over-the-counter medications and supplements vary widely when it comes to safety during conception and pregnancy, so your best bet is to read labels carefully and to speak with your provider to determine whether they're safe to continue using.

A 2018 study led by the Boston University School of Public Health found that marijuana use in men and women does not seem to decrease chances of getting pregnant. ACOG, however, states that there are "concerns regarding impaired neurodevelopment [in babies], as well as maternal and fetal exposure to the adverse effects of smoking," and advises hopeful parents to quit their use of marijuana. A 2017 study found that using marijuana during pregnancy increased the risk of newborn illness and death.

Many women also wonder about the safety of cannabidiol, or CBD. The trouble is, CBD is relatively new to the mainstream, which means we don't know a lot about its impact on conception and pregnancy. If you are taking CBD, I'd suggest talking to your provider about it, so they can help weigh the potential risks and benefits.

There are, of course, many other illicit drugs out there. They should not be used when you are pregnant. They can be very risky (or even deadly).

If you use drugs and want to quit, there are a lot of options to support you. Seek out a provider who can meet your specific needs and think of all the ways you and your little one will benefit.

Men's Wellness Matters, Too

Encourage your partner or sperm donor to consult his health practitioner to support his overall wellness. A man can increase sperm motility and count by taking steps to keep his testicles healthy. This includes not wearing tight pants, not going into hot tubs, and not keeping a cell phone or other wireless devices near the testicles. As I mentioned, men might choose to stop smoking or stop using recreational drugs, including all forms of marijuana. Though research is always evolving here, past studies have found that vitamins and supplements such as vitamin C, vitamin E, carnitine, zinc, folate, L-arginine,

and coenzyme Q10 may contribute to improved sperm counts.

Rest Up!

Sleep (or lack thereof) is a big focus of pregnancy, early parenthood, and believe it or not, conception! Researchers found that women who get more than 8 hours of sleep per night have a 20 percent higher level of follicle-stimulating hormone (FSH), which encourages ovarian follicles to grow before releasing an egg. Adequate sleep can also contribute to healthier levels of many other hormones involved in conception, and it decreases stress, which can help as well.

If you have sleep issues, check out "Insomnia" on page 440. The suggestions there may help! You can also consider seeking treatment, which may improve your chances of getting pregnant. All sorts of herbal remedies, therapies, and over-the-counter and prescription sleep aids are available, but make sure to consult your provider.

And this goes for men, too: Getting less than 6 hours of sleep per night can make them a bit less fertile. Let's hear it for early bedtime.

Chart Your Cycle

In chapter 3, we'll talk about how to chart your cycle, and it can be a good idea to start a few months before you want to become pregnant, if possible. Keeping track of your period provides a ton of useful information about what your body is up to, and it is most helpful when you have details to look back on so that you can better predict what's to come.

Eliminate Environmental Pollutants

Over the past decade or so, there has been a lot more attention on reproductive toxins.

There are chemicals in our air, water, and industrially made products that can interact with our hormones and change how they function. They are known as endocrine disrupting chemicals (EDCs), and they can make it harder to get pregnant and cause lower sperm counts. In some cases, they can be passed on to a fetus through the placenta and cause health issues, either immediately or later on.

Minimizing exposure to these harmful chemicals can be difficult because the more common and affordable products on the market are more likely to have them. And often we cannot control our exposure to the pollutants in our environment.

So much of this is just unavoidable. The goal, then, is to do the best we can, when we can: staying up-to-date with new findings, advocating for policies that support increased access to healthier options, and choosing less-dangerous products when we are able.

A major medical organization called the International Federation of Gynecology and Obstetrics (FIGO) has launched a campaign to help women make lifestyle changes that can protect their health and the health of their future children. Some ways to do this include:

- Minimize your use of plastic food containers. Whenever you can, try to store food in stainless steel or glass containers. (I save empty glass containers—like jelly and sauce jars—wash them, and then use them to store leftovers.)

- Be aware of bisphenol A (BPA), which might be present in canned food and children's bottles and cups.

WANT TO MAKE YOUR OWN HOUSEHOLD CLEANER?

In a spray bottle, mix:

$1/2$ cup distilled white vinegar

1 cup water

1 tsp. castile or dish soap

Lemon juice or essential oils for scent, if desired

(Just don't spray vinegar on marble, granite, quartz, or unsealed grout.)

- Ask your dentist to avoid plastic-based tooth sealants (which may contain BPA).

Evaluate your personal cosmetics, soaps, shampoos, and household cleaners for parabens and phthalates because these chemicals can change how estrogen functions in your body. Try to choose products that specifically advertise that they are free of parabens and phthalates. Or make your own! This goes for any trips to the nail salon: Use toxin-free polishes or go au naturel. The Environmental Working Group website is a great resource for evaluating the ingredients of your products.

Choosing organic produce, grains, dairy, and meat is awesome for avoiding pesticides and herbicides. Unfortunately, the organic stuff can be difficult to find and expensive to buy.

The Environmental Working Group puts out a yearly list of the Dirty Dozen™ foods, a list of twelve foods that are most important to try to find organic when possible because the nonorganic versions contain the highest levels of chemicals of all the fruits and vegetables. The current list from 2019 includes:

1 Strawberries
2 Spinach
3 Kale
4 Nectarines
5 Apples
6 Grapes

7 Peaches
8 Cherries
9 Pears
10 Tomatoes
11 Celery
12 Potatoes

In contrast, the Clean 15™ list names the fifteen safest produce items to eat if buying organic is not possible. The 2019 list includes:

1 Avocado
2 Sweet corn
3 Pineapple
4 Frozen sweet peas
5 Onion
6 Papaya
7 Eggplant
8 Asparagus

9 Kiwi
10 Cabbage
11 Cauliflower
12 Cantaloupe
13 Broccoli
14 Mushrooms
15 Honeydew melon

Finally, take precautions to reduce air pollutants in your home. New furniture or carpets can emit EDCs. You can avoid this by choosing used household items or new items that are made from all-natural materials. You'll also want to try your best to keep your indoor air free of tobacco smoke, car exhaust, paint fumes, industrial emissions, and wildfire smoke. A few effective ways to do this include not wearing shoes in the house, filling your house with plants, using low-VOC (or no-VOC) paint, and purchasing or borrowing a standing HEPA air purifier or opening your windows if the outdoor air quality is safe.

We can't guarantee a toxin-free life anymore in this day and age, but we can trust that if we make the best choices possible, our bodies will be as resilient as they can be.

nourish

Let's Shift the Dialogue

So often when we talk about "eating healthy," we go first to things we are going to remove from our lives, and it can feel a bit like punishment. But your body is about to create and carry life completely from scratch. Let that sink in for a moment. A little baby is about to depend on your body for shelter, safety, comfort, and growth. A body that can do *that* should be revered, not deprived.

So, can we shift the dialogue together?

Let's stop "watching what we eat" and start focusing on food that nourishes our bodies and our souls. And sometimes our souls need ice cream.

Let's think about nourishment as a way to celebrate and honor our bodies and the amazing work they do.

You with me? Yes! Let's do this.

Following are a few ways to start.

Nourish Yourself with Superfoods

Now is the time to start preparing your body to grow a baby with good, balanced nutrition. Choose foods that reflect the magnitude of the work you are about to do—delicious, nutrient-dense foods that energize and nourish you as you nourish your baby. If you're anxious to get started, check out "Eating for Fertility" on page 42!

Move Toward a Healthy Body Mass Index

Can I tell you something? I hate diets for three reasons:

1 Diets are not fun.
2 Diets are not fun. Not a typo; this one bears repeating.
3 Diets are about depriving your body

instead of nurturing and supporting your body.

Before we dive in here, it's important to note that weight is a tricky thing, to put it mildly. First, there is growing skepticism around the idea of an ideal weight, as human bodies vary so much. Also, being "overweight" or "underweight" is rarely as simple as having too many or not enough pounds on a body. There is often a web of underlying physical and emotional issues that contribute. "Weight" is also an incredibly triggering word for many women, with social implications and a deeply embedded stigma.

You are about to ask your body to do the most powerful and awe-inspiring thing imaginable: grow a baby. This is, therefore, a time to honor your body and all the beauty that comes with it, not to name its flaws with shame and doubt—even though our society unfortunately does a good job of leading us down that path.

We can take small steps toward changing cultural attitudes around body shame by focusing on our own personal attitude, and by shifting our mindset, a little every day, to get closer to one that celebrates our bodies rather than degrades them.

Instead of saying to yourself, "Ugh, if I don't exercise and lose this weight now, I am going to have even more baby weight to lose postpartum," try saying, "I am going to dance in my living room for 20 minutes today because dancing always makes my body feel good."

Instead of ridiculing yourself for having the second helping of dessert last night, try saying, "That cheesecake was delicious, but today I feel like my body needs some leafy greens and tea."

Let us please be nice to ourselves and our bodies.

With all that in mind, let's look at some research findings about the impact of weight on fertility.

Scientists have found that it takes women with a body mass index (BMI) of over 25 or under 19 longer to become pregnant. A BMI over 25 may make a woman three times more likely to experience infertility. One explanation for this is that having a BMI over 25 can change the way something called your hypothalamic-pituitary-ovarian (HPO) axis makes and distributes hormones, which can change ovulation and the menstrual cycle, thus making it harder to get pregnant.

The good news: A woman with a BMI over 25 who moves toward a healthier BMI by reducing her calories and starting to exercise will significantly improve her chances of getting pregnant.

Women who have a BMI of less than 19 also have lower rates of fertility. If your BMI is under the normal range, you may not ovulate regularly, have a period, or store enough fat to produce adequate hormones. Increasing and maintaining your BMI can be hard, so it may be helpful to work with your provider or nutritionist to make a plan.

You can find your body mass index easily by using a free online BMI calculator. Once you've calculated your number, you can refer to the following chart to see which category you're in.

BODY MASS INDEX (BMI)	
Underweight	Less than 18.5
Ideal weight	18.5 to 24.9
Overweight	25 to 29.9
Obese	30 or higher

move

Being pregnant and having a baby is hard work, and you want to be as strong and fit as possible so that you can rock this. That's why it's so important to exercise and move your body during pregnancy.

The key to working out prepregnancy is to exercise, but not to overexercise. Women who exercise more than 60 minutes per day can have a higher risk of not ovulating, but women who exercise 30 to 60 minutes per day actually have improved fertility. This goes for males as well: Studies have linked strenuous exercise to not-so-great swimming abilities in sperm.

The best way I have ever heard healthy exercise described was this: "Move your body in a way that feels good." I love this perspective because it focuses on the enjoyment of the activity, not just the "get healthy and lose weight" aspect of it.

Do you have a favorite way to get your heart pumping or break a sweat? Yoga, running, hiking, Zumba, Pilates—whatever it is, go you!

We will also guide you through specific movement techniques that will help your body stay strong and healthy through pregnancy, birth, and postpartum. If you are excited to start learning, you can jump to "Lift and Wrap" on page 31!

love AND VILLAGE

If you are in a relationship and will travel the road of conception, pregnancy, and parenthood with a partner, taking steps to prepare for the upheaval—the joyful and the wild—can help create a strong foundation upon which to grow, together.

Mama, I promise this is not one of those "Oh, you have *no* idea what you are getting yourself into" moments. You are a smart woman, and you know that this is a big deal. The point here is to encourage you to have honest and open dialogues with your partner about what your desires and expectations are—and to intentionally continue that conversation as your story unfolds.

Chrissy Powers, a marriage and family therapist, says that our ideas of what parenthood will be like are often romanticized, and this can cause a great deal of stress on a relationship. Of course, becoming a parent is one of the greatest gifts in this world and can bring so much joy and love. But it can be difficult to fully comprehend the magnitude of this endeavor and its impact on your relationship before you are *in* it. Powers, herself a mama of three, says that "unmet expectations can cause discord."

You are the star of this show, but remember that your partner's experience and concerns

SOMEONE TO LEAN ON

In this book, I'll often refer to your pregnancy or labor partner—the main person you will rely on for support during this upcoming journey. It may be your significant other, or it may be your best friend or a family member. Who has the calmest energy? Who do you know you can rely on? Who will be so thrilled to experience this phase of your life with you, who will celebrate the Wonder Woman that you are, and who will stay connected to your child in their life?

That's your person.

also need to be considered. When differences arise, do your best to listen without judgment and make sure to acknowledge their point of view.

A few questions to consider now might be:

- For female/male relationships: Do we want to just stop using birth control and see what happens, or would we prefer to be a bit more methodical about timing sex?

- If we know that we will need assisted reproductive therapies to get pregnant, which methods are best for us and which do we prefer? How do we feel about the methods that are available to us?

- How will we feel if pregnancy happens right away? And if it doesn't?

- What is our plan for when (not if) we have disagreements along this journey? Do we want to consider seeing a therapist to help with existing issues (which we all have) and to assist us when new ones arise?

- What aspects of our relationship are most important to us? How can we hold on to those pieces as we begin this next adventure together?

One idea to help you and your partner bond over this experience is to make any necessary lifestyle changes together. In addition to improving your chances of conception if your partner is male, getting healthy together will certainly help when you have an active baby crawling around. It will also help you feel like the burden does not rest solely on your shoulders—because it doesn't! Incorporate a daily walk together or take turns cooking healthy meals for each other. Bonus points for when this continues through pregnancy and parenthood!

The Impact of TTC on Your Village

This is also a great time to think about your village—the friends, family members, and community who will support you moving forward. Think about how wonderful it will be for your child to grow up in the embrace of a loving network of people. And for you—well, your village is priceless.

When do you want to start connecting with your village around this momentous time in your life? Deciding to have a baby usually doesn't come with a public announcement. In fact, many women tend to keep the news to themselves. Of course, this is a very personal matter, but women do talk about feeling isolated and lonely because they aren't sharing yet.

A few ideas to consider:

- Do you want to ask around to see if any of your friends might also be trying to conceive around this time? If so, would you feel comfortable sharing this experience with them?

- Do you want to ask your mom or sisters about their experiences trying to conceive? Sometimes fertility issues can be hereditary. For example, early menopause may be linked to decreased egg reserves at a younger age. If your mother went through menopause early, you might too. Do remember, though, that women getting pregnant today are often older than our mothers and grandmothers were when they conceived. In fact, in 2015, for the first time, the number of women who got pregnant in their 30s surpassed the number in their 20s. So, don't assume you're genetically like your mom. And don't rely on her history alone to predict your fertility.

If you will be a single parent, among the strong 23 percent of mamas in the US who are single, your village will likely be your rock. Who is in that village? How can you ensure that you will have frequent and meaningful contact with your village? Do you want someone to come to your prenatal appointments with you? And your birth?

work

There are many aspects of work to consider when planning for your pregnancy. Here are five questions to think about and possibly address during your planning:

1 If you plan to try to conceive by monitoring your ovulation and timing sex or insemination (see chapter 3, "How to Conceive," for more on this), will your work schedule (and your partner's) allow for this? For example, do you frequently travel for work, potentially taking you away from your partner during your fertile window? If so, is there a way to shift your schedule?

2 If your journey to parenthood will involve fertility treatments, does your work schedule allow you to adhere to a fairly rigid schedule of appointments and ultrasounds? If not, can you make any changes now?

3 Are you exposed to toxins in your workplace, and if so, is there a way to minimize that? Examples might be paint fumes if you are an interior designer, bleach if you are a hairstylist, or any number of chemicals if you work in a lab. What precautions can you take as you start your conception journey to reduce your level of contact with potential toxins?

4 Are there work conditions that might make it harder for you to take care of your hard-at-work body? For example, when I was pregnant with my daughter, I was working 12-hour shifts on a very busy hospital unit in New York City. Bathroom and rest breaks were not easy to come by. Luckily, I had phenomenal co-workers to cover for me while I took breaks, but I had to remember to ask. What can you do now and in the months to come to improve your working conditions?

5 If you own your company or manage people at work, is there anyone you can delegate tasks to in the event you need to take a day off (for conception or dealing-with-symptoms purposes)?

You may already be wondering about planning for work-related factors further down the road. To read about planning for maternity leave, see "Work" on pages 136 and 171, and for financial planning for a baby, see "Work" on page 136. Throughout this book, we also suggest many ways to acquire goods and services that are low-cost or free.

My sincere hope is that you never have to deal with workplace discrimination during your pregnancy journey. Unfortunately, many employers may deny time off for employees; refuse to make reasonable accommodations; or make unlawful changes to an employee's title, working hours, or benefits once they become aware of a pregnancy. If you encounter these issues in your workplace, visit the US Equal Employment Opportunity Commission website (eeoc.gov) for information.

gather

- ○ Items to include in your meditation nook, such as candles, symbolic objects, cherished photos, flowers, and so on
- ○ Notebook or journal for writing your thoughts during each month's reflection
- ○ Prenatal vitamins
- ○ Vinegar, castile soap, and lemons or essential oils and a spray bottle (if you want to make your own cleaning spray)
- ○ Items to keep you safe at work (for example, face masks or gloves)

todo

- ○ Apply for health insurance if you do not already have it.
- ○ Call your health insurance company to verify pregnancy-related coverage.
- ○ Schedule a preconception visit with your health-care provider.
- ○ Schedule a dentist appointment.
- ○ Start taking prenatal vitamins.
- ○ Consider lifestyle changes you'd like to make.
- ○ Stop taking birth control (if that is part of your plan).
- ○ Set up a meditation nook in your home (or in your workplace, if you can—why not?).
- ○ Take a nap!

remember

Try to find a few moments of mindfulness every day. Observe what comes up without judgment and nurture your mind with gentleness and love.

The Extraordinary Anatomy of Pregnancy and Birth

My body is
astonishing.

FROM DIANA

So, you've decided that you want to have a baby (*yay!*). The next thing to do is to consider how you are going to make that baby. In order to do that, it helps to understand the (amazingly cool) anatomy involved.

If you are already pregnant, this chapter is for you, too! In fact, we will be coming back to these pages throughout your pregnancy journey. After all, it has likely been a while since you studied anatomy, and pregnancy brings the subject front and center. If you are feeling a bit unsure of how it all works, you are not alone.

Let's look at all the ways your body is adapted for pregnancy and birth. The more you know about how all your parts work together, the better you will be able to understand what's happening at your appointments and during your birth. In the immediate term, getting a grasp of anatomy will assist you with the exercises in the "Move" sections of this book, which are intended to help you prepare for the physical task of birthing and your recovery afterward.

Ultimately, it is about understanding just how incredible your body is so that you can honor and celebrate yourself throughout this journey.

xo,

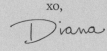

P.S. I also want to take a moment to acknowledge women with disabilities. First, please know that many women with disabilities have healthy and beautiful pregnancies. And, yet, there are also many circumstances that can make your experience more challenging, such as facilities that are not accessible, or health-care team members that are not as helpful and supportive as they should be. And there will be unique medical considerations based on your personal circumstances. This journey can feel like a lonely one—and one that is perpetually uphill—and I want you to know that I see you.

My biggest piece of advice for you is to communicate and advocate. Let your team know exactly what you need, ask as many questions as you need to, and trust yourself—you deserve to feel nurtured and listened to throughout this entire adventure.

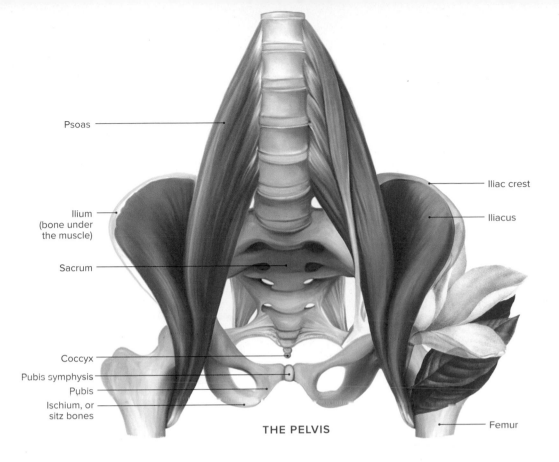

Psoas

Ilium
(bone under
the muscle)

Sacrum

Coccyx

Pubis symphysis

Pubis

Ischium, or
sitz bones

Iliac crest

Iliacus

Femur

THE PELVIS

PELVIS

Your pelvis has some pretty special features that make pregnancy and birth possible.

Bones

To start, a female pelvis is wider than a male's. Those hips don't lie, mama.

The bony structure that makes up your hips and bottom is known as your pelvic girdle. On each side of the pelvic girdle, you have several bones: the ilium (the broadest part and what you feel when you put your hands on your hips), the pubis (in the front, just above the vulva), and the ischium (also called the "sitz bones" because it's what you sit on). The sacrum is the lowest part of your back. It has a triangular shape and is made of fused spinal vertebrae. At the bottom of

the sacrum is the coccyx, or tailbone. All of these bones are held together at joints made of cartilage. One of the more noticeable of these joints is the pubis symphysis, which connects the two pubis bones and can sometimes get sore during pregnancy (see "Pelvic Girdle Pain" on page 465). Ligaments surround the pelvis offering additional support. Throughout pregnancy, the hormone relaxin will be at work relaxin' those ligaments to allow your pelvis to widen for birth. This is why you may develop the (adorable) pregnancy waddle, why you are more prone to injury when you are pregnant, and why your balance becomes less steady as your pregnancy progresses.

Your pelvis expands and contracts—amazing, but true. Stand up and place one hand on your

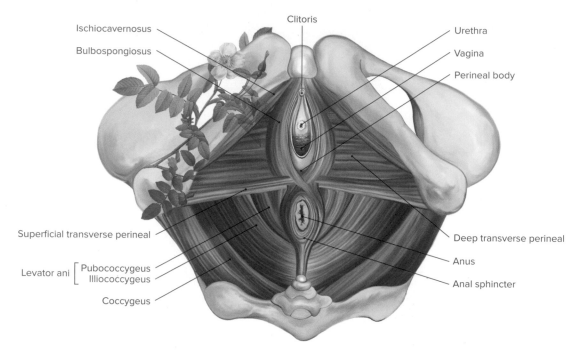

Ischiocavernosus

Bulbospongiosus

Clitoris

Urethra

Vagina

Perineal body

Superficial transverse perineal

Deep transverse perineal

Levator ani [Pubococcygeus
Illiococcygeus

Anus

Anal sphincter

Coccygeus

THE PELVIC FLOOR

pubic bone and the other on your sacrum. Lean back slightly and then lean forward. Can you feel how there is a bit more space between your hands when you lean forward?

If you were to squeeze a pelvis inward at the hips, you'd see the top flex inward and the bottom flex outward, much like a clothespin. (We'll come back to this when we talk about using the hip squeeze on page 290.)

Pelvic Muscles

Two main muscle pairs support the pelvis: the psoas and the iliacus. The psoas pair begins at the middle of the back and sweeps around each side from the spine over the pelvis to attach to the top of the thigh bone (femur).

The psoas supports our organs diagonally, like a shelf. When the uterus is large during the third trimester, the flexible psoas is essential for allowing the baby to descend into the birth canal.

The psoas is connected to the same tendon as the iliacus muscle pair. The iliacus spreads from the top of the thigh over the rim of the pelvis. Together, they form a part of your hip flexor muscle group, responsible for moving your legs up toward your torso, helping you squat, and yes, helping you position yourself to push out a baby.

Pelvic Floor

Three layers of muscle come up into the lower part of the pelvis to contract around the uterus, urethra, and rectum. When your pelvic floor muscles are in good shape, it is easier to birth, you have better control over going to the

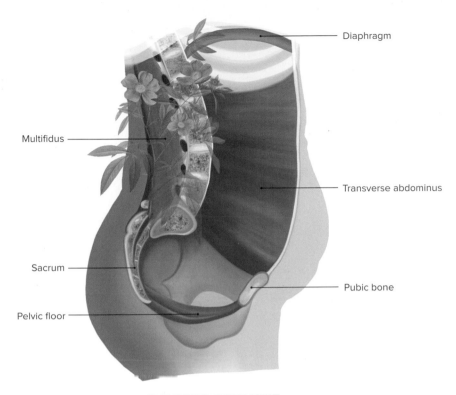

Diaphragm

Multifidus

Transverse abdominus

Sacrum

Pubic bone

Pelvic floor

THE INNER CORE UNIT

bathroom, and you will be less prone to injury in pregnancy.

The pelvic floor muscles sit inside your pelvis—much like a hammock of strong fibers—attaching from the sitz bones (also called sit bones), tailbone, and frontal pubic bone. You can imagine your pelvic floor muscles as one of those crane claw arcade games (where the claw comes down and you try to pick up a stuffed animal with it). The way the claw comes together and up as it tries to pick up the toy is very similar to how your pelvic floor muscles work when they tighten.

THE INNER CORE MUSCLES

Think of your inner core as a unit of inner muscles in your abdomen and back,

underneath the exterior layer of abdominal muscles that is sometimes called the six-pack. Your inner core unit is the foundation of your strength.

Pre- and postnatal exercise specialist Brooke Cates, who will be taking you through the "Move" sections in this book, teaches women to visualize their inner core unit as a box. Your diaphragm muscle is the top of the box, your pelvic floor is the bottom, and the transverse abdominal muscles make up the front, back, and sides. Another way to think of the transverse abdominal muscles is as a corset that wraps around your core and spans from the top of the pelvis up to the bottom four vertebrae of the rib cage.

The multifidus muscle lines the spine on either side and accompanies the transverse abdominal muscle in the back of the box.

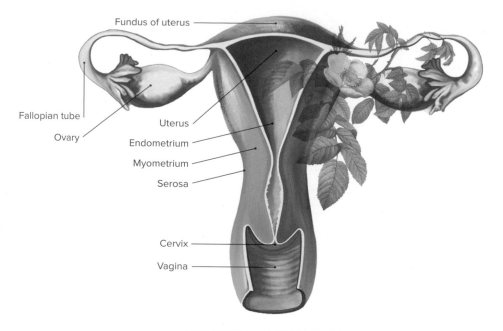

Fundus of uterus

Fallopian tube

Ovary

Uterus

Endometrium

Myometrium

Serosa

Cervix

Vagina

THE REPRODUCTIVE ORGANS

THE REPRODUCTIVE ORGANS

Ovaries

Ovaries are small but mighty organs. They sit in your lower abdomen, house your eggs, and make hormones that contribute to the menstrual cycle and fertility. Inside the ovaries, a cohort of follicles starts to develop. Inside one of the follicles is the egg that will fully mature and eventually be released from the follicle when it opens (or ruptures). We'll talk more about this in chapter 3.

Fallopian Tubes

Fallopian tubes connect the ovaries to the uterus. They are also where the sperm usually meets and fertilizes the egg, transforming it into a zygote. Fallopian tubes are lined with tiny hair-like structures called cilia, which nudge the egg or zygote forward on its journey to the uterus.

Uterus

The uterus is a hollow (powerful, amazing, superhero) organ that cradles your baby as they grow and then ushers them out into the world during labor. It is made of three layers:

Endometrium   As the innermost layer and lining of the uterus, the endometrium has much to do with supporting the growth of your pregnancy. It is where the fertilized egg burrows in after fertilization, and it is where the placenta anchors and starts to develop.

When you are not pregnant, the endometrium grows thick with blood and tissue during each menstrual cycle, and then sheds it in the form of your period.

Myometrium   The myometrium is the middle layer of the uterus. It is the thickest layer and is

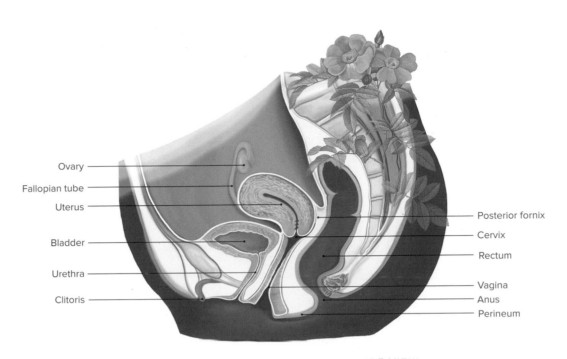

THE REPRODUCTIVE ORGANS, SIDE VIEW

Ovary

Fallopian tube

Uterus

Bladder

Urethra

Clitoris

Posterior fornix

Cervix

Rectum

Vagina

Anus

Perineum

made of smooth muscle. This is the powerhouse of the uterus that is responsible for contractions during labor (and also cramping during menstruation). It has a system of nerves running through it that respond to hormones and other chemical messages in your body.

Serosa or Perimetrium   The serosa is the outermost layer, made of epithelial cells (which is also what skin is made of). It serves to separate the uterus from the other organs in the body.

When you are not pregnant, the uterus sits nestled in your pelvis and is about 3 to 4 inches tall, roughly the size of your fist. By the end of pregnancy, your uterus will have grown to the size of a watermelon. (*Whoa!*)

The fallopian tubes feed into the uterus toward the top like two straws. The very top

of the uterus is called the fundus, and at the bottom is your cervix.

Cervix

The cervix is the opening of the uterus. This is the part that is swabbed during a pap smear (see page 453) and the part that softens, effaces (thins), and dilates (opens) in labor to release your baby. The cervix looks like the stretchy neck of a balloon.

The cervix does three things when you are in labor:

1   **It softens.** Tap your chin. That's about the firmness of your cervix when you are not in labor. Now tap your cheek. That's how soft it will get.

2   **It effaces, or thins and shortens.** We measure this in percentages. Throughout

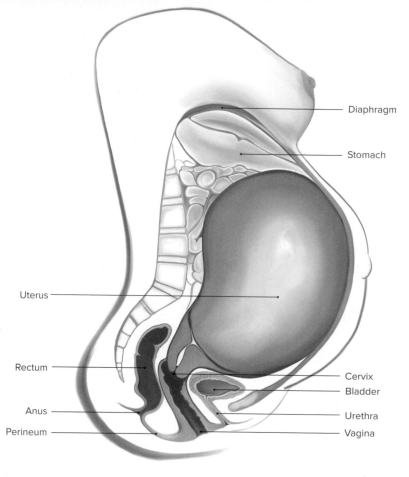

Diaphragm

Stomach

Uterus

Rectum

Cervix

Bladder

Anus

Urethra

Perineum

Vagina

THE PREGNANT BODY

pregnancy, you are likely 0 percent effaced. When your cervix has thinned halfway, it is 50 percent effaced, and when it is as thin as paper, it is 100 percent effaced.

3 **It dilates, or opens.** Before labor, your cervix is "closed." Of note, some women do start to dilate before they are in labor, especially if they have had vaginal births before. As labor progresses, your cervix gradually opens. We measure this in centimeters. A "fully dilated" cervix is 10 centimeters wide—about the diameter of an average-size bagel.

Vagina

The vagina is the canal that leads from the uterus to the outside of the body, lined with muscles and nerves. The cervix sits in the top of the vagina, at the deepest part. The vagina is kind of like a J-shaped tube, except that it is made of many folds of tissues, called rugae, that allow the canal to expand and stretch.

The vaginal fornices are the deepest, cave-like parts of the vagina that surround the neck of the cervix.

Vulva and Perineum

The vulva is made of all the external parts

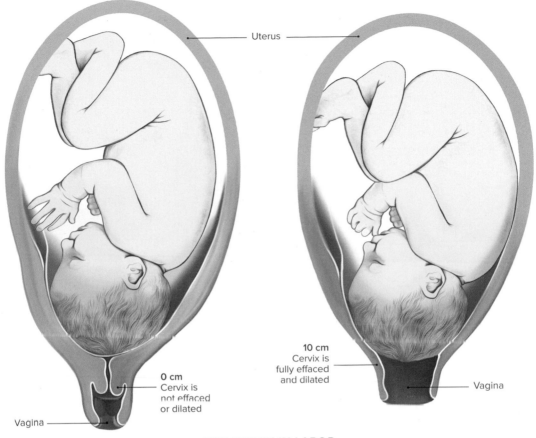

Uterus

0 cm
Cervix is not effaced or dilated

Vagina

10 cm
Cervix is fully effaced and dilated

Vagina

THE CERVIX IN LABOR

of your reproductive system. There are two sets of lips—the inner, smaller labia called labia minora, and the outer, larger labia, called labia majora.

At the apex of the vulva is the clitoris, the part that is responsible for pleasure and orgasms. Only a small portion of the clitoris can actually be seen. The entire clitoris is embedded 4 inches deep and contains 4,000 nerve endings—yup, really!

On the other side of the vagina is the anus. This is the opening to the rectum.

The perineum is the area between the vagina and the rectum.

ENVISIONING THE CERVIX

In Spanish, the cervix is often called *el cuello de la matriz*, meaning "the neck of the uterus." Come to think of it, the cervix does kind of resemble a turtleneck. Many people also like to think of the cervix as a flower bud that blooms over the course of labor.

Normally, the cervix is about 3 to 5 centimeters long, and when you are in labor, its real magic begins.

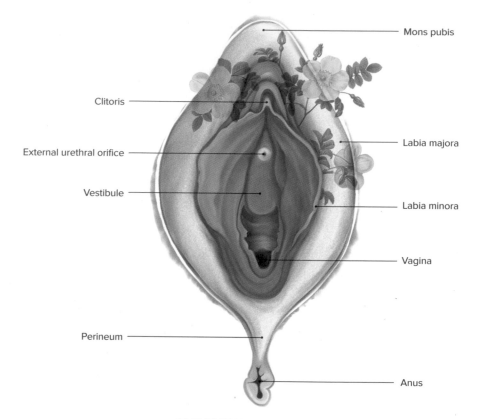

Mons pubis

Clitoris

External urethral orifice

Vestibule

Labia majora

Labia minora

Vagina

Perineum

Anus

THE VULVA AND PERINEUM

HORMONES

During birth, your body is orchestrating a complex biochemical operation that depends on a balance between hormones that help your labor progress and hormones that promote pain relief and provide an extra dose of energy.

There are several hormones involved in labor and birth:

Estrogen   Helps the uterus contract effectively during labor.

Progesterone   Supports your uterine lining in pregnancy to help with implantation and the maintenance of a healthy pregnancy.

Oxytocin   The love hormone. It is what your body releases when you fall in love, when you have an orgasm, and when you nurse your baby, and it is the hormone that causes contractions. Oxytocin is also responsible for helping your uterus contract again after the baby is born, which decreases the amount of blood loss. Oxytocin also facilitates mother-baby bonding— the head-over-heels-in-love feeling that surges through you when you snuggle with your baby.

Cortisol   Known as the stress hormone. As the baby reaches maximum capacity for your uterus, your body begins to release cortisol. This triggers a surge of estrogen, which "tells" the progesterone (which has been preventing contractions ever since you became pregnant) to calm down so that the uterus can start to contract.

Prostaglandin   Helps to soften your cervix.

Relaxin   Relaxes the muscles of your pelvis to allow more room for the baby to move through.

Adrenaline and Noradrenaline   Give you the extra dose of mama-bear energy to power through labor and push your baby out.

Endorphins   Feel-good hormones that help you cope with labor and encourage bonding with your baby.

Prolactin   Nicknamed the "mothering hormone," prepares your body for breastfeeding.

It also, very welcomingly, provides feelings of peace and contentment.

move

Lift and Wrap

To help you understand how your inner core and pelvic floor work, let's do our first guided movement. As mentioned earlier, Brooke Cates, who is a pre- and postnatal exercise specialist, core rehabilitation specialist, and holistic health coach, will provide guidance in the "Move" sections throughout this book. Be sure to check with your provider before trying any new movements or exercises to make sure they are appropriate for your specific situation.

We are going to spend a lot of time during your pregnancy journey concentrating on your core, which is the abdominal area and center of your

PELVIC ANATOMY

Historically, Western obstetrical medicine has focused on the shape of the pelvis of mostly white women of European origin. A groundbreaking 2018 study of hundreds of women's skeletons from across the globe reveals that the shape of pelvises has evolved greatly across the human race. The findings showed that sub-Saharan African populations tend to have deeper birth canals, while Native American women have wider pelvic openings. The pelvic shapes of Asian, European, and North African populations vary between these two extremes.

Yet a surprising finding of the study was that the different pelvic structures were formed by random mutations. There was no particular reason for the pelvis to change shape: It just did, as populations migrated out of Africa over the past 50,000 years. While some pelvises are narrower in different parts and wider in others, the birthing experience isn't necessarily determined by what shape pelvis a woman has. While issues related to a woman's pelvic shape do arise, they are rare. Because so many changes happen to the ligaments and musculature around the pelvis during pregnancy, the bones tend to move in an optimal way to let the baby pass through.

body. Your core will take on significant physical changes as your baby grows, so preparing for the job ahead can set you up in substantial ways. Connecting to the core optimally now and in the months to come can help you prevent common pregnancy-related injuries while keeping you as comfortable as possible in your pregnant body.

Often when we exercise, we only focus on (or connect with) one aspect of the core (if at all). Connecting to all of the parts of your core takes dedication at first, but shifting what it means to engage your core will change the way you strengthen your core for life—not just during pregnancy.

Practice

The following movement is called the lift and wrap, and we'll come back to it again and again.

FEMALE GENITAL MUTILATION

It is estimated that 513,000 girls and women living in the US have had, or are at risk of having, female genital mutilation or cutting (FGM/C). Women who have had genital alterations may be missing parts of their anatomy, which can impact the sensations and experience of birth. If you have experienced FGM/C, you may have specific concerns regarding your birth. You are entitled to respectful and sensitive care. There are providers who have extensive experience working with women who have had FGM/C, so you can absolutely ask to discuss this before deciding if a provider is right for you.

You may have heard of Kegel exercises, for which you clench the muscles of your vagina as if you were trying to hold in pee. The lift and wrap takes Kegel exercises further: You'll be using your entire inner core "box."

The "lift" refers to your pelvic floor muscles.

From a neutral position, begin to exhale as you draw your pelvic floor muscles in toward the center and upward (just like the lifting claw mentioned on page 25). If you want, you can gently insert a finger into your vagina. You should feel the vagina tighten around your finger equally on all sides (many women don't at first. Don't worry; you'll get there).

The "wrap" refers to the transverse abdominal muscles (the sides, back, and front of the box). Remember the muscles that act like a corset? Think now about tightening that corset all the way around as you draw your pelvic floor muscle upward so that your entire core is activated.

This is the way your core should engage in all exercise and any daily movement that requires core recruitment.

Tips for Success

- Place a hand on your abdomen and feel the core pull away from the palm as you exhale and engage.

- Allow your exhalation to be slow and controlled as you begin. This will ensure a deep connection versus a speedy, superficial one.

- Pay attention to other muscles that seem to fire and try to turn them off by relaxing them over time, isolating the engagement to the pelvic floor and core.

- Apply this new core activation to all core-specific exercises. Feel how engaged your core is. Notice how much harder core-specific activity becomes when you start tapping into deeper muscles. You will begin to witness a huge shift in the effectiveness of all abdominal exercises.

remember

The female body is complex and beautiful. Knowing more about your body can help with every stage of conception, pregnancy, and birth. And it allows you to fully participate in decision-making as you progress through this phase of your life. See if you can spend a few moments every day simply reflecting on all the wonder that is your body.

How to Conceive

This time
is sacred, and
I am marvelous.

How did you learn about how babies are made?

Confession: I didn't fully understand the female reproductive system and menstrual cycle until I learned about them in midwifery school. Yes, when I was younger, my parents had "the talk" with me, and yes, my middle school gym teacher explained the concept of puberty to us—a conversation I forcefully blocked out the minute it was over.

But the truth is that for all its beauty, the female body is mysterious, and most women find themselves with at least some questions. Our current sex-ed system can leave something to be desired (though of course, there are some fabulous programs out there). It's also often not inclusive of the many ways that people grow their families now, with the options of adoption, insemination, in vitro fertilization, and surrogacy.

This chapter will reintroduce you to the basics of reproduction, aka making babies. We'll also touch on the many ways that babies can be made with the help of assisted reproductive technology.

If you're part of the LGBTQ+ community or a single mom, advanced reproductive medicine may be a part of your family planning experience. Your route to conception will require many decisions and may involve known or anonymous sperm donors, egg donors, or gestational carriers who may or may not become a part of your family in the future.

When we talk about conception, we must understand that the process is different for every woman. For some, it is easy and fun. Others find it stressful and, at times, heartbreaking. And woven within that are the very real socioeconomic factors that have a profound impact on what this path will look and feel like. Being focused on your process is completely normal! But understanding what other women in our communities, and around the globe, may go through on this journey is important as well. After all, we are talking about giving birth to the next generation of world-changers. We need to be in this together.

However it happens, conception is incredible.

xo,

Diana

UNDERSTANDING THE MENSTRUAL CYCLE AND OVULATION

First, let's take a closer look at the amazingness that is the female reproductive system.

The Menstrual Cycle

The menstrual cycle usually lasts from 21 to 35 days, and it's normal for this number to vary from month to month.

Your cycle is made up of two phases: the follicular phase (before you ovulate) and the luteal (loo-tea-uhl) phase (after you ovulate).

All month long, the endometrium grows with specialized tissue and blood so that if you become pregnant, the fertilized egg has an optimal place to implant (burrow) and start to grow. If you don't become pregnant, that blood and tissue sheds. This is your period.

The first day of your period is day 1 of your cycle. Periods last about 3 to 7 days. The cramping you may experience during your period is your uterus contracting to release the blood and tissue. These are related to the contractions that happen when you give birth, but we'll talk about those in a few chapters ahead.

The follicular or first phase of your menstrual cycle is named after the oh-so-important follicle-stimulating hormone (FSH). FSH is produced by the pituitary gland, in your brain, and its job is to make the follicles in your ovaries grow. What are follicles? They are fluid-filled sacs storing the immature eggs. While several follicles grow each cycle, one (or sometimes more) will eventually become dominant, and that follicle will release the egg during ovulation.

As the follicles grow, and the eggs inside them mature, they produce and release estrogen, which helps make the uterine blood lining and causes some changes in your cervical mucus, which eases the sperm's journey (more on this soon).

When your estrogen level reaches a certain tipping point, your luteinizing hormone (LH) will surge. This causes the egg from the dominant follicle to be released. Hurray! Ovulation. You may be able to feel ovulation as a minor pain in your lower abdomen (called mittelschmerz), but many women don't.

Now you've probably heard that you ovulate on day 14 of your cycle. And you might! Sometimes. Confused? Mother Nature is tricky like that.

The follicular phase (leading up to ovulation) varies in length for many women. So, one month you may ovulate on day 13 and then the next month on day 16. And this can be very normal. What does not usually change is the length of the luteal phase after ovulation. This is why charting your cycles is so important: It is how you will learn about *your* cycles.

After the egg is released through ovulation, it survives for 12 to 24 hours. If a sperm reaches the egg during that window, pregnancy is a distinct possibility. If the egg is fertilized by a sperm (*woohoo!*), that's conception, and DNA from the egg and sperm will do their spiraling dance, uniquely combining to make your baby. Over the course of 5 to 6 days, the fertilized egg travels through your fallopian tube toward the uterus. The follicle that the egg first burst from is now called a corpus luteum, and it releases estrogen and progesterone to help make the uterus an even nicer place for a fertilized egg to grow.

When the fertilized egg arrives in your uterus, it will burrow itself into your uterine lining (this is called implantation and can sometimes cause a bit of spotting). The cells that are developing into your placenta start to secrete human chorionic gonadotropin (hCG), the hormone that pregnancy tests detect.

If the egg is not fertilized after ovulation, the corpus luteum will shrink, which decreases the amount of hormones it releases. This hormonal drop triggers your period.

Monitoring Your Ovulation

Tracking your ovulation, otherwise known as charting, can increase the odds of conception each month because it helps you time intercourse or insemination to occur during the fairly narrow window of fertility—when your egg can become fertilized.

Before we get into the *how*, let's first discuss whether you want or need to chart your cycles. This is a personal decision and depends on several factors. If you will be using fertility treatments, you will likely monitor your cycles and ovulation as part of the treatment plan. If you will be trying to conceive through intercourse, you can choose whether you want to track your cycles.

Here's my take: Charting your cycles can be incredibly empowering. It can create a deeper understanding and appreciation of your body, and (midwife-nerd alert) it is *fascinating*.

But just because I am a cycle geek doesn't mean you have to be. In fact, you may really dislike the process, and that is fine!

If you don't already track your cycles, take a moment and check in with yourself. How will keeping on top of your ovulation make you feel, and what are your needs and desires for this period of time? Following are some things to consider.

You may choose to chart if:

- You want to understand your cycles and fertility signs.

- You are hoping to get pregnant quickly or on a specific schedule.
- You think you will feel a sense of control—and therefore stress relief—from knowing when to time sex.
- You might like to continue charting after your pregnancy, perhaps for birth control purposes.
- You are using fertility treatments.

You may choose *not* to chart if:

- You feel that it will cause you more stress.
- You prefer to take a "wait and see" approach.
- You just don't see yourself being that organized.

If you decide that tracking is for you, let's dive into how to do it. If you're not interested in this tracking process at the moment, feel free to skip to "Fertile Period" on page 40.

How to Track Your Cycles

The first step is deciding where you are going to track your findings. There are many apps out there, or you can record data on a paper chart or spreadsheet. Visit mother.ly/becomingmama for a printable fertility chart that gives you space to record cervical mucus, basal temperature, cervical position, your period, ovulation, sexual activity, pregnancy test results, and other symptoms. (*Whoa!*)

Something very important to note: Research has found that apps that only use information about your cycle length to predict ovulation are not reliable, since cycles can vary so much between women. To get the best results, learn to notice your body's signals in addition to paying attention to a calendar.

The following sections tell you what you are going to look for.

Cervical Mucus   Cervixes naturally have discharge: fluid that leaks from the cervix and eventually out of the vagina. This is normal and healthy—and a key aspect of getting pregnant.

This discharge is called cervical mucus (and is much like the mucus we have in our noses). Its purpose is to help sperm travel up through the opening in the cervix and into the uterus and fallopian tubes where it will meet the egg and hopefully fertilize it.

Cervical mucus changes as your monthly cycle progresses. Starting on cycle day 1, when your period starts, all you likely see is the blood of your period. When your period ends, you will have a few days without mucus.

As ovulation approaches, your cervical mucus production will start to pick up. It will start out as dry or sticky, and yellowish or white, and get progressively watery (in color and consistency). Just before ovulation starts, the mucus will be at its most slippery: Many compare it to uncooked egg whites. If you take some mucus between your thumb and pointer finger, it will likely stretch between them as you slowly move them away from each other. This type of cervical mucus is sperm friendly in that it's easy for sperm to swim through it to their final destination. This egg-white mucus will last through ovulation and will then start to get white and sticky again as you approach the time of your period.

To check your cervical mucus, you can simply pay attention to any discharge you see on your underwear or when you wipe after going to the bathroom. Or you can gently insert clean fingers into your vagina and then look at your fingers to see what the mucus looks like.

When your cervical mucus is closest to the egg-white consistency, it is the best time for sex or sperm transfer.

Changes in Basal Temperature   Checking your body temperature before you get out of bed can help you learn a lot about your cycle. The average waking body temperature in the weeks before ovulation is about 97.0–97.5 degrees Fahrenheit. After ovulation, it heads upward to about 97.6–98.6 degrees Fahrenheit. It will remain elevated until you get your period and it drops back down, or it will stay high because your uterus is now baking a baby! (18 days of a high temperature is usually the magic number.)

Use a basal thermometer, which can be found at your local pharmacy. These are accurate to 0.1 degrees, unlike normal thermometers, which are accurate to within about 0.2 degrees. Basal thermometers allow you to note very small shifts in temperature. You can check your temperature in your mouth, your vagina, or your rectum, but stay consistent. (Need I say it? Once a rectal thermometer, *always* a rectal thermometer.) Check your temperature before you get out of bed in the morning and after getting at least 3 hours of sleep. It works best if you take your temp and record it at the same time each day. Of note, this can be tricky for people who work varying schedules. If this is the case for you, it's especially wise to pair basal body temperature recording with other methods of assessing ovulation, since using temperature alone may be less reliable.

Here's the thing about basal body temperature. It gives us more information looking backward than it does looking forward. You'll only know you've ovulated after the fact. By the time you've seen a temperature rise, you've already ovulated. But by charting for several months in a row, you'll begin to see your pattern: "Oh, wow, my temp rises each month between day 15 and 17, so I must ovulate on day 14 to 16!"

Cervical Position   Around the time of ovulation, your cervix will become higher, softer, and more open (as opposed to low, firm, and closed). With clean hands, you can insert a finger into your vagina to feel for your cervix and begin to chart your findings. Don't be afraid to ask your women's health-care provider to teach you how to do this at your next visit.

Once you've plotted all your findings on a fertility chart or app, you'll be able to see what your amazing body is up to. And soon enough, you'll be able to apply the tracking skills you're developing at this stage to charting the poopy diapers and nap schedules of your darling little baby.

Ovulation Predictor Kits   Ovulation predictor kits can be purchased at most pharmacies as well as online. The tests range from very simple dollar-store strips to advanced machines. The purpose of these tests is to help you figure out when you are ovulating by testing the level of luteinizing hormone in your urine or saliva. There are wearable devices that can help as well by using your pulse rate or temperature when you sleep to see where you are in your cycle, and the research on their efficacy is promising!

However, some providers don't recommend using ovulation predictor kits right away because they worry that we might become too reliant on the (not-foolproof) technology. If you miss the subtle physical body signs described above, you might miss your window of fertility. There is also variation in how the urine-based tests detect your LH surges, so these tests are not guaranteed. It does seem that accuracy picks up when women use urine-based tests combined with checking for cervical mucus. So, if you are up for doing both, that might be your best bet!

Now that you know how to determine when you are ovulating, let's talk about what to do about it.

Fertile Period

Each month, conception can happen during your fertile window, which is about 5 days long, based on how long eggs and sperm can survive in your body. Once released from the ovary, an egg can survive for 12 to 24 hours. To become fertilized, it needs to meet the sperm during that window of time. Luckily, healthy sperm can survive in your body for up to 5 days. Fertilization can only happen when the sperm and the egg are alive in your body at the same time. (This is why knowing when you ovulate can improve the odds of conception.)

Since sperm can live in your body for up to 5 days, if sex or insemination happens within the 4 days before ovulation, there is a good chance the sperm will be alive and waiting for the egg when it releases. Sperm can also be introduced into your body in the 12 to 24 hours after you ovulate and still have the chance of meeting a healthy, living egg.

For example, say you ovulate on Thursday at 11:00 p.m. Having sex or an insemination on Friday means the sperm can possibly meet the egg during that 12- to 24-hour window when the egg is released and able to be fertilized.

But if you had sex or an insemination on Thursday (or Wednesday, or maybe even Tuesday or Monday), the sperm may still be alive and waiting for the egg when it's released on Thursday night. So if you are going to ovulate in the next few days, you can increase the chances of having living sperm ready to fertilize your egg by having sex or completing an insemination.

Timing Sex and Insemination

So, how often should you have sex when you want to get pregnant?

One of the simplest strategies here is to have sex every other day, all month long.

If you are tracking ovulation, and your partner's sperm count is healthy, having sex every day during your fertile window will increase the odds that sperm is waiting for your egg when it releases. Your provider will guide you if your partner has been diagnosed with a low sperm count: Often the recommendation is that you have sex every other day in this case, to give the sperm a chance to build up.

Sperm is healthiest when men ejaculate every 2 to 3 days, so your partner or sperm donor may not want to wait too many days between orgasms—lucky guy.

If you are planning a pregnancy through insemination or fertility measures, your provider will help you determine which days are best for insemination and may recommend a few days before and after the day of ovulation to increase the chances. This is what women who do at home intravaginal inseminations often do as well (see "Intravaginal Insemination (IVI)" on page 48).

If you are in your early 30s or younger, it can be normal to take up to 12 months to get pregnant.

BRINGING SEXY BACK

Sex for a purpose might be a new thing for your partnership, and it may feel a bit, well, unsexy. So to the extent that you want to, infuse a little extra magic into your sex life. This is not a business transaction, and it doesn't have to be timed perfectly to the minute! Get creative and be yourself!

It is also worth noting that many couples really enjoy this time. For example, having unprotected sex to try to make a baby after years or even decades of trying to avoid pregnancy can feel like a whole different sexual experience!

Here are the comments of some Motherly mamas:

"Trying to conceive, we felt very little stress and mostly fun. I actually miss that life stage. Excitement. Anticipation. Hope. Connection." KATE

"It definitely got less fun the longer it took and the more I thought something must be wrong with me. We finally conceived on a day I hadn't tested or even looked at the calendar. We were just enjoying each other after being apart a few weeks due to travel. My advice would be to try to have moments where you're not worried or tracking because those are really important to stay connected, and you never know!" ALLISON

Other tips:

- Avoid lubrication, or find a sperm-friendly lubricant since regular ones can decrease sperm motility.

- Stay horizontal for about 15 minutes after sex or insemination when possible. (Though be sure you pee right after this to decrease the risk of developing a urinary tract infection, which can happen after intercourse.)

- Do what you can to keep the experience fun and playful. If you will be conceiving through sex, you may be having more sex than usual during this phase of your life. See if you can also view it as a way to connect more closely with your partner, as opposed to having it feel like another item on the to-do list.

Remember that open communication can be a total game changer here. Tell your partner how you are feeling and listen to what they are going through as well. It's all valid, and so important to talk about.

If you'd like to track your fertility signs, visit mother.ly/becomingmama to download a free chart.

nourish

Eating for Fertility

The connection between what we eat and fertility has long been studied, yet the conclusions are far from concrete. While there may be ways we can improve our chances of getting pregnant by being mindful of what we eat, it is extremely important to note that infertility can be multifactorial.

There are many women who do everything "right" and still struggle with infertility. To imply that, one, women are to blame for fertility issues, and two, lifestyle changes are possible and accessible for everyone is to grossly discount the real experiences of women in our society. Dietary suggestions are one aspect of a complex web of factors, and we must maintain a broad and holistic view.

With the above caveats in mind, here are three changes you can make to your diet that may boost your fertility:

1 **Decrease fast-food intake.** A 2018 study found that reducing the number of times you eat fast food per week—or cutting it out altogether—can impact fertility. The less fast food we consume, the lower the chance of infertility. This is likely because fast food contains higher levels of unhealthy fats and sugar, which can impact conception.

2 **Consume less sugar.** We can get very specific about this one. Drinking one or more sugar-sweetened drinks per day can decrease both male and female fertility. So opt for unsweetened beverages when possible.

3 **Eat more fruits.** The same study on fast food found that women who ate three or more servings of fruit per day tended to get pregnant faster. While fruit does contain sugar, it is naturally occurring and is digested along with the fiber in the plant, meaning that its impact on your blood sugar is less than if you eat refined sugar with no fiber.

Changes do not always have to be drastic. In fact, many of these studies found that even small changes made an impact. Do what you can, when you can.

THE 2-WEEK WAIT

The 2-week wait is the time between when you ovulate and when your period is due—and when you can take a pregnancy test (more on pregnancy tests in chapter 5). Let me tell you, if you're excited to get pregnant, those 2 weeks are some of the longest weeks you will ever experience. Every minute feels like a year as you wait and wait and wait. You may find that you are constantly assessing your body for pregnancy symptoms: *Was that a cramp? Do my areolas look darker? I swear I just felt nauseous.*

If this is you, know that you are totally normal. I mean, you are waiting for life-changing information. It is understandable (to say the least) that you might be a little on edge.

I am not going to tell you not to think about it (because that might be impossible), and I am definitely not going to tell you to stay relaxed (because *hello, unhelpful comment of the year*). What I will encourage you to do is to reflect and listen to yourself. If researching "signs of pregnancy" makes you tense or worried, avoid the temptation. If thoughts are swirling around your mind, and you just have to get them out, talk to your partner or a trusted friend. Do not force yourself to act in a way that doesn't serve you. Your mind and body hold a lot of wisdom. Honor them and yourself.

The 2 weeks will pass, I promise. And I am rooting for you!

In the meantime, see if you can get hyperfocused on self-care. Get some extra sleep, eat well and hydrate, and stay active doing the things you love. Spend time connecting to your partner or a friend. And through it all, take lots of deep breaths. Remind yourself that no matter what that test says in 2 weeks, this is part of your journey to becoming mama.

IF YOU DIDN'T GET PREGNANT THIS MONTH

You spent all month thinking about it, timed your sex or inseminations around ovulation, and made it through the 2-week wait. But instead of getting a positive pregnancy test, you got your period.

This can be so disappointing.

The moment you decide that you want to get pregnant, it seems like it's the only thing you can think about, which makes a negative pregnancy test all the more discouraging.

I wish I could hug you, but since I can't, following are a few thoughts to get you through.

You Are Not Alone

Most people do not get pregnant in any given month they are trying to conceive. While statistics do not make the disappointment you may feel any less difficult, they can offer insight that not getting pregnant right away does not mean that something is wrong.

What you are experiencing is challenging, but common.

We Are Learning More and More

Fertility is a hugely studied field, and women who are trying to get pregnant are benefiting from tons of new information.

For example, historically women have been told that there is a precipitous drop in fertility that happens after age 35. But after examining the results of studies including 58,000 women, Marinus Eijkemans and colleagues wrote that their "findings challenge the unsubstantiated pessimism regarding the possibility of natural conception after age 35 years." In other words, there was a decline in fertility, but it may not be as extreme as we once thought.

Sarah Bjorkman, MD, counsels her patients that there's a slight decline in fertility starting at age 32 and a more significant decline after age 37. She strongly encourages women to speak with their providers as soon as they start thinking about planning for a baby to optimize their chances of success, whenever they are ready.

Keep in mind that even well-done studies can only go so far in helping you anticipate your own experience. They are based on large populations and may or may not reflect what is happening for you specifically. To get a better picture, I encourage you to talk to your provider for a personalized interpretation of your fertility.

Reassess Your Strategy

While a negative pregnancy test is no reason to panic, it's always good to spend some time making sure your current "strategy" is working for you.

If you are having sex or using insemination at home to get pregnant, pay particular attention to signs of ovulation and the timing of intercourse or inseminations. You can always check in with your health-care provider for tips catered specifically to you.

If you are already getting fertility treatments, your provider will help you reassess and make sure the methods being used are still the best choices for you.

Nurture Your Relationship

Babies bring joy, but baby-making doesn't always feel that way. Scheduled sex and insemination appointments don't always scream romance. And when they don't result in a pregnancy, it can be that much more difficult.

Have an open conversation with your partner about how you are both feeling. Marriage and family therapist Chrissy Powers encourages couples to stay in dialogue throughout the process of getting pregnant because your thoughts and emotions may continually change. Try to remember that you are in this together and that understanding each other more fully will strengthen your bond.

Find Your Village

Many women decide to keep their attempts at conception a secret, and of course, that is completely fine. But if you feel comfortable bringing it up, you may be surprised to learn that there are others in your circle who are going through the same thing.

Research finds that receiving support from other women who are TTC, along with compassion from family and your partner, can significantly improve your experience.

If you don't have a local village, look online. There are social media groups that can offer tremendous support, and of course there is your TTC Motherly village at mother.ly /becomingmama.

It may be difficult to be around people who are getting pregnant when you are dealing with negative pregnancy tests. If you find yourself feeling jealous or resentful, don't worry. It's normal and completely understandable. If you need to take a little break from hanging out with those people, honor that need. Just do your best to not be consumed by it—not for their sake, but for yours.

Be Gentle with Yourself

It's so easy to get swept up in the potential for self-judgment and shame. Please hear me when I say that you haven't done anything wrong. It reminds me of Julia Roberts in the movie *Notting Hill*: You're just a girl, standing in front of some sperm, asking them to make you pregnant. This is still a wildly exciting time in your life.

So, take a break from thinking about it. Indulge in your favorite food, put on a pair of fuzzy socks, and watch movies all day.

Be kind to yourself. Because you are amazing.

Most women I know do not relish getting their period. Our society generally doesn't do a great job of empowering women's natural cycles. "Periods are gross" is the underlying message we receive from a young age. Plus, they can be uncomfortable and inconvenient, and we tend to face them with a feeling of "ugh." For a woman who is trying to get pregnant, periods can be particularly upsetting because in addition to the annoyance, there is the knowledge that conception didn't happen that month.

Grieving the arrival of your period in this phase of your life is normal, natural, and completely okay. Sometimes though, reframing how we think about periods can help us to get through the disappointment that they can bring.

Some women have found it helpful to have a plan in place for day 1 of their cycle. If you anticipate that day as a miserable one, why not deliberately make it something to look forward to instead? Maybe you can find a way to spend some time alone, letting out your disappointment and then restoring yourself any way that feels right. Lounge around and read an indulgent book. Spend the afternoon outside or go out for dinner. Gather with other women for connection or support. Do what makes you feel whole and centered. The promise of your period is that the cycle is starting again, and the possibility of new life is renewed.

Know When to Get Help

If you are reading this for the first time, it's likely that you are not in need of assistance. However, at some point, you may decide to consult with health professionals who can advise you about other measures to increase your fertility.

In women age 35 and under (who are using intercourse to get pregnant), infertility is diagnosed when pregnancy has not occurred after 12 or more months of regular, unprotected sex. For women over 35, infertility is diagnosed after 6 months. About 1 out of every 9 women and 1 of every 11 men have a fertility issue, and it can impact every aspect of their lives.

I spoke with Dr. Aimee Eyvazzadeh, an ob-gyn who specializes in reproductive endocrinology and infertility. She says that she wishes more women would seek help sooner for their fertility concerns, and she advocates for preventative fertility measures like hormone testing and egg freezing. She feels that we need to change the messaging that women receive: If you are worried about your fertility, discuss it with your provider or meet with a specialist. Many insurance plans will cover the diagnostic tests for infertility.

FERTILITY TREATMENT AND TECHNOLOGIES

Using advanced reproductive technology (ART), in which sperm meets egg without traditional heterosexual sex, is an increasingly popular option for straight and gay couples, as well as for single people. Aside from infertility challenges, many prospective parents often need to consider other methods and involve outside parties such as gestational carriers or gamete donors to have a baby.

If you are in the position of seeking treatment for infertility, you probably know that various paths can end up being quite expensive, sometimes prohibitively so. For example, in vitro fertilization requires harvesting eggs and combining them with sperm in a petri dish to make embryos. The embryos are then implanted in the uterus over successive menstrual cycles until the process succeeds or the embryos run out. In 2019, this process could cost between $10,000 and $15,000 each cycle. This doesn't include the cost of preparatory fertility drugs. (We'll cover other treatment options in just a bit.) Unfortunately, most insurance companies in the US do not cover fertility treatments, although a few do because of legislation that varies by state. Some private companies and universities also offer fertility treatment coverage, so definitely check with yours to see what their policies are.

While it's encouraging that the trend seems to be toward providing more resources for families using assisted reproductive technology, there is so much more that needs to be done to ensure that everyone who wants to has their best shot at having a family.

Many people end up using savings, borrowing from their retirement accounts, asking friends and family for assistance (directly or via crowdfunding sources), or taking out private loans to finance needed fertility treatments. It's not an easy process, for sure, and it can take an emotional and financial toll. None of the options is guaranteed, but the statistics paint a positive picture for those who are able to avail themselves of the medical route.

Fertility Screening Panels

A good place to start exploring your fertility options is a thorough fertility screening, as Dr. Eyvazzadeh recommends. Gaining a complete understanding of your physiology and hormone levels can help you feel more empowered and also provides valuable information for creating a treatment plan.

A fertility screening can include the following tests:

Ultrasound   A routine pelvic exam has the potential to miss some of the most common issues that could be affecting your fertility. Conditions like fibroids or ovarian cysts can't always be felt. An ultrasound will help your provider see the size, shape, and position of the uterus and determine if anatomical issues are affecting your fertility. It's simple and will offer more detail than a manual exam. It involves your provider placing an ultrasound probe into your vagina, which will magnify any potential issues. The ultrasound will also allow your medical team to see how many follicles are present in your ovaries, known as your antral follicle count, which is a good indicator of your ovarian reserve, or how many eggs you are carrying.

Hormone Tests   Hormones are created in your endocrine glands and act as chemical messengers that control a lot of bodily functions, including hunger, energy levels, and your reproductive system. They also influence your emotions and mood. Think about how you might get irritable or weepy just before you get your period. That's due to fluctuating hormone levels.

The hormones critical to your fertility that are generally tested are anti-Mullerian hormone (on blood tests, this shows up as AMH), which can signal how many eggs you may have left; follicle-stimulating hormone (FSH), which gets made in the pituitary gland and once per cycle triggers your ovaries to release an egg; and estradiol (E2), which starts a hormonal chain reaction leading to ovulation. Age is still the best indicator of your egg quality and ability to get pregnant naturally, but these tests can provide you and your doctor some data points in your ability to conceive.

Genetic Testing   We inherit genes from each of our parents and pass them on to our children. Our genes determine the majority of our traits, including the color of our hair and eyes, the diseases we may get, and also how our reproductive systems behave. By way of a simple blood draw, there are now multiple reproductive gene tests that will reveal genetic variants linked to common diseases related to infertility. Your fertility provider can also offer you an extended carrier screening panel to test both your eggs and the sperm of your partner or donor to make sure they don't share common mutations.

Tubal Testing   Often fertility challenges can arise when one or both of your fallopian tubes are blocked. This is known as tubal factor infertility because the egg can't be transported down the tube. Your provider can perform a tubal evaluation called a hysterosalpingogram, or HSG, where a small amount of nontoxic dye is pushed through the uterus and tubes to see if blockages exist. (Blockages may come up if you've had sexually transmitted infections, endometriosis, or abdominal surgeries. Sometimes blockages can be cleared.) This is

the cause of infertility in 25 to 30 percent of women, who rarely know they have it because it doesn't usually present with symptoms.

Semen Analysis   It's essential to remember that both sperm and egg play a role in fertility. Yes, the old cliché "It takes two to tango" is accurate! A thorough semen analysis is part of routine fertility screening if your partner is male.

Remember that it's not just women who are having children at older ages now; so are men. There is ample research showing that as men age, their sperm develops more genetic problems. One is DNA fragmentation, which is the amount of damaged DNA in a sperm sample. The field of epigenetics, which is the study of gene expression, is helping medical professionals and researchers understand the way that the changes in sperm DNA influence fertilization, embryo quality, and miscarriage as well as neurodevelopmental diseases in children like autism, schizophrenia, dyslexia, and bipolar disorder. For these reasons, if you're using donated sperm, it may be a good idea to choose a donor in his 20s or 30s.

The plus side for men, however, is that if a semen analysis does show DNA fragmentation, they have the opportunity to improve their sperm quality through lifestyle and dietary changes. A health-care provider can offer more insight and guidance as necessary.

Once your fertility provider gains a solid understanding of your situation, many options can help you get on the route to a healthy pregnancy. Here's an overview.

Fertility Medicines
Prescription drugs may be one of the first options to investigate, especially if your

practitioner identifies that your ovulation is irregular or unpredictable. Clomid and Letrozole are oral medications that are most commonly used. There are many others out there depending on what your hormonal screening shows, but one thing to note is that most of these are administered via injections that influence hormone production. And yes, you have to give them to yourself or have someone give them to you, which can take some getting used to! It's worth noting that use of these medications comes with a higher likelihood of carrying multiples.

Intrauterine Insemination (IUI)

IUI can help when you have had trouble conceiving with your partner or if you're trying to conceive with donor sperm. IUI is a less invasive and generally lower cost option than in vitro fertilization (IVF).

Intrauterine insemination increases the chances of connection between sperm and egg by bypassing the cervix. Your provider inserts a long and skinny plastic tube in the vagina and through your cervix, placing the sperm (which has had dead and suboptimal material removed, sometimes referred to as "washed and spun") directly into the uterus. This is a fairly simple procedure, and most women find that it does not cause too much discomfort. This can happen during natural ovulation if you time your cycles. Ovulation can also be induced by first taking hormones to stimulate egg growth and then getting a shot of human chorionic gonadotropin (hCG) to time your ovulation for the day of insemination. IUI has been found to be slightly more effective than ICI (see the next section, "Intracervical Insemination (ICI)").

Intracervical Insemination (ICI)

In ICI, the sperm is placed close to the cervix via a small tube rather than directly into the uterus, and the sperm does not have to be washed and spun.

Intravaginal Insemination (IVI)

In this case, the sperm is placed into the vagina with a syringe (also known as the "turkey baster method"). While it's not as efficient as IUI or ICI, many people choose this method because you can do it at home with the help of your partner—or even by yourself. This might be a good choice for you if you are hoping to avoid the clinic setting and looking for a conception process that feels more intimate and personal.

In Vitro Fertilization (IVF)

In vitro fertilization is a more invasive series of procedures than any of the methods above, but it increases the chances of getting pregnant. If you are not using frozen eggs, donor eggs, or your own frozen embryos, the first phase of IVF begins by stimulating the growth of eggs with hormonal injections. The eggs are then removed through a procedure, and egg and sperm are brought together in a petri dish to achieve fertilization. The embryos are screened for genetic problems, and then the most viable one or two are placed back inside the woman's uterus at the ideal time, about 3 to 6 days after the egg is fertilized. Depending on how many embryos you choose to implant, IVF can carry a higher likelihood of twins or multiples.

Donor Eggs and Embryos

Donated eggs can be fertilized by the sperm of your partner or someone known to you and then implanted via IVF. Additionally, some fertility clinics offer programs in which people who have gone through IVF treatment can donate frozen unused embryos. You usually have the opportunity to see the medical history of the donors and choose an embryo that will be implanted in your uterus.

Surrogacy and Gestational Carriers

Surrogacy is when a woman agrees to carry a pregnancy for a person or couple until birth. There are two types of surrogacy. In traditional surrogacy, the surrogate woman is artificially inseminated with the sperm (her egg becomes fertilized), and in gestational carrying, an embryo is implanted via IVF (your egg or a donated egg). If you are interested in exploring these options, there are organizations that can support you and assist in arriving at a legal agreement that protects everyone involved.

Complementary Medicine

Many women also seek out complementary medicine and lifestyle changes to achieve their pregnancy goals, either as a first step or in conjunction with fertility specialists. Reproductive nutritionists, functional medicine doctors, and acupuncturists all have specialized practices encouraging fertility for their patients. If this is of interest, you can search for a professional in your area with fertility expertise or ask your provider for a recommendation.

Adoption

Adoption is a beautiful way to grow a family. If you are interested in learning more, you can start by reaching out to a local adoption agency or speaking with a local group that supports adoptive parents.

gather

- ○ App or notebook to record fertility signs
- ○ Basal thermometer
- ○ Ovulation kit or wearable ovulation tracker, if using
- ○ Sperm-friendly lubrication

to do

- ○ Decide if you want to chart your cycles, and if so, start!
- ○ Consider dietary changes to make.
- ○ Identify your support team (medical and social).
- ○ Look into your insurance coverage and determine fertility treatment coverage, if applicable.
- ○ Schedule an appointment with a fertility specialist if appropriate.

remember

We are lucky to live in a time when so many options exist for people to get pregnant, and so many resources and supportive organizations are available to assist your fertility experience. Your individual path to motherhood has so much beauty in it. Now, beauty does not mean perfection: It can be messy, confusing, and overwhelming. But so is life. Ultimately, no matter how you are doing it, you are the epicenter of a journey that can create a new little life. How powerful is that?

Take care of yourself and take care of each other. *You've got this.*

Miscarriage and Loss

You were
in the world
but bricfly, but
in my heart
forever.

Oh, my darling.

Though I am not sure of the details that led you to this chapter in the book, I am fairly sure you wish you weren't here right now.

No matter the reason that brings you here, your heart is heavy, and your mind is consumed.

I want nothing more than to be able to cocoon you in comfort and surround you with love. And you, well, *you* want so many things that seem impossibly out of reach right now. Answers, the ability to sleep, eyes that don't feel swollen from crying, a glimpse into the future that feels light instead of dark.

Most, if not all, of those things will happen in time. In these heartbreaking moments, and in many challenging moments of life, I remember this idea from Ajahn Chah, a Thai Buddhist monk: *Right now, it's like this.*

And it's okay to be *in* it. The sadness, the anger, the resentment, the disappointment—whatever emotions are ripping through you right now. No emotion is wrong or unjustified. In fact, you don't need to *justify* anything you are feeling.

This loss is a part of your motherhood journey. Because motherhood is all of it. It is daydreaming of your future children when you're a little girl. It's the shock and joy of a positive pregnancy test. It is the bitter, heart-wrenching agony of a miscarriage. It is grief and healing. It is hope. And ultimately, it is love.

So, if it feels right (and only if it feels right), go ahead and love the pregnancy that ended. And love yourself, deeply.

The reasons you find yourself in these pages are yours to know. The grief that you feel right now feels lonely and all-encompassing. But in that grief, you are connected to women across generations and continents who are on this journey with you. While you heal, know that we are all holding you.

xo,

Diana

P.S. Sometimes miscarriage comes with other feelings, besides sadness. Perhaps your pregnancy was unplanned, and you were feeling ambivalent or upset about it, and maybe contemplating your options. It is possible that for you, miscarriage comes as a relief, which may make you feel good, or guilty, or both. I want to make sure you know that we are holding space for you, too. There is no one set of emotions that are valid during a miscarriage. They are all valid, and you are worthy. So, use the pieces of this chapter that are helpful to you, and be gentle with yourself as you go through your own healing journey.

WHAT IS MISCARRIAGE?

A miscarriage is the spontaneous end of a pregnancy before the 20th week. From 11 to 22 percent of clinically recognized pregnancies end in miscarriage. However, many embryos are formed and don't progress beyond the first few days (this is called a chemical pregnancy). They are released during a normal menstrual flow, so this percentage is likely higher.

The commonality of miscarriage does not make yours any less hard to bear, but please know that you are not alone.

SIGNS AND SYMPTOMS OF MISCARRIAGE

Little is scarier when you are pregnant than seeing a smear of vaginal blood. If you have come to this section of the book, there is a chance that is what happened to you.

Spotting is fairly common during pregnancy and can have several causes. It occurs in about 25 percent of pregnancies. (See "Spotting and Vaginal Bleeding" on page 447 to learn more about its causes.)

Other symptoms of miscarriage may be:

- Pain or cramping in the abdomen or lower back
- Fluid, foul smelling discharge, or tissue expelled from the vagina
- Fever, chills, or body aches

If you have any of these symptoms, it is always a good idea to call your doctor or midwife. If your pregnancy is early, and you don't yet have a provider, that is okay (and normal). You can call the person you see for regular gynecologic care, or you can go to an emergency room.

WHY DOES MISCARRIAGE HAPPEN?

It is human nature to crave answers, especially in the time of grief and loss. One reassuring aspect of miscarriage is that it is almost always due to factors outside of your control. Multiple studies have revealed that in healthy women, miscarriage is *not* correlated with too much exercise, having sex, or having a job that involves straining, lifting, or night shifts.

Miscarriage may have the following causes.

Genetic or Chromosomal Abnormality One theory about the cause of miscarriage is that the embryo or fetus reaches a point where an abnormality prevents them from continuing to develop. Some theorize that the abnormality is somehow detected by the woman's body, which then initiates a miscarriage to stop a potentially dangerous or unviable pregnancy.

Traumatic Life Events There are studies that show that women who experience negative events, such as the death of a spouse or parent, a situation of war or scarcity, or violent experiences, have a higher risk of miscarriage. But please note that everyday worries and stress at work are not linked to increased risk.

Other Physiological Responses Scientists are researching the origins of miscarriage, which may also include immune, autoimmune, or other microbiological factors.

WHAT HAPPENS?

If you are concerned that you may be having a miscarriage, the first thing to do is call your provider. They may suggest that you come into the office or possibly head to the emergency room.

I want to stop for a moment to address something that more than a few women have shared with me over the years regarding medical staff's attitude toward miscarriage (this may be your own care team or the ones you meet in the ER). Most medical providers out there are genuinely good, caring people who will treat you with the empathy and compassion that you deserve during this awful event. It is my sincere hope that that is your experience.

I need to brace you for the fact, however, that this is not always the case. Sometimes women feel as though they don't receive the emotional support they need from the nurses, the doctor or midwife, and sometimes the front office staff. This can be quite hurtful.

Here is likely what is going on behind the scenes:

- They are busy. This is not an excuse, but it can explain why they may have difficulty tapping into their more nurturing side.

- Their job is to make sure you get the treatment that you need to stay safe. They cannot save the pregnancy, and sometimes this message comes across in a way that feels clinical and insensitive.

- They may be a bit desensitized. Miscarriage is common, and over the years, medical workers tend to build emotional defenses (knowingly or not) to prevent themselves from burning out. What this means for you is that you get a provider who does not seem sympathetic about your loss, and that can hurt.

Let me be clear: None of this is okay. You deserve as much warmth and attention as you want during this time. Truly, this is a "them" thing, not a "you" thing. Whatever emotions you're experiencing are the *right* emotions for you, even if they are not reflected back by your health-care team. Please do not let the attitude of others make you question your own thoughts and feelings.

Consider bringing a support person with you to your appointment or ER visit—someone you trust to provide the right amount of love, no matter what.

When you arrive in the office or ER, the providers will likely do a pelvic exam, an ultrasound (usually using a transvaginal wand that is placed inside your vagina), and blood tests to determine your levels of hCG. If tissue from the pregnancy has come out, and you have had miscarriages in the past, they may also ask if you want the tissue tested. This may reveal whether the miscarriage is caused by chromosomal abnormalities, which would prompt future discussions with a fertility specialist (if desired). Although tissue sampling is usually recommended after a repeat miscarriage, it isn't usually done for the first one (see "Recurrent Miscarriages" on page 64 for more information).

Depending on your specific circumstances, your provider will recommend a treatment plan or present options to choose from. In addition to the physical and medical factors, there is a ton to consider from a personal and emotional level as well. Talk to your provider about it all. Read the quotes that follow from members of the Motherly community who share how they went about making the decision that worked best for them.

Expectant Management
This means allowing the process to happen

naturally on its own. From 60 to 85 percent of miscarriages require no interventions, through a process that can take 2 to 6 weeks. Expectant management is usually only offered if the loss occurs in the first trimester, as it can involve less risk at this early stage of pregnancy.

What you may experience: moderate to heavy bleeding with cramping. You may also see some blood clots or pieces of tissue come out or even the recognizable fetus and placenta.* Your provider will ask you to report bleeding that is so heavy it saturates a pad in an hour or two, fever, chills, light-headedness, and any other concerns immediately. You may be given pain medication to help with the cramping.

It's important to note that expectant management does not always work, and some women end up needing to have medical or surgical treatment as well.

You might choose expectant management if:

- You prefer not to take medications or have surgeries.
- You want the process to feel as "unclinical" as possible.
- You are comfortable with some uncertainty around the length of time this phase will take.

*If you choose expectant or at-home medical management, you may want to consider what it will be like for you to potentially see tissue from the pregnancy, which may or may not look like an embryo or fetus. As with every aspect of this experience, there is no right or wrong way to feel or cope. Whether or not you choose to look, and what you choose to do with the tissue, is completely up to you. It may come out on your pad or in the toilet, or perhaps you'd like to bury the tissue in

The expectant management route allowed me to process my grief in a much more tangible way. I felt physically, emotionally, and spiritually connected to the process, and I think I moved through my grief in a healthier way than when I had my D&C."

CATHERINE

"I decided to take the oral medication because I didn't want to have surgery, but the idea of going home and just waiting for the miscarriage to pass on its own was more than I could take." ANIYAH

"My provider and I decided it was probably best not to wait for things to progress naturally, since it hadn't yet passed on its own. The idea of taking medication sounded anxiety-inducing and potentially traumatic for me. Although more invasive, I liked that the D&C meant that the miscarriage would be resolved in a short procedure. It also made me feel better that my OB would perform it and that I would be under the supervision of medical professionals instead of dealing with this by myself at home." MAURA

a garden or other place that is meaningful to you. Some funeral homes offer cremation services for miscarriages. If you belong to a spiritual community, a leader may be able to offer suggestions as well.

Medical Management

You may be given a vaginal suppository or oral medication called misoprostol (or Cytotec), which helps the uterus release its contents. About 71 percent of women will have completed miscarriage within 3 days of taking the medication. Some women will need to take another dose. For about 15 percent of women, medical management does not remove everything, and surgery is required. Some providers also recommend another medication taken before the misoprostol, called mifepristone. Sometimes an injection of a medication called methotrexate is used, especially in the case of an ectopic pregnancy (page 57).

What you may experience: symptoms similar to those listed under "Expectant Management" (above). Medications can also cause diarrhea and nausea.

You might choose medical management if:

- You prefer to avoid surgery.
- You prefer for the process to move along without the waiting period.

Surgical Management

Doctors can perform a procedure to empty the tissue from the uterus. This is called a dilation and curettage (D&C). Surgical management may be recommended when women have dangerous symptoms, such as an infection or severe bleeding, the pregnancy is further along, expectant or medical management has not been successful, or the woman prefers it. Some forms of D&Cs can happen in the office setting, under local anesthesia. During a D&C, the cervix is slightly dilated (opened), and an instrument called a curette is used to remove the miscarried pregnancy. Your provider may also use a small vacuum to remove the tissue (this is sometimes referred to as a dilation and evacuation, or D&E).

What you may experience: D&Cs and D&Es are relatively short procedures, usually lasting less than 30 minutes. After it is over, and depending on what type of anesthesia you receive, you may stay in the clinic or hospital for several hours for monitoring. You will likely have a small amount of bleeding and some moderate cramping. You can ask for pain medication if this is the case.

You might choose surgical management if:

- You prefer for the process to move along without the waiting period.

- You don't want the uncertainty that expectant or medical management can come with. The risk that not all the tissue would be removed during a surgery is only about 1 percent.

Many hospitals and clinics have options for parents who wish to bury or cremate the remains of the pregnancy. If this is of interest, let your provider know, or ask to speak with a social worker.

TYPE OF LOSS

There are a lot of medical terms used to describe miscarriage and loss and the various

SENSITIVE TERMS

The medical term for miscarriage is "abortion." You may see it written as threatened, spontaneous, missed, incomplete, or complete abortion. (The medical term for pregnancies that are not continued by choice is "termination" or "induced abortion.")

courses it can take. If you feel called to learn more about your specific type of loss, you can begin here. If reading through these descriptions will be triggering and you prefer to skip over them, I'll see you again on page 59, "Recovery After Miscarriage."

It is important to remember that "type of loss" and "emotions experienced" happen independently of each other. No ranking exists to qualify which type of loss is harder than another. Your experience is your experience.

Miscarriage

A miscarriage, or spontaneous abortion, is when a pregnancy stops developing and the embryo or fetus dies before the 20th week of pregnancy.

Threatened Miscarriage

When a woman has vaginal bleeding, but a miscarriage has not yet been diagnosed, she is usually given the diagnosis of "threatened miscarriage." This is upsetting wording, no doubt. Vaginal bleeding can have many causes and does not always mean impending miscarriage. There can be other benign causes, such as bleeding that may happen right when the embryo implants in the uterine wall. (For more on vaginal bleeding, see "Spotting and Vaginal Bleeding" on page 447.)

Chemical Pregnancy

Chemical pregnancies are miscarriages that occur very early, usually just around the time of your period. They likely account for about half of all miscarriages. In fact, many women do not even realize that they were pregnant in the first place because the bleeding looks like a period. Women today are likely more aware of their chemical pregnancies than in generations past because pregnancy tests are so advanced and can detect pregnancy hormones very early.

Ectopic Pregnancy

An ectopic pregnancy is a rare complication (occurring in less than 1 percent of pregnancies) in which a fertilized egg implants in a location outside of the uterus. The most common site is a fallopian tube—which is why they are sometimes referred to as "tubal pregnancies"—but they can also occur in the ovaries, cervix, or abdomen.

If an ectopic pregnancy occurs, the embryo will grow, possibly causing the fallopian tube to burst, which is a serious condition.

Just like other forms of miscarriage, an ectopic pregnancy is challenging because, for a period of time, your body is tricked into thinking it is a healthy pregnancy. You may get a positive pregnancy test and experience early pregnancy symptoms, like nausea and tiredness. As the embryo grows, though, it may start to cause some additional symptoms:

- Vaginal bleeding (spotting or severe)
- Pelvic pressure or pain
- Shoulder pain
- Dizziness
- Difficulty breathing or blue lips and nails
- Confusion
- Sweaty, clammy skin
- Restlessness

Any of these symptoms warrant immediate medical attention.

The provider will likely suggest a vaginal ultrasound to diagnose what is going on. If they find an ectopic pregnancy, the growing tissue will need to be removed as quickly as possible to prevent more complications. They may suggest a medication given by injection, or it may require surgery to remove the embryo. The tube it was growing in can sometimes be repaired, though sometimes it needs to be removed.

Women may be more likely to have an ectopic pregnancy if:

- They have had one before.
- They have had pelvic inflammatory disease (PID).
- They have an IUD in place or have had a tubal ligation surgery.
- They smoke.
- The pregnancy was conceived using IVF.

Yet just like miscarriage, it often happens with no rhyme or reason.

Blighted Ovum

This type of miscarriage is also called anembryonic. In an anembryonic pregnancy, an egg is fertilized and attaches to the uterine lining. The gestational sac begins to develop, but the embryo inside does not. This is usually caused by a problematic chromosome.

Molar Pregnancy

Also called a hydatidiform mole or gestational trophoblastic disease, molar pregnancies are rare (about 1 in 1,000 women will experience it). Sometimes a problem can occur at the time of fertilization, which causes the cells that normally grow into the placenta to develop into abnormal tissue. Women can have a complete molar pregnancy, in which the abnormal placenta cells are the only parts of the pregnancy that grow, or a partial molar pregnancy, in which some abnormal placenta cells grow while other parts are normal, possibly even including a developing embryo. Molar pregnancies can become dangerous for the woman, as they can invade the uterine muscles and can also become a type of cancer, though this is incredibly rare.

Molar pregnancies may end on their own and be passed from the body, or they may require intervention, such as medication or a D&C. Historically, the medical community has suggested monitoring your pregnancy hormone levels for a period of time after a molar pregnancy and waiting about a year before trying to conceive again. The theory was that a resurgence of hCG could trigger the abnormal cells to start growing again. However, more current research is showing that women may not need to wait that long, so definitely speak with your provider about this if you've experienced a molar pregnancy.

Missed Miscarriage

In a missed miscarriage, the embryo or fetus is not living, but the signs or symptoms that can accompany a miscarriage are not present. They are usually diagnosed during an ultrasound or blood work.

For some, a painful aspect of a missed miscarriage is that, through no fault of your own, there was a period of time when you were not aware that the pregnancy was lost. Women have described feeling guilty and questioning why their bodies or intuition didn't let them know that something had happened. Some women feel uncomfortable with the idea that they have been carrying a lost pregnancy, embryo, or fetus for a period of time. Any of these feelings are valid.

Please know, though, that the "miss" is not on you. For reasons beyond your control, there was no way for you to know.

Treatment for a missed miscarriage (medical management or surgery) is often needed unless your provider determines it is safe to wait to see if it passes on its own. Your preference here is, of course, important as well.

Incomplete Miscarriage

In an incomplete miscarriage, the pregnancy has stopped progressing and starts to leave the body through bleeding and tissue passage, but some tissue remains in the uterus. This means that medical intervention is usually necessary to complete the process.

It can be difficult to come to terms with the idea of a miscarriage, only to find out that there is still more you need to go through to complete the process.

Septic Miscarriage

In rare circumstances, tissue from the miscarriage can become infected. If the bacteria migrate to the bloodstream, it is possible to develop a whole-body infection, known as sepsis. A woman with sepsis might have a fever (temperature of 100.4 degrees Fahrenheit or greater), chills, foul-smelling vaginal discharge, prolonged bleeding, and pain in the lower abdomen. These are emergency symptoms that require immediate medical attention. Treatment will likely involve surgery to remove the infected tissue and antibiotics to treat the infection.

RECOVERY AFTER MISCARRIAGE

The physical and emotional recovery from a miscarriage go hand in hand, and of

MISCARRIAGE AFTER AN INDUCED ABORTION

ACOG states that women who have had an induced abortion are not at an increased risk of future fertility issues or pregnancy complications. If you have had an induced abortion, this miscarriage may come with additional emotions, but please hear me—every pregnancy is its own entity. Try to focus on your needs in the here and now, without judgment.

course everyone's process will be different. Following are some things you might be wondering about.

Bleeding

Most women find that they bleed for a few days to a week or so after the tissue has left the uterus. If you bleed for longer than 2 weeks or bleed heavily—filling a pad in an hour or two—call your provider. If you are using expectant management you will likely have heavy bleeding, but you should still call with this amount of bleeding because it is possible that you will need emergency treatment. Many providers will recommend that you avoid using tampons during this time to prevent irritation or infection.

Hormones

Your hCG (pregnancy hormone) level will gradually decrease during and following a miscarriage, but the rate depends on how far along the pregnancy was, if the miscarriage is complete or still in process, and which (if any) treatment measures were used.

Return of Period

Most women find that their period returns about 4 to 6 weeks after their miscarriage. It may take a few months for your cycles to return to normal.

Lactation

Depending on how far along your pregnancy was, you may find that your breasts lactate, or leak breast milk, after a miscarriage. This can certainly be a difficult and painful reminder of your loss.

If you experience lactation, you can try these measures of relief:

- Wear a supportive bra without underwire.

- Apply cold washcloths to your breasts to relieve discomfort.

- Put a head of cabbage in your refrigerator and place its leaves in your bra.

- Talk to your doctor or midwife about taking pain medication, like ibuprofen.

- Be mindful of the development of a painful, red, warm breast lump, especially one that comes with a fever. If you develop this, it could be a plugged duct, or mastitis. Reach out to your provider for support.

Some women decide to donate their breast milk after a pregnancy loss. If this is of interest to you, look up the organization Human Milk Banking Association of North America for more info.

Body Weight

It is possible that your pregnancy came with some weight gain, and its lingering after a miscarriage may feel burdensome. To the extent that you can, release any feelings of self-critique. Give yourself time to grieve, even if that means indulging in some comfort food.

There is usually no such thing as immediately "bouncing back," and the pressure to do so is unfair, especially in this phase of your life. We can *reflect* on our past, of course, but we can't go back to change it. We only have the present time and can only move forward—when we are ready. So, if you don't feel like bouncing back right now, don't.

The caveat I will share is that sometimes resuming activities like exercise and healthy

A NOTE FOR PARTNERS ON MISCARRIAGE

This loss is your loss too. Yes, your partner is the one who is going through the physical trauma of this loss, so she will need your support. Just remember that your feelings are entirely valid as well. The days of confining cultural expectations are on their way out, so please feel what you need to feel.

Research has shown that when partners "perform caring acts" and engage in sharing and talking about the experience after a miscarriage, the connection between the couple improves. So, if you can, tell her how you feel. Leave her a note in the morning to tell her you are proud of her. Cook dinner for her or drop off her favorite snack for lunchtime at work. And remember that her healing will not be linear, so be as patient as you can.

eating can help you heal in restorative ways and find the peace and acceptance that you may be craving. It's also important to remember that sometimes weight gain and overeating can be a sign of depression, which you are likely at a higher risk for during this difficult time. If you feel that you are depressed, do not hesitate to reach out to a therapist.

nourish

Nourishment After Loss

In order to rebuild and recover, your body needs healing nourishment.

Keep food simple. Aim for whole foods that require minimal preparation and have higher nutrition content. Include the following:

Protein for Rebuilding Try to incorporate a source of protein with each meal and snack to optimize rebuilding in the body. Examples of protein-rich foods include eggs, nuts/nut butter and seeds, yogurt, cheeses, beans, lean meats, poultry, and seafood.

Easy-to-Digest Foods Warm and cooked (as opposed to raw) foods can be therapeutic to your body and soul and promote healing. This might include bone broths, soups, or stews. These foods can also be easier on your body to digest and process during this delicate time.

Nourishing Fats Including healthy fats in meals and snacks can also help your body better absorb nutrients and promote satiety after eating. Avoid the more unhealthy vegetable oils, such as canola oil, safflower oil, and corn oil, and focus on grass-fed butter, extra-virgin olive oil, coconut oil, and animal-based fats.

Water to Stay Hydrated Replenishing fluids is also critical to recovery from a miscarriage. Drinking 10 cups of non-sugar, non-juice, and non-caffeinated fluids per day is your goal. This might include warm herbal teas, such as red raspberry leaf tea, which is a natural herb that can help the uterus strengthen and heal.

Of note, some providers do not recommend red raspberry leaf tea in early pregnancy (we just don't know that much about it yet). If you plan to start trying to conceive soon after a miscarriage, discontinue drinking it or speak with your provider for their take.

RETURNING TO YOUR DAILY LIFE

You may be anxious to return to a sense of normalcy after this unexpected experience. If your bleeding has stopped, you are feeling well enough, and there are no medical contraindications, you can slowly start to resume the things that make you feel whole.

Recovery does not happen in a straight line. It varies by day, or even by the hour. So, try to include some flexibility and grace into your schedule and routine. If you get to the gym and simply can't go in, it's okay. You can try again tomorrow (or the day after that). If you planned a coffee date with your best friend but wake up and find that the idea of sitting in a crowded restaurant feels like too much, ask them to come over and watch a movie with you instead.

move

Most providers will recommend that you wait a few weeks after a miscarriage to resume any exercise routines, though it's best to speak with them to understand their specific recommendations for you. As with everything, take it slow and listen to your body. If something hurts, if you start bleeding, or if you have any other concerns, call your doctor or midwife right away.

love
AND VILLAGE

Times of grief and stress can bring couples closer together, or they can put a strain on relationships. One of the keys is to remember that each person involved is grieving in their own way. It can feel frustrating if your partner is handling the grief differently than you are; for example, if you are calm, but they are bursting into tears often. To the extent that you can, extend the gentleness that you are treating yourself with to your partner. And talk about it, as often as it feels right.

In 2016, researchers looked into the impact that miscarriage has on male partners. They found that men tend to feel many of the same upsetting emotions that women do during and after a miscarriage but demonstrate their feelings differently—and perhaps for a shorter period of time than women. Many said that during the healing process from a miscarriage, they felt it was their job to "support and protect" their partners and lighten the load by running errands, taking care of the household, and so on. Men also found that social expectations put pressure on them to act strong or hide their emotions—despite their sadness.

For same-sex partners of women who have miscarried, the loss can be amplified if medical staff do not recognize the partner's parental role and that it is often harder for same-sex partners to become pregnant.

One of the keys to going through a miscarriage as a couple is communication. One of

you may be inclined to try to move on quickly, while the other may want to talk about it often. The couples who can find harmony in how they communicate about the loss tend to be more satisfied in their relationships, so try to have the conversation. For example:

Babe, I can foresee myself needing to talk about this to process what I am feeling, but I also want to be respectful of your needs. Can we find a designated time every day to spend some time chatting? It will help me to know that we've set aside a few minutes to talk, so I don't have to worry about initiating the conversation every time.

Returning to sex is a personal decision, and only you and your partner know what is right. The medical community has routinely encouraged women to wait at least 1 to 2 weeks after a miscarriage before having intercourse, but ACOG states that this is not based on evidence. So, talk to your provider about the best plan for you.

Have a conversation with your partner about how you are feeling and let them know that you may need to stop or take a break if unexpected or difficult emotions come up for you. And remember that they may have their own process to go through as well.

If pregnancy is a possibility, be sure to have a birth control plan in place if your provider recommends that you wait a period of time before trying again.

Sharing About Your Loss

Miscarriage has rarely been a topic of public discussion, and a stigma has developed around it. In recent years, thankfully, this is changing. So many women are coming forward with their stories and creating a more understanding environment around loss. Right now, or when you have healed, you can decide how and if you want to speak about your experience. But know that there is camaraderie out there, if you want it. Whether you read a memoir that touches on loss, connect with a friend who has gone through it, or find a local support group, you may find tremendous comfort in shared experiences.

If you are part of a spiritual or religious community, you might find solace in focusing on those beliefs and speaking with a trusted leader within the organization.

Your village loves you and wants to do right by you; they just don't always know how. As a culture, we do not tend to be comfortable with silence, especially when it comes to sad events like a miscarriage. We want to fill the void and make it better. This is well intentioned, but it has the potential to make things feel worse for you. You might hear comments like:

"It wasn't meant to be."

"At least now you know you're able to get pregnant. There will be another baby soon."

"The best thing to do is get on with your life and move on."

"It could have been worse. You were only x weeks along. Someone I know lost her pregnancy at xx weeks!"

These comments may resonate with you, and that's great. Or you may find them off-putting, which is also totally fine. The point is that you do not have to mold your

healing process to fit into other people's ideas or story.

Here is my advice: Think about the people in your life who you know will give you the support you need. To the extent that you can, increase your time with them and decrease your time with the people who tend to bring you down. Also, think about what might be helpful and ask for it. It is perfectly fine to say, "Listen, I want to spend time with you, but I don't feel like talking. Can you just come over and sit next to me?"

It is not possible to control all of your interactions entirely, as you know. Before you leave home in the morning, try this little mindfulness practice:

Close your eyes and take a deep breath. Imagine a protective layer forming around you. It can be a sort of fog, a warm light, or maybe a cloak or blanket wrapping around you. This is your force field. Remind yourself that you can't control what people say, but you don't have to absorb the messages that don't serve you. Let them bounce off your force field.

One other issue to be aware of is how you may feel when you are around pregnant women or new parents. If you find yourself having to fake a smile—or unable to find one at all—you do not have to feel guilty. Grace, a Motherly community member, said:

We lost our babies [in September]. In the last three months, I've watched several of my friends announce their pregnancies or have their babies. I'm happy for them— how can I not be?—but I'm resentful that they get to keep their babies while I didn't. I think about it all the time, but it only really hits me every so often. When it does, it knocks me down, and it takes some work to get back up again.

Prepare yourself for how you might want to respond if this happens to you. It is okay to decline an invitation to a baby shower. You might also consider having a conversation or sending a message to your pregnant friends or family members that says something like this:

I am sincerely happy for you and wish you all the joy and love in the world. I want to let you know that I am going through a grieving process right now, so I may be a little out of touch for a while. I am not avoiding you. I just know that I need to

focus on my own healing before I can turn my attention outward. I will reach out as soon as I am ready!

Motherhood During a Miscarriage

If you have a child, there are some additional challenges to going through a miscarriage. It can be hard to grieve when you are in the midst of busy #momlife, and of course, there may be questions from your kiddo if they are aware of what happened—which is totally normal. Dr. Claire Nicogossian is a licensed clinical psychologist who has had a miscarriage—and a subsequent "rainbow baby" (see "The Rainbow Baby" on page 66)—and is passionate about supporting other women who have had losses. She recommends following your child's lead. They are likely going to have a lot of questions. Remember that they are curious and trying to process. If you don't know the answer, it is okay to say, "I don't know. What do you think?" Responding with love is all they need.

Therapy

Many women choose to see a therapist to help them process their emotions, and it can be really helpful. You can start by asking your primary care provider or a few trusted friends if they have local professionals that they recommend. Or go to a website like psychologytoday.com to find someone. Many therapists have sliding fee scales, and many insurance plans will cover a certain number of behavioral health sessions each year, so check with your insurer.

Recurrent Miscarriages

When a woman has two or more miscarriages, it is called recurrent miscarriage. Recurrent miscarriage is rare, happening to only about 1 percent of women. After three miscarriages, providers will usually recommend testing to look for the possible cause, though more than half of the time a cause cannot be identified. Testing may include blood tests, a pelvic exam, or ultrasounds.

Recurrent miscarriages can be caused by chromosomal abnormalities of the developing embryo. Sometimes women and men produce eggs or sperm that are more prone to problems, and some women may have structural issues or chronic illness that can lead to miscarriage, such as uterine fibroids, adhesions, a septate uterus (uterus with a partial "wall" in the middle), autoimmune disorders, or polycystic ovary syndrome.

The treatment for recurrent miscarriages depends largely on the cause, if discovered. Chromosomal issues can be addressed by in vitro fertilization (IVF) and/or using donor sperm or donor eggs. Problems with the uterus or cervix may be fixed with surgery. And treatment plans can be developed to address underlying illnesses.

Miscarriage as a Part of Life

A miscarriage can feel like the most isolating event of your life. But it is also one of the ties that bind us. We don't talk about miscarriage enough, but we all know its impact. So many women have had them, and those who haven't know someone (or several people) who have. From women we pass on the street to those we interact with on a professional or social level to close friends and family, miscarriage is all around us.

But so too is love.

The profound human experience you are going through connects you to so many women—past, present, and future—who know what it is to feel this loss. There is a global village of women holding space for you.

Some women are comforted by finding a special way to honor their lost pregnancy, embryo, or fetus. (This is certainly a personal decision, and if it doesn't feel right, that's completely okay.) If it does, here are a few ideas:

- A ceremony or funeral with friends and family

- Plant a tree in memory of the loss

- Purchase or make a piece of memorial jewelry

- Get a symbolic tattoo

- Create a rock garden

- Make a scrapbook with photos and sentimental items

- Commemorate a significant day of this journey (such as the day you found out you were pregnant, the pregnancy's due date, the day the pregnancy was lost) with a yearly tradition

Work

Work after a miscarriage can be therapeutic, and difficult. You may relish the chance to be distracted and back in your routine. But it can be tough if you are with a customer, nannying a toddler, or in a meeting and are suddenly overcome with emotion and tears. Consider these ideas:

- If you have a compassionate boss or co-worker, do you want to let them know what's going on, so they can provide necessary support?

- Do you want to have a story ready to go should you start crying or find the need to step out of the room? (A little fib is okay here if you don't want to share, I promise.)

While many women have chosen to keep their losses quiet, know that you certainly don't have to. You might also consider speaking openly at work about your miscarriage: telling everyone what happened, crying when you need to cry, or taking a mental health day if that is available to you. When you think about it, it is *quite* unfair that women have to carry the trauma of miscarriage and are also expected to be discreet and secretive in order to "act professional" in an attempt to protect others from having uncomfortable feelings. Our society wants us to hide our vulnerability, but that is what makes us the most human and alive.

Your whole self is valuable. You don't need to hide any of it.

In sharing, you might also inspire others around you to feel more comfortable to share about their losses, which would be a huge shift in the right direction.

This decision is of course yours to make. Being a part of this culture shift is not your responsibility in these moments if you don't want it to be. Your primary focus is you. The rest will fall into place.

THE RAINBOW BABY

You may or may not be thinking about trying to get pregnant again. As with everything else you are dealing with, this is such a personal decision. Some women start trying again as soon as they are able, while others need more time to heal. Only you can know what feels right for you.

ACOG states that while the general recommendation is for women to wait for several cycles before trying to conceive again, we don't actually have much research to support this. The recommendation is so that your uterus has time to heal, your hormones can reregulate, and you can accurately figure out your due date. If you don't have a period before conceiving again, it can be hard to tell the baby's due date without an ultrasound. Consider speaking with your provider about what you want and ask for suggestions based on your situation.

Of note, a 2010 study of over thirty thousand women found that women who conceived again within the first 6 months of having a miscarriage tended to have better outcomes than those who waited longer.

Another huge factor, of course, is your level of readiness. Whether you are anxious to conceive, need more time, or prefer not to try at all is completely up you. You may also need to pull together the financing for another round of reproductive assistance.

If you do become pregnant with a rainbow baby (the term for a baby born after a miscarriage because after the storm comes beauty), the following words from Dr. Claire Nicogossian may be helpful.

Here are five things to know about your pregnancy with your rainbow baby:

1 For many, the process of grief is a journey never completely done. Grief isn't something a person can work through methodically like a list in a

timely, structured way. Grief is messy, unpredictable, raw, and uniquely expressed. It can show up in surprising ways when a woman becomes pregnant after a loss: crying in the market when walking by a baby, trying to hide physical signs of showing so you can keep the secret of being pregnant just a little longer, being preoccupied with worries about something going wrong with this pregnancy. If you experience grief that catches you off guard when you're pregnant, this is entirely normal. Be gentle with yourself and let go of any judgment. Grieving the baby you lost and feeling excited about the new pregnancy can coexist. Allow yourself to experience the roller coaster of emotions you may have without judging yourself or thinking it should be a certain way. Instead, accept what you are feeling and move through the grief as it happens.

2 Worry is not uncommon during pregnancy, and for mamas who've had a loss, anxiety can be off-the-charts intense, often overshadowing joy. If you're experiencing significant worry during your pregnancy, or when worry gets in the way of everyday activities or prevents you from sleeping, eating, taking care of your family, or functioning at work, it is time to get support. Reach out to your provider or therapist and discuss how you are feeling and how worry is impacting you and your pregnancy. There is help: Talk about it.

3 Many women feel cautiously connected to their next pregnancy after experiencing loss. These feelings are totally understandable. Being tentatively connected has a lot to do with self-protection: not wanting to be hurt again should something happen to this pregnancy. Be kind to yourself if you notice feelings of disconnection, protection, and fear. If any of these feelings persist or become disruptive to your everyday functioning, please reach out and talk to your provider.

4 Feelings of guilt during pregnancy after a loss can catch some mamas off guard. You may notice feeling guilty at times for being happy, excited, or connected to the new pregnancy. Positive feelings during pregnancy can be stressful because there may be simultaneous fears of being disloyal or forgetting the baby you lost because you feel happy. Here's what I want you to know: You can feel happy for the new baby and sad for the baby you lost. You can feel both emotions. Just observe them and understand that a mother's heart is vast enough to feel a complex range of emotions, from guilt to joy and everything in between.

5 Any mama who has experienced loss knows in her heart that no other pregnancy or child can replace the one she lost. And so, there is a bittersweetness to pregnancy after a loss: gratitude, excitement, anticipation, as well as sadness and anger. As you move through your pregnancy and welcome a new baby, there may be a strange feeling of wondering: Would this new baby even be here if I hadn't lost my other baby? Many mamas experience these thoughts and feelings. What I have seen be helpful for some mamas is to find a way

to honor and remember the baby who was lost, a concrete gesture of keeping the lost baby part of the family.

It cannot be emphasized enough that you are not alone. Here's what Motherly's community members want you to know:

"I want other women who have suffered a miscarriage to know how common it is. I felt so isolated following my first loss. And although the second miscarriage was just as awful, knowing I wasn't alone in what I was going through made it easier to talk about it and my feelings with my friends and family." KATE

"It definitely helped to know that it's common. But I was mad and upset that no one wanted to talk to me about it. I really wanted to talk about it out loud, but everyone around me would tiptoe around the subject or pretend it never happened. I wanted validation that the baby I lost was real for me, and just because I miscarried doesn't mean it magically disappeared and doesn't exist anymore. I felt like everyone just swept it under the rug and moved on." SYLVIE

"I wish people would realize that it's all a process. It's messy, and it's hard, and there's no right or wrong way of doing it. Just because you're told there's no heartbeat, it doesn't end there. You'll doubt yourself. You'll probably blame yourself. You'll grieve and sometimes feel silly about it because you never met the baby, or held them, but it's still a loss of that life that you expected to have once the baby was born. It's mourning the future you thought you'd have and what they could have been like. It's sometimes wondering if the little girl or the little boy you see at the store looks like what your baby would have been like. There will be reminders and memories that will hurt, but it's important to let yourself feel them. Cry when you need to. Grieve as much as you need to. And if you don't need to, that's fine too. We all handle it differently." MITZI

"We're talking about trying again. It's hard now that we've lost the innocence of a relatively complication-free first pregnancy; we know what the risks are and what can happen. We know now that not every pregnancy ends in a baby. It's knocked us over and challenged everything we thought our lives would be.

"I'm not over it. I never will be. But one thing I've learned, and I hope other moms will benefit from, is that you don't get better. You get stronger. You learn how to take it a minute, an hour, a day at a time. You learn to take care of yourself. Hopefully, you can have others around to take care of the little everyday things so that you can focus on dealing with the one impossible thing. Our families were there to take care of those little things, and it meant the world." GRACE

pause AND REFLECT

Written for you by Catherine Keating, a yoga instructor, author, and mom of two who has experienced two miscarriages.

Find a comfortable position for your body, either lying down or sitting up. If you are lying down, allow your body to sink into the floor. If you are sitting, be sure either your feet or sitz bones are connected to the floor beneath you. Notice that the earth is supporting you.

Begin with your breath. Place one hand on your heart space and the other on your lower belly, your womb, and begin breathing deeply and completely. On the inhalation, allow your heart to lift your hand; then allow your lower belly, your womb, to lift your other hand. Exhale. Sink deeper and deeper into the earth. Allow Mama Earth to hold you.

Let any feelings that arise come through without judgment. Every feeling is valid; every emotion is sacred.

Inhale. Exhale.

You are safe. You are loved. You are nourished.

Stay connected with your breath; remain present with each inhalation and exhalation.

Start breathing in and out from your heart space. Feel or envision a warm glow around your heart. Feel it expand and retract on each breath.

After a few breaths in this way, send your golden glow to your womb space. Inhale and allow for a greater expansive warmth. Think to yourself, "I am loved."

Exhale and feel the warmth radiate throughout your body, extending down past your feet and all the way up through the belly, heart, throat, face, and out of the top of the head. Think to yourself, "I am whole."

As you continue to breathe, invite this warmth or glow to become a softness that settles into the spaces of your heart and your womb. Notice if you are holding any breath, tension, or negative thoughts in these areas. Breathe love into the spaces. With each inhalation, repeat internally, "I am here." And with each exhalation repeat internally, "I am loved."

In this place, a relaxed position with a warm loving glow growing from your heart to your womb and back again, know this truth: Love, all love, is present, always. Your baby's love is still here. Love is still here.

Love never disappears. Love is an energy that may change forms, but never disappears.

Listen for any messages that might come to you and return to your breath. Become aware, again, of your inhalations and exhalations. Allow your chest to rise and fall. Come back into your body. Wiggle your fingers and toes; stretch like a cat waking up from a nap.

Know you are loved.

And know you can return to this place at any time.

Love is never broken.

remember

Your loss has become part of your journey. You may decide that this is the end of your pregnancy journey, that it's just too painful to try again. Or you may need some time before you're ready to try again. Or you may be ready right now. Whatever you decide is the right path for you *is* the right path for you.

Finding Out You Are Pregnant and Your First Weeks of Pregnancy

Welcome to motherhood; it begins now.

Have you heard the expression "Today is the first day of the rest of your life"? Well, wel-come to the rest of *your* life. You will always be you, a strong woman with her own goals, passions, and importance in the world. But now that (rock star) woman is becoming a mama, and everything is about to change.

I say that not to scare you—even though the thought of it is, well, scary—but rather to prepare and empower you. This is all a lot to take in—this massive, life-changing news that your baby is on their way and that you are on your way to becoming a mama. It can seem hard to believe. This is real. Although it feels like a lot is happening *to* you right now, you are actually in a position of serious influence.

You have the power to cocoon yourself in a village that nurtures you. If you have a part-ner, expecting a child together will connect you deeply—talk about an adventure! But it can also cause some rifts along the way. Open communication will help you find ways to lean on each other as you grow into this new chapter together.

This is also a perfect time to look at your community at large. Maybe you'll reconnect with those who are physically far away, find a supportive online group, or find a new mom club around the corner. And don't forget about all the professional resources you may have available: From lactation consultants to yoga instructors, they are there to build you up so that you can harvest all of your inner awesome-sauce (yup, I went there).

You have the power to explore and redefine your professional and personal life. Pregnancy and motherhood often inspire us to reassess priorities and goals in new ways, big and small. What will the next months be like for you at work, wherever work happens for you? Can you make any adjustments in your daily grind that will allow you to *grind* a little less and rest a little more? *Psst: Close to 50 percent of our Motherly community told us that they made career changes as they transitioned into motherhood, something we'll talk about in more detail in a few chapters.*

And you have the power to change the world. Really, you do. That little baby you are growing so carefully is about to become a member of our global human community. Right now, they're busy making you feel kinda nauseous. But before you know it, your precious baby is going to be a citizen of this world, bringing their voice, thoughts, and love into it and making it a better place to be. How powerful is that?

We come to this moment with our own unique stories—from *how* we got pregnant to the events that led us to this moment, from our ancestral and family lineages to the deeply individual and intimate emotions we experience every day. What a personal and universal phenomenon that no matter how we got here and what our stories look like, we are united by the fact that much of what we go through is the same.

Take a few deep breaths and try to feel the connections you have gained—to your baby, and to mothers around the world, past and present.

Welcome to motherhood. It begins now, and we are so happy to have you here.

xo,

Diana

Throughout this journey, I will guide you through specific areas to reflect on. For this reflection, try being still and present for a few minutes. Focus on your breath. Breathe in deeply through your nose and feel your lungs fill with air while your belly expands. Exhale and feel your muscles loosen, sending tightness and stress out with your breath.

Our world is full of so much noise. It easily infiltrates our bodies and our minds, leaving us feeling frenzied. It can be so hard to connect with our bodies when the world around us demands so much.

But if we can carve out a few precious moments of refuge, we can reground and recenter.

See if you can find a way to reclaim your roots and your balance.

Think about how you can create your own sanctuary—even if it's nothing more than a calming mantra or image that you focus on as you breathe deeply.

- In what areas of your life do you feel frenzied and less connected than you'd like to be?
- Where might you have an opportunity to slow down each day, if only for a few minutes?
- What will it feel like to be still for a few minutes?
- How can you create a habit of retreating from the noise?

ALL ABOUT PREGNANCY TESTS

One of the first rites of passage of modern motherhood is seeing the positive sign on a pregnancy test. It's a simple signal, but there is a lot going on to make it appear.

From the moment the fertilized egg attaches to your uterine lining—about a week after conception—your placenta starts to form. Your placenta is an incredible organ

THE PLACENTA IN SOUTHEAST ASIA

The placenta holds a great deal of cultural value around the world. In Southeast Asia, the word for placenta means "jacket" in the Hmong language—the very first item to keep the baby warm and protected. In this culture, when a baby is born, the placenta is often buried. When the person dies, it is believed that their soul travels to the placenta burial site so that they can put their jacket back on before they can comfortably leave this world.

with the sole purpose of supporting your pregnancy and helping your baby grow.

Your placenta will do many important things for your baby throughout your pregnancy (we'll talk more about them when the placenta ups its workload in the second trimester). Right now, though, it is making the oh-so-important hormone human chorionic gonadotropin (hCG).

This hormone is present when you are pregnant to help protect and support your pregnancy and developing embryo by maintaining the other necessary hormones (like estrogen and progesterone) and by telling your body not to have a period.

Your hCG level will continue to rise through most of your first trimester, roughly doubling every 2 to 3 days. Pregnancy tests work by detecting the hCG present in your body, either in your blood or in your urine.

When to Take a Pregnancy Test

As mentioned in chapter 3, the 2-week wait can seem painfully slow. So, if you are yearning to take a pregnancy test, I totally get it, especially since many brands advertise detecting pregnancies very early.

Here is the thing though: By taking tests early, you may be increasing your odds for upset in two ways. First, it may just be too early to tell. Seeing a negative test is hard, so you may not want to go through that until the result actually means something; a negative pregnancy test today may be a positive test tomorrow. The tests are also expensive. Second, and sadly, some pregnancies end very early in what is known as a chemical pregnancy (see "Chemical Pregnancy" on page 57 for more). There is a chance that a pregnancy detected by a very early positive test can just end, and that might be a heartbreaking experience to go through.

Of course, this decision is yours to make. I encourage you to think through the possible scenarios and how they would make you feel as you decide what to do.

Urine Tests

Store-bought pregnancy tests (aka "pee-on-a-stick" tests) can usually start to detect the hCG hormone in your urine when it reaches 20 milliunits, or sometimes even lower, which happens around or just before your missed period. This is usually about 12 to 16 days after you ovulate and conceive.

Store-bought, or over-the-counter (OTC), pregnancy tests vary, as do, of course, women's bodies. Some women will get a positive pregnancy test days before their missed period, while others have to wait longer. This can be a super-stressful period of time, but try to remember that those little sticks are just, well, little sticks. They are an important tool, yes, but ultimately your body is in charge of the pregnancy.

Blood Tests

Blood tests (also called quantitative pregnancy tests) have to be ordered by a health-care provider and are usually used for women who may have a high-risk pregnancy or have undergone fertility treatments. They may also be used if there is a concern about miscarriage.

Blood tests are more sensitive than urine tests. They can detect very small amounts of hCG, starting around 1 week after ovulation. With these tests, an hCG value greater than 5 milliunits is considered a positive pregnancy test. In a healthy pregnancy, the hCG value will double approximately every 2 to 3 days.

HCG VALUES BY WEEKS SINCE LMP	
Weeks	hCG Value Range
4	5–426 mIU/mL
5	18–7,340 mIU/mL
6	1,080–56,500 mIU/mL
7 to 8	7,650–229,000 mIU/mL
9 to 12	25,700–288,000 mIU/mL
13 to 16	13,300–254,000 mIU/mL
17 to 24	4,060–165,400 mIU/mL
25 to 40	3,640–117,000 mIU/mL

The hCG levels in blood pregnancy tests vary a lot. A test done at 4 weeks may show an hCG level of anywhere from 5 to 400 milliunits, and a test at 8 weeks may show an hCG level of anywhere from 7,000 to over 200,000 milliunits. That's a huge range!

That's why just one blood draw value doesn't tell us much about whether a pregnancy is progressing normally. We need a few numbers to compare to see if and how the number is increasing. If you are using blood tests to check on your pregnancy, your health-care provider will probably order two tests, 2 to 3 days apart.

For example, if a woman's hCG on Monday is 15 milliunits, we would expect that it would reach 30 milliunits by Wednesday or Thursday.

It is important to note that because these tests are so sensitive, it is possible to get a false positive—a test that says you are pregnant when you are not. This can happen if, for example, you have had a recent miscarriage and some of the hCG hormone from that pregnancy is still in your blood. Your healthcare provider will help you assess the results as they apply to you and your scenario.

Ultrasounds

Ultrasounds use high-frequency sound waves to make images of things inside the human body—like a uterus and a developing embryo. Transabdominal ultrasounds are done by placing a plastic transducer (also called a wand) on your belly with some gel (to help the sound waves travel into your body). Transvaginal ultrasounds are done by placing a lubricated probe in your vagina.

During early pregnancy, a transvaginal ultrasound may be used to:

- Detect a pregnancy
- Determine how far along a pregnancy is
- See how many embryos are growing (single baby, twins, or more)
- Find the location of the pregnancy (for more information on ectopic pregnancies, which occur outside the uterus, see page 57)
- Check for a heartbeat
- Monitor how an embryo is growing
- Assess the pregnancy if there is a concern for miscarriage
- Look at maternal organs and structures in the pelvis

At about the 5-week mark, ultrasounds can show the beginning of a developing pregnancy, called the gestational sac. Starting at around 6 or 7 weeks, a heartbeat can usually be detected in a healthy pregnancy.

A NOTE FOR THE MAMA WHO IS FEELING NERVOUS

The existence of all this pregnancy detection technology is both awesome and challenging. We have access to a lot of information, which can help us but also make us nervous about all of the things that could potentially go wrong.

Everyone feels differently about this. You may not be comfortable with lots of different tests and may prefer to take a wait-and-see approach. As long as there is no medical risk to just lying low and watching, that is completely acceptable.

Or perhaps you are nervous and craving the information that can come from these early tests. That is normal (and understandable)

GROWING BABY TERMINOLOGY

Your growing baby will have different technical names throughout pregnancy:

Zygote Immediately after fertilization until day 5, an egg that has been fertilized by sperm

Blastocyst Five days after fertilization, dividing cells that implant in your uterine lining

Embryo Weeks 5 through 10

Fetus Week 11 through birth

Newborn Birth to about 2 months old (the cutest, softest thing you could ever imagine)

as well. This "thing" you are going through is a big deal! And we all come into pregnancy with our individual experiences and personalities, which impact how we feel.

It is also important to know that obstetric practices and providers have different protocols. Some may offer an ultrasound and blood work to confirm pregnancies very early, while others don't routinely offer those tests at all.

Generally speaking, more invasive tests (like the blood test) are reserved for when they are medically necessary. This comes from a variety of reasons: insurance rules, financial concerns, and not wanting to expose people to tests they don't "need."

It is also worth considering the research around potential risks of some of these tests. ACOG states that there are no known long-term dangers posed by having frequent and early ultrasounds but acknowledges that this could change one day as research progresses. If you are concerned about ultrasounds, you can check with your provider about any recent findings and let them know that you prefer to minimize or pass on ultrasounds.

And in the case of early pregnancy loss, unfortunately, tests cannot change the outcome.

But that doesn't mean they are not valuable: Your emotional well-being is important.

Wherever you are on the nervousness spectrum is okay. You may find that speaking openly with a few trusted friends or family members about their experiences can be helpful in sorting through your thoughts. And of course, talk with your care provider to help you make the best choice for you. If an extra blood test or an ultrasound would make you feel better, there is value in that. Do not be afraid to ask for what you need.

This is a lot, I know. There is no one right way to feel, and chances are you're experiencing a lot of different thoughts and emotions right now.

Mama, you are not alone in this.

Your journey through pregnancy and parenthood will be full of tiny—and huge—decisions, just like this one.

Should I ask for an early ultrasound if available? Should I get an epidural? Should I return to my job after the baby is here? Should I say yes to sleepaway camp? (That decision will be here before you know it, by the way.)

I hate to say it, but these answers will rarely come easily. We have access to so much information, and there can be so much noise out there, that it can be hard to know what the right thing to do is.

So here is my advice, for now and for always: Ask for opinions, look for research, and then do your very best to tune out the noise and listen to your heart. We all make mistakes; we all change our minds. But if you make these decisions from a place of love, you're doing it right.

One more thing: If you are having fears around the possibility of miscarriage, you are not alone. You can turn to page 57 to learn more about miscarriage and then to "A Note for the Mama Who Is Feeling Nervous" on page 75 to read about the common, significant, and distressing fear of loss—and how to cope.

WHOA, YOU'RE PREGNANT!

This moment is bound to come with tons of emotions.

Take some time to reflect on what those emotions are—without judgment. We receive so many messages, outward or subconscious, about how we should feel about pregnancy, babies, and motherhood. But that doesn't mean there is one right feeling. Chances are that in any given day you are having many different emotions and thoughts about it. And it's also okay if you are not having powerful emotions about the pregnancy yet.

It's all okay.

Here's how some Motherly mamas felt when they first found out they were pregnant:

"I was so happy because I had always hoped to be a mom, but I also felt overwhelmed with the idea of being responsible for another human being. I also felt scared because I wanted so badly to have a healthy pregnancy and a healthy baby."   JENNIFER

"I didn't feel pregnant. I was expecting some sudden change or something that would make me feel different all of a sudden. And then the morning sickness made it worse because I just felt constantly sick (but still not pregnant), and no one knows yet, so it's just an awkward stage of pregnancy. Once I felt [the] baby moving, that was when I really started feeling motherly."   JULI

"I was terrified. We had decided we would try, and it happened very quickly. Finances, lifestyle changes, how it would work in an apartment, the fact we had no close family to help, everything. It was overwhelming for both me and my partner."   LIZETTE

It's okay if you are nervous. It's okay if you can't stop crying. Or smiling. Or both. It's okay if you're unsure.

It's all okay.

None of it dictates what kind of mother you're going to be. So, don't resist the feelings that are coming up for you: There is wisdom in all of it.

If Getting Pregnant Has Been a Long Process

Becoming pregnant after experiencing a miscarriage or loss, a long road of trying to conceive, or undergoing fertility treatments can come with a unique and difficult assortment of emotional responses. Some women feel conflicted. They always imagined this moment and how happy they'd feel, and yet they are now finding that they are having trouble embracing the joyful aspects of being newly pregnant. This in turn makes them feel guilty. *This is what I wanted. I should be happy right now.*

Psst: If you are pregnant after a miscarriage, turn to page 66 to read some advice about the rainbow baby journey.

You may also feel extra anxious about the health of the pregnancy. When you've experienced struggle and sorrow, the pain and stress can be hard to forget. It's only natural to feel almost desperate to avoid that again.

Or maybe you feel just fine!

It's all understandable. The essential piece is that you continue to take care of *you*. Research has found that incorporating relaxation exercises into your daily routine can significantly reduce your level of anxiety. You might also consider meeting with a mental health therapist to help you cope.

Carolyn Wagner, a Chicago-area therapist who specializes in maternal mental health, advises that a history of infertility is a risk factor for perinatal mood and anxiety disorders (PMADs). She says it is super-important to understand that just because the pregnancy was hard fought and very much wanted, it can still be a difficult adjustment.

"There may be extra anxiety due to a history of pregnancy or infant loss, or heightened worry because it took so long to get pregnant: What if we lose this pregnancy and then it takes forever to get pregnant again? If there was any kind of fertility treatment, all of the extra hormones could add to the difficulty," she says.

Moms in this situation can first and foremost give themselves permission to feel whatever feelings are coming up, Wagner urges. "You can be grateful for your pregnancy *and* hate morning sickness or wonder if you have what it takes to be a mom *and* question what you were ever thinking doing this as you pass another sleepless night. You can be grateful for your pregnancy *and* sometimes think maybe this was a mistake. Whatever you're feeling is absolutely okay. Make sure that you're continuing to take care of yourself, whether that's getting exercise, spending time with friends, taking a nap, or reading a good book. So much attention is focused on the baby growing inside you, but you need care, too."

Wagner also says, "Find a provider that you trust, whether it's an OB or a midwife, and call them when you have a question or something doesn't feel right. If they know your long journey to pregnancy and are the right fit for you, they'll understand that you may need a little more reassurance and will happily provide it." It can be so tempting to scour the Internet for answers, but if you find that it stresses you out, give yourself permission to let it go.

It's also useful to add a doula to your team if you are able. Doulas are not just there for labor and delivery; they are your partner through your entire pregnancy (more on doulas on page 92). Surrounding yourself with as much care and support as possible is essential both now and once the baby arrives.

If Pregnancy Comes as a Surprise

Surprise pregnancies are very common. Almost 50 percent of pregnancies in the US, and 40 percent of pregnancies in the world, each year are unplanned.

Many women with unplanned pregnancies immediately start thinking about the events of the past few weeks—such as drinking alcohol, smoking, getting an X-ray—and worrying that their developing baby is at risk.

TRAUMA-INFORMED CARE

Women who have experienced trauma may find that pregnancy, birth, and the health care that comes with them can be triggering and possibly emotionally distressing. Know that you have the right to care that makes you feel safe and is understanding of your needs. Survivors often report that in the context of prenatal care, the following aspects are important to them:

- Clear communication, with language that does not remind them of past trauma
- Control over who is in the room during pelvic exams and bodily exposure

Don't hesitate to speak candidly with your provider about your needs and consider that working with a therapist through this time may be particularly helpful.

If this is you:

- You didn't know, so don't feel guilty!

- Many medical professionals agree on the "all or none phenomenon" in those very early weeks of pregnancy (after conception, before the positive pregnancy test). This means that the action in question will either cause a very early miscarriage or do nothing at all. In other words, if the drinks you had at your cousin's wedding 3 days before you found out you were pregnant were going to harm the pregnancy, they would have already done so, and your pregnancy would not have progressed to this point. If this pregnancy does end in miscarriage, it's likely not because of that night of drinking, but rather an unavoidable problem within the pregnancy (such as an unpreventable genetic abnormality).

So, try not to worry, and just avoid alcohol and other harmful substances from now on (for more on what to avoid, see "Nourish" on page 80).

Women who have unplanned pregnancies have a slightly higher risk of experiencing "psychological distress" during the baby's first year of life. I think it's a good idea for all women to seek a mental health therapist during pregnancy, but this may be even more important if you have a surprise pregnancy. Preemptive emotional TLC can go a long way.

Financial instability, relationship distress, or a lack of social support can also make mood disorders more likely if the pregnancy was unexpected.

"If the pregnancy is causing strain in your relationship (or if the relationship distress predates the pregnancy), now is the time to get into couples counseling to see what can be worked through and to learn new and better ways to communicate," therapist Carolyn Wagner says.

In the case of financial trouble, Wagner says it's a good idea to find out what community resources are available, including the Special Supplemental Nutrition Program for Women, Infants, and Children (WIC), specialized health insurance for women during pregnancy and postpartum, food benefits, and assistance with newborn essentials. "Even if these aren't pressing needs, it's always good to know what is available, as it can help ease some of the anxiety."

If You Find Out You Are Pregnant Late into Your Pregnancy

About 1 out of every 475 women will not know they are pregnant until they have reached the end of their pregnancy. That's more common than we might think!

When we see these stories on TV (often sensationalized!), we are often quick to think, "How could that happen?" But the truth is that there are many reasons that this could occur: a history of irregular menstrual cycles, the absence of pregnancy symptoms, and failed birth control, just to name a few.

So, if you are starting this journey well into your pregnancy, you are not alone. The most important step is to start getting prenatal care right away so that your provider can get you all caught up with necessary testing and medical assessments. Also, depending on "how pregnant you are," you may have less time to prepare emotionally and logistically for your birth and for meeting your baby, which can feel overwhelming. But take heart. Your body has been doing the work of growing your baby all along and will continue to do so. Take a few deep breaths and jump onto this wild ride.

nourish

Foods to Avoid

Now is a great time to start taking prenatal vitamins if you haven't already! Check out page 8 for the latest info to help you choose the best vitamins for you.

While you are increasing the amount of nourishing foods in your diet, you may also want to consider cutting some foods out. There are foods that we generally recommend avoiding during pregnancy. But a quick note first: There are people who choose not to adhere to these guidelines, based on two things. First, these rules are fairly new. When I was pregnant with my first, I followed the rules to the letter but was often reminded by my mom and mother-in-law that none of this existed when they were pregnant, and their kids turned out just fine. Second, women all over the world continue to eat the foods on this list and have healthy pregnancies. It is important to note that when you are pregnant, your immune system is not quite as strong as it normally is, so you may be more susceptible to certain kinds of bacteria (like those potentially found in the "avoid" list).

My personal decision was to follow the guidelines because I realized that, ultimately, I would be less stressed if I did. I knew that if I ate something on the "avoid" list I would experience a slight but constant worry, so leaving the foods out just felt easier for me. Remember that you can always check in with your provider about specific questions you have related to foods.

Registered Dietician Nutritionist Crystal Karges lists the following foods that are usually on the "avoid" list during pregnancy:

- Raw/unpasteurized foods, including dairy, seafood (like sushi, oysters, and mussels), raw eggs (and foods that contain raw eggs like cookie dough and salad dressings), and meats

- Deli meats, unless heated per the FDA guidelines (see next column)

- Unwashed produce (fruits and veggies are essential to a balanced diet, but make sure you're washing them well before eating)

- Precut fruit that's been sitting out, and fresh-squeezed juice, as it may not be pasteurized

- Sprouts

- Soft cheeses, including brie and gorgonzola (if you can see the mold on it, it's best to avoid it)

- High-mercury fish, including swordfish, king mackerel, tilefish, and shark

- Leftovers that have been unrefrigerated for longer than a couple of hours

- Alcohol (there is no amount of alcohol that is known to be safe during pregnancy; pass on the drinks while pregnant, mama, to keep you and your little one safe)

The FDA recommends cooking meats to the following internal temperature in pregnancy (always use a clean thermometer when testing, especially if testing multiple times):

- Beef, pork, lamb, veal: 145 degrees Fahrenheit
- Ground meat: 160 degrees Fahrenheit
- Poultry (whole and ground): 165 degrees Fahrenheit
- Fish: 145 degrees Fahrenheit

A few other tips:

- Be careful with poultry that is stuffed, as bacteria can grow in the stuffing.
- Beware of the picnic: Foods that have been sitting outside for some time may spoil, especially in the heat.
- When in doubt, throw it out.

gather

- ○ Pregnancy tests
- ○ Prenatal vitamins
- ○ A list of the foods to avoid to carry with you or hang on your fridge

to do

- ○ Start taking prenatal vitamins if you haven't already.
- ○ Practice meditating using the reflection in this chapter.
- ○ Consider how you will share the pregnancy news with your partner or closest allies.

remember

There is a saying among women who have had a challenging conception journey or for those who are scared to lose a pregnancy: "Today, I am pregnant." If it feels right, take a few moments every day to remind yourself that today, you are in fact pregnant. You might find it beneficial to try to grasp on to and celebrate that phrase each day.

Choosing a Birthplace and Provider

This is my birth.

It may seem impossibly early to start thinking about giving birth. However, where you give birth can dictate who your health-care provider is throughout your pregnancy, so before you make your first prenatal appointment, you may want to give it some thought. (But don't worry too much. If you decide in a few months that you'd like to make a change, it's usually possible.)

Choosing your birth provider and location can be a tricky thing. Well-intentioned people in your life may start to give you their advice about where you "should" give birth. This noise can sometimes make it hard to listen to your own head and heart. If you have a trusted friend to talk to, they might be a great place to start. Maybe hearing their story will help you get some clarity on what you want.

Ultimately, though, this is *your* birth, and you have to do what feels right for *you*.

So, take some time and really get reflective and honest with yourself:

- What do you think will be most important to you during the course of your prenatal care and during your birth?
- What vibe do you want during your appointments? How about during your birth?
- What will make you feel safest while you are in labor?

These answers may come easily, or you may need to sit with these questions for a bit. When feelings do arise, trust them. Your intuition knows what she's talking about!

Research shows that choosing a birthing place that makes you happy can improve your mood and well-being throughout your pregnancy. Trust yourself and your judgment, and do what is right for you, while taking into account your and your baby's safety.

xo,

Diana

BIRTHPLACE

There are usually three options available for giving birth: hospitals, birth centers, and your home.

To start, it can be helpful to consider the following questions. Remember that all of your answers can change in the next 9 months. Birth plans are made to be refined! But it's always good to have a starting point:

- What do you want the overall experience and "vibe" to be like at your birth?

- Do you have any medical conditions that may require additional support during your pregnancy and birth?

- Do you expect to have a low-risk or high-risk pregnancy?

- How do you think you will want to cope with labor and birth? Epidural or other medications? No medications? Undecided? (See chapter 22, "Pain and Coping Techniques.")

- How do medical settings make you feel? Comforted? Or nervous?

- What types of settings do you have access to?

- What settings does your insurance cover and how much, if any, are you able to afford to pay out of pocket for uncovered expenses?

- If your family is LGBTQ+ or you are concerned that you may be treated in a different way from other patients, it's important to look into the organization's approach or to get a reference from friends. Consider whether the staff have received sensitivity training, if they regularly provide services for families like yours, and if you generally feel like you will be treated well at the facility.

Depending on where you live, you may not have much choice of setting, but it's still a good idea to ask these questions and consider what is important to you.

If your current women's health-care provider attends births, and you like them and where they practice, you can go right ahead and keep seeing them. But some women use this time to reevaluate their desires and concerns and think about choosing someone new.

Hospitals

Most women in the US (about 98 percent) give birth in hospitals. Yet the small percentage of births happening outside of hospitals is on the rise. More women choosing home birth and birth centers for labor is providing more choice around birth practices, and it's also putting pressure on hospitals to incorporate more woman- and family-centered models of care. Hospitals all over the country are offering amenities and choices that allow women and their families to feel empowered, respected, and well cared for.

In a hospital, you have nearly immediate access to a wide range of medical interventions including continuous monitoring, pain medications, and advanced emergency equipment. An operating room is available should a Cesarean section become necessary.

This also means that intervention rates are the highest in hospitals. For example, over 50 percent of women giving birth in hospitals get epidurals. While low-intervention births are definitely an option in hospitals, you and your labor support team may have to advocate to get one, simply because they may be less common there than at a birth center. Most hospitals do allow for walking around the labor unit if it is safe to do so, but women who are being continually monitored must generally stay in their rooms (or near them in the case of portable monitors). Some hospitals have bathtubs and showers to labor or give birth in, which can greatly increase your comfort level.

In a hospital, you can often be attended by an obstetrician (MD or DO), midwife, family doctor, or a combination of these (more on these roles soon). A hospital birth may be recommended if:

- You have a chronic medical condition that may require special monitoring or support during labor.
- Your pregnancy is high risk (pregnant with multiples, complications, and so on).
- Your baby will likely need immediate after-birth care in a neonatal intensive care unit (NICU).
- There is a high likelihood that you will need a Cesarean section, or you are having a planned Cesarean.
- You would like the option to have an epidural.
- You feel more comfortable in a hospital setting, regardless of the items mentioned above.
- It is the only option covered by your insurance.

QUESTIONS TO ASK YOUR POTENTIAL BIRTHING PLACE

It can be helpful to ask to take a tour of a prospective birthing place. Here are some questions to ask on your tour:

- What labor coping tools do you have here?
- I am planning to have an unmedicated birth/ medicated birth/vaginal birth after Cesarean (VBAC). How would you support that here?
- What is your intervention rate (consider things like Cesarean sections, inductions, and episiotomies)?
- How many people are allowed in the labor room with me? Can my older child attend the birth?
- What follow-up support do you have for parents after we go home?

- What makes your setting unique?
- Is there a number I call to let you know that I am in labor and on my way?
- Where should we park?
- Where should we check in and what documents do I need to have with me?
- Can you walk me through the steps I'll take from arriving at the hospital to being brought to my labor room?
- What is the postpartum experience like?
- Are the rooms private or shared?
- Can my partner or a family member spend the night with me?
- Can all of baby's care happen in my room?
- Can you tell me about your neonatal intensive care unit (NICU) if applicable?

When choosing a hospital, it may also be important to consider the NICU within that hospital. About 7 percent of babies spend some time in the NICU after they are born.

There are four levels of nursery and NICU care available:

- Level I: newborn nursery
- Level II: special care nursery
- Level III: NICU
- Level IV: regional NICU

Women who are anticipating a low-risk pregnancy and birth can usually safely deliver in a level I or II hospital, while women whose babies may have more complications and risks may choose to deliver in a hospital with a higher level NICU. (For more information about NICUs, see "When Your Baby Needs NICU Care" on page 477.)

One other consideration when choosing a hospital is that some institutions have religious affiliations that may govern philosophies of care. It is fine for you to inquire about what this means for your experience.

Birth Centers

Birth centers provide family-centered care to women during their pregnancy and birth in a location designed to feel more homelike than a hospital might. Some are physically connected to hospitals, while others are in a free-standing building near a hospital.

When a woman gives birth in a birth center, she usually is not connected to the continuous monitor, but rather receives intermittent monitoring or auscultation (listening). (For a detailed description of monitoring, see "Fetal Monitoring: Continuous Versus Intermittent"

on page 305.) She will have a room in the center and may be able to walk freely around the center and its grounds. Some birth centers have bathtubs and showers to labor or give birth in.

Research has found that birth centers are a safe option for women with low-risk pregnancies and that women who labor in birth centers tend to have fewer interventions and Cesarean sections.

Birth centers are stocked with medical equipment, such as oxygen, Pitocin (a drug used to control bleeding in the event of a postpartum hemorrhage; see "Postpartum Hemorrhage: Warning Signs" on page 350) and other medications, intubation trays, and more. This means they are ready to handle an emergency if it comes up. Some birth centers offer pain medications, but not epidurals. If interventions are needed, women are usually transferred to a hospital.

A birth center birth might be for you if:

- You do not have a medical condition that may require special monitoring or support during labor.

- You are expecting a low-risk pregnancy and birth.

- You know you do not want to have an epidural.

- You do not think you'll feel comfortable in the medical setting of a hospital but also do not feel comfortable giving birth at home (or are not able to).

- Your insurance covers it, or you can pay for uncovered expenses out of pocket.

Home Birth

A home birth takes place in your (or perhaps another person's) home. Home births are usually attended by midwives, though some doctors do attend them as well.

Home births make up the smallest percentage of births in the US—less than 1 percent. But it was completely different in the last century. In 1938, 50 percent of babies were born in the home! It's also more common around the world. For example, up to 20 percent of women in the Netherlands give birth at home. While home birth rates dropped dramatically in the US during the mid-1900s, they are now on the rise as women and providers advocate for increased birthing options.

In general, home births involve fewer interventions. The safety of home birth has long been discussed. According to ACOG, "High-quality evidence that can inform this debate is limited. To date, there have been no adequate randomized clinical trials of planned home birth." There are many variables that can determine the safety of home birth, and it's very hard to account for all of them when doing studies like this. For example, the American College of Nurse-Midwives (ACNM) states that it can be hard to confirm results, as many are based on the review of birth certificates, which "have limitations that confound the results, such as no differentiation between planned and unplanned home birth or type of provider."

Here is what the leading organizations have to say about home birth:

ACOG states that while they believe hospitals and in-hospital birthing centers to be the safest place to have a baby, women should be supported when they choose home birth in the presence of "a certified nurse-midwife, certified midwife, or midwife whose education and licensure meet International Confederation of Midwives' Global Standards for Midwifery Education." The American Academy of Pediatrics (AAP) agrees with ACOG. They state that some studies have found an increased risk of infant mortality and decreased APGAR scores (see "The APGAR Score" on page 273) in home births.

ACNM states that "International and US research results support the conclusion that planned home birth with an educated, skilled attendant can be a safe, satisfying, cost-effective care option for healthy, low-risk women who want to give birth at home." The Midwives Alliance of North America (MANA) agrees, stating that a "home birth study from the MANA Statistics Dataset shows that planned home birth with skilled midwives is safe for low-risk pregnancies."

So, what's a mama to do?

Meet with providers, and ask a lot of questions. This is a great time to get multiple opinions—talk to an ob-gyn and a home birth midwife, and maybe even hospital and birth center midwifery practices. They can more accurately assess the details that are specific to you and give you a personalized recommendation about the appropriateness of having a home birth.

Of note, ACOG estimates that one-fourth of home births are unattended, meaning that there is no midwife or doctor present to assist with the birth. These births consist of the rare didn't-make-it-to-the-hospital-in-time births but also include people who choose to go it alone on purpose. The latter of these options can be quite risky, as birth can turn dangerous on a moment's notice, and is therefore not recommended by any of the leading professional organizations.

A home birth might be for you if:

- You do not have a medical condition that may require special monitoring or support during labor.
- You are expecting a low-risk pregnancy and birth.
- You know you do not want to have any pain medication.
- You feel more comfortable or safer at home than you do in any medical environment.
- You want your other child or children and/or a large group of people to attend your birth.
- Your insurance covers it, or you can pay for the uncovered expenses.
- You live close enough to a hospital to transfer, should the need arise.

A note on home birth safety: The professional attending the birth brings emergency supplies and equipment with them (such as oxygen and Pitocin). And if needed, the laboring woman will be transferred to a nearby hospital (either by car or ambulance, depending on the seriousness of the situation).

BIRTH ATTENDANT

You'll also need to choose a provider who will take care of you during your pregnancy, birth, and postpartum period.

Obstetrician

Obstetrician-gynecologists (ob-gyns) are physicians who specialize in pregnancy and labor and delivery care. In addition, they also provide gynecological care to nonpregnant women. Some have further training in high-risk pregnancies. Ob-gyns can be medical doctors (MDs) or doctors of osteopathy (DOs). Both types of doctors are licensed physicians and have received similar education, but their approach to patient care may be different. DOs receive additional training in the musculoskeletal system (bones and muscles) and often incorporate that knowledge into their treatment of all parts of the body, including during pregnancy care.

Family Physician

Family physicians are doctors who care for the entire family, and this sometimes includes care during pregnancy and birth. They usually care for low-risk pregnancies, though this is not always the case. You'll find them attending births in hospitals and in homes.

Midwife

The word "midwife" comes from Middle English and means "with woman." Midwives provide holistic care and support to women through pregnancy, birth, and the postpartum period. They also care for nonpregnant women. A few things to know:

- Midwives attend births in hospitals, birth centers, or homes.

- Midwifery care often results in fewer medical interventions, though you absolutely can still have an epidural, ultrasounds, and other procedures with a midwife.

- Midwives usually care for low-risk pregnancies independently. If you require additional medical interventions during your pregnancy or birth, your midwife can often collaborate with a physician, or you can be transferred completely to the care of an obstetrician.

DISCRIMINATION AND DISPARITIES IN MATERNAL HEALTH

Maternal health in the US is in a state of crisis: Women and babies of color experience a disproportionate number of complications related to pregnancy and birth.

The infant mortality and preterm delivery rates are higher, and there is a higher risk for pregnancy-related illnesses and complications. The reasons behind these inequities are historical, with chronic systemic racism and routine discrimination at the forefront.

New York Times reporter Erica Green, as a black woman living in the Baltimore area, shared her personal story of racism following the birth of her second child. While her first birth was wonderful, her second birth experience (a repeat, planned Cesarean section) was just the opposite. She felt that the nursing and medical team in the postpartum unit did not address her pain adequately and made her feel like her requests for medication were part of drug-seeking behavior rather than the reasonable needs of a woman who just had major abdominal surgery. Green said that the staff also made an assumption regarding her socioeconomic status: They asked her if she was interested in WIC (the Special Supplemental Nutrition Program for Women, Infants, and Children) several times, and though she declined each time, they continued to leave the paperwork "just in case."

Deeply hurt by the experience, Green says that it caught her completely off guard. But then she started to see media coverage about the disparate treatment of black women, including celebrities, that had led to emotional and physical trauma after giving birth.

"It is not something we talk about. People prepared me for all kinds of things, but no one told me I might face discrimination." She is now determined to share her story so that women of color can be on alert and advocate for themselves if necessary.

"I wish I knew that this was a more common experience so that I could see the warning signs. I just assumed that I was going to be treated respectfully and like any other woman postpartum. . . . It was humiliating and paralyzing to feel stereotyped," Green says. "I felt ashamed by my inability to stand up for myself and what I needed. I felt so disempowered. The shame is what bothers me the most."

The impact of this crisis is profound. And it is time to say "enough."

Throughout this book, you will be alerted to complications that women of color and LGBTQ+ people are particularly vulnerable to so that you can be on alert for yourself or be an advocate for other women. But this book is just scratching the surface. It is the responsibility of every single one of us not only to be aware of the issue, but to look for the inherent inequalities that exist all around us and speak out against them, so that the babies we are growing today can have a better world tomorrow.

If you experience discrimination of any kind during your pregnancy, you can reach out to the patient advocacy department of your medical institution, the Health and Human Services' Office for Civil Rights (hhs.gov), a local discrimination attorney in your area, or the Council on Patient Safety in Women's Health Care (safehealthcareforeverywoman.org).

Midwives have relationships with obstetricians: The specifics vary by state, but in all cases, midwives can consult and collaborate with doctors and transfer care should a patient need additional medical support that is beyond the scope of a midwife.

When choosing a midwife keep in mind that there are a variety of ways that midwives are trained:

- A certified nurse-midwife (CNM) is a registered nurse (RN) who has graduated from an accredited nurse midwifery program. Most have a graduate degree in midwifery, nursing, or public health. CNMs must pass a national certification exam from the American Midwifery Certification Board (AMCB).

- A certified midwife (CM) has a college degree (often in a health-related field) but is not an RN. CMs have attended a graduate-level midwifery program and have passed the same certification exam as CNMs.

- A certified professional midwife (CPM) receives training from educational programs or through apprenticeship. Most receive certification from the Midwifery Education Accreditation Council (MEAC).

- Traditional midwives are midwives who have received training through apprenticeship. They are typically not certified or licensed.

For more information on midwifery, refer to the American College of Nurse-Midwives (ACNM) and the Midwives Alliance of North America (MANA).

Questions to Ask a Potential Provider

- Where do you deliver babies?

- How many years have you been practicing?

- Do you work with anyone else? What are the chances that *you* will be the person who delivers my baby, versus someone else? Can I meet that person (those people) if someone else may deliver the baby?

- Will you see me for each visit, or is there a team of people I might see?

- What is the Cesarean section rate at the place you attend births? What is *your* Cesarean section rate?

- How many laboring women do you care for at a time, on average?

- I would like an unmedicated/medicated birth. How do you feel about that?

- I would like a water birth. Is that a possibility with you?

- I am nervous about _____. What are your thoughts about it?

- How do you feel about working with doulas?

- I am LGBTQ+. Have you had experience working within the queer community?

- I am a survivor of violence. How will you help me to feel safe while giving birth?

- What other types of professionals will I have access to during my pregnancy (lactation consultant, nutritionist, geneticist, and so on)?

For midwives specifically:

- Are you licensed by the state?

- Under what circumstances would you need to collaborate with a physician for my care, or would I need to transfer completely to physician care?

- Do you have privileges at the hospital I would be transferred to (for home and birth center births). Will you be able to continue to be my provider if we transfer?

OTHER PROFESSIONALS

It may seem early to start thinking about all the people you might interact with during the next 9 months, but I want to plant the seed now because these experts can have a significant impact on your pregnancy, often right from the beginning.

Doulas

Doulas are birth professionals who provide labor and birth support to women and families. Through their experience and training, they become experts in physical and emotional labor coping skills. Most are not medical professionals, so they do not perform medical assessments or procedures.

About 6 percent of women in the US currently use doulas, though that number is increasing. A large review of research found that doulas have a profound impact on labor: Women with continuous labor support are less likely to have Cesarean sections and other medical interventions, need less pain medication, and report being more satisfied with their birth experience.

A 2017 study in Iran published in the *Global Journal of Health Science* compared the anxiety levels and labor pain of 150 first-time mothers who had doula support to those who didn't. The results showed that mothers who worked with doulas benefited by experiencing less anxiety and less pain during labor.

Dr. Amy Gilliland, who has done extensive research on the relationship between doulas and mothers, attributes these positive reactions to attachment. Moms tend to feel vulnerable during labor, so a doula becomes a secure and comforting base. This attachment in the form of soothing touch and extended eye contact allows for a drop in stress hormones and a surge in oxytocin in both the mother and the doula.

Some women may wonder why their birth partner is not enough. It turns out that the team effort between doula and partner actually enhances this relationship because the doula's knowledge and experience can help calm the birth partner's nerves, too. A 2008 study published in the journal *Birth* found that when a woman had the support of both a partner and a doula, her risk of Cesarean decreased in comparison with women who labored just with a partner.

Unfortunately, doulas are not currently covered by most insurance policies in the US, so if you choose to use a doula, you will likely have to pay out of pocket. While there is no doubt that the investment is a good one, it's simply not an option for a lot of people. There are volunteer doulas and doulas-in-training who may be able to work with you for a reduced fee. Your medical provider might be able to point you in their direction.

Deciding to use a doula is, of course, a personal decision as well as a financial one. You may not feel comfortable with the idea of someone outside of your family being in your birth room. If you are on the fence, consider meeting with a doula to chat through your concerns. It may help you make the decision either way.

If you decide to work with a doula, most women start the meeting and interview process in their second trimester, though it's never too early or too late to start (just be aware that some doulas book up well in advance).

Interview questions for your doula:

- Are you certified? (Note: This is not a requirement for doulas.)
- I am thinking about an unmedicated birth/getting an epidural. Do you support women who make that choice?
- Who is your backup doula, and can I meet them?
- How many times will we meet during my pregnancy?
- When are you officially on call for my birth?
- What happens if I go into preterm labor?
- What happens if my labor is long?
- What coping skills do you like to use at births?
- What happens if I need a Cesarean section?
- I am LGBTQ+. Have you had experience working within the queer community?
- What is your fee structure?

Of note, some doulas offer services for women who have a miscarriage or termination; this support can be invaluable. Additionally, postpartum doulas can have a tremendous impact in the first weeks of motherhood. For more on postpartum doulas, see "Postpartum Doulas and Newborn Care Specialists" on page 339.

Chiropractors

Chiropractors are doctors within the complementary branch of medicine. The basic theory of this one-hundred-year-old specialty is that when the musculoskeletal system is in alignment, the body will have a better ability to heal itself from illness and pain. Chiropractors use hands-on techniques to manipulate the spine into alignment, which appears to be safe during pregnancy when done by a chiropractor with prenatal training and expertise.

As your belly grows, you may find that you are experiencing new (or worsening) aches and pains in your back and throughout your body. A chiropractor might be able to help. Some women also report that routine chiropractic care helps their baby get into a better position for birth, and research backs this up. If (many weeks from now) your baby is breech, you might also visit a chiropractor who can perform something called the Webster technique to help your baby flip into the head-down position (more on breech babies on page 198).

Do check with your health insurance provider to see if chiropractic care is covered. If not, be sure you know how much your practitioner will charge you. Many provide services on a sliding fee scale to accommodate different income levels.

Acupuncturists

Acupuncture is a form of traditional Chinese medicine that has existed for thousands of years. Acupuncturists place tiny needles into specific parts of the body to rebalance the flow of energy (known as qi). People seek acupuncture care for a vast number of reasons, including fertility and pregnancy discomfort. Research has found that when done by a qualified practitioner it is safe for pregnant women.

If you've never had acupuncture before, the idea of someone sticking needles into your body may not strike you as a great way to spend an afternoon. But women report wonderful results including decreased pelvic and back pain, decreased depressive symptoms, and labor pain management. And if I may add a personal note, my pain threshold is not high, so it took me a long time to try acupuncture. When I finally did, I found that the needles barely hurt (if at all), and I always feel great after a session.

In addition, a form of acupuncture called moxibustion may also be effective in turning a breech baby to the head-down position.

Again, seek prior authorization with your health insurance provider or ask about sliding fee scales if paying for treatment out of pocket is financially prohibitive for you.

Massage Therapists

Massage therapists use a series of techniques to rub and knead muscles, tendons, and ligaments to break up scar tissue, improve relaxation, and reduce pain. It is generally considered safe to get massaged while pregnant when done by a therapist who is certified in prenatal massage, but check with your midwife or doctor to be sure.

The benefits can be quite remarkable: decreased depression and anxiety, less stress, less pain during pregnancy, and maybe even shorter labors! Um, yes please?

Kymberlie Berrien, massage therapist and doula, notes that massage can work preventatively as well, reducing the impact of common

pregnancy symptoms like back and pelvic pain. Berrien advises that when you choose a therapist, look for someone with extensive prenatal experience is certified by an independent and nationally recognized program.

Prenatal massage is often covered by flexible spending accounts (FSA) and health savings accounts (HSA). Some states also cover it under group health plans. Berrien has clients who put massage gift certificates in their baby registries and says that some massage schools offer programs where students give massages, observed by instructors, at a reduced rate. There are also many self-massage techniques you can learn that can be quite effective at relieving muscle pain and improving relaxation (see "Massage" on page 292).

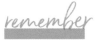

remember

Choosing your birthplace and provider is an important step in setting the tone for your pregnancy and birth. You have a choice. You deserve to be treated with respect and compassion. And on behalf of all providers out there, we are so honored to be on this journey with you.

PART II

Pregnancy
Month by Month

DEAR MAMA,

As co-founders we are united in a common mission for Motherly, but as mamas, we are completely different women.

Jill is a total planner—when it came to expecting her first child and the fact that a brand new person would be coming into her life, she was ON it during her pregnancy. She read ahead, made lists, and did everything she could to feel more in control and less anxious about what was happening to her and her baby.

Liz took her pregnancies *One. Day. At. A.Time*. She was obsessed with knowing what her body and baby were up to at each exact moment and deeply craved ways to connect with her experience and bond with her baby in the present moment. The future seemed too hard to wrap her mind around. Today was what fueled her.

In a lot of ways, we could not be more different from each other, yet we are bound together by our intense love of motherhood, our children, and oh yes, Motherly.

The way that you choose to approach your pregnancy is entirely up to you—there is no right or wrong way to mark this journey. You can, and should, approach pregnancy *your way*. That means you should feel empowered to make your own choices about things like genetic testing, finding out your baby's sex (or not), and deciding how and when you announce your pregnancy at work. But sometimes, pregnancy makes decisions for you—and almost every woman experiences some kind of curveball she didn't see coming.

In our cases, Liz was diagnosed with hyperemesis gravidarum (a severe form of morning sickness that left her bedridden for the first trimester) during three of her pregnancies. Jill experienced pregnancy-induced hypothyroidism that caused significant swelling and weight gain and created risk for her and her baby. Both experiences were not chosen (and to be honest, we'd much rather not have experienced them.). Yet even in these challenging moments, we learned more about the power and resilience within us as women than any pregnancy textbook could ever reveal.

And we hope you find your power on this path, too.

As the unsolicited advice begins, and as your pregnancy journey unfolds, mama *you do you*. We invite you to forge your own path. This is the time to nurture your identity, not lose it. These coming months will give you the opportunity to discover who you are, and who you are becoming as a mama. It will provide opportunity for pure joy and profound challenge. Just like motherhood.

And if no one has told you lately, let us be the ones to do the honor: You are doing incredible work. You can do this. You've got this.

xo,

Jill + Liz

Month 2

WEEKS 5–8

Today,
I am pregnant.

FROM DIANA

Welcome to being pregnant, and it's already month 2!

As a midwife, I am in awe of the beauty of pregnancy. I am astonished by what a woman's body can do.

But life is complex, and nothing is ever just one thing. Something that is innately beautiful can also have its rough spots. There are times when pregnancy is hard, and the beauty feels further away from our grasp. The symptoms, the decisions, *giving birth*—all wildly beautiful and difficult at the same time.

These first weeks of pregnancy are no exception. You have all the feelings of wonder and excitement, but under it all is a dreadful thought: What if I lose the pregnancy?

For some women, this is an omnipresent fear. For others, it's an occasional flashing thought in their minds. No matter what, it makes this phase of pregnancy, well, hard.

You may not have told many people about your pregnancy, and your first prenatal appointment probably isn't for at least a few weeks, so there is a good chance you are feeling alone in your worry.

Mama, I wish that I could do more to ease your weary heart.

I can give you the statistics. From 11 to 22 percent of clinically recognized pregnancies (presence of a positive pregnancy test) end in miscarriage. This means that 78 to 89 percent do not. That's a lot! Yet I know that while numbers make you feel a little better, you can't shake the thought of, "Fine, but what if I am not in that 78 percent?" I am so sorry that I can't make that better.

What I can do is remind you that you are not alone. There are thousands of other women around the world who are sharing your concerns at this very moment. Being nervous does not make you overly sensitive; it makes you normal, and it makes you a mama.

- Don't be afraid to embrace this pregnancy, if you are ready to. Sometimes fighting the joy can make the fear worse.
- Talk to a few trusted friends or family members. You might be surprised to learn that they've gone through the same thing.
- Be gentle with yourself.

I am sending you a big, enveloping hug. And I hope you can be comforted by some simple, true words: "Today, I am pregnant."

xo,

Diana

Pregnancy is a time of planning and looking to the future, and we'll do all of that together in this book. But first, let's take some time to look back.

Think back on the timeline of your life and all the lives that came before yours. There have been millions of moments, events, meetings, and departures that have led you to *this* moment, right now, the one where you are newly pregnant with your baby.

All the steps that you have taken—and all of your ancestors before you—have influenced the here and now.

Can you recall any course-defining moments in your life?

What does it mean for you to be pregnant right now, in this moment of history?

What is the ancestral significance of your pregnancy?

What does it mean for you to be creating a new generation in your ancestral line?

Take a deep breath and place your feet on the floor or ground (you can even take your shoes off, if you want).

Feel the earth underneath you, supporting you and your budding baby.

Imagine your feet as roots, connecting you to the earth.

Connecting you even deeper to the generations and generations of people who have come before you.

Women have been growing, giving birth to, and raising babies since the dawn of humanity. Their journeys were not easy; yet they persevered, always guided by fierce and powerful love for their children. You are joining that mighty lineage of mama-warriors.

When the experience gets hard, when you doubt yourself, think back on everything that happened to put you right here, with this baby inside you. You are never alone in this.

bonding
WITH YOUR BABY

You are starting the work of growing your baby, and it is quite a lot of work! You'll experience an array of physical and emotional changes, and you'll see almost all aspects of your life start to change as you begin your transition into becoming this baby's mama.

This month of pregnancy is a unique one in that it is possible that you (and perhaps a few people close to you) are the only ones who know that you are pregnant.

And it feels a bit surreal! The world is continuing on totally normally, and many people in the course of your days don't have a clue of what's going on inside you. When you look down at your belly, you can't see any difference. And yet, your entire world has changed, and a million tiny (but huge) things are happening inside your body.

This is your time to just marvel at it all. Spend some moments every day in the quiet, secret revelry of being newly pregnant with your baby. This time is just for you two (or three or four). The world will know soon enough, and your attention will quickly become more outwardly focused as you go to all your prenatal visits, celebrate with friends and family, and hear all of their (well-meaning) advice and ideas.

But for now, it's just you, a mama and her sweet baby, starting this journey together.

See if you can take a few moments every day to just be with your baby. Take some calming breaths, place your hand on your pubic bone, and send your loving vibes into your pelvis where your baby is nestled, taking it all in.

Symptoms
YOU MIGHT FEEL

- Bloating
- Breast soreness/ tenderness
- Nausea and vomiting
- Sensitivity to smells
- Skin darkening

- Fatigue
- Spotting
- Frequent urination

To learn more about the symptoms that are impacting you—and how to deal—turn to the "Symptom Checker" on page 429. Remember, your provider is your first stop for any symptoms that concern you, so don't hesitate to reach out to them.

prenatal
VISIT THIS MONTH

Many women can expect to have one visit with their provider during their second month of pregnancy.

Your first prenatal appointment is a big one and is often the longest one you'll have during your pregnancy. The first visit usually happens between 8 and 12 weeks, though this can vary depending on the provider and your specific health needs.

Here is what you can anticipate at that first visit: First and foremost, you'll figure out the window of time when your baby may make their grand entrance. Your due date is calculated by using the first day of your last period (also called your last menstrual period, LMP). To be exact, it is 280 days from your LMP. If you want to get math-y with it, here's the equation:

- Remember the day that your last period started.
- Subtract 3 months.
- Add 7 days.

For example, if your LMP was September 20:

- Subtract 3 months from September and get June.
- Add 7 days to 20 and get 27.
- Your baby is due on June 27!

We are also big fans of plug-in-the-date apps, or simply asking your provider to help you figure it out.

Psst: Since pregnancy is 40 weeks, and there are roughly 4 weeks in a month, you are actually pregnant for almost 10 months, not 9. Sorry! We promise to make them as fun as possible for you!

And don't worry. It's common for women not to know when their LMP was. If that's the case, your doctor or midwife will likely recommend an ultrasound to help determine how far along you are.

Lots of Questions

Your doctor or midwife will want to know all about you to help guide you through the healthiest pregnancy possible. They'll ask about your overall health and family history and any medical problems, past surgeries, or medications that you might be taking. With that information, they will be able to help you make decisions about additional specialists

---

PREGNANCY IS DIVIDED INTO THREE TRIMESTERS

First trimester: weeks 1–12
Second trimester: weeks 13–27
Third trimester: weeks 28–40

Some consider the first trimester to end after week 12, while others say it's after week 13. In this guide we'll be using 12, but 13 is great, too, if that works best for you.

you may need to see during your pregnancy, which medications you can safely continue to use and which you should discontinue, and more. They will ask about any previous pregnancies as well.

If your partner is male or if you are using the sperm of a known donor, your provider will ask some questions about their history as well. For example, it's good to be aware of any genetic conditions that run in his family that may be passed along to your baby. If the sperm came from a sperm bank, then you will likely have information on hand about your donor's medical history, though not all sperm banks do extensive testing yet.

It is also possible that you don't know the medical history of the person the sperm came from, and that's okay. Your baby's development will be monitored, and if concerns come up, your provider will help you address them. You can always choose to do further testing after the baby is born, and DNA testing during pregnancy is available as well.

There will likely be some pretty personal questions too: your social and sexual relationships, whether you've had any sexually transmitted infections (for more info on this, check out "Sexually Transmitted Infections During Pregnancy" on page 470), where you work and live, if you drink alcohol and smoke.

IS THIS ABUSE?

Talking about violence and abuse is never easy, but it is so common, so we must talk about it. A lot.

Almost 25 percent of women in the US have experienced violence from an intimate partner, and the risk may increase during pregnancy and the postpartum period. If you feel unsafe in any way, there is help for you.

In addition to the immediate consequences, sadness, injury, and even death, it has been found that women who experience violence are more likely to have postpartum depression after the baby arrives.

Violence comes in many forms. Honestly, if you are thinking to yourself, "Is this abuse?" there is a good chance it is. Violence includes:

- Hitting, kicking, biting, pushing, and any other form of physical contact causing you pain or injury

- Forcing you to have sex or perform sexual acts against your will
- Verbal insults
- Threats
- Withholding finances, food, and other necessities from you
- Preventing you from leaving your home

Please know that this is not on you. This is not your fault. And you deserve to be treated well. Leaving an abusive situation is a thousand times easier said than done, but you can do it—for both you and your future child.

The National Domestic Violence Hotline (thehotline.org) is a wonderful resource, with options to call or chat silently online. You can also walk into a local emergency room or tell your provider that you need help.

It may start to feel like when your parents interrogated you as a teenager.

Again, all of this is to help you be as healthy as possible and to make sure the care they provide is tailored to your specific needs. I know this can feel a bit uncomfortable, but remember, they are sworn to keep your information confidential. It may make you feel uneasy, but know that this is their job. They ask these questions many times a day (and have heard all kinds of answers), so it's pretty rare that something you say will surprise them.

This is also a valuable time to discuss any psychological conditions with your provider. Therapist Carolyn Wagner says, "Preexisting mental illness can not only get worse during pregnancy due to changes in hormones and increased stress, but certain mental illnesses also increase your risk of developing more significant perinatal mood and anxiety disorders."

"For example, women who have bipolar disorder prior to pregnancy are at much greater risk of developing postpartum psychosis," she explains.

If you are currently on medication, you'll need to confirm that it is safe for pregnancy, and if not, work with your prescriber to discuss the possibility of transitioning to a different medication for the duration of your pregnancy.

"During pregnancy, it can be helpful to seek out a therapist who can support you as you navigate all of the physical and emotional changes," Wagner advises. "This is also a great opportunity to establish a relationship with a therapist whom you can continue with postpartum. You can work together to create a good postpartum plan that includes plenty of social support and help that allows for maximum rest and sleep time."

What Else Will Happen at This Month's Prenatal Visit

A physical exam. This will include the standard listening to your heart and lungs, a breast exam, and possibly a pelvic exam.

Did you just shudder a little bit? Yeah, I know. Let's stay with this for a minute.

Confession: Part of the reason I became a midwife was because I disliked pelvic exams so much. The cold exam table, that paper gown, having to make small talk with someone you don't really know while they place something called a *spec-u-lum* in your *va-gi-na*—not the ideal way to spend your morning.

It can also be uncomfortable, both physically and mentally.

So, I am truly with you on this. But let's make it better.

First, your vagina. A lot of people think of vaginas as a tube, almost like a paper towel roll, that they picture stretching during sex, pelvic exams, and of course, birth. But as discussed in chapter 2, the vaginal walls are actually made of numerous small folds, called rugae. Have you ever wondered how the vagina can sometimes feel so small, yet it can expand to allow a baby to pass through? It's due in part to the rugae, which are like pleats all along the inside of the vagina. When they unfold under the pressure of a baby's body, the birth canal enlarges. These rugae expand as the baby passes through, to allow more room.

Here are a few tricks to make speculum and pelvic exams easier:

- Bring your bottom all the way to the end of the exam table, just before it feels like you might slide off.

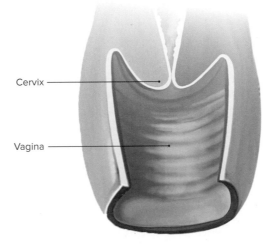

VAGINAL FOLDS

- Make your hands into fists and place them under your bottom so that your bottom is raised up off the table.

- Place your feet on the foot rests (yes, I purposefully did not call them "stirrups" because you are getting a pelvic exam, not riding a horse), and when you are ready, let your knees fall out to the side like a butterfly.

- Wiggle your toes and unclench your jaw: Both of these things will help you relax the muscles in your pelvis, which will make it less uncomfortable.

- Most providers try to use distracting chitchat, so you can engage with them if you'd like. If not, repeat a calming mantra to yourself in your head. "I am safe" or "relaxed and light" work well for this scenario.

The pelvic exam is done to assess the health of your vagina, cervix, uterus, and ovaries (see diagram and description of anatomy on page 26). Your provider will also be able to feel the size of your uterus, which is already growing.

So, these are important reasons to perform a pelvic exam, but if pelvic exams make you too uncomfortable, let your provider know.

Pap smears and tests for sexually transmitted infections are routinely done in early pregnancy. For more info on Pap smears, see page 453, and for sexually transmitted infections, see page 470.

There are also a number of additional tests that may be run at the first prenatal visit. These include:

- Blood work
  - Complete blood count (CBC) (page 453)
  - Blood type (page 452) and Rhesus factor screening (page 178)
  - Syphilis test (page 473)
  - HIV and AIDs tests (page 473)
  - Rubella immunity (page 453)
  - Hepatitis test (page 472)
  - Carrier testing for genetic diseases (page 452)

- Urinalysis and culture

- Blood pressure check (Blood pressure will be an important indicator of health through pregnancy and postpartum. For more on this, see "High Blood Pressure (Hypertension)" on page 462.)

- Weight check, and maybe height at this first visit

- Dating ultrasound (Don't worry; this has nothing to do with match.com! Some providers perform transvaginal ultrasounds at the first visit to see how far

TAKING CARE OF YOUR VAGINA DURING PREGNANCY

In the next 9 months, you are going to spend a lot of time thinking about your reproductive organs (and we are certainly going to talk about them a lot in this book). So, let's start with how to take care of your vagina.

My friend in midwifery school used to say that the vagina is a rainforest. Vaginas, like rainforests, involve a complex system that generally does a phenomenal job of taking care of itself. When the system is tampered with too much, problems can arise. So, vaginal health is often about simple and gentle care.

Some helpful tips on care of your vagina:

- Vaginal discharge is normal, and you may find yourself with more during pregnancy. It should be clear or whitish, and without a fishy odor. See "Bacterial Vaginosis (BV)" on page 458, "Yeast Infections" on page 469, and "Sexually Transmitted Infections During Pregnancy" on page 470 to learn more about healthy versus unhealthy discharge.

- One of the most important things to do is give up douching. Douching can lead to a temporary "fresh" feeling but ultimately creates an imbalance of bacteria and yeast, which can lead to infections.

- Clean your pelvic area with mild soap and water, and no need to scrub hard or internally. Again, your vagina takes care of itself.

- When possible, choose cotton underwear because it is more breathable: Vaginas like to breathe. And spending time without any bottoms on at all is a good idea too (let's hear it for naked sleeping!).

- Consider your pubic hair maintenance. Some women choose to shave or wax some or all of their pubic hair. Of course, this is 100 percent up to you. I will say that removing pubic hair can lead to infections, inflamed hair follicles, and irritation, especially when you are pregnant and skin tends to be more sensitive. Also, please don't feel that you have to do it for the sake of your provider and your upcoming pelvic exam (and later for your birth). I promise you we don't even notice.

- Never feel embarrassed to ask your midwife or doctor questions about your pelvic health. They are not embarrassed to talk about it (ahem, clearly).

along you are and assess the overall health of the pregnancy, though oftentimes this is not needed or done. For more details, see "Ultrasound" on page 457.)

- Genetic screenings (Your provider may start to talk about genetic screening options. If you'd like to learn more now, visit "Genetic Screening" on page 117.)

Questions to Ask Your Provider

If this is your first visit with your provider, you're probably bubbling over with questions. Some to consider might be:

- How might my personal and family history (and that of my partner or sperm donor, if applicable) impact my pregnancy and birth? Are there any precautions I should take because of them?

- When will I have my first ultrasound?

- I have been running/swimming/doing yoga. Is it okay to keep doing it?

- What changes should I make to my routine?

- What foods should I avoid eating?

- Is it safe for me to have sex?

- I have been having the following symptoms: _____. Is that normal?

- Can I take my existing medications and supplements?

- What medications/over-the-counter remedies should I avoid?

- Are there any other medical providers I should set up an appointment with now?

- What should I do if I have a question or concern between visits?

- Are there any educational or support resources in our community that you recommend?

And of course, "Will my life ever be *normal* again?"

Psst: We can answer that last one for you. The answer is "no." This is your new normal! But in the best way possible.

WEEK 5

Your baby, currently called an embryo, is 0.6 millimeters long—the size of a sunflower seed and the shape of a peanut shell (aw, little peanut!).

In a few weeks, your baby will start to more resemble a teeny tiny human, but even now some of their most intense development is occurring, especially related to the nervous system.

They have three layers (ectoderm, mesoderm, and endoderm), which will grow into all the different parts of your baby's body. The ectoderm will become the baby's nervous system (parts like eyes, ears, and brain); the mesoderm will become bones, muscles, and the circulatory system (like the heart); and the endoderm will become some of the baby's organs (like their liver).

Baby's umbilical cord is currently just a short connector to the rapidly growing

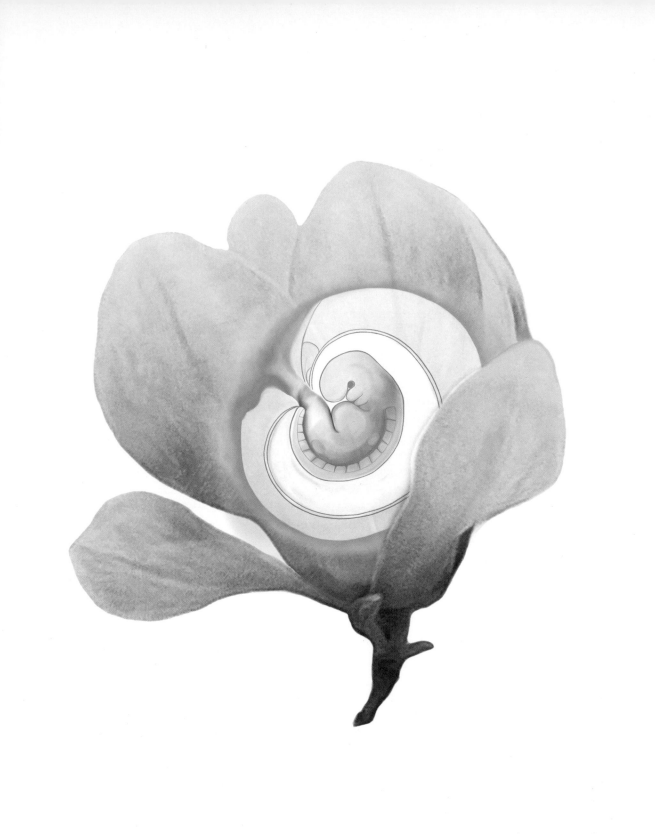

WEEKS 5–8

placenta, but it will eventually extend to from 18 to 23 inches, completing its length in week 28.

You have developed a solid mucus plug that will sit in the cervix throughout the pregnancy, protecting the uterus from infection.

nourish

Hydration

In this early part of your pregnancy, you are likely still soaking in the fact that your body is now home to your growing baby. The weight of this can feel overwhelming at times, and you undoubtedly want to do all the right things to create the healthiest pregnancy possible—for you and your babe.

The good news is that your body is fully capable of doing what is needed to grow your baby healthy and strong without much of your conscious involvement.

The "Nourish" section for each month of pregnancy will focus on the most important nutrients to get. But before we do that, let's spend some time here on the simplest—yet probably most overlooked—aspect of prenatal wellness: hydration.

During pregnancy, aim to drink at least ten 8-ounce glasses of fluid (mostly water) per day.

Seven ways hydration can help you during pregnancy:

1 **It improves blood flow.** During pregnancy, your blood volume increases significantly. And since blood contains water, adequate fluid in your body will help blood flow tremendously.

2 **It increases your brain power.** Optimal hydration can help your brain work to its full capacity (which, let's face it, can get difficult as #pregnancybrain takes effect).

3 **It improves body performance.** Hydration can help you perform physical tasks better (for example, ahem, labor!).

4 **It helps you sweat.** While it may not always feel pleasant, sweating is an oh-so-important bodily function that helps us to cool down when we are hot, something that happens a lot during pregnancy. Not only will sweating keep you more comfortable, but it will also help support a safer body temperature for your baby to grow in.

5 **It helps you poop.** Yup. Constipation is a common pregnancy symptom and complication, but good water intake can definitely help prevent it. (It will also help prevent urinary tract infections.)

6 **It decreases nonlabor contractions.** When a uterus gets dehydrated, it often responds by contracting. Staying hydrated can prevent this and help your uterus have more powerful "real" contractions when it is time.

7 **It can decrease headaches.** Many pregnant women suffer from headaches, and hydration can help prevent them.

Now, drinking all that water can feel like a burden at first, though your body will start to crave it quickly. To make hydration more palatable, squeeze some fresh fruit into your water: berries, cucumber, lemon, or lime—anything goes. One word of caution though: Avoid precut or presliced fruit here. It has a higher likelihood of being contaminated by listeria and has likely been handled by many people before making it into your water glass. It will be safer to cut it yourself.

Coconut water is also a great way to get some hydration and extra electrolytes: Just be mindful of sugar intake.

Lastly, consider starting a water log. If you have a daily planner, draw ten circles on each day and fill them in as you drink.

move

Lift and Wrap in Everyday Life

The way we move in daily life is just as important (if not even more so) than exercise for the health of our core.

Did you know that learning to use your core in a healthy way during pregnancy can decrease your chances of developing diastasis recti (see page 357), incontinence (see page 354), and umbilical hernias (see page 461)? Your belly is growing every day, and learning how to continue daily movements while protecting the core is a vital tool in the prevention of injury. Even if you don't have time to work out, incorporating the lift and wrap into your daily life will help you get stronger. (Cool, huh?)

Practice

Add the lift and wrap core concept (from page 31) to daily actions and movements such as:

- Laughing
- Coughing
- Sneezing
- Reclining into a chair or couch
- Picking up anything over 10 to 15 pounds

Tips for Success

- When performing any of the daily activities or actions listed here, think about a gentle and supportive lift and wrap upon the movement or action. The idea is to correctly use the entire inner core unit when doing each of these.

- To check in on your core's strength and natural tendency, place a hand on your abdomen and cough. Does your core pulse toward the spine or push outward into your palm? After you learn to use this technique and get comfortable with it, your core will slightly engage, or turn on, and move toward the spine instead of moving outward.

- All of this can seem overwhelming in the beginning. The more you do this and build the awareness, the more it will start to happen automatically. You won't have to pay this much attention to your inner core forever: This is just a season.

WEEK 6

Your baby is the size of a sweet pea, about 0.098 inches (less than one-tenth of an inch) long. This is an exciting week for your baby (and you)! Week 6 is when the heartbeat may be visible for the first time on an ultrasound (sometimes it takes a bit longer to be able to see the heartbeat, though, which can be normal).

Your baby's heart is beating at about 110 beats per minute, a number that will increase to 120–160 beats per minute in the coming weeks.

Little buds have formed where the arms will soon start to grow.

At 6 weeks, you might also be able to tell if you are carrying twins (or more!)—though not always.

Your uterus is starting to enlarge a tiny bit, but for now, baby still rests snugly inside your pelvis.

love
AND VILLAGE

Assembling Your Pregnancy Village

Huge moments—like the one you are in right now—cause us to step back and examine who our nearest and dearest are and what roles they play in our lives. A lot can shift in your closest relationships throughout this motherhood journey, so it's important to be prepared.

So, in this hugest-of-huge experiences in your life, who is in your village? And are you ready to tell your village that you are pregnant? (Hint: There is no right answer.)

If you have a partner, it's likely that they know. What about your parents, family (immediate and extended), your partner's family, friends, co-workers (wow, you are popular!)?

Here are a few things you can consider when deciding when, and to whom, to announce this exciting news:

- Are you ready to share the news, or does it need to stay private longer?

- How will each of these people make you feel? Do they tend to comfort and nurture you? Or are they a bit more of the stress-inducing type (said lovingly, of course)? How will their energy impact you?

- Are they good at keeping secrets?

- Is there information some people could give you that would help you right now? For example, maybe your sister just had a baby and can give you some great advice.

- Does anyone *need* to know to help keep you safe? (For example, when I was pregnant with my first child, I was an oncology nurse and had to give chemotherapy, which I couldn't do while pregnant. So, I told a few close colleagues at work who could prepare my patients' chemo for me.)

The other thing to consider, which doesn't feel great to think about, is what happens if you have a miscarriage? Theoretically, you'll have to tell all the people who know about your pregnancy the news about the loss, which may be a conversation you don't want to have. If that's the case, you might consider waiting until the start of your second trimester, when the miscarriage risk drops dramatically.

When we asked our Motherly community, the majority of the mamas told us that they announced their pregnancy to their partner immediately, a few close friends and their parents within a few weeks of finding out, and then made it "social media official" around 12 or 13 weeks. Sooner or later, the baby bump will announce itself.

Murphy's Law suggests that you will find out that you are pregnant 2 days before your best friend's wedding (or family reunion, or beach trip, or any other event where there may be social drinking). And even in your day-to-day life, it can be hard to keep such big news a secret!

Most women don't start showing (having a visible baby bump) until after 12 weeks (and some not until much later), but that is not always the case. Bloating can also make you feel as though you are showing early as well.

Here are a few of my favorite tricks for hiding the news, if that's what you decide to do:

- Flowy tops are your best go-to fashion.

- Use a hair elastic to keep your pants fastened. Thread one end through the buttonhole, twist it into a figure eight, and loop both ends around the button.

- Cranberry juice and seltzers look a lot like cranberry and vodkas—with antioxidants too!

You may also want to come up with answers to the "Why aren't you drinking?" and "Why are you so tired?" questions ahead of time. Close friends and family may still call you out, so it's good to be prepared.

On the flip side, you may be bursting at the seams to share the news. Sometimes all the "don't tell until your second trimester" advice can feel a bit like raining on your parade. If you are excited and ready to shout from the rooftops, go for it!

WEEK 7

Your little one is the size of a blueberry, about one-third of an inch long. Not only does baby now have a more developed brain—that is gaining about one hundred cells per minute—they also have a liver and lung buds. The face is starting to define itself. Spaces for the nose, eyes, and mouth have developed.

Little legs and arms are starting to grow from your baby's torso, and with this, your baby is actually starting to look like, well, a baby!

work

Reminder: You are still very much a woman; you just so happen to also be pregnant. You will continue to be a star at work, at home, and everywhere in between. It's just a little harder to shine when you aren't sleeping well and can't keep your lunch down.

This is a great time to think about how you are going to make it through, and dare I say, thrive, in your day-to-day life.

First, if you have not had a chance to read the section on staying safe at work, you can check it out on page 18. You may also want to review the earlier tips on keeping the pregnancy a secret, just in case a co-worker happy hour is in your near future. Lastly, if you need to tell your co-workers and boss you are pregnant now, skip ahead to page 137 for some tips.

Beyond that, let's focus on two things this month: decluttering your calendar and planning for self-care.

Declutter Your Calendar

Raise your hand if your work, social, and home life leave you exhausted by the end of the week. The truth, dear mama, is that motherhood will only add to the busyness.

Unless, of course, you intentionally unbusy yourself.

This is a challenging thing to do! We tend to take on projects and say "yes" to more than we can manage before we even have time to reflect on the stuff that is filling up our time.

So, look at your calendar closely. For every scheduled item on there, ask yourself these questions:

- Do I have to do this?
- Does this make me happy?
- Do I look forward to this?

If the answer to those questions is "no," consider giving yourself permission to cut that item. By intentionally unbusying your days, you'll have more time to rest, and you know, grow a human. And when that human arrives, your habit will be a lifestyle that will benefit you and your baby a hundred times over.

Plan for Self-Care

Just like a cluttered calendar, self-care can get away from us quickly if we do not purposefully add it into our days. Once again, motherhood makes this even harder.

So, start now.

Make a conscious effort this month of getting into the habit of weaving self-care into the tapestry of your day. That means:

- Listening to your body when it has a need (like rest, hydration, nourishment, and quiet).

- Tuning in to your patterns so that you can start to anticipate the need for self-care before you are burned out (for example, "When I travel more than 2 hours from home, I know I feel extra tired the next day, so I will start to build a day of rest in to my future trips.").

- Pinpointing three to five activities that feel nurturing (napping, taking a bath,

walking, chatting with a friend, having a healthy meal, petting your dog, having sex—anything goes!).

- Letting go of the guilt. If you ask most moms, they'll tell you that when you enter motherhood, you get two things: a baby and guilt ("mom guilt," to be specific). Many women start to feel guilty about taking care of themselves when they become moms. There seems to be this sense that the baby should take absolute priority, all the time. While your priorities will certainly shift, and your baby will need almost constant attention, you deserve to stay high on your priority list as well. You don't stop mattering the moment you bring a child into this world.

You are now the trunk of your family's tree. To have healthy branches and twigs, it is essential that the trunk be healthy. You are allowed and encouraged to prioritize yourself on this entire journey.

So why not get into the habit now?

WEEK 8

Your baby is the size of a raspberry, about 0.67 inches long. All four chambers of the heart are now working to pump blood through the baby's body. Their eyes are starting to move from the side of the face to the front. The ears are also moving into position but will remain lower on the head for a bit longer.

Ready for this? You're growing your baby's hands this week! Right now, they look like little paddles, but can you imagine the first time those tiny hands grab yours?

You may notice that your breasts are changing. They may be filling out a bit, and your areolas might be getting darker and bigger. This is in preparation for potential breastfeeding. Babies see in contrast, so the more difference in color between the areola and your surrounding skin, the easier it is for baby to know where to go! As you get closer to giving birth, your areolas also have a different pH than the surrounding skin, making it easier for a sensitive infant nose to locate.

gather

- ○ Water bottle
- ○ Maternity clothing that you can wear through pregnancy and into the postpartum period:
  - Several tops that open in the front and allow access for breastfeeding and room for growing breasts
  - Flexible-waistband pants and skirts
  - Loose-fitting dresses
  - Leggings with maternity waistbands
  - Compression socks
  - Comfortable shoes (sometimes pregnancy causes feet to expand and stretch out, so you may even need to go up a size in footwear)

to do

- ○ Reflect: What does it mean for you to be creating a new generation in your ancestral line?
- ○ Ask your family members about their medical and pregnancy histories, if available.

- ○ Schedule your prenatal appointment.
- ○ Schedule a visit with a mental health therapist if it feels right.
- ○ Start or continue taking prenatal vitamins.
- ○ Drink ten 8-ounce glasses of water a day.
- ○ Practice the lift and wrap in your daily movements.
- ○ Define who is in your pregnancy village.
- ○ Ensure your work safety.
- ○ Declutter your calendar.

And above everything else:
- ○ Marvel in the wonder of it all.

remember

Remember to breathe. Feel the earth underneath you, supporting you and your budding baby. You are grounded by the generations of women who have become mothers before you and connected to women around the world who are becoming mothers with you.

You've got this.

Month 3

My body
is growing
a human.

Your body is incredible.

There is nothing else in this world that can do what your body is doing right now. It is growing an intricately complex human life, with no instruction manual. It just knows what to do and is doing it beautifully.

Pregnancy is a time to revere your body.

But that doesn't always come easily: Your shape is morphing in ways you never expected and making you feel pretty uncomfortable. It is understandable and common to feel confused—and even betrayed—by your body these days. You are trying hard to keep your nausea at bay. You are going to bed at 8:00 p.m. for the first time since elementary school. You are doing so much to try to feel better, and yet your biology continues to rebel and leaves you feeling powerless.

But therein lies your power.

The discomforts of pregnancy are reminders of how powerfully your body is working.

If your pregnancy symptoms seem to have taken over, remember that your body is doing everything it can to nurture and protect your baby. You don't have to enjoy the symptoms, or even be grateful for them. You are allowed to cry, moan, and complain about them. But if you can, try to remember that you are building a human being—from scratch!—and allow yourself to feel a sense of awe and some tremendous pride, even if you feel kinda yucky.

The "Symptom Checker," on page 429, has ideas on how to deal with all the symptoms you may be feeling. Never hesitate to also check in with your provider to see what's normal and what's not.

Take heart, mama. I know you might not feel good right now. I know you have moments where you feel unsettled. I wish I could wrap you in a cloak of deep rest and your favorite comfort food (but only the ones that don't make you nauseous). Know that this too shall pass and that you are rocking this.

xo,

Diana

WHAT IT REALLY FEELS LIKE

You are not alone in your symptoms. Here are what a few Motherly mamas experienced as they started their pregnancy journey:

"Exhaustion and nausea for me! Both had a big impact on my life, physically and emotionally, too. I generally loved being pregnant but struggled emotionally in that first trimester just handling life and parenting and work when I was running on what felt like empty. This new juggle can feel a little isolating if you haven't made your pregnancy 'public' to your community yet. It can be overwhelming fighting the lack of energy, plus the sickness and headaches at work, when you aren't yet comfortable sharing your pregnancy news. I found it so vital to lean on my partner and the close friends and family members who I'd shared early news with for emotional support during that time."
                                    JACQUI

"I remember lying down in my cubicle at work one day because I just needed to shut my eyes for 5 minutes. I could not stay awake to watch a movie or do anything fun with my husband. Also, I could take a nap during the day and still be so tired and ready for bed by 9:00!"
                                    BRITTANY

"I had exhaustion, nausea, and headaches. I definitely had a shorter fuse and felt irritated a lot of the time. Since it was my second pregnancy, and I had a toddler, friends would let me come over and fall asleep on their couches while they watched my toddler, and my husband understood that dinner was not going to happen every night unless we ordered pizza. We ordered a lot of pizza!"
                                    JUSTINE

pause
AND REFLECT

The symptoms of pregnancy can make it hard to appreciate your body and can even make it feel like you are at odds with it. *Come on, body! Help a mama out here!*

But let's see if you can take a few moments to focus on all that is good in your body. Your body is working so hard right now: She deserves a lot of love.

Think about your feet and your legs. The idea that pregnancy can cause your feet to grow is indeed true. Researchers have found that during a first pregnancy, a woman's arches become flatter, and her foot size increases. Your feet and your legs will support you, your growing belly, and your changing body as you advance through your pregnancy. They will continue to be there for you as you pace the floor in early labor, as you carry your baby for the first time, and through a million other moments of motherhood.

Think about your pelvis. Already the seat of your power, it's now sheltering your baby through their most delicate developments. Soon your baby will grow and rise higher in your abdomen, and your pelvis will slowly start expanding to make room for your baby to pass through when they are ready to be born.

Think about your digestive system. Your GI tract is slowing down, and in the process absorbing more nutrients to send to your growing baby and expelling the things not needed. Your tummy may not be acting like a friend these weeks, but trust that it is acting as a guardian.

Think about your breasts. Your breasts go through a second puberty of sorts during pregnancy to prepare for the possibility of breastfeeding. They are preparing to provide the nourishment your baby needs, and in doing so, provide the love, safety, and reassurance little ones crave.

Think about your brain. Your brain's structure will change during pregnancy. By the time your baby is born, your brain will have less grey matter, which scientists think helps new mothers respond to their newborns' needs with more attention and concern.

Think about your heart. Your heart is busy beating for two, pumping an increasing blood volume through your body every day, supporting your body's intense work. And your heart is prepping to fall in love. It may have already happened or may take a few weeks after birth, but trust me, mama, your heart is the most powerful of all.

bonding WITH YOUR BABY

This is a special time because you may still be keeping baby's presence a secret from your outer circles, and baby's home is still mostly hidden from view. But soon your belly will expand, and you will symbolize new life to everyone who sees you.

For now, though, your baby is still like a dream: a very powerful presence, but not filling your day-to-day reality. Give yourself permission to feel that presence and daydream about your future child. Start imagining what it will feel like to hold them and respond to their cries. It's not too early to ask what names this little person might like to be called and what qualities you hope they embody.

As you tap into the emerging energy of your little one, pay attention to any insights that pop up. This is the beginning of your mother's intuition, a new quality that you are uniquely positioned to acquire over the next months. Allowing yourself to attune to baby will set you up for a wonderful connection that will last a lifetime.

Symptoms YOU MIGHT FEEL

- Breast soreness/tenderness
- Constipation
- Cramping
- Fatigue
- Frequent urination
- Nausea and vomiting
- Nipple and areola darkening and enlarging
- Sensitivity to smell
- Spotting

To learn more about the symptoms that are impacting you—and how to deal—turn to the "Symptom Checker" on page 429. Remember, your provider is your first stop for any symptoms that concern you, so don't hesitate to reach out to them.

prenatal VISIT THIS MONTH

Most women can expect to have one visit during their third month of pregnancy, which may include:

- Blood pressure check
- Weight check
- Urine sample
- Follow-up on lab results from your last appointment

If this visit falls around or after the 12-week mark, get ready for some excitement in the form of one of the most amazing sounds you have ever heard.

At 12 weeks, your baby—and therefore your uterus—has usually grown enough to emerge above your pelvis (instead of being snuggled down inside it).

This means that with the use of a Doppler ultrasound (a handheld machine that detects the sound of blood moving through vessels), you may be able to hear your baby's heartbeat, though it is also possible that you'll need to wait a few more weeks to hear it, which can be totally normal.

The heart rate will be around 110 to 160 beats per minute, and the heartbeat sounds like a tiny train or galloping horse.

Brace yourself. This is a big one.

Genetic Screening

You will also have the opportunity to make some decisions about genetic screening and testing.

Noninvasive prenatal testing (NIPT), also called cell-free fetal DNA testing, can be done between weeks 10 and 20. It assesses the chances of chromosomal abnormalities, such as Down syndrome (trisomy 21), Patau syndrome (trisomy 13), Edwards syndrome (trisomy 18), and certain single-gene disorders associated with abnormalities of the skeleton, bones, or heart. This test can also determine the sex of your baby if you'd like to know.

The first-trimester combined screening is an optional test that is offered between 11 and 14 weeks. The test involves taking a blood sample from you along with an ultrasound that looks at certain aspects of the baby's development.

Neither of these screenings is diagnostic. This means that the results are not definitive ("The baby does or does not have Down syndrome") but rather a prediction of chance ("There is a higher or lower than normal chance that the baby could have Down syndrome").

If tests come back indicating that there is a high chance of abnormality, your provider may recommend a chorionic villus sampling

(CVS) or amniocentesis. They are more invasive but can give a definitive yes or no result.

Again, these tests are optional. Remember in chapter 5 when we talked about pregnancy being the start of making all these parenting decisions? Here it is again. There is no right answer, except for the one that feels right for you.

To read more about what these tests involve, see "Noninvasive Prenatal Testing (NIPT) and Multiple Marker Screening" and "Chorionic Villus Sampling (CVS)" on page 455 and "Amniocentesis" on page 454. For some general ideas on what to consider when deciding if these tests are right for you, see "Prenatal Tests" on page 452. And know that genetics is a quickly evolving field, so new findings and tests could come out at any time.

Questions to Ask Your Provider

- Did all the results come back from my last appointment, and how does everything look?
- I am having a hard time coping with _____ symptoms. Can we discuss some options?
- Can we talk through the chromosomal testing, so I can make an informed choice?

TWINS, TRIPLETS, AND BEYOND

Multiple pregnancy can arise in two different ways. It can be the result of more than one egg getting fertilized, which produces fraternal multiples. It can also occur when a fertilized egg divides and grants the exact same DNA to all of the babies who then develop into identical multiples.

Multiples are much more common these days because women are delaying childbearing until their late 20s and 30s, when multiples are more likely to occur. Couples or individuals who use assisted reproductive technologies are also more likely to conceive twins and multiples.

If you're pregnant with more than one baby, chances are good that everything will go well. But there are certain aspects of the experience that will be different. You will likely gain more weight and have more checkup appointments, and you'll be more likely to deliver early and deliver through a C-section. Multiple pregnancies may increase the risk of some complications. To read about those, see "Multiple Babies" on page 464.

If you feel ready, there are some other "complications" of having multiples that we should probably discuss:

- Overabundance of love. One baby is wonderful. Two or more babies . . . I mean . . . come on.

- The comments, oh, the comments. "Are they identical?" "Can you tell them apart?"

"You have your hands full!" "Ugh, twins. I can't even imagine." Don't worry, you'll be able to laugh these off soon.

- Volume. Getting to live with their built-in BFF means that there will almost always be something hilarious to laugh at, a story to tell, and games to play. This means your home will pretty much always be loud, but oh, so filled with joy.

- Multiple-mama bonding. Some of the tightest mom friendships I have ever seen are between moms of multiples. Find your village and know that they are going to support you so much.

- Chaos. But the greatest kind ever. Things are going to be unpredictable and wild and silly and intense. But mama, it's the best. And you are going to rock it.

WEEK 9

Your baby is the size of a grape, about 0.87 inches long. Your baby's embryonic tail has disappeared, and all their essential organs are growing! Their toes are becoming distinct, and their arms start to bend at the elbows. Your baby also has nipples! And eyelids! What a busy little bee.

You may notice more weight gain at this time, most often due to retaining fluids and your increasing blood volume.

A little-known fact is that your respiratory system changes during pregnancy because the positions of your ribs and diaphragm shift. By this week, your lung capacity has increased to provide more oxygen to the baby. It may make you short of breath at first, but you are actually breathing more efficiently.

nourish

Eating When You're Nauseous

As you've likely started to discover, growing your baby is no easy feat—physically or mentally. You may be dealing with overwhelming nausea and fatigue as your body adapts to the changes happening to support your little one. The thought of food and eating may be more than you can handle at this point.

If food is feeling complicated, remember to keep it simple by bringing it back to basics. Focus on getting in whole foods in their natural form. Minimizing your intake of processed foods will help you maximize nutrient density. Focus on fruits, vegetables, nuts, seeds, legumes, whole grains, meat, fish, poultry, avocados, and unprocessed oils (like extra-virgin olive oil).

If it's hard for you to pronounce some of the ingredients listed on a food label, it's more likely to be a processed food with lower nutrient quality.

While your nutrition may feel like it's less than ideal, or food is just hard to keep down, your body is still doing exactly what it needs to do to support a healthy baby. Do the best you can, but no need to feel guilty if you just can't stomach much these days.

Trust your body as the best guide for what you need to help you navigate nausea, morning sickness, and fatigue. Eating small, frequent meals and snacks can also be easier on your body and digestive system. Eat slowly and mindfully when possible and avoid drinking too much liquid at mealtimes.

Consider incorporating foods that may help soothe these symptoms and provide morning sickness relief, such as:

- Ginger (including ginger ale and ginger chews)
- Peppermint tea
- Whole-grain breads
- Salted crackers
- Dry cereal (fortified)

move

Diaphragmatic Breathing

This is a great time to introduce diaphragmatic breathing to your pregnancy. This form of breathing provides endless benefits to you, your core, and your baby throughout pregnancy, during birth, and for life. We adults tend to breathe shallowly (thank you, stress), without a ton of thought on how we breathe throughout the day.

Repatterning your breath doesn't happen overnight, but its benefits during your pregnancy are too good to ignore. Breathing with your diaphragm instead of your chest can:

GINGER TEA RECIPE

For soothing relief, make your own homemade ginger tea to help keep the nausea at bay.

Take fresh ginger that has been peeled and cut into a 1-inch cube and steep it in 8 oz. hot water for about 5 minutes. Sweeten with a drizzle of honey and a squeeze of fresh lemon juice.

- Aid digestion

- Calm the body and mind

- Turn on your parasympathetic nervous system (which slows and relaxes the body and helps you move through discomfort with more ease)

- Deliver oxygen and blood flow to organs and muscles more efficiently

- Optimize how your inner core muscles work together (think of the "box" we introduced on page 25)

- Provide a supportive form of breathing to assist you in your labor and birth process

Practice

Find a comfortable position—like sitting or lying on your back—to begin. Place one palm on the side of your rib cage and the other between the bottom of the rib cage and your belly button.

Begin to breathe as you normally would and witness where the movement is taking place. Now it's time to shift the awareness and the breath.

Inhale as you imagine filling your rib cage with your breath, allowing the ribs to expand out to the sides into the palm on the rib cage. Notice that this breath also enables the upper abdomen to rise ever so slightly into the other palm.

Exhale and notice your body and palms move back inward, as the rib cage and upper abdomen fall back toward neutral.

Continue taking slow, steady, deep breaths as you focus on the movement happening beneath each palm.

Once you begin to understand the concept of this form of breathing, and your body is responding with ease, shift your awareness to your pelvic floor.

Remember that the pelvic floor muscles play a vital role in diaphragmatic breathing. Just as your rib cage and abdomen rise and fall with each breath, so should your pelvic floor muscles. In fact, they follow the exact same pattern. As the rib cage and belly rise (ever so gently), your pelvic floor muscles should relax, soften, or lengthen down toward your vagina. As the rib cage and belly fall back to neutral, your pelvic floor muscles should rise back to neutral.

See if you can make this form of breath your new normal. The more you breathe this way in everyday life and during cardio-based workouts, the more you are building the optimal foundation for your entire body.

Tips for Success

- Be patient. It's potentially been a while since you have spent this much time focusing on your breathing, and it can take time to repattern even something as simple as breath.

- If you find that the majority of your breath resides in your chest rising and falling, place one palm on your chest and one on the side of your rib cage. Breathe into the palm on the rib cage and try to keep the palm on the chest as still as possible (the chest can rise ever so slightly in the last portion of your inhale).

- If connecting to your pelvic floor seems foreign to you, you may find the following technique helpful: Try placing your

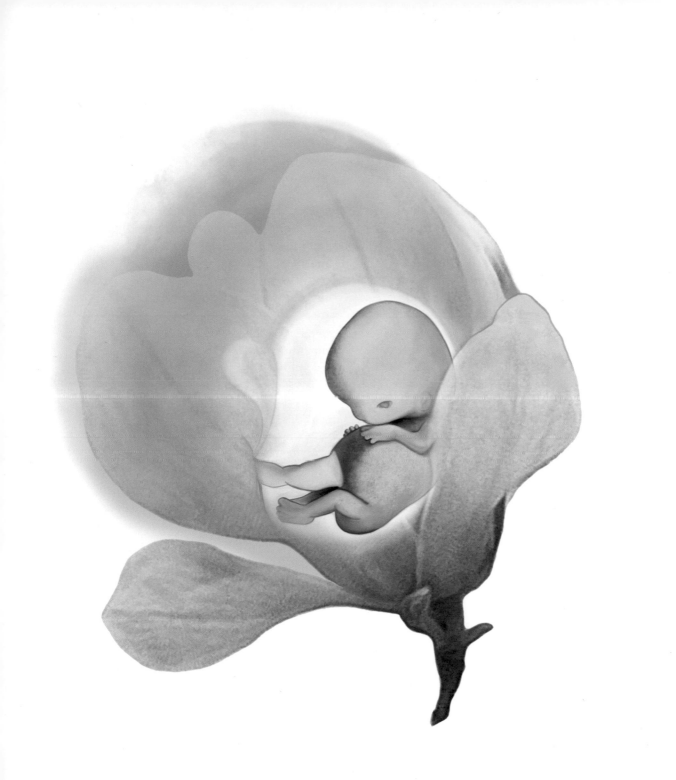

WEEKS 9–12

index finger on your perineum (the place between your vagina and anus). Now imagine breathing into that place and try to connect with the subtle movement that happens in this area when you inhale and lengthen downward and exhale and rebound upward. You may be able to better understand the connection now.

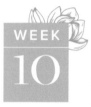

WEEK 10

Your baby is the size of a prune, about 1.2 inches long. Their fingernails are visible, they have elbows and knees, and they are kicking their legs and moving all over the place, though you still won't be able to feel your little prune move for a while (usually around the 20-week mark).

love AND VILLAGE

Sex During Pregnancy

Let's talk about sex.

If you find yourself with many (many) questions about sex and intimacy during pregnancy, you are not alone! In early pregnancy, women who know that they are pregnant have less sex than women who don't know they are pregnant. In other words, knowing we're pregnant changes how we relate to sex.

Safety of Sex in Pregnancy

Every woman and every pregnancy is different, so this is one that you should run by your provider to make sure they can account for your specific circumstances.

Generally speaking, it is safe to have sex during pregnancy. This includes vaginal and anal penetration, oral sex, fingering, breast stimulation, using sex toys, masturbation, and having orgasms. Get it, girl.

A quick note about orgasms: The hormone oxytocin is known as the love hormone. It is released when you fall in love and when you have an orgasm, and it is the hormone that makes your uterus contract in labor. In fact, your uterus also contracts a bit when you orgasm, but this is not likely to harm your baby in a healthy pregnancy.

Your baby is safely tucked in your uterus, away from your vagina and anything that goes into it. They are cushioned by your (superhero-strong) uterus, amniotic fluid, and your body's tissues, so they are not going to get hit with a penis, fingers, or a sex toy (as much as romantic comedies like to mock this!).

Developing inside your cervix is something called a mucus plug, which is, in fact, made of mucus, like what's running out your nose when you have a cold. Your mucus plug helps prevent bacteria from entering through your cervix and into your uterus.

As far as the worry about jostling the baby with the movement of sex, it's likely that the baby is rocked to sleep by it (how sweet). And maybe you will be too, depending on how strong your pregnancy fatigue is!

As your belly continues to grow, you may have to get a bit creative when it comes to positions. You can expect it to be awkward, but it should not hurt; if it does, stop and readjust, or check with your provider. Using water-based lubrication can help as well.

There are some instances when your doctor or midwife will advise you not to have sex and orgasms. Some of these reasons may include:

- If you have a history of, or are at risk for, preterm labor (see "Preterm Labor and Premature Babies" on page 242)

- If your placenta is growing close to your cervix (see "Placenta Previa" and "Low-Lying Placenta" on page 474)

- If you or your partner has an untreated sexually transmitted infection (see "Sexually Transmitted Infections During Pregnancy" on page 470)

- If your water has broken (see "Water Breaking" on page 239)

If you are having oral sex, it is important that your partner not blow into your vagina, as this could lead to an amniotic fluid embolism (see "Amniotic Fluid Embolism (AFE)" on page 477).

You are more at risk for a urinary tract infection (UTI) when you are pregnant. Sex can lead to UTIs because the bacteria from the anus travels into the urethra. Take some extra precautions to prevent this by:

- Peeing immediately following sex, and always wiping from front to back
- Avoiding going from anal penetration to vaginal penetration without thoroughly cleaning the penis/fingers/toy first

Be cautious with rough sex and activities that could lead to injury (including tears) in your vagina and surrounding areas, where bacteria could enter and cause infections.

What About Your Sex Drive or Lack Thereof?

Some women find that pregnancy makes them way more "in the mood" than they used to be. Higher levels of estrogen can bump up your sex drive, as can oxytocin later in pregnancy. Oxytocin is the l-o-v-e hormone, after all.

Your vagina and clitoris are also getting a lot more blood flow these days, which makes them more sensitive to touch and more lubricated.

A NOTE FOR PARTNERS ON PREGNANCY SYMPTOMS

For partners and supportive friends and family members, it can be tough to watch the person you love feel uncomfortable, especially when there is not much you can do to make her feel better. If you are feeling helpless, know that research has found that women who have high levels of social support (like that of a partner, friend, or family member) in their first trimester experience major benefits: improved quality of life, less depression, and even babies born at a healthier birth weight! In other words, your loving and caring presence makes a difference.

Here are some ideas to try:

- Tell her that she is doing a fantastic job.
- Bring her a plate of crackers and jelly in the morning to help keep her nausea at bay.
- Rub her back to help her fall asleep.

None of these are revolutionary acts, but they will mean the world to her.

Your growing breasts and nipples may respond to sensation differently now, as well. And have you seen yourself recently? You are a glowing, sexy, gorgeous woman. Own it!

In short, some women find that they have some of the best sex of their lives during these 9 months.

You may also find that the idea of sex is, well, the least sexy thing you can think of right now.

This is going to vary a lot, of course. Women often find that their desire for and enjoyment of sex changes throughout pregnancy. You may be very in the mood in the beginning and then find that you have absolutely no desire later on, or vice versa. A growing belly can make positioning a bit awkward, and the symptoms of pregnancy can make it harder to feel revved up.

Psst: Sometimes decreased libido can be a warning sign of depression. Just pay attention to how you are feeling and consider speaking to a therapist if you are worried.

Remember this: your body, your rules. Listen to the wisdom of your body. If it wants sex, go for it. If it needs Netflix and sleep, go for that. Keep in mind that there are a lot of ways to connect with your partner beyond sex.

Your baby is the size of a lime, about 1.6 inches long. Previously called an embryo, your baby has officially graduated to fetus status! Cap and gown well deserved. They will technically be identified as a fetus until they are born, when they will be called a newborn, an infant, and all the adorable nicknames you develop for them.

Your baby's little eyebrows are developing, and they have started to pee! This urine helps make up the amniotic fluid, which the baby swallows to help develop the lungs. We're not sure who thought drinking pee was a great idea, but it seems to work just fine for these little ones.

In another week or so, your uterus will grow beyond the pelvis, and you may be noticing the need to loosen your pants a bit or transition to maternity wear (if you haven't done so already).

work

For many mamas, this month is all about survival mode, especially when it comes to work. Whether it's getting through the day without throwing up on your desk or staying awake so your toddler doesn't destroy the entire house, it can be a real doozy.

If you are working outside the home, you may decide this is the time to tell your workplace your news, simply because hiding it is too hard. If so, jump ahead to page 137 where we go into this at length.

Whether or not you are ready to spill the beans, here are some tips from the Motherly community about how to survive these next weeks:

"[Think] about setting up a discreet nap situation at work and where to put extra snacks at your desk."   JESSICA

"I got by on candied ginger, sipping on ginger ale, and eating arrowroot crackers all day. Also with a lot of grace from my employer."   MARY

"I survived by telling my boss super-early (before I told my parents), took nausea medication prescribed by my doctor, and asked to work from home." LIZ

WEEK 12 Your baby is the size of a plum, about 2.1 inches long. Your baby's reflexes have started to develop, they can suck their thumb, and they are beginning to grasp with those tiny fingers.

Baby is beginning to yawn. (Is there anything cuter than a newborn baby's exaggerated yawn? Becoming human is *exhausting*.) Baby's eyes move closer together this week, and the chin is much more distinguished.

At 12 weeks, you may be able to hear your baby's heartbeat with a Doppler ultrasound, though it's not uncommon to have to wait a few more weeks for this.

Around week 12, your placenta (which has been growing along with your baby) is cranking and ready to support your baby's needs (more on placentas on page 166).

gather

○ Crackers, peppermint, and anything else that soothes your symptoms
○ Ginger (peeled and cubed), honey, and lemon for DIY nausea tea
○ Lubrication for intercourse

to do

○ Reflect on the power of your body.
○ Schedule your next prenatal appointment.
○ Consider your options for genetic testing.

○ Visit the "Symptom Checker" on page 429 to get ideas for coping with any discomforts.
○ Ask your provider if it is safe to have sex (only, of course, if you want to have sex).
○ Set up your work environment to help you cope with symptoms.
○ Practice diaphragmatic breathing.

remember

The discomforts of pregnancy are reminders of how powerfully your body is working.

Month 4

WEEKS 13–17

Release the *not enoughs*, the *can'ts*, and the *doubts*.

note FROM DIANA

Something remarkable happens in your second trimester.

Maybe it's the easing of those first-trimester symptoms. Maybe it's that you start to see your (swoon-worthy) bump. Or maybe it's that you can detect those first fluttering kicks (*so* soon, I promise!).

Whatever the cause, the second trimester is a magical one because suddenly you actually *feel* pregnant.

You continue to wrap your mind around the enormity of it all, but perhaps for the first time, you have these thoughts of "Wait. I am pregnant. I am going to have a baby."

See? Magic.

While you spend the first trimester focused inward, you will tend to shift to a more outward focus in the second trimester, both in the direction your belly starts to grow and in the way you navigate the world. Your village likely knows that you are pregnant by now. You will begin to think about how having a baby may change your relationships. You might have to consider what this means for work and your career. You may even begin to think about the gear, nursery design, and registries (so fun!).

In essence, you are traveling further down your path toward motherhood. You begin this trimester with a baby the size of a lemon. When you end this trimester, your baby will be the size of a large eggplant, you will feel them move all day long, and you will be thinking about birth plans and names.

Welcome to your second trimester.

It's getting real, mama.

xo,

Diana

P.S. A lot of women find that they feel their best during the second trimester. Those first-trimester yuckies start to fade, but the "whoa, there is a big baby in here" feelings of the third trimester have not yet set in. If you do feel well, try to spend some time being mindful of all that is good.

The second trimester is when pregnancy transitions from a concept to a reality. You can feel your baby in your womb and imagine that one day you will be this precious baby's mother.

You likely already have some ideas about what this means and what type of mother you want to be. Next month, we'll delve into the core values that will guide you every day as a mom.

But before we can do that, we must do the (sometimes challenging) work of clearing space for those values, of letting go of that which does not serve us.

We all have our insecurities, right? The muck that prevents us from seeing ourselves as we are. It's the part of us that feels "not enough": the knot in your stomach that makes you question your intuition, or the voice in your head that says you're not up to the task of being somebody's mother (*you are*), or the fear you feel thinking about how you'll handle labor and birth (*you can do this*).

Take a few moments and sit with your muck, even though it makes you uncomfortable. Write it down: a sentence for each uncomfortable thought.

And then, let it go. You can tear up the page, even.

Release the not enoughs, the can'ts, and the doubts. These are not truths. We absorb these nontruths as we go through our days, and they become so ingrained in our minds that we start to believe them as real.

But this is the real story: You are more than enough. You can. You will.

Spend some time this month quieting the nontruths. When you feel one of them creeping in, which you will, thank it for the opportunity it's provided, and then send it away again. Soon, they will start to come with less frequency and less urgency. And then you'll have more room for the good stuff.

And remember, therapists are available to help you work through anything that comes up.

POSTPARTUM RECOVERY IN CHINA

It's never too early to start thinking about your postpartum period. Imagine giving birth to your baby and immediately becoming the center of pampering attention for a full month. Someone is with you 24/7 to take care of you and your newborn, so you can rest, eat nourishing foods, feed your baby, and recover from childbirth.

Sounds pretty nice, right?

Mary Sabo, doctor of acupuncture and Chinese medicine, writes of the tradition of "Sitting the Month," or *Zuo Yuezi* in Chinese medicine. Thousands of years ago in the Chinese Han dynasty, it was recognized that the month directly after childbirth is crucial to the future health of the mother and newborn. This program has become a tradition in Chinese culture and involves rules for the month following childbirth, some of which are still followed as closely as they were two thousand years ago. Women may be encouraged to avoid contact with wind and cold; they eat bland, warmed foods; and they only rest, eat, sleep, and feed the baby. For the first 30 days, they may have no visitors and no entertainment! While some of this tradition has evolved, the old wisdom about what promotes the healing process still rings true.

bonding
WITH YOUR BABY

One of the movements that infants respond to positively is rhythmic rocking. Most parents seem to know this intuitively and use a rocking or swaying motion, along with physical touch and carrying, to help relax and soothe crying babies. But they might not realize that there are many neurological and developmental benefits to rocking a baby. Because you are stimulating their inner ear's vestibular system, this aids in developing the parts of the brain dealing with motor skills and coordination. Even at this early, pre-birth stage, you can gently rock in a chair and begin the relaxation response for your tiny one. Try spending a few minutes in a rocking chair or rocking on a yoga mat on the floor. Imagine your baby responding blissfully (and sleepily!).

Symptoms
YOU MIGHT FEEL

- Back pain/ache
- Bleeding gums
- Bleeding nose
- Congestion
- Constipation
- Fetal movement
- Groin pain
- Headaches
- Heartburn or reflux
- Hemorrhoids
- Linea nigra
- Vaginal discharge

To learn more about the symptoms that are impacting you—and how to deal—turn to the "Symptom Checker" on page 429. Remember, your provider is your first stop for any symptoms that concern you, so don't hesitate to reach out to them.

prenatal
VISIT THIS MONTH

Most women can expect to have one visit during their fourth month of pregnancy, which may include:

- Blood pressure check
- Weight check
- Urine sample
- Listening to the baby's heartbeat
- Follow-up on lab results from your last appointment

Your midwife or doctor will now palpate (feel) your abdomen to measure your uterus's growth (and your baby's, of course) at every visit. At 12 weeks, the top of your uterus is just above the top of your pubic bone, and every week after this, it climbs about another centimeter more. Your provider will place their hands on your belly and gently press to feel where the top of your uterus is.

If it has been recommended, you may choose to have an amniocentesis done between weeks 15 and 20. An amniocentesis diagnoses chromosomal abnormalities, including Down syndrome, and neural tube defects like spina bifida.

Just like the previous genetic testing we discussed, amniocentesis is an optional test, but it is more invasive because the provider must extract your amniotic fluid. Depending on factors like the results of previous screening tests, family history, and your age, your provider may or may not recommend one, but ultimately, it is up to you.

For more information on what's involved, jump to "Amniocentesis" on page 454.

The multiple marker screening, also known as the triple or quad screening, is an optional blood test that assesses the chance that the baby may have a chromosomal abnormality, such as Down syndrome. This screening can be done between weeks 15 and 20. For more information on this test, see "Noninvasive Prenatal Testing (NIPT) and Multiple Marker Screening" on page 455.

Question to Ask Your Provider

- Can we talk about the amniocentesis and the multiple marker screening and if they might be a good idea for me?

WEEK

13

Your baby is the size of a peach, about 2.9 inches long. There are nails on your baby's fingers and toes. Your little one hiccups (to learn more about hiccuping, see "Baby Hiccups" on page 429), makes sucking motions, stretches their arms and legs, and can touch their face. (*So cute!*)

Baby is producing their own white blood cells now, though they can't yet fight off an infection without your help. They're also getting sweat glands and the tiniest strands of hair. At this point, the baby has a more clearly defined neck, allowing them to bob their head up and down slightly.

nourish

Cravings

Welcome to the second trimester, mama! Hopefully, you'll find that symptoms associated with morning sickness subside during this time, though for some, nausea might continue to persist (and if it does, keep going with the tips from last month). Many women worry that their nutrition has been less than ideal going into the second trimester, but rest assured that your body is fully capable of doing what is needed to grow your healthy baby.

This month's reflection is about shedding self-limiting thoughts. With that, I hope you will begin to trust yourself and your body more.

QUICKENING

When you start to feel your baby's movement will depend on a few factors. If this is your first baby, you'll likely feel it later, at around 20 weeks, though it can be earlier or later. If it's your second baby, you may feel movement earlier. If your placenta is toward the front of your belly (known as an anterior placenta), you may have to wait a bit longer to feel the movements since it provides a buffer.

Many cultures designate this moment, called quickening, as the first major milestone of a pregnancy. In the days before pregnancy tests, this was a reliable sign that a new life was on its way. Women often say that the first movements feel like a goldfish bumping up against the side of its tank or the flutter of butterfly wings. Other women put it a little more bluntly: "It feels like gas."

Your baby is already moving a lot; you just can't always feel it. But when you do, there are simply no words. Enjoy, mama! This experience is one of the well-deserved delights for all the hard work you've put into growing this baby!

SMALL, FREQUENT MEALS

Your appetite may fluctuate as you transition into the second trimester, and that is entirely normal. Eating small, frequent meals consistently can help ensure that you are getting the necessary nutrients to support your pregnancy.

As your energy levels and appetite gradually improve, tune into your body to decipher what she needs to grow your baby. You may begin to notice cravings for certain foods or food combinations—even things that you wouldn't usually eat or even think to put together! This may be your body's way of getting essential nutrients that might be needed in more significant quantities.

For example, if you are craving salty foods, it sometimes means that your body is dehydrated! Get yourself a big glass of water, sip it all down, and then see how you feel. Oftentimes, this will make the craving go away. Another delicious idea for when you crave salt is to bake sweet potato spears and drizzle them with olive oil and sea salt for a salty crunch. Added bonus: Sweet potatoes can stabilize your blood sugar, which can help you avoid postmeal energy crashes.

Speaking of sugar, another way your body might let you know it needs some energy is by activating your sweet tooth. Respond by making a refreshing smoothie with a handful of sweet frozen berries and spinach. Sweet-tooth cravings can be used to your benefit by opting for a nutrient-dense treat, like dark chocolate covered almonds or low-sugar frozen yogurt for added calcium and probiotics.

Remember, cravings are an important clue to pay attention to during pregnancy. Your job is to find nourishing ways of satisfying those cravings that are healthy and sustainable for pregnancy. (And the occasional splurge never hurt anyone!)

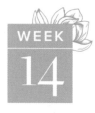

WEEK 14

Your baby is the size of a lemon (but much sweeter!), about 3.4 inches long. Your little one has developed the ability to make facial expressions. Though baby still can't fully open their eyelids, they are able to perceive light. It is commonly said that if you shine a flashlight at your belly, the baby will move away from the beam. Baby's first game of tag, perhaps?

move

The Belly Pump

If you've been working on your diaphragmatic breathing (see page 119), it's now time to take it to the next level, to add even more strength and connection to your changing core.

The belly pump is the exercise component of diaphragmatic breathing. It is almost exactly like the diaphragmatic breathing technique, but on the exhale, we create an intentional activation of the pelvic floor and transverse abdominal muscles (the body's natural corset, which is responsible for the stability of the pelvis and spine).

HOW TO WEAR A SEAT BELT WHILE PREGNANT

Wearing a seat belt during pregnancy is more important than ever: You are now driving or riding for two! When you strap yourself in, place the shoulder belt against your shoulder, center it between your breasts, and then place it down the side (not on top) of your belly. The lap belt should sit snugly under your belly bump.

It's very similar to concepts that have been used by pelvic floor physical therapists for years in helping women heal from pregnancy injuries.

When applying the belly pump to your pregnancy, you can expect the following:

- Decreased low back pain. The transverse abdominal muscles are responsible for stability of the spine and pelvis. Implementing techniques like the belly pump helps strengthen these muscles to support the growing belly and extra weight being placed on the spine. This will ultimately lead to less back pain. (*Yes, please!*)

- An intentional strengthening of your core even as your belly grows. Commonly, women are told to avoid crunches and other traditional abdominal exercises during pregnancy. Techniques like the belly pump allow women to maintain optimal strength of the core while pregnant.

- Decreased chance of pelvic pain, pelvic floor injury (such as prolapse), and incontinence. With each inhale and exhale, the diaphragm, pelvic floor, and transverse abdominal muscles work in concert with one another as they are intended. Through this, you can bring more balance to the pelvic floor. And more balance means fewer chances of these injuries.

- A better understanding of how to use the muscles of the inner core when it comes time to push during birth.

- A stronger connection to your core for life.

Practice

Find a comfortable position. Place one palm on the side of your rib cage and the other between the bottom of the rib cage and your belly button. Begin to breathe as you normally would and witness where the movement is taking place.

Inhale, filling the rib cage and belly with a gentle breath. The rib cage and belly will naturally expand, and the pelvic floor will soften. This is the same as in your diaphragmatic breath.

As you exhale, make a *sssss* sound. This will help you connect deeper to the pelvic floor and corset muscles. With this exhale, start engaging and lifting the pelvic floor muscles

GARDENING DURING PREGNANCY

Wondering about whether you can cultivate your green thumb while you grow your sweet bump? In general, the answer is "yes," with some safety guidelines.

The main concern is exposure to a parasite that causes a disease called toxoplasmosis (which can cause serious complications; see "Toxoplasmosis" on page 468 for more on this one). The parasite is spread when cats and other animals use your yard as a bathroom, which is not something we can generally control.

To keep yourself safe, always wear gloves when you garden, don't touch your face or hair with your gloves, and wash your hands thoroughly when you are done.

Also consider whether plants have been sprayed with pesticides recently, and if so, make sure to avoid being near them.

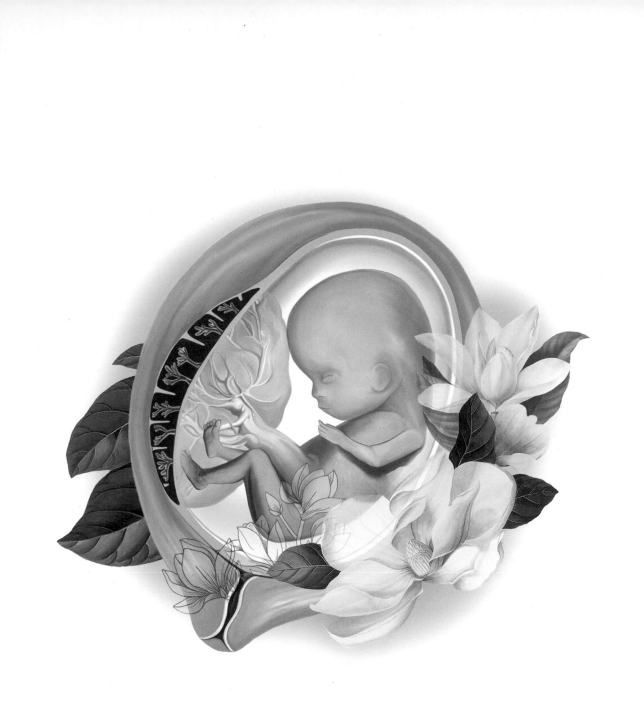

WEEKS 13–17

(the crane claw movement described on page 25) as you then layer onto the pelvic engagement with a wrapping of your abdomen as if you were tightening a corset around your torso. You can imagine this activation moving up the core with your exhale. Your pelvic floor engages, then hip bones draw together, next the midsection wraps toward the belly button, and at the end of your sssss exhale, your rib cage knits together toward the center.

Take your time, allowing your breath to be deep and expansive, yet slow and controlled.

Tips for Success

- The core engagement that happens with the belly pump is the same as lift and wrap mentioned on page 31.

- Use the sssss sound to connect deeper to the core muscles. Try it without the sssss sound to feel the difference.

- Always begin your exhale and engagement with the pelvic floor and end with the knitting of the rib cage. Think about zipping up tightly from the bottom.

- Try to connect to the full softening and lengthening of the pelvic floor on the inhale, just as you do with diaphragmatic breathing.

- As always, talk with your provider if you have concerns.

WEEK 15

Your baby is the size of an apple, about 4 inches long. All four adorable inches of the baby are on the grow! Your baby has fragile skin at this point, and blood vessels are easily seen through it, showing the fantastic intricacies of their body's development. The umbilical cord is still getting thicker and longer. Its job is to deliver nutrients to the baby through oxygenated blood while recycling waste and low-oxygen blood back to you to process and eliminate.

Your breasts are starting to make colostrum, aka liquid gold—the very first type of breast milk your baby will receive if you choose to nurse or pump. (To learn more about colostrum, jump to "Breast Milk" on page 393.)

love AND VILLAGE

Now is a good time to start shaping what your family culture will look like. You and your partner, co-parent, or someone else significant in baby's life can spend some time writing down answers to these questions. You don't need to agree on everything now, and you may only reach agreement once you know how your particular family functions. The point is just to begin the conversation and to start taking steps toward feeling rooted in your family's needs and desires.

- What do you appreciate most about how you were parented?

- What would you change about how you were parented?

- Describe the qualities that you would like to embody as a parent.

- How do you anticipate wanting to bond with your baby and child?

- Imagine that your baby is now a feisty 3-year-old. They are developing a habit of not listening to you and pushing back when you make requests. How would you approach this issue? What type of behavior modification will you use as a family?

- What structure or institutions will guide your child's education and spiritual or religious life?

- Who else can you depend on to help you with your child?

Parenting is all about flexibility, and many of the answers you give here will change—perhaps often. That is absolutely to be expected. The goal, though, is to stay focused on what matters most to you and your growing family.

A NOTE FOR PARTNERS ON DEPRESSION

Did you know that more than 10 percent of soon-to-be fathers experience depression and anxiety during their partners' pregnancies? This may be higher if mama is also depressed. There is also some research into female partners' responses as well, showing that the emotional toll of pregnancy isn't just on the pregnant mom, especially given the potential for added concerns among same-sex couples such as discrimination and lack of support (from policies, workplaces, and so on).

This matters for a few reasons. First, of course, is that you deserve to feel good, simple as that. Expecting a baby is stressful for everyone, and having depression or anxiety on top of that normal stress only makes it harder.

Second, depression impacts your relationship with your partner.

And third, new parents with depression tend to have a harder time bonding with and parenting their new babies.

The good news is that depression and anxiety respond well to treatment. Reach out to your health-care provider or a therapist. It's confidential, and whether you begin taking a mood medication, embark on a course of behavioral therapy, or both, almost all patients gain some relief from their symptoms.

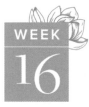

WEEK 16

Your baby is the size of an avocado, about 4.6 inches long. This week, the baby's size almost equals that of the placenta. Their taste buds are formed, and they are able to perceive different tastes in the amniotic fluid (more on this in "Week 21"). The baby is double the size they were just 4 weeks ago, and their tiny muscles are building up strength. Watch out, you may be able to start feeling those muscles aiming a kick your way very soon!

Navigating work and pregnancy are front and center for a lot of women. About 56 percent of pregnant women are employed full time, and 82 percent of first-time pregnant women who are employed work until the very end of their pregnancies. The dynamics of navigating the workplace while pregnant present a host of potential issues, some psychological, some social, some physical. We hear from Motherly readers that they are very concerned about how to communicate about the pregnancy, especially with their managers and bosses.

Many women who are employed outside the home decide to tell their employers their pregnancy news when their second trimester starts. Depending on your boss, co-workers, and general work culture, this can either be a breeze or make you feel like you're walking into the principal's office again. Keep in mind that if you plan to take federal leave under the Family and Medical Leave Act (FMLA), you must give them at least 30 days' notice.

Don't worry; we've got expert tips on how to handle this with grace and ease.

If you are feeling a bit nervous, you must remember that you have not done anything wrong by becoming pregnant. It's reasonable to expect that your workplace will respond professionally, respectfully, and even compassionately, and most do. If they do not, that is their problem, not yours, to be blunt. Take a deep breath and walk in there with your head high (and your bump bumping).

How to Tell Your Workplace You Are Pregnant in Six Steps

1 **Do your research.** Try to find out your company's official policy on pregnancy and maternity leave, so you can go into the conversation knowledgeable and confident.

> "I was so nervous to tell my male bosses. Specifically, I was stressed that they would look at me differently, not take me as seriously, not give me new clients/projects, and assume I wasn't coming back to work despite my insistence that I was. It ended up being completely fine, and they were happy for me and understanding."
> ELLI

> "It was so stressful having to tell my supervisor. It's almost like you feel like you're letting them down knowing that you will be out of the office for months. I had to keep telling myself, 'You're having a baby. This is the most amazing thing ever!' In the end, there was no need for me to be stressed anyway!"
> MARISA

> "I resented the fact that I had to tell my co-workers and clients and come up with a whole action plan for when I would be out of the office, while my partner didn't have to deal with any of that. He got all the congrats and well wishes. I got more work to do. No one asked him to take less time off or if he was going to return to work ASAP."
> JACKIE

> "The first pregnancy, I felt bad because I had just transferred to that location 2 months prior, after trying to get transferred there for years. They were really supportive. I had to tell them early because I was working in a pharmacy, and there are a few medications that I couldn't handle while pregnant."
> CASSIE

EMPLOYMENT AND PROTECTIONS

In the US, we have basic protections for pregnant women under both federal and state law. We're not the parental utopia of Scandinavia, but we aren't left totally out in the cold. If you are employed, you may be able to combine all of your company's time off, which includes sick days, vacation days, personal days, and any applicable maternity leave, when planning for your postpartum time off.

The Family and Medical Leave Act (FMLA)

This law entitles you to 12 weeks of unpaid maternity leave and a guaranteed return to your job, if your company offers it and if you are eligible. The US Department of Labor (DOL) website (dol.gov) details which criteria make companies and employees eligible. Your employer may also be responsible for paying some portion of your health insurance while you are out. However (and unfortunately), if you are one of the employees in your company who falls in the top 10 percent of wage earners, your company is not required to hold your job for you since they can likely demonstrate that your absence will be detrimental to the company.

Short-Term Disability (STD)

This benefit program is run by the DOL and operated by your state. It provides financial support for your maternity leave from your employer, your union, or the state welfare system. You can get coverage under this policy for some part of your salary for 6 weeks. You must have contributed a certain amount to the system before you are able to collect benefits, however, so check with the DOL about requirements. For moms who are self-employed or perform contract work, private disability payments are also available from private insurers. Again, these have to be set up for a significant amount of time before you can be paid from them.

The Pregnancy Discrimination Act (PDA)

This law states that discrimination against women who are pregnant qualifies as sex discrimination, and it outlaws discrimination against employees because of "pregnancy, childbirth, or related medical conditions." So you can't be fired, demoted, or passed over for promotion because of your pregnancy. In companies with fifteen or more employees, pregnant women must be treated similarly to any employee who has a medical condition that impacts their ability to work. This means that your employer must make accommodations for you if you are unable to perform some duties because of your pregnancy. It's not extra money, but it is a solid protection for keeping your job. Unfortunately, this law doesn't apply to very small companies.

Protections During Hiring

Are you in the process of applying for a new job while you are pregnant? The PDA protects you, too. Companies cannot turn you down just because you are pregnant (even if you have a pregnancy complication).

2 **Know the laws.** A clear understanding of your rights will help you feel confident if the conversation should turn sour. See "Employment and Protections" on page 138 for an overview of the relevant regulations.

3 **Consider the future.** It may seem early to make the "work or stay home with the baby" decision, but it is a good idea to start thinking about it now because your boss will likely ask you when you make your announcement. Don't sign any official agreements yet, as you want to have the flexibility to change your mind. Do have something concrete to say if they ask, such as, "I plan to use our company's policy of 6 weeks off and will likely then use 12 weeks of FMLA to extend the leave to 18 weeks. After that, I plan to come back full time." Again, this can change. But your boss will likely go into planning mode and will appreciate that you've thought ahead about it, too. Equally important, this will put you in more of a position of power. Stating what you want firmly, in the beginning, will decrease the chances that your boss will impose their wants on you. If you are unsure what the future holds but want to start thinking about it, jump to "Work" on page 171.

4 **Create your plan of attack.** Experts advise telling your boss before anyone else at work. You want them to hear it first from you, not a co-worker. That said, if there is someone you trust at work who has gone through this before, you might gain a lot of insight by chatting with them first.

5 **Schedule a meeting.** It's best to avoid the "Oh hey, by the way" conversation in the elevator. Get a meeting locked on the calendar when you can talk, undisturbed and undistracted.

6 **Be brief, polite, and if you need to, be brave.** Remember, you haven't done anything wrong or anything worth apologizing for (so no stammering out, "I'm so sorry, but . . ."). Be your charming and polite self, but stand tall and proud.

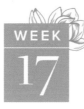

WEEK 17

Baby is the size of an onion, about 5.1 inches long. Their practice breathing begins

GETTING PARENTAL LEAVE AS AN LGBTQ+ PARENT

Many LGBTQ+ families do not receive fair treatment when it comes to paid and unpaid leave to support birthing partners and infants, especially if they work hourly wage jobs that do not qualify for FMLA. Unfortunately, our laws have not caught up with our social reality, forcing LGBTQ+ families to get very creative when it comes to taking time off to care for loved ones.

The good news is that there are private companies that are striving to do better, even if the law does not require them to do so. If your company does not, it may be worth looking into others that do.

You may also consider speaking with a family law attorney who can advise you of your options.

around now, so baby actively inhales and exhales the amniotic fluid through their lungs, which now have an extended network of branches.

Your baby is starting to fill out a bit, the precursor to those swoon-worthy chubby baby rolls. At this point, the baby already has a unique set of fingerprints.

gather

○ Information on your company's maternity leave program, if applicable

○ Information on your FMLA eligibility

to do

○ Reflect: Release the *not enoughs*, the *can'ts*, and the *doubts*.

○ Schedule your next prenatal appointment.

MATERNITY LEAVE AROUND THE WORLD

Following is a glimpse of maternity leave policies in some countries around the world:

- Australia: 18 weeks with 42 percent of salary
- Bulgaria: 58 weeks with 78 percent of salary
- Chile: 18 weeks with 100 percent of salary
- Ghana: 12 weeks with 100 percent of salary
- Greece: 43 weeks with 54 percent of salary
- Israel: 14 weeks with 100 percent of salary
- Mexico: 12 weeks with 100 percent of salary
- South Korea: 13 weeks with 79 percent of salary
- United Kingdom: 39 weeks with 30 percent of salary

○ Schedule an amniocentesis or a chromosomal screening if you and your provider have decided to do this.

○ Practice the belly pump.

○ Discuss parenting goals with your partner or village members.

○ Consider what you might like maternity leave to look like, if applicable.

○ Schedule a meeting with human resources, your employer, and/or your employees to share the news of your pregnancy and begin planning for leave.

remember

Our brains are very good at tricking us into believing all the negative thoughts about ourselves. Mama, they are simply not true. It takes practice, but eventually, you will be able to recognize and dismiss the untruths and embrace the pure and simple fact: You are amazing.

Month 5

Focus on becoming unapologetically you.

FROM DIANA

Oh hey, halfway point, I see you!

Can you believe that this month you are crossing the 20-week mark?

At the end of your fifth month of pregnancy, you will be closer to the end of your pregnancy than to the beginning. Which means: *It's time to start talking about birth!*

Here are a few items to start with. First, if you are thinking about taking a birth class, now is a great time to start looking, as they tend to fill up. You can ask your provider and local moms if they have one to recommend. Remember, Motherly offers an online birth class (taught by me!), and we'd love for you to join us—mother.ly/becomingmama.

When choosing a birth class, consider the following points:

- Who teaches it? What is their experience level, certification, philosophy, and approach? Do you feel welcomed by and comfortable with the instructor?

- Does it cater to the type of birth you want? (See chapter 25, "Birth Plans," if you're excited to read ahead.) For example, if you want to have a home birth, will they cover the info you need to know? And if you are planning to have an epidural, will they walk you through that process and provide specific coping skills for you?

- What are the costs, schedule, and location?

Second, if you have the budget and are thinking of hiring a doula, start making some calls. Doulas book clients several months out, so if you start looking for one now, there will be a better chance they are available. For more, see "Doulas" on page 92.

Last, focus on you. We are going to dive into birth in the coming chapters (hooray!). This is not just anyone's birth; *you* are the center of this universe.

Mama, this is your birth. Ask friends and families for their stories if you want. Consult with your doctor or midwife, of course. But don't forget to listen to your heart and instincts and embrace the possibility that your story will shift and change as it unfolds.

I want you to focus on becoming unapologetically you. Get grounded in that, and the rest will come naturally.

xo,

Diana

Last month, you spent time clearing away the ideas that do not serve you. Now, let's delve into what does.

Your task this month is to define your values. Your lines in the sand. Your truths.

What matters most to you?

Establishing your values will allow you to do two things:

- Maintain your connection to the woman you were before motherhood
- Guide you through parenting every day

Your values are your compass, your own North Star.

When your values are vague or undefined, it's easy to lose sight of them. You'll be pulled in directions that don't feel right and make choices that don't feel authentic.

But when your values are clear and strong, decisions will be pure and come naturally.

This doesn't mean you won't make mistakes; motherhood is full of them. What it means though, is that you'll never question your motives. When you parent from your values and your heart, you can trust that your intentions were right, even if the outcome is not.

Ask your partner and those who may help you raise your baby to do this exercise as well. It is okay if your values are different. It may even be helpful if they are. Be sure not to try to change your values in an attempt to match anyone else's. They'll lose their shine if you do.

So, mama, what are *your* values?

Figuring this out may be harder than you think.

Tiffany Han, writer, speaker, artist, and life coach, believes wholeheartedly in the importance of value identification and works with her clients to help them home in on theirs. To help get you started, Han has shared her comprehensive list of values with us.

Take a look at all the values on the following page (with a pen in hand). Cross off the ones that do not resonate. Then, make a list of all that remain and start ranking them. Can you narrow it down to twenty? How about ten? What would your top, number one, value be?

I did this exercise not long ago, and it has been an absolute game changer. (My number one value is trust. Who knew?)

After you have defined your values, think about how they apply to the following questions:

- What excites you about becoming a mother?
- What kind of mother would you like to be?
- What do you want to give to your child?
- How can you create space in your life to nurture a child?
- How will you focus in on your values on the really tough days?
- When your child is grown, what would you like them to say about how you raised them?

Write your answers down and keep them in a safe place. You can return to them whenever you need to in order to remind yourself of your values or to revise them as your family life unfolds.

bonding
WITH YOUR BABY

It is during this month that you will likely be offered the anatomy scan, an ultrasound usually done around 20 weeks, in which your baby's entire body is checked to make sure all is progressing well. It's also a time for you to sneak a peek at this darling being who is usually hidden from view. You may choose to find out whether you're having a girl or a boy at this time.

What's amazing about the opportunity of this diagnostic tool is that these are some of the most jaw-dropping images you will

LIST OF VALUES

Abundance	Delight	Intuition	Progress
Acclaim	Determination	Inventiveness	Prosperity
Accomplishment	Devotion	Joy	Quality
Achievement	Diligence	Kindness	Reliability
Action	Discipline	Knowledge	Reputation
Adventure	Ease	Leadership	Resourcefulness
Affection	Effectiveness	Logic	Respect
Agreeableness	Efficiency	Love	Responsibility
Alignment	Elegance	Loyalty	Romance
Ambition	Enthusiasm	Luxury	Safety
Analysis	Equality	Mastery	Security
Artistry	Excellence	Mindfulness	Self-expression
Authenticity	Expression	Mischief	Self-reliance
Balance	Fairness	Moderation	Sensuality
Beauty	Faith	Money	Service
Bravery	Family	Nature	Sincerity
Calm	Flexibility	Order	Social justice
Caution	Flow	Organization	Spirituality
Choice	Freedom	Originality	Spontaneity
Collaboration	Fun	Passion	Stability
Comfort	Function	Patience	Status
Commitment	Generosity	Peace	Strength of character
Communication	Grace	Perseverance	Structure
Compassion	Happiness	Physical strength	Style
Confidence	Harmony	Playfulness	Success
Connection	Hope	Pleasure	Temperance
Consistency	Humility	Popularity	Thoroughness
Control	Humor	Power	Trust
Conviction	Independence	Presence	Truth
Creativity	Ingenuity	Prestige	Wealth
Curiosity	Innovation	Problem-solving	Wisdom
Dedication	Integrity	Productivity	

ever see. To this day, I still remember the shape of my daughter's leg as I saw her kick the side of my belly on the ultrasound screen. Now, when she's running on the soccer field, I often reflect back on my first view of her powerful kicks!

You and your partner can clear some time right after the ultrasound to reflect on what you saw, what struck you, and what you learned about the shape of your special one. Use this moment to connect to baby's potential growth and to your mutual feelings about raising this child. Yes, their shape is already set; their bones and tissues and vessels are all complete. But they can still become *anything*. What does this mean to you?

Symptoms YOU MIGHT FEEL

- Back pain/ache
- Bleeding gums
- Bleeding nose
- Congestion
- Constipation
- Fetal movement
- Frequent urination
- Gas
- Groin pain
- Headaches
- Heartburn or reflux
- Hemorrhoids
- Spider veins
- Swelling
- Vaginal discharge

To learn more about the symptoms that are impacting you—and how to deal—turn to the "Symptom Checker" on page 429. Remember, your provider is your first stop for any symptoms that concern you, so don't hesitate to reach out to them.

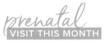

prenatal VISIT THIS MONTH

Most women can expect to have one visit during their fifth month of pregnancy, which may include:

READ AHEAD

Whether you've seen your baby on an ultrasound or started to feel the kicks, the idea that you are about to have a newborn may be starting to feel real. If you want to start prepping now, chapter 28, "Your Baby and Bonding," is packed with information on what the first 3 months of your baby's life will be like. (*So exciting!*)

The halfway milestone is a great time to start learning about birth. The first step is to understand the anatomy of your body, which allows all of this work to happen in the first place! If you haven't yet, read chapter 2, "The Extraordinary Anatomy of Pregnancy and Birth," and then you can learn about labor in chapter 17, "Going into Labor."

- Blood pressure check
- Weight check
- Urine sample
- Listening to the baby's heartbeat
- Follow-up on lab results from your last appointment

When you reach the 20th week of pregnancy, the top of your uterus is usually at the level of your belly button (when you are lying flat on your back). After this point, your midwife or doctor may no longer just feel with their hands. They will likely use a tape measure to assess your uterus and baby's growth at each visit. They'll hold one end at the top of your pubic bone and then measure how many centimeters to the top of your uterus. This is

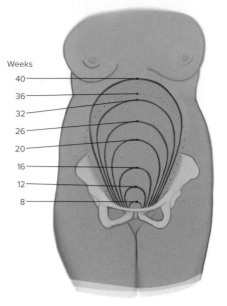

Weeks
40
36
32
26
20
16
12
8

CHECKING FUNDAL HEIGHT

called your fundal height (the fundus is the uppermost part of your uterus).

Mother Nature, being the crafty lady that she is, made this easy: Roughly speaking, each week of pregnancy equals another centimeter of uterus growth. At 22 weeks, the top of your uterus will be about 22 centimeters from the top of your pubic bone. This definitely varies, though, depending on your body structure, how many babies you are growing, and more. Your provider will let you know if there is reason to worry.

As mentioned, the big event of this month will likely be your anatomy scan. The ultrasound will also look at your placenta and its location, the umbilical cord, and your uterus, ovaries, and cervix.

For more details on this ultrasound, see "Anatomy Scan" on page 457.

Questions to Ask Your Provider

- Is there a birth class you recommend?
- Is there a doula you recommend?

- Do I have any special nutritional needs at this stage?

Also ask about any and all symptoms that you have been experiencing.

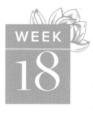

WEEK 18 Your baby is the size of a bell pepper, about 5.6 inches long. Your baby's genitals, which were indistinguishable as one sex or another in early embryonic development, are now likely visible on ultrasound.

As baby flexes their arms and legs, you may be able to feel the movement.

You may notice that your nipples and areolas are getting a little darker in color while also developing tiny glands for lubrication, called Montgomery's tubercles. These produce oil that baby is attracted to by scent.

Eat Small Meals and Boost Your Protein!

While you're busy between appointments and preparing for baby, remember that nourishing your body well still needs to be a priority. Small, frequent meals throughout the day can help prevent the risk of heartburn, which can become more of a concern as your baby gets bigger and bigger.

Pregnancy also puts an increased demand on the body for protein and iron, so be sure to include plenty of foods that are naturally higher in these areas: fish, chicken, dairy, and high-quality non-deli meats. And don't forget that legumes, fortified cereals, and dark, leafy green vegetables also have lots of protein.

While they are super-common, the food products with "high protein" labels that mostly contain processed soy sources may not be the best for pregnant women. Some studies have found that the soy protein isolates in manufactured bars, drinks, supplements, and cookies can impact your thyroid function. Real, whole foods are the best way to go. If you get a significant amount of your protein from soy, aim for organic and minimally processed versions when possible.

One other key reason to make sure you're getting enough protein is that it can prevent swelling. When you have high blood protein levels, salt and water are better maintained inside your blood vessels. When your blood protein levels drop, fluid can leak out of the vessels and cause swelling in your feet and legs. If you experience swelling, try upping the quantity of protein that you eat over a day or two and see if the symptom improves.

A note on salt: While we often hear of the importance of low-sodium diets, current

MEDITERRANEAN CHICKPEA SALAD

Ingredients for the Red Wine Vinaigrette
1/2 cup extra virgin olive oil
1/4 cup red wine vinegar
1/4 cup water
1 large lemon, juiced
1/2 tsp. garlic, minced
1/4 tsp. dried basil
1/4 tsp. dried oregano
1/2 tsp. sea salt
Ground pepper to taste

Ingredients for Salad
2 14-oz. cans chickpeas, drained and rinsed
3 medium avocados, cubed
1.5 lbs. tomatoes, chopped
1.5 lbs. cucumbers, chopped
1/2 medium red onion, finely chopped
1/2 cup fresh herbs (parsley, cilantro, and/or dill), finely chopped
Optional add-ins: Cooked chicken, crumbled pasteurized feta cheese, sunflower or pumpkin seeds

Directions

1 Add all vinaigrette ingredients to a small bowl and stir gently to combine.

2 Add the vinaigrette to the bottom of four glass jars. In a large bowl, combine the chickpeas, avocado, tomatoes, cucumbers, red onion, and chicken and cheese (if using). Divide evenly between the jars, top with fresh herbs and seeds (if using), and seal with an airtight lid.

3 Store in the refrigerator. When ready to enjoy, shake or stir well and serve!

MEAL PREPPING

As your appetite and energy improve, take some time each week to do some basic meal prepping, so you have healthier choices available throughout the week. This might include planning out meals; batch cooking vegetables, proteins, and grains; washing and slicing produce; and more.

research does not suggest that pregnant women should restrict their sodium intake in an effort to avoid hypertensive issues or swelling. In fact, sodium is a crucial nutrient during pregnancy. That said, if you have chronic medical concerns, your provider will help you find the right prenatal diet that addresses your needs.

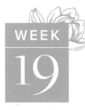

WEEK 19

Your baby is the size of a mango, about 6 inches long. Their senses are all starting to develop, and they can hear your voice! Find your favorite children's book for your partner to read your baby their first bedtime story, sing some lullabies, or tell your little one about your day.

Vernix is forming on your baby's skin. Vernix is a wax-like goo that coats your baby in utero. It helps keep them warm and protects their skin, especially from the increasing amount of urine in the amniotic fluid. The vernix sometimes dissolves as the pregnancy reaches the due date, though some babies are still covered in it at birth. While your baby will likely not cut their first milk teeth until they are half a year old, they now

have all twenty teeth buds. Even their adult teeth are starting to form, but these won't erupt for another 6 years at least.

move

Squats

As your pregnancy progresses, see if you can work in some daily squats! Squats are vital for increasing core and glute strength (aka your butt) and can help prepare your body for the birthing experience. Some women may even choose to give birth while squatting, so practicing now can only help.

Don't hesitate to hold on to a stable object to help maintain your balance.

Practice

Think about all the ways in which you may perform a squat naturally throughout your day. When you catch yourself squatting, perfect your form and think about it as a functional form of exercise.

Pick 2 to 3 days a week where you build on to your squats, challenging yourself to do ten one day, fifteen another, and so on.

Find your diaphragmatic breath (see page 119) with your squats. Inhale as you lower and exhale as you rise. You can even replace the diaphragmatic breathing with a belly pump (see page 132) while squatting, for some extra pelvic floor and core love.

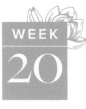

WEEK 20

Your baby is the size of a banana, about 10 inches long! Fine, soft hair called lanugo has started to form on your

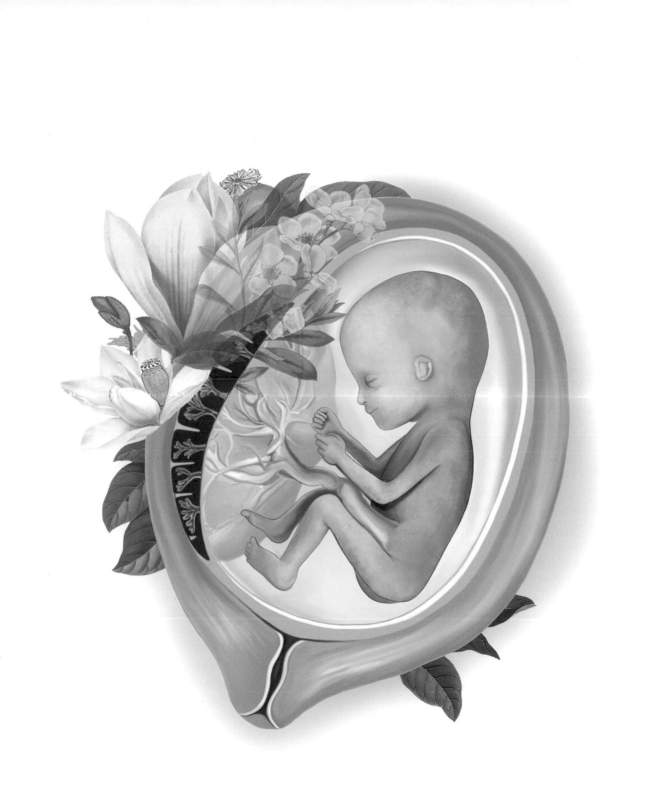

WEEKS 18–22

little one's wrinkly skin. This hair serves to keep them warm in the womb. They may shed it as they approach their due date, or they may be born with it.

Their nervous system is maturing rapidly, and they are responding to newly fused nerve pathways for touch sensations, temperature, and pain.

BMI AND PREGNANCY

Pregnancy can pose unique challenges for women with BMIs over 25, which is about half of all pregnant women. Evidence suggests that the risk of experiencing some complications increases when your BMI is greater than 25, such as gestational diabetes, high blood pressure, and blood clots. This is, of course, important for you to know so that you can be on the lookout for potentially worrisome signs. There is a fine line, though, between education and making someone feel bad. Unfortunately, a significant number of pregnant women report feeling stigmatized by their health-care team regarding their weight.

Mama, you are not alone. Listen to their medical counsel, of course, but also know that you are worthy of respect. If you feel like you are not getting it, please don't hesitate to advocate for yourself or bring along someone who can support you. Remember also that pregnancy is multidisciplinary. If your provider makes suggestions regarding your weight, take advantage of other team members who can help: nutritionists, social workers, prenatal-certified fitness experts, and therapists.

Baby is starting to produce meconium, its unique brand of poop. It's made up of old cells, mucus, bile, and amniotic fluid. You will see meconium in the first days of your baby's life: It looks like dark green or black tar.

love AND VILLAGE

People love a woman with a bump, almost as much as they love a mama with a new baby. Family members, friends, co-workers, and that random lady on the train all seem to be flocking to you right now. They want to touch your belly, tell you their birth stories, ask you millions of questions, and give you their advice. If you're LGBTQ+, you may be getting even more questions about how the baby was conceived, some of which may be very uncomfortable and intrusive.

How this makes you feel is up to you. Here's what some Motherly mamas said about it:

"I received lots of unsolicited advice, but for the most part, it was fine. I tried to keep an open mind and remember that they were genuinely trying to help. It was only stressful when people were persistent with advice that I disagreed with. I really don't like conflict, and having to openly disagree with people about something they wholeheartedly believed in was difficult." VALERIE

"Surprisingly, I didn't get much unsolicited advice at all. I did get a lot of 'just wait' comments that upset me. I still get those types of comments about whatever stage my baby is in. You think teething is bad? Just wait 'til she cuts molars. You think 1-year-olds are a handful? Just wait 'til the terrible 2s, and on and on." SHARRY

"I figured most people were just trying to make a connection, even if sometimes it wasn't appropriate or agreeable." CORAL

Storytelling is one of the greatest enduring acts of humans. Across cultures and throughout time, people have used stories to share knowledge and build connections, and motherhood has always been a central theme. Our ancestors gathered around fires and told each other tales of birth and babies. Ancient midwives taught their daughters and granddaughters all they knew through words and stories.

Today, we are less likely to gather around a fire than we are around a glowing smartphone, but the primal instinct is still the same. Stories equal compassion, concern, and safety.

When your loved ones (and strangers) share their stories and advice, they are using the most ancient form of communication to express their attention and care. It comes from a place of love.

That doesn't mean you have to love it.

Do not be afraid to trust yourself in the face of all the words coming at you these days. Absorb only as much as is helpful to you, and then either tune it out or ask people to stop.

You might say: "Thanks for wanting to share your birth story! I can't wait to hear it after

WHEN YOU ARE PREGNANT WITH A GIRL, YOU EMBODY THREE GENERATIONS!

Eating well is always important, and possibly even more so when you're pregnant with a girl. When you're pregnant with a girl, there's a direct connection between what you eat and her future health. Girl babies may be born with their lifetime supply of eggs*, while boys will continually make new sperm after they hit puberty. Nearing 20 weeks of pregnancy, the reproductive organs of the female baby are already formed, and that includes millions of immature eggs inside her wee ovaries. Think about what that means. Way back when your grandmother was pregnant with your mom, the egg that went on to make you was already inside your future mother! That's three generations wrapped up into one beautiful woman at the same time!

Researchers have now found that what you eat can have a direct effect on the mitochondrial DNA present in your baby girl's unfertilized eggs. Mitochondria are the powerhouses of cells, supplying energy for metabolism and other biochemical processes. They have their own sets of genes, inherited only from eggs, not sperm, which allow metabolic problems to be passed along through generations.

Eating foods high in fat and sugar can therefore predispose her to metabolic problems that cause obesity, heart disease, and type 2 diabetes.

So, mama, you aren't just eating for yourself and baby; you are also eating for your grandbaby. How powerful are you!

*Recent research has called the long-standing belief that women do not produce new eggs into question: It appears that we might! Still, the eggs that your daughter does have now will be with her for a while. Even if we do make new eggs, the importance of the ones we are born with endures.

Thinking about getting a tattoo and joining the inked mama club? (I don't think this exists, but if you find out that it does, please invite me.) You might consider waiting until after your baby is born, or even until after you are done breastfeeding. While most tattoo artists and shops use clean and safe equipment and techniques, there is a risk of being exposed to disease. There is also some concern about how the body processes fresh ink and whether it poses health concerns. It is likely best to avoid the risk, just in case. (If you already have a tattoo, there's no need to worry.)

Besides, waiting until after your baby is born may offer you a wealth of additional inspiration for a new design!

CAR SEATS: NEW OR USED?

The American Academy of Pediatrics recommends buying new car seats when possible because it is difficult to know the true history of a car seat. Once a car seat has been in a crash, it is usually no longer usable and must be discarded because it may not protect your child properly. Car seats also have expiration dates. And there is the possibility that a car seat has been altered in some way or has been subject to a recall. If you do get a used car seat, be sure to look into all of these factors. If you are unsure, it is best to leave it and find another one.

I've given birth, but I find that right now, stories are making me feel a bit stressed, so I am choosing to wait to hear them."

Or you could say: "You have so many good insights into [parenthood topic]. It's a little overwhelming for me to listen to them right now, but if questions come up later, I know exactly who I am going to come to for ideas!"

WEEK 21

Your baby is the size of a carrot, about 10.5 inches long. By this point, your baby's movements have turned from flutters to kicks and jabs.

Babies can start to taste around this point in pregnancy! The flavors from the foods you eat seep into the amniotic fluid, which your baby swallows and tastes. Experts theorize that by exposing your baby to lots of unique flavors in utero, you may be setting them up to appreciate varied tastes when they are out in the world.

work

There is nothing like expecting a baby to make you feel like a full-fledged adult. The idea of being responsible for a new tiny human can be daunting! But if you can take some time now to figure it out, you can spend all your post-birth time cuddling with your baby.

Health Insurance

Having a baby is considered a "life-changing event" by insurance companies—um, yeah, to say the least. What that really means, though, is that you may have the option to make changes to your insurance policy that you couldn't make otherwise.

If you've got private health insurance, your baby should be covered on your plan after they are born. You will need to call your insurance company after their birth to have them added to your plan, usually within 30 days of their birth (call your company to confirm).

Now is a good time to investigate what your insurance coverage is, as well as which pediatric care providers you will be able to go to. If the available options don't feel right, you may be able to switch plans.

You may also be eligible to apply for health insurance through the Affordable Care Act (go to healthcare.gov for more info on this).

Medicaid can provide low-cost or free health care for people and families that meet certain criteria for income, family size, and a few other factors. The programs vary by state, so your best bet is to go to your state's Medicaid web site for more details and an application.

Life Insurance

Life insurance is an insurance policy that will provide financial security to your children should something happen to you. There is a wide range of policy types and costs, but an insurance agent or specialist will be able to help you find the one that works best for you, if you're interested.

Wills and Trusts

A will or trust is a legal document that outlines what should happen to your property and dependents (like your baby) in the event that something happens to you. In addition to specifying where your money and belongings should go, you'll be able to state who will become the guardian(s) of your children.

This is an unpleasant thing to consider, of course, but once it's written, you don't have to think about it again (unless you decide to change it). And despite the discomfort of going through this exercise, you are giving your family an incredible gift in creating this plan. You can also write a "do-it-yourself will" without the help of a professional. However, be aware the laws vary by state, especially when it comes to guardianship, so it may be advantageous to seek legal guidance for this one.

Financial Planning

Bola Sokunbi, a money expert and certified financial education instructor, teaches that spending some time thinking about your post-baby finances now can greatly improve your quality of life moving forward by making your finances more stable and decreasing the stress that comes from money worries.

She finds that women often overlook this aspect of parenthood, telling themselves, "I'll figure it out later." But that can be a stressful thing to have to deal with after the baby arrives.

A few big questions that can help you get started:

- Do you plan to move to accommodate your growing family?

- Will you be employed outside of the home, and if so, who will care for your child while you are working?

- What supplies do you anticipate needing to buy? Can you get hand-me-downs, or will you need to buy most things new? (See "Gather" on page 173 for our comprehensive list.)

- Do you plan to breast- or formula feed (or both)? (See chapter 29, "Breastfeeding" and chapter 30, "Pumping and Bottle-Feeding.")

- What kind of diapers do you plan to use? (See "Diapers, Diapers, Diapers" on page 368.)

These decisions will likely have a financial impact worth considering.

When you have your answers, set up a spreadsheet or download an accounting software program and spend some time researching what your expenses will be in your baby's first year of life. Set aside some money each month to cover these expenses, starting now. Sokunbi says you can even set up different accounts for different goals, to really help distinguish them from each other.

Things to consider include:

- Moving and housing costs
- Childcare
- Formula and other feeding supplies
- Diapers and wipes
- Clothing
- Baby gear
- Health insurance premium and co-pays
- Unexpected costs that may come up

When it comes to baby gear, Sokunbi advises keeping your lists simple and realistic. She says it's common for new moms to want to give baby everything, so they splurge for brand-new, organic, top-of-the-line stuff. But that way of life is just not sustainable for so many of us. Instead, work within your existing income and choose the products that will work financially over the long term. Consider the fact that babies don't really wear out

clothing or furniture, so it makes more sense to get secondhand items whenever possible.

Put the pricey items on a gift registry if you can. For example, diapers and diaper services can become a costly regular expense. Wouldn't it be awesome to be gifted a supply that will last a while?

In addition to saving for the day-to-day essentials, Sokunbi states that it's important to start or continue to save for long-term goals, when possible (retirement, college, vacations, and so on). For many people, this type of saving will slow way down with a baby in the mix, but that doesn't mean you have to stop. Even if it's a small amount, it will add up and will help keep you focused on your goals. Once you've adjusted to #momlife, you can always rev up saving again.

It's also essential to always be looking ahead, past the next 12 months. Sokunbi recommends looking at your overall plan every 4 to 6 months and adjusting the budget as necessary. Before you know it, you'll be considering day care, preschool, school systems, after-school activities, summer camps, holiday presents, and back-to-school shopping—all things that potentially require money.

If you feel overwhelmed by this, know that it's normal and don't be afraid to reach out for help. There are financial experts who do exactly this for a living (like Sokunbi!), as well as websites and apps, many of which are free.

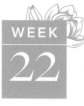

WEEK 22

Your baby is the size of a papaya, about 10.9 inches long. Like an insulated electric cord, your baby's neurons are developing a protective sheath made from a fatty layer called myelin. This allows neurons to carry signals without interfering with one another, allowing impulses (information) to move around the brain efficiently.

Now your sleepy baby has distinct periods of activity and rest and may even react to loud sounds like your dog barking or your fave workout music playing. (*Aw!*)

gather

- ○ Spreadsheet or financial planning program, or app for establishing and maintaining your budget
- ○ Breast pads (in case you start leaking breast milk soon; more on this on page 392)
- ○ Formula and other feeding supplies, diapers and wipes, clothing, and a car seat

Psst: If you are excited to get shopping or setting up your registry, check out our full recommended list on page 173.

to do

- ○ Reflect: What are your values?
- ○ Look for a birth class, if interested.
- ○ If opting for a doula, start looking for potential candidates.
- ○ Schedule your next prenatal appointment.
- ○ Eat small meals and boost your protein!
- ○ Practice squats.
- ○ Check on health insurance for your baby.
- ○ Consider life insurance and a will or trust.
- ○ Start planning your financial future.
- ○ If you haven't already, read chapter 2, "The Extraordinary Anatomy of Pregnancy and Birth." Then read chapter 17, "Going into Labor," and chapter 28, "Your Baby and Bonding."

remember

You defined those values for a reason, mama. Now is the time to hold on to them tightly.

Month 6

Mothcrhood
will make me
even stronger.

I am rarely at a loss for words, but at this moment, I am struggling. That is because I am trying to express what it means to become a mother—an experience so earth-shatteringly profound that words fall far short in doing it justice.

Becoming a mother means simultaneously accessing your highest self and your most primal self. You'll also touch on your deepest fears and feelings of overwhelm and face some of the most raw and challenging moments you will ever know.

It means discovering parts of yourself you never knew existed, having emotions you never knew were possible, and experiencing a love so profound that it makes you levitate.

Your body and brain physically change. Your DNA changes. Your schedule, relationships, priorities, and goals all change.

Motherhood changes *almost* everything.

Almost.

While life as you know it will be quite different, *you* are not going anywhere. The values you identified last month and the things that light you up will be your constant. You will continue to be the woman that you are.

Be proud of that woman.

Trust that woman.

You've made it through every challenge you ever faced by being you, getting stronger at every turn.

If "little-girl you" could see you right now, how proud and in awe would she be? (Answer: very.)

And that strength you have now? It just keeps growing, mama.

xo,

Diana

Tiffany Dufu is an author, public speaker, consultant, and activist and has dedicated her career to advancing women and girls. I spoke with her about the challenges that so many women face when they become mothers: How can I be a mom *and* have a career that I love?

Dufu believes that women are wonderful at taking their unique talents and gifts and turning them into careers. She finds that women having babies today are ahead of the curve. "This is the first generation to assume that livelihood and the ability to do good in the world can go hand in hand," she said.

In other words, you are amazing.

If pregnancy brings the desire to switch focus in some capacity, you are not alone. Many women decide to make changes to their careers as they transition into motherhood. This may mean switching jobs, leaving the paid workforce, decreasing hours, increasing hours, starting your own business, amping up your hobby to become a side gig: The list goes on and on.

Most women also find that this is a time of refocusing priorities in general, beyond career.

Dufu recommends that before any of this, though, you get very clear on what matters most to you.

When she asks women what matters most to them, they almost always say something like family, career, spirituality, and health. And then she asks them to go deeper, "But what do you hope to achieve in relation to those areas of your life?" Your answer will help you create a filter through which everything passes.

Dufu shared her own answers: Instead of saying her priorities are her career, her relationship, and her children, she said that she strives to advance women and girls, nurture a healthy partnership with her husband, and help her children to become conscious, global citizens.

"Unless you are clear about what matters most to you, you are not in the driver's seat. You are living someone else's story," Dufu says.

From the time we are born, we absorb thousands of subtle (and not so subtle) messages about how we *should* exist in the world, and motherhood is perhaps at the forefront of this. How many times have you heard the expression "good mom"? These two simple words carry a tremendous burden of expectation—expectations that we did not set for ourselves but that were instead set for us by the society we live in. Dufu gives the example of being present for your baby's first steps. In order to be a "good mom," we have this idea that we *must* be there to see them, "despite the fact that no one can remember who was there with them when they took their first steps," she stated. We have adopted the pressures that society puts on us without having a say in it.

So, ask yourself what truly matters to you and get clarity on why you are here.

When you have it, answer these questions:

- How can I best achieve this?
- What are the things that only I can do? What are the things that I do best?

Dufu gives another example of kids' birthday parties. She felt, as some moms do, a lot of pressure to be the one always RSVPing, buying the gifts, and standing around socializing over pizza—all the things she thought made her a "good mom." But then she realized that (a) she didn't like all that, but her husband did, and (b) kids' birthday parties did not advance her

MICROCHIMERISM

Recent biological science has shown us that not every cell in our body is our own. While we learn in science classes that we are unique individuals with our own distinct DNA, new findings reveal that we are all carrying DNA from other family members.

Most of us have at least a few cells from our mothers. Yet surprisingly, we can also carry cells from our maternal grandmothers and possibly older siblings! How is this possible? It's a recently discovered phenomenon called microchimerism.

Throughout pregnancy, maternal and fetal cells mingle, crossing the placenta and blood-brain barrier. Mothers' cells start living in their fetuses, and they continue to do so after the baby is born. Because they are stem cells, microchimeric cells are able to grow and thrive and can even stay in the mother's and the baby's body for decades, possibly even a lifetime.

So, for you, this means that you already have parts of your baby incorporated into your body, and vice versa. Six percent of the mother's DNA in the third trimester can actually be from her baby!

Reflect on what this could mean for you. Not only are you made up of past generations, but you are made up of your baby. You are not a single, solitary, isolated self. You bear the imprint and signature of others, and not just physiologically. The people who surround us help make up who we are mentally, emotionally, and every other way.

What do you value about being intimately connected—forever—to another being who needs you?

purpose of raising and nurturing conscious, global citizens.

So, she stopped going. She forwards the invitation to her husband, and sometimes the kids go, and sometimes they don't. Dufu feels empathy when her kids miss a party and are sad about it, but she has given herself full permission not to feel guilty. And this has changed her self-perception.

By getting clear on her priorities, Dufu gives herself permission to "drop the ball" (which is the title of her fabulous book) without guilt and to focus on the aspects of her that "separate her from the world" and truly matter.

And so, mama, I ask: What matters to you?

bonding WITH YOUR BABY

Recent studies have shown that unborn babies can interact socially beginning around 14 weeks of gestation. How do we know this? By looking at developing twins with ultrasonography, a high-resolution internal organ imaging technique. Even at this early stage, it appears that there is a need for human connection, because the twins studied were continually reaching out for contact with one another. They were observed stroking one another's head and back, and they did so with more force and intention than when they touched their own bodies. (*This is the cutest thing I have ever heard of.*)

For moms having twins or multiples, this is wonderful to imagine, and even to feel. For moms with solo babies, it just means that your touch is most certainly appreciated and felt by baby. So, don't feel self-conscious about reaching out to touch, rub, massage, and gently press on your belly.

Symptoms

- Baby hiccups
- Back pain/ache
- Constipation
- Frequent urination
- Groin pain
- Heartburn or reflux
- Hemorrhoids
- Itching
- Leg cramps
- Snoring
- Swelling
- Varicose veins

To learn more about the symptoms that are impacting you—and how to deal—turn to the "Symptom Checker" on page 429. Remember, your provider is your first stop for any symptoms that concern you, so don't hesitate to reach out to them.

prenatal
VISIT THIS MONTH

Most women can expect to have one visit during their sixth month of pregnancy, which may include:

- Blood pressure check
- Weight check
- Urine sample
- Listening to the baby's heartbeat
- Belly measuring and fundal height check
- Glucose challenge test
- Follow-up on lab results from your last appointment

Testing for Gestational Diabetes Mellitus (GDM)

The American Diabetes Association recommends that between weeks 24 and 28, women be screened for gestational diabetes mellitus (GDM), though women who are at higher risk are often also checked earlier. Gestational diabetes occurs when a woman has a higher-than-normal amount of glucose (sugar) in her blood during pregnancy. In gestational diabetes, hormones made by the placenta make it

TRAVELING WHILE PREGNANT

Wondering if it's safe to travel during this phase of pregnancy? Generally, yes, but it does depend on your specific scenario. Spoiler alert: Ask your provider. Here are a few things to consider:

- Ensure that your travel destination does not have any infectious threats, such as Zika virus (see "Zika" on page 469). The CDC has an awesome website that will give you information about travel health: cdc.gov/travel.

- When possible, ensure that your travel destination has a nearby hospital with a NICU in the event that you go into labor, and your baby needs extra medical care.

- If you are planning to take a flight, there is an increased risk of developing a deep vein thrombosis (see page 459). There are certain conditions that might make that risk greater as well. Most providers advise that when a pregnant woman of normal risk plans to fly, she should wear compression stockings, get up and walk often or do calf exercises (at least every 30 minutes), and drink plenty of water. Talk to your provider about their specific recommendations.

- Check in with your airline because they may have specific rules about travel limits and may also require a letter from your provider.

harder for the body to manage insulin, which is what moves glucose from the blood into the body to be made into energy. This means that there is more glucose in the bloodstream—and therefore more glucose going to your baby.

We worry about gestational diabetes because if left untreated, it can lead to some complications for both mom and baby. It is relatively common. From 2 to 10 percent of pregnant women will develop it. So, routine screening is recommended.

GDM may run in families, so it might be interesting to ask your family members if they had it. Of note, women who have immigrated to the US seem to be at a higher risk for developing GDM.

Here is what happens during the glucose challenge test (GCT): You'll drink a bottle of sugar-loaded liquid (it tastes like unfizzy soda, usually orange) that contains 50 grams

of glucose, wait 1 hour, and then have your blood drawn. You don't need to do anything special to prep for this test, though anecdotally, some people advise not eating a ton of carbs or sugar the night before or morning of.

If the result of your blood glucose (sugar) level is normal, you're in the clear! If the number is elevated, your provider will likely recommend a definitive test, which is unfortunately even less fun than the screening. For this test, called a glucose tolerance test (or GTT), you will need to fast the night before (ugh). When you arrive at the clinic, you will have your blood drawn, after which you will drink the sugary stuff again (this time with 100 grams of glucose). You will then have your blood drawn again, once per hour, over the course of 3 hours. The result of this test will show definitively if you have gestational diabetes or not.

These are the current testing guidelines from the American College of Obstetricians and Gynecologists, but some practices do it a bit differently, so make sure to ask what your specific plan will be.

For some women, the oral glucose test is more than an annoyance: It may make you feel nauseous, or you may not feel comfortable ingesting the orange drink. If this is you, let your provider know because there may be a workaround. For example, it is possible that having 28 jelly beans or 10 Twizzlers instead of the sugary drink may yield similar results—and would likely be easier to stomach. This is not yet a well-proven alternative, but it is worth a conversation for sure.

Understand that tests are not perfect, and there are cases of women being incorrectly diagnosed. If you are concerned about the test, definitely speak with your provider. See "Gestational Diabetes Mellitus (GDM)" on page 460 to read about possible treatment.

READ AHEAD

Labor is divided into four stages, and this is a great time to get to know what they entail! Spend some time this month reading chapters 18–21, about the wonder that is labor.

EXPECTING A BABY IN FINLAND

The Finnish government sends expectant mothers a box of baby items while they are pregnant. And, the box contains a mattress, and can be used as the babies' first bed!

Questions to Ask Your Provider

- What type of testing for gestational diabetes do you recommend in your practice?
- What do you think about cord blood banking?
- I am thinking of traveling to _____. Is it safe?

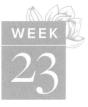

WEEK 23

Your baby is the size of a grapefruit when all curled up and measures about 11.4 inches long when they're stretched out.

Their (adorable) face is well formed at this point, with eyebrows and the cutest little eyelashes. Baby's skin is starting to develop tough

CORD BLOOD BANKING

When your baby is born, you have the option to bank their cord blood. Cord blood contains stem cells, which have the potential to cure diseases such as cancers (leukemias and lymphomas) and anemias, and the list will likely grow as research continues. It can also be used for research (when donated).

If you choose to bank the blood, it is removed from the umbilical cord with a needle at the time of birth (it doesn't cause any pain) and then saved in a cord blood bank. You have the option to bank your cells in a private bank (where the cells are reserved for you, or possibly a family member) or donate them to a public bank, where they may be used by someone else (much like when you donate regular blood).

There are a few important factors to note about private cord blood banks:

- Private banks are less regulated than public banks.

- The American Society for Blood and Marrow Transplantation reports that stem cells from private banks are rarely used—only about one deposit in several thousand.

- Private cord blood banking can be expensive, ranging in cost from $1,350 to $2,300 or more at the time of collection, plus a yearly banking fee. Public banking is a donation and therefore free.

For these reasons, the American Academy of Pediatrics released the following statement:

Public cord blood banking is the preferred method of collecting, processing, and using cord blood cells for use in transplantation in infants and children.... There is a more limited role of private cord blood banking with families with a known fatal illness that can be rescued by a healthy cord blood transplant within the family.

If you are considering cord blood banking, your provider can help you make the best decision based on your personal and family history. Be sure to talk with them before your birth, as you may need time to order a banking kit.

Visit bethematch.org to find a public bank near you to begin the process.

PETS

Do you already have a baby of the furry nature (or scaled or feathered) at home? You may be wondering how that impacts your pregnancy and life with a newborn. During your pregnancy, you'll need to take a few extra precautions:

- Be careful of bigger animals jumping on your belly, and avoid activities where you could get knocked over by an animal (walking a not-so-good-on-a-leash dog, visiting dog parks, riding horses, and so on).

- Take your pets to the vet to ensure they are healthy.

- Do not change cat litter boxes or clean the cages of your rodent, reptile, or amphibian friends, as you could touch or breathe in some dangerous bacteria.

- Keep animals away from your face.

- If you have a cat, keeping them indoors can decrease the risk that they get illnesses that can make you and the baby sick.

- Avoid bites, and if you are bit, report it to your provider right away.

- Wash your hands after contact with all animals.

Unfortunately, many experts recommend that pregnant women avoid rodent pets, and that reptile and amphibian pets (snakes, turtles, and so on) not be present in homes with babies and children younger than 5, due to the risk of salmonella. It can be devastating to have to say goodbye to a pet, I know, but the risks may just be too great. See if you have a friend or family member who can adopt them, turn to your local animal rescue center for relocation support, or ask your veterinarian for tips.

Healthy birds are generally considered safe to have during pregnancy and infancy, but check with your vet and health-care provider to make sure.

Good news: Research finds that when babies spend time with dogs and farm animals during their first year of life, they are less likely to develop asthma later on! Babies who live with cats end up with fewer respiratory infections, as do babies who live with dogs, who also get fewer ear infections.

Many suspect that our smart animal friends understand when we are pregnant. When the baby is born, bring your pet the baby's hat or blanket, so they can get used to the smell. Introduce them slowly, and chances are they will become fast friends.

If you are worried that your particular animal may be aggressive with your baby, start talking to your vet now about possible training and behavioral interventions.

keratin, which will turn into sturdy palms and soles as well as fingernails and toenails.

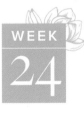

Stabilize Blood Sugar

The "rules" of what you should do to have a healthy pregnancy can feel overwhelming at times, but understand that there is not a one-size-fits-all approach for you or your baby's health and wellness. Try to look at your pregnancy and road to becoming a mother from a more holistic lens: You are not just what you eat or how much weight you gain or the birth plan you have in mind. You are the sum of many beautiful parts that are uniquely woven together to make the mother that your baby needs.

With your gestational diabetes testing this month (and perhaps a diagnosis of gestational diabetes), there is a big emphasis placed on sugar. So, let's focus on building meals and snacks that include a combination of complex carbohydrates that are high in fiber, along with protein and healthy fats. This combination of macronutrients can help keep your blood sugar stable throughout the day and prevent energy crashes. Eating small, frequent meals throughout the day can also be an effective strategy for helping your body balance your blood sugar levels.

Here are some examples of easy meals and snacks that are optimized with a healthy balance of fats, protein, and complex carbs for keeping your energy levels up and blood sugar stable:

- Fresh berries with cottage cheese
- Apple slices with peanut or almond butter
- Whole-grain crackers with sliced cheese and veggies
- Hummus with carrot, celery, and bell pepper slices
- Quesadilla with one small corn tortilla and cheese with avocado and full-fat sour cream
- Nut butter on sprouted whole-grain bread
- Milk with a handful of mixed nuts, like almonds and walnuts
- Low-sugar, full-fat Greek yogurt with mixed berries and nuts
- Apple with string cheese
- Whole-grain tortilla chips with beans and cheese
- Smoothie with 1/2 cup plain Greek yogurt, 1/4 cup berries, and 1 cup unsweetened almond milk

If you are diagnosed with gestational diabetes, your provider can help you figure out the best diet for you.

WEEK 24

From head to foot, your baby is the size of an ear of corn, about 11.8 inches long. The twenty-fourth week is a huge milestone for your baby in that they are now considered "viable." If they were to be born, there is a significant chance that they would survive (with substantial medical support). This can be a big relief! Of course, we hope your baby continues to bake for another 16 weeks, but it is encouraging to know that every week that passes means better odds and outcome for them.

Their memory functions are getting started, and brain electrical activity now looks similar to that of newborns. Let's hope they are

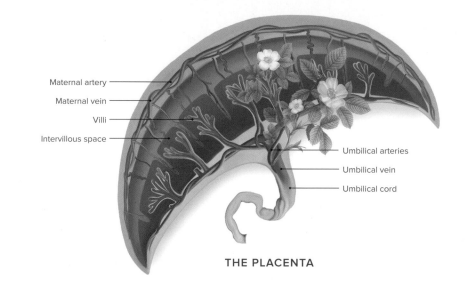

Maternal artery

Maternal vein

Villi

Intervillous space

Umbilical arteries

Umbilical vein

Umbilical cord

THE PLACENTA

YOUR AMAZING PLACENTA

You probably have some inkling that your placenta is amazing, but it really, truly is.

No other organ grows in the human body for such a short period of time, and with such a generalized purpose. Scientists still have a lot of studying to do to understand how the placenta is able to implant in the uterine wall and regulate so many body functions.

While nourishing the fetus with vital nutrients, proteins, fats, and carbohydrates, the placenta also performs the function of the future lungs, exchanging oxygen for carbon dioxide. It siphons off baby's cellular waste, regulates baby's temperature, and helps fight infections and strengthen immunity. It grows and expands along with the baby until the thirty-fourth week, when it reaches maturity at about 2 pounds. During the last part of the pregnancy, the placenta begins aging, until it begins to manufacture the hormones that trigger the birth process.

If you are pregnant with multiple babies, they may each have their own placenta, or they may share one, depending on if your babies developed from separate eggs or from one egg that split.

Unfortunately, the placenta has often been treated as an afterthought (it's called "afterbirth," after all). Yet it is a wondrous part of our bodies that deserves more attention! If you have a vaginal birth, your labor will not stop once the baby is born. Contractions will continue, the placenta will detach from the uterine wall, and you'll give a few little pushes to deliver it (more on this in chapter 20).

If you are up for it, request to see the placenta once it's out: It is very cool to see. The side that attaches to the uterus will be bumpy and a bit bloody, and the side that faces baby is magical. The umbilical cord forms the trunk of a tree of blood vessels that radiate out to the perimeter like so many rivers and streams. Some have proposed that the structure is the original "tree of life" that is prominent in so many cultural traditions.

For more info about what can be done with your placenta after birth, see "What do you want to do with your placenta" on page 326.

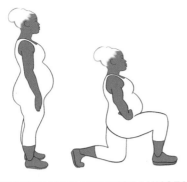

ALTERNATING REVERSE LUNGES

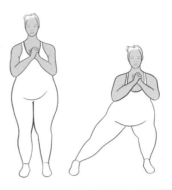

ALTERNATING SIDE LUNGES

getting started with a lifelong meditation habit in there!

Lunges

This is a great time to start practicing lunges (with your provider's blessing, of course). Not only does lunging help with muscle strength, it can help during birth, too! If your labor slows down, or if your baby's position is not ideal, your provider may encourage you to do some lunges to move your pelvis in ways that may help.

Practice

There are two types of lunges to focus on: alternating reverse lunges and alternating side lunges.

To do alternating reverse lunges, stand with your feet hip-width apart and your hands on your hips. Step one leg back directly behind you and lower yourself into a lunge. Ensure that your front leg does not go past a 90-degree angle. Hold this pose for a moment and then return to neutral. Repeat on the other side.

Try 10 reps of this and then rest. See if you can gradually build to three sets of 10 reps, three times per week.

To do alternating side lunges, stand with your feet hip-width apart. Step one leg out to the side, and lunge, ensuring that your knee does not extend farther to the side than your foot. Keep your gaze forward and maintain an upright posture. Return to center and repeat on the other side.

Try 10 reps of this and then rest. See if you can gradually build to three sets of 10 reps, three times per week.

WEEK 25

Your baby is the size of a rutabaga when curled up and about 13.6 inches long when stretched out.

Your baby is currently very lean. However, they will now start storing fat. In particular, brown fat, which provides fuel for after the birth and keeps them warm, is accumulating on their shoulders and back.

Baby's red blood cells were previously only created in the liver but are now produced in their bone marrow, meaning that baby is getting just a bit more independent from you. That growing supply of red blood cells means that they will soon be able to carry their own nutrients to every cell instead of relying on the placental supply.

You may notice that your center of gravity has shifted, so be aware of your posture and any developing back pain. Yes, it's time to hold any and all stair railings!

love AND VILLAGE

In chapter 7, we chatted about assembling your pregnancy village (see "Assembling Your Pregnancy Village" on page 109). Now it's time to think about your motherhood village.

Humans crave connection and community, and it is never more vital than in motherhood.

Studies find that when women have positive social connections during those early months of motherhood, they can experience less stress and even less depression. Despite the addition of an adorable connected-at-the-hip-buddy-for-life (aka your baby), many new moms report feeling unexpectedly isolated as they transition to parenthood. It is possible that you'll take a maternity leave or experience a career adjustment. You will likely find that your social life changes: The 2:00 a.m. last call at the bar gets traded in for the 2:00 a.m. call for a fresh diaper.

There is also an element of self-doubt that can creep in and shake your confidence.

BABY SHOWERS

Parties to celebrate the arrival of a baby, as well as a woman's transition to becoming a mother, have been around for a long time. Some believe the tradition dates back to ancient Egypt, when mothers and their new babies were welcomed back into the public eye after a period of seclusion.

The classic shower, surrounding the expectant mom and showering her with gifts (and cupcakes) will never get old. But if this isn't your style, there are lots of other ideas to think about.

Some parents prefer the idea of a couples' shower, where the pregnant mama and her partner are the stars of the show. And that show can happen anywhere: your house, a bar, a restaurant. Anything goes. Social media has no shortage of inspiration if you are interested in having a gender reveal party, in which

the boy or girl announcement is made to party guests.

I also love mother blessing ceremonies, which are inspired by the Navajo Blessing Way. In this heartfelt and moving ceremony, people gather with the pregnant woman to offer her blessings, good thoughts, and love centered around her impending birth.

There is also the concept of a post-birth celebration. You may be planning a bris (religious celebration when circumcision is done), a naming ceremony, or a "sip and see," where friends come over for refreshments and casually meet and celebrate the baby. In addition to the possible cultural and religious reasons behind this, the concept of people coming together to support you while you are healing from birth sounds pretty awesome to us—especially if they come with food and the desire to fold some laundry.

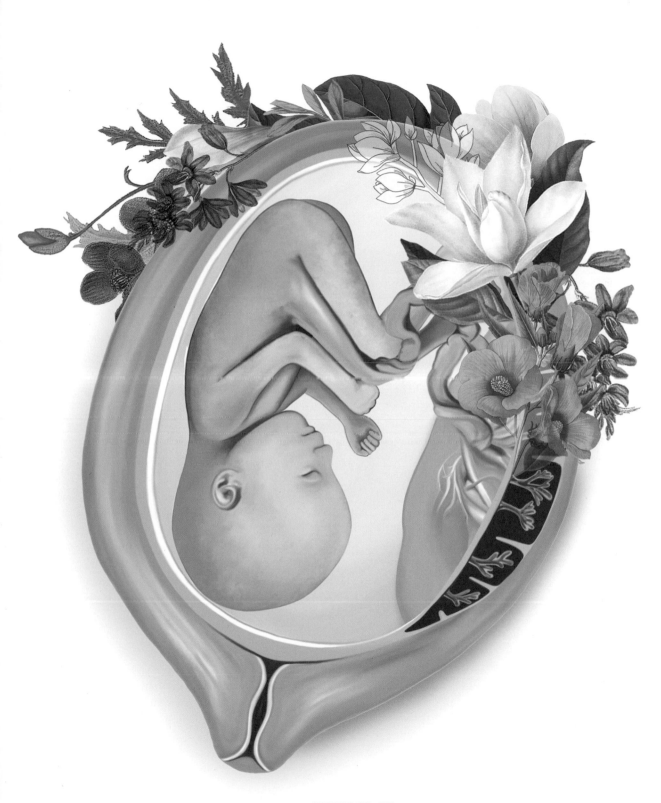

WEEKS 23–27

A supportive village can change everything. There is remarkable power generated when a few trusted allies surround you in a force field of love and positivity—and create a space for real, honest talk—as you make this huge transition. You can find new moms' groups online, through Facebook, Meetup, and other social sites, and you can also ask your provider to connect you. And Motherly cannot wait to lavish you in support and nurturing. Don't forget to visit us at mother.ly /becomingmama.

Spend some time this month reflecting on that force field:

- What do you anticipate your needs will be?

- What are the things you need to feel a sense of wellness now? These could be sleep, camaraderie, time outdoors, having a clean house, laughing, reading, or time alone. The things that matter to you now will continue to matter post-baby.

- Who in your current village can support you in making self-care a priority?

- Do you think you'll want company while you are on maternity leave? Who do think you'll want to hang out with the most?

- If this is not your first baby, who would be happy to entertain your toddler for a few hours, so you can take a breather?

- Who makes the best lasagna?

- And who can call you up out of the blue and say, "Hey, you are awesome."

Think now about what you may want and then assemble your dream squad.

Motherly mamas shared that their most significant advice for brand-new moms was to reach out, ask for help, and find your squad:

"Make it a priority to connect with others. Join the hospital moms' group. Join the playdate Facebook group. This really helped drive the message home for me that I am not alone and that there are others out there having the same baby joys and struggles as me. It's so good to connect with others to share both the laughter and the tears."   RACHEL

"Don't hesitate to ask, anything and everything! Find a few moms you trust, or whose parenting style you admire, and reach out. And don't say no to the friend who will bring you coffee and not laugh at you in your hospital-grade mesh panties! Don't say no to the friend who offers to hold sweet baby, so you can shower, nap, check things off your list. Enjoy the help!"   DIANE

"Ask for help and never be ashamed or guilty for it. I remember crying on the first nights at home because I didn't know how I would stay awake to breastfeed. I was so tired. I asked my husband to just sit with me and help me stay awake."   SARAH

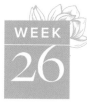

WEEK 26 Your baby is the size of a head of lettuce when curled up, about 14 inches long when stretched, and can finally open their tiny little eyes.

They can make a fist, grasp the umbilical cord (like a little toy!), and explore their body and environment with their increasingly coordinated hands.

Baby's brain is still pretty smooth-textured on the outside but is starting to develop cerebral folds and wrinkles. Keep eating that fat and protein to help baby get even more brainy!

work

After spending time last month looking at your finances and insurance, you might better be able to answer the question of what you will do after the baby arrives.

No matter what the answer is, you will be "working," that's for sure! It's just a matter of where. Researchers have found that stay-at-home mothers spend an average of 98 hours working per week and that their workload would garner a salary of $143,000 per year outside the home. Um, hello.

In Motherly's 2018 State of Motherhood Survey of 5,700 mothers in the US, we learned the following about work and motherhood:

- About 70 percent of those surveyed are employed (53 percent full time, 17 percent part time).

- Most employed mothers choose to work outside the home for financial reasons, though many also do so because they enjoy their work.

- About 50 percent of women made changes to their work upon becoming mothers

(working more or fewer hours, leaving or changing their jobs, and so on).

- Most women with partners said that their partner's work hours have either stayed the same or scaled up since becoming a parent.

- Most mothers who are not currently employed outside the home plan to return to employment at some point in the future.

Women are more educated today than in previous generations, and for the first time in history, more so than men. Women have more options than ever before as well. And there are growing opportunities for people to partake in flexible employment options, freelance jobs, and remote work positions. Increasingly, women are running their own businesses, allowing them full control over their schedules and working lives.

It's also important to note that life is more expensive, even when inflation is factored in. Consider, for instance, the power of $10 over the past 30 years. According to the Bureau of Labor Statistics Consumer Price Index, prices in 2018 are 113.02 percent higher than in 1988. That means that $10 in 1988 had the purchasing power of $21.30 in 2018. In very literal terms, you could buy two packs of high-quality diapers in 1988 for what it costs to buy one today. That has a huge effect on a household budget! When you factor in that just from 2000 to 2015, the price of food went up 45.7 percent and housing went up 59 percent, it means that for most families, it's more challenging to live on just one income.

Since the mid-1960s, the incidence of women working outside the home has continued to increase. In heterosexual relationships between 2010 and 2014 there was a 37 percent increase in relationships where the father stayed home and the mother was the breadwinner.

So, the typical question "Are you going to keep working or stay home?" is not so simple anymore. Plus, about a quarter of all moms are now single parents, most of whom will be rocking a job and new mamahood.

In a study on how American culture views "staying at home" versus "working" for mothers, academics Elizabeth Paré and Heather Dillaway wrote, "Motherhood and paid work are intimately intertwined and most women maintain both social roles simultaneously, negotiating the boundaries of each every day. Most women cannot even decide to be a 'stay-at-home' mother or a 'working' mother. The public (outside the home) and private (within the home) do not separate easily in the life of a mother or paid worker."

Motherly mamas agree: About 78 percent said they have mixed feelings about the trade-offs that come with combining motherhood and work.

So, what does all this mean for you?

Money expert Bola Sokunbi advises women not to make hasty decisions about possible career shifts, especially right after having a baby. New motherhood can involve a complicated adjustment, and it may be beneficial to just *be* for a while before making any big changes.

When you do start the process of making the decision, now or after the baby comes, Sokunbi says to consider the following:

- Create a budget to figure out how much money you need to have in the household (refer to page 153 for budget help). This will allow you to see if making a change to your employment status is possible and what your financial needs will allow for.

- Don't forget about commute time! When you don't have a child at home, a commute is an annoyance, but easier to deal with. When you do have a baby, long commutes often mean increased needs for childcare and of course the potential for emotional impact (for everyone in the family) of being away longer.

- Before quitting, think about asking for an additional month of maternity leave. Perhaps that extra time will make the idea of going back to work more appealing or easier to process.

- If you do quit your job, plan first, whether this means securing an alternative job or saving up as necessary.

- Keep in mind the unfair reality that many women face: Stepping out of the labor force for an extended time isn't only about sacrificing a paycheck. You might also pass up benefits, health care, promotions, mentoring, retirement savings, and more, so it's important to take the full picture into account.

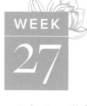

WEEK 27

Your baby is the size of a head of cauliflower when curled up, about 14.4 inches long stretched out.

Baby is still flipping up and down and sideways and doesn't seem to be settling down any one way.

There's seriously nothing like feeling your baby move inside of you. And while they're exploring your womb, your baby is developing tactile sensation and muscle tone (*so cool!*), but whoa, baby, could you "explore" a little bit more gently?

gather

It's time to start thinking about what items you'd like to have for baby. Perhaps you are getting ready for a baby shower or a Blessing Way ceremony in which you will receive gifts (or visiting your sister who is ready to give you #allthehandmedowns), and it's great to offer your friends and family a list of items that you know you want.

Motherly has assembled this list of starter items that you're sure to use. To see our favorite items, visit Motherly's Essential Baby Registry at mother.ly/st/registry.

- ◯ Diapers
- ◯ Wipes
- ◯ Diaper rash ointment
- ◯ Place for diaper changes (table, pad or towel on the floor, or other location)
- ◯ Crib or bassinet for sleep, and mattress (Confirm that crib meets current safety guidelines. For example, older cribs had sides that could drop down. These are very dangerous and not recommended!)
- ◯ Sheets and mattress protector
- ◯ Baby monitor(s)
- ◯ Gentle baby-safe laundry detergent
- ◯ Baby soap and shampoo
- ◯ Baby lotion
- ◯ Towels (baby towels are cute, but grown-up towels work just fine)
- ◯ Hairbrush
- ◯ Nail clipper or file

ONESIE MAGIC

It took me no less than *three* children to learn the following tidbit about onesies, so I really want you to know now! Most onesies are designed with little slits on either shoulder. The reason for the slits is so that you can take the onesie off by pulling it down their body instead of up and over their head. You will understand the beauty of this the first time your baby has a poop explosion (aka blowout) up the entire back of their onesie!

- ◯ Fan for baby's room
- ◯ Stroller
- ◯ Car seat (see "Car Seats: New or Used?" on page 152 for comments on used car seats)
- ◯ Place for baby to play while contained (like a Pack n' Play)
- ◯ Breast pump and milk storage bags (if applicable)
- ◯ Bottles and formula (if applicable)
- ◯ Nursing pillow
- ◯ Newborn thermometer
- ◯ First aid kit
- ◯ Suction bulb (the one that hospitals give you is the best, IMO)
- ◯ Diaper bag
- ◯ High chair
- ◯ Bibs
- ◯ Onesies
- ◯ Safe sleep swaddles
- ◯ Bouncer
- ◯ Playmat
- ◯ Toys
- ◯ Teethers
- ◯ Pacifier

○ Baby carrier

○ Safety gates and babyproofing items (see "Babyproofing" on page 378 for ideas)

to do

○ Reflect: What matters to you?

○ Schedule your next prenatal appointment.

○ Think about how to stabilize your blood sugar with smart snacks.

○ Practice the alternating reverse lunge and the alternating side lunge.

○ Call your insurance company to see if they cover breast pumps and begin the process of getting yours.

○ Read about the stages of labor in chapters 18, 19, 20, and 21.

remember

"Unless you are clear about what matters most to you, you are not in the driver's seat. You are living someone else's story."

TIFFANY DUFU

Month 7

WEEKS 28–31

I am growing the
next generation.

Maybe it seems like you just took your pregnancy test yesterday, or perhaps you wish you could just fast-forward through to the final birth scene. Either way, you know that you're getting closer to the big day. This is it. The third and last trimester: *Can you believe it?*

Your body has gone through some phenomenal shifts to support the growth of your baby (who is the size of an eggplant!) and to prepare for labor and birth, which is not far away.

You have been reflecting on the other aspects of your life that will change. From your relationships and village to your resources and time, you have been hard at work prepping your life for this new person.

You have been busy. Please do not underestimate everything you've done and be sure to take some time to celebrate how amazing you are. Afternoon nap well deserved!

At the start of your second trimester, we talked about how pregnancy starts to feel real. Now that you are at the start of your third trimester, the idea of giving birth starts to feel real. And that is incredibly exciting and intense at the same time.

You have worked on solidifying your values and clarifying how you want to maintain your identity as a woman as you become a mama. Now it's time to use that insight to guide you as you wrap your mind around birth.

Next month, we are going to focus on the fears that may come up (and how to manage them), but of course, feel free to jump to page 191 if you need to hear about it now.

For the next few weeks, we will concentrate on developing your birth preferences (your birth plan) and learning about all the coping skills that are available to you.

Also remember, because I haven't said it for a bit: *You've got this.*

xo,

Diana

P.S. A lot of women really enjoy their second trimester but find that as they round into the third trimester, they start to experience more discomfort. Don't forget that you can take a look at the "Symptom Checker" on page 429 to learn about anything you might be experiencing and to pick up some tips for feeling a bit better.

Your baby is wrapped up in you (and you are already wrapped around their little fingers). You are each other's worlds. That won't change after your baby is living outside of you. You will continue to be home to your baby, even as they grow and become more independent.

In those first weeks and months, they will want nothing else but to be curled up on your chest, as they try to make sense of the world they have just joined.

As they learn to crawl, walk, and run, the thrill of their newfound freedom will be cradled by their deeply seated knowledge that mama is right there with them, to cheer them on when they feel unsure and to catch them when they fall.

The years will pass by, and slowly but surely—on a foundation of your love and strength—they will spread their wings as they embark on their inevitable, bittersweet, and beautiful objective of flying away.

But you will always be home base. Always.

Very soon, your baby will be joining the outside world as its newest and tiniest citizen.

They are in our bellies and our arms but briefly, but their mark on our communities and societies will be profound.

Reflect for a moment on the magnitude of what you are doing. You are growing a new being who will become an adult with a unique and significant influence on the universe.

What do you imagine their interests will be? Will they be like yours, or totally different?

What will light their heart ablaze?

What will make them smile and laugh?

What injustices will they claim as theirs to dismantle?

Who will they love?

How will you foster their growth into the person they will become?

Parenting is a collection of tiny moments, many of which feel insignificant when we are in them. The decisions to let them eat cereal for dinner once in a while (or regularly!), or to let them stay home from school even though we know their belly doesn't really hurt, or the thousands of other parenting "imperfections" we see in ourselves will not impact their ability to change the world when they are grown.

Because all of your actions and decisions will come from a place of love, your child will always feel that from you, even when they are grown and away.

Through the collection of tiny moments that is motherhood, you are about to change the world.

How amazing are you?

bonding
WITH YOUR BABY

What do you envision doing with your baby when they are born? Will you go on a daily walk? Perhaps cuddling up with each other and a pile of books will be your thing. Or maybe mommy-and-me yoga?

Psst: Your baby will love to do pretty much anything with you, so pick the activity that brings you the most joy.

Think about how you'll spend intentional time connecting with your baby, and start now. Take a daily bonding walk while your baby is still inside you. Make note of a beautiful tree you pass and how it changes with the seasons as your pregnancy progresses. Imagine that one day you'll be saying to your child, "We walked by this tree every day from the time you were just the size of an eggplant!"

Or maybe it will be, "No matter how busy our lives get, I always make time for a mini yoga session with my little one on Saturday mornings."

Whatever activity you choose, your baby will feel the relaxing, soothing effects of it even while still in utero, and the bonding effects will last you both a lifetime.

- Baby hiccups
- Backache
- Braxton-Hicks contractions
- Constipation
- Fatigue
- Hemorrhoids
- Hot flashes
- Itching
- Leg cramps
- Shortness of breath
- Sleep challenges

KICK COUNTS

During this third trimester, it's a good idea to do a kick count every day. There are a number of techniques to do this, and you can also ask your provider. One way is to pick the same time every day and lie on your left side with your hands on your belly. See how long it takes for your baby to move ten times. The period of time should be roughly the same every day. If suddenly it takes much longer, it may be a sign of potential problems and an indication to call your provider.

Of note, on rare occasions babies let us know that something is wrong by moving too much. If your baby suddenly starts to move significantly more than they normally do, call your provider right away. Hyperactivity can indicate compression of the umbilical cord, and you want to have immediate attention if that is the case.

- Frequent urination
- Getting full quickly
- Groin pain
- Heartburn or reflux
- Heart rate increase
- Snoring
- Stretch marks
- Swelling
- Vaginal discharge
- Varicose veins

To learn more about the symptoms that are impacting you—and how to deal—turn to the "Symptom Checker" on page 429. Remember, your provider is your first stop for any symptoms that concern you, so don't hesitate to reach out to them.

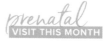

prenatal
VISIT THIS MONTH

It is likely that you will start having prenatal checkups every 2 weeks now instead of every 4 weeks. This is to ensure that your baby is continuing to grow at a healthy pace, to make sure all of your questions are answered, and to keep a closer eye on the usual data points, such as your blood pressure and urinalysis.

At these visits, you can expect:

- Blood pressure check
- Weight check
- Urine sample
- Listening to the baby's heartbeat
- Belly measuring and fundal height check
- Follow-up on lab results from your last appointment
- Rh immune globulin (RhIG) injection, if applicable (Wait, what's RhIG? Read on below.)

About Rhesus (Rh) Factor

Back when you had your first prenatal visit, one of the tests done was checking your blood type and antibody status.

If you are among the 15 percent of people who have a negative blood type (A–, B–, AB–, O–), week 28 is an important one for you.

Having an Rh-negative blood type means that your blood cells are lacking a protein called Rhesus factor (more commonly called Rh factor). Being Rh-negative is not usually a big deal, except when you are pregnant.

In the making of your baby, the egg and the sperm each contributed to the Rh factor of the baby's genetic makeup. If both genes are negative, your baby is Rh-negative: no health concerns here at all. But if the sperm's genetic contribution is positive, it wins, meaning that your baby is Rh-positive.

Here is the concern: If your Rh-positive baby's blood mixes with your blood, your body's immune system will think this Rh-positive blood is a threat. Your immune system will, therefore, mount a defense against the baby's blood in the form of antibodies. These defense antibodies can cross the placenta and lead to a condition known as Rh incompatibility in which the baby can become very ill with anemia and, potentially, more serious complications.

Most commonly, the mixing of your blood and the baby's blood does not occur until the birth process. Additionally, these antibodies take some time to develop. This is why most women who are pregnant for the first time are not at risk of passing these defense antibodies to their fetuses.

However, these antibodies can also develop as a result of amniocentesis, chorionic villus sampling (CVS), bleeding during pregnancy, abdominal trauma, external cephalic version (ECV) (see "Baby Positions" on page 198), and miscarriage.

Once developed, these antibodies stay in your blood. So, what's an Rh-negative

READ AHEAD

Now that you know what will happen during labor, it is time to start thinking about what you want your labor to be like. This month, read chapter 22, "Pain and Coping Techniques." This is a great time to hop on a birth ball and start practicing the skills you'll learn there (said figuratively; no actual hopping, please).

mother to do? Rh immune globulin (RhIG)! At 28 weeks, you will be offered RhIG, which is an injection given to an Rh-negative woman that prevents the body from making antibodies (RhoGAM and Rhophylac are two commonly used RhIG brand names in the US). You will also be offered RhIG for the examples mentioned above. Prior to receiving the injection, you will have a blood test to confirm that you have not already produced Rh antibodies because RhIG is not effective if you already have antibodies in your blood.

After your baby has been born, they will have their blood type tested. If they are Rh-positive, you will be offered RhIG again. This will prevent Rh antibodies from forming that may impact a future pregnancy.

Now, there are people who are concerned about using RhIG products. They are derived from blood products, which means there is a (very small) risk of virus transmission. As with all forms of medication, there is a risk of side effects. Mamas worry about potential impacts on their unborn babies. Lastly, there is a chance that the RhIG is given unnecessarily (if your baby is Rh-negative).

Ultimately, most providers recommend that the benefits of RhIG outweigh the risks. But as always, if you are worried, talk to your provider and get the best advice for you.

Tdap Vaccine

ACOG recommends that all pregnant women receive the Tdap vaccine between weeks 27 and 36 of pregnancy (even if you have been vaccinated recently). The Tdap vaccine protects against tetanus, diphtheria, and pertussis (pertussis being the one we're most concerned about here).

Pertussis is also known as whooping cough, and it can cause very severe infections in young babies (who cannot be vaccinated against it until they are 2 months old). When you get the vaccine, you build antibodies against pertussis that you pass to your baby through the umbilical cord, which helps protect them once they are born. It is also recommended that those who will care for the baby be vaccinated, to decrease the risk of pertussis transmission to the baby.

Questions to Ask Your Provider

- How do you suggest I count fetal movements?
- Do I need the RhIG (RhoGAM) injection?
- Can I preschedule the visits for the rest of my pregnancy?

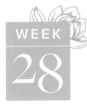

WEEK 28 Your baby is the size of an eggplant, about 14.8 inches long. Your baby's eyesight is really improving. The baby is blinking and sensing light.

Their head continues to grow bigger to accommodate the growing brain that is continuously adding brain cells. (They're super-smart; we can already tell.)

The baby could see a palm reader this week because creases are now visible on their chubby little hands.

nourish

Glycine for Growth

Your body continues working hard to grow your baby in this final stretch, and it can be exhausting. Many women find that they get hungrier in this trimester, and for good reason! At this point in your pregnancy, your blood volume has increased by almost 50 percent, your breasts are preparing to make milk, and your uterus is stretching to accommodate your growing baby (who is getting heavier every day).

Not to mention, your baby is starting to gain weight rapidly in this later stage of pregnancy as they continue to develop their bones, organs, connective tissues, and muscles.

So, let's focus on food that will keep you feeling energized and that will continue to support the growth spurt your baby is going through in this trimester.

This is the time to home in on the nutrient called glycine. Glycine is an essential amino acid that will help your body build new connective tissue. Your body depends on glycine to help support your stretching skin and growing uterus, and your baby also needs this nutrient to form their DNA.

The good news is that you can easily get this crucial nutrient in your diet through natural, whole foods. Bone broths and slow-cooked meats are some of the richest sources of collagen and gelatin, which naturally provide glycine. Here are some nutritious foods that will help you up your glycine intake to help support your body (and your baby) through this final trimester of pregnancy:

- Slow-cooked pork (carnitas)
- Chicken and vegetable soup made with bone broth
- Skin-on, bone-in poultry, like chicken thighs
- Bacon or sausage (with no added nitrates)
- Ground beef (grass-fed whenever possible)
- Beef pot roast, slow-cooked with root vegetables

If you have a plant-based or vegetarian diet, try adding in shiitake mushrooms, legumes, and seaweed, all of which contain glycine.

As another option, you can also use a powdered collagen supplement or pure gelatin powder, which can be mixed into other foods and drinks to boost your glycine intake.

Another important thing happening in this trimester is your baby's rapidly accelerating brain growth. To support this, remember to eat your omega-3 fatty acids, which are naturally found in fatty fishes like salmon, sardines, and mackerel; grass-fed beef and butter; as well as pasture-raised eggs, nuts, seeds, and seaweed. Eat up, mama!

move

Inner Thigh Squeezes
As your pregnancy progresses, it can be common for women to experience some level of pelvic pain associated with the natural changes occurring in the body. If you happen to be one of these women, you don't

SOUND SLEEP
Women who report significant sleep difficulty during pregnancy have been found to be more at risk for developing postpartum anxiety and depression. If sleep is an issue for you, talk to your provider and consider connecting with a mental health therapist. You can start preventative measures now and have an established relationship should you need emotional support later.

PREGNANCY TRADITION IN INDIA
In parts of India, starting in the seventh month of pregnancy, women sometimes wear glass bangles so that the baby can hear them and be comforted by the sound.

have to spend the remainder of your pregnancy uncomfortable or in pain. Here are some simple exercises that can both prevent and reverse signs of common pelvic issues such as pelvic girdle pain (see page 465), symphysis pubis dysfunction (see page 465), and sacroiliac joint dysfunction (see page 465). As always, do check with your provider first.

Practice
To perform inner thigh squeezes with a yoga block or small inflatable ball, lie on your back or sit up straight in a chair. Place a foam block or small ball between your legs, just above the knee. Squeeze the ball, engaging your inner thighs as you exhale and engage

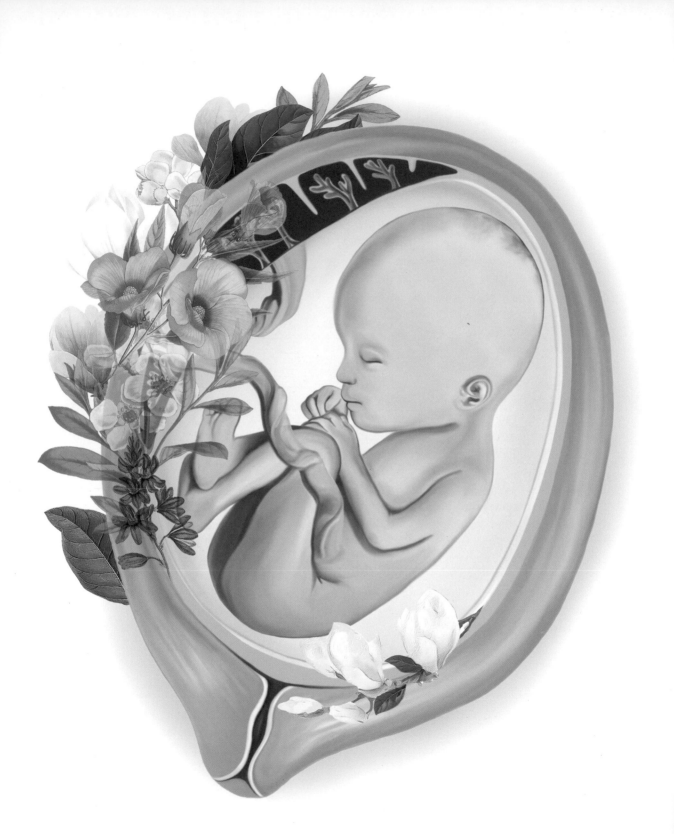

WEEKS 28–31

your pelvic floor and tighten your core at the same time. Do this for 30 to 60 seconds, 3 times in a row, with 30 to 60 seconds in between, several times per week.

Don't forget the belly pump from page 132 to help keep your pelvis strong and healthy.

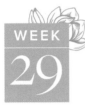

WEEK 29

Your baby is the size of a butternut squash, about 15.2 inches long, and things are getting real. Baby's preparing to breathe outside of the womb by producing a substance called surfactant that helps the air sacs in the lungs expand.

We can't wait for you to hear those sweet first cries!

love
AND VILLAGE

We are delving into birth preparations this month, and a huge part of that is assembling your birth support team—the people (beyond your provider) who will be with you when you are in labor.

The first part of this, of course, is deciding who you want to invite to your birthing place.

- If you have a partner, will they be with you during labor?
- Friends or family members?
- Your other children? (See "Bringing a Child to Your Birth" on page 185 for a few tips.)
- What about a doula? (See "Doulas" on page 92 for more info.)

It is also important to think about who will not be in the room with you. Remember,

NAMING YOUR BABY

Have you picked a name for your baby yet? This can be such a fun and meaningful thing to do, though if you find it stressful, you're not alone.

Psst: We love name articles at Motherly. Come on over for some serious inspiration (mother.ly/becomingmama).

Here are a few things to consider:

- Do you want the name to have a special meaning, or will you choose something based just on liking it?
- Are there family names (or variations of them) that are important to you?
- Will you decide their name before you meet them, or do you want to spend some time with them and then choose what suits them?
- Do you care if the name is trendy or popular?
- How do you feel about names with difficult spellings or pronunciations?
- Does the name you like have a nickname? How do you feel about it?
- What will the baby's initials be?
- Will your baby have a middle name?
- And what about their last name? Will you, for example, combine your and your partner's last names? Hyphen or no hyphen?

Ack, it's so much!

Here is the thing though: Within a matter of days, your baby's name will just *be*. People will stop asking (and commenting), and your baby and their name will become one. You will choose the perfect name for your baby. We love it already.

this is your birth. Not your mom's or your mother-in-law's. Not your best friend's. Not your partner's cousin's babysitter's. And yet, all of these people probably want to come to your birth.

They love you, and they are so excited for you. It's beautiful to have such an active village, but at the risk of sounding curt, you don't owe those (beautiful) people anything, at least not in this setting.

When considering who will be present at your birth, think about who will best contribute to the energy you want in the room. If someone always makes you feel calm and safe, they might be a terrific presence. If someone tends to leave you feeling anxious and uneasy or has a habit of

A NOTE FOR PARTNERS ON STAYING IN THE ZONE

Giving birth is an intuitive process. We don't *tell* our uterus to contract; it just does. Certainly, the whole brain is involved in giving birth to a baby. But there is no denying that birth tunes in a mama to her intuitive, emotional, rhythmic mind.

Often when a woman is in labor, we take her out of that space. Seemingly simple questions like, "What time did your contractions start?" or "What is your phone number?" require a fair amount of analytic power to think about and answer, and she can feel she's been taken "out of the zone."

My husband loves golf, and so (somehow) I have found myself watching the occasional tournament. As the players approach the last few holes, I always notice how laser-focused they become. They rarely talk, and they don't acknowledge the fans. They totally remind me of women in labor. It's not that they can't talk; they just really don't want to. They are deeply in the zone and know that staying there is critically important to maintaining the focus and rhythm to get to the end.

And so, dear labor partner, one of your most significant responsibilities will be to help her remain in her intuitive mind—the zone—as much as possible. If you can track and communicate information for her, she can stay in her flow.

Psst: Don't worry, mama. Again, it's not that you won't be able to think and speak. Labor does not touch your ability to analyze, intellectualize, or get your brainy-ness on. It's just lovely when you don't have to.

This also applies when helping her find ways to cope with labor. For example, because you will have discussed and practiced coping skills (ahem), you know that she really loves the idea of getting into the shower when she is in labor. So, when the time comes, instead of saying, "What do you want to do now?" (a well-intentioned question that unintentionally brings her into analyzing her situation), you could try, "How about a shower?"

If she doesn't want to take one, she'll let you know. But it may feel a bit gentler on her hard-at-work brain when you guide her through her birth preferences. Keep in mind that letting her lead is going to be best, and she may want to diverge from the original plan. Don't take it personally if she is not considering your feelings at this point.

being overzealous with judgment or unwanted advice, maybe don't invite them.

Psst: If your partner's cousin's babysitter gets persistent, try this: "We've already reached capacity in the birth room, so we can't have you there. But could you come over after we get home? There is no one I'd trust more to hold the baby while I get a postpartum nap in, and your amazing chicken potpie is just what I'll be craving!"

It's also important to find out how many support people your birthplace will allow in the room with you—for example, many hospitals have a two-person limit.

Once you have decided who your support team is, start the birth talk! Let them know what your birth preferences are, the vibe you want in the room, what coping skills you like, and all the other details that will allow them to help you have your best birth possible. We will talk about birth plans next month, but if you are excited to get started, go ahead and jump to chapter 25 now!

If there is someone in your life who makes you feel unsafe, you might consider letting your birth team and providers know. Most hospitals have security officers posted at all times, and if you give them a heads-up, they can be extra-vigilant on your behalf.

WEEK 30

Your baby is the size of a head of cabbage when curled up, about 15.7 inches when stretched out!

Kind of adorable news: Your baby is proportioned like a newborn, has all their external features, and weighs almost 3 pounds! From here on out, your baby is going to gain

BRINGING A CHILD TO YOUR BIRTH

Inviting your child to your birth can lead to one of the most beautiful experiences you will ever have. Children may be amazed by the process and feel so special and empowered to be there.

If this is something you are interested in, speak with your provider to find out if it is allowed at your birthing place. It is also an excellent idea to have an extra support person there whose only role is to care for the child, so if they need a snack, need to leave the room, and so on, your primary support person can stay with you while the child's support person tends to their needs.

You will also want to prepare them for what they will see. Birth illustrations and videos (that have been prescreened by you) are a great place to start. Lastly, talk to them about the noises they will hear: "Mommy might be yelling or grunting a lot." Let them know that this is because you are working very hard.

One way that we often tell parents to practice hearing the noise of labor is to have the child "help" your partner or a friend move something heavy. Set a box full of books or toys on the floor and have your partner demonstrate pushing the box while making noises of exertion. "See how when we work hard, we sometimes make big noises to help us feel strong? That's just like what mommy will be doing when she works to bring the baby out."

READ AHEAD

Interventions may become a part of your birth story. If you want to learn more about them, read chapter 23, "Interventions," and chapter 24, "Cesarean Births."

about half a pound per week until the end of pregnancy.

At the start of this week, your baby is swimming in a pint and a half of amniotic fluid.

As they continue to grow and take up more space inside your uterus, the amount of fluid will decrease.

Finding Childcare

No matter where you plan to work post-birth (see "Work" on page 171 for a recap), it is almost guaranteed that you will need some form of childcare—someone to safeguard your baby— at some point. Whether it is to return to the paid workforce, run an errand, or have a few moments of quiet, reinforcements are essential, so now is a good time to start the process of defining your needs and seeking support.

For many, childcare is a family affair. In fact, 60 percent of grandparents take some role in caring for their grandchildren. You may have family nearby, or even live in a multigenerational home where your parents will be involved in childcare.

If support from family members isn't an option (which for many, it's not) couples spend an average of 25.6 percent of their income on childcare; this jumps to 52.7 percent for single parents.

Compare this to European countries where childcare is subsidized by the government. In Denmark, for example, couples spend an average of 10.7 percent of their income on childcare and singles an average of 2.9 percent.

However, if you ask many American parents about childcare, chances are their shoulders will immediately tense up; they will take a deep breath and exhale with an "ugh." Unless they have family around and willing to assist, finding childcare is notoriously stressful, and often expensive, depending on the scenario. Bottom line: You are not alone in this experience.

With a little knowledge and some dedicated time, you will find the perfect person or place for your little one. Every family has their own needs, means, concerns, and desires, so try to focus on what works best for you.

When looking for the right childcare arrangement, here are some factors to keep in mind:

- Do you trust them? Gut feelings are valid.

- Do they have the appropriate credentials (CPR, first-aid training, and so on)?

- Can they provide a background check? It is possible that you will need to do this on your own. Search online for a local or national company to help you get started.

- Will this arrangement provide the necessary support for your family's schedule?

- Will they honor your family rules/values?

- Do you agree with their style of childcare and discipline?

- Are there any cultural considerations?

- What do their social media profiles look like? Is there anything on there that concerns you?

- Will they provide references you can contact?

- If applicable, are they familiar with LGBTQ+ families and their needs?

Following are the most common childcare options that parents choose from. Keep in mind that this is a very personal decision, and you can always reassess and change your mind.

Family Members or Friends This can be a great option if you have family or friends nearby. The positive aspects are that it is likely someone you know well and trust, and there is often a financial advantage. The potential downside is that it can be tricky to navigate "philosophical differences." For example, you have decided you're going to pick the baby up every time they cry, but your mother says they need to learn to soothe themselves.

Co-op If you have several friends with similarly aged children, forming a child-care co-op can be beautiful. You will come together and decide on a shift schedule, and then each adult will be responsible for watching the group of children during their shift. This is often a free option, as everyone gets the same benefit.

Co-ops are not without their pitfalls. For one thing, watching a group of children is demanding, and simply not everyone's cup of tea. Clear expectations are going to be what helps a group like this succeed. Make sure that

READ AHEAD

Are you planning to breastfeed? Bottle-feed? Both? We've got you! Read chapter 29, "Breastfeeding," and chapter 30, "Pumping and Bottle-Feeding," to learn more about both.

BABYMOONS

Babymoons are the "about to become parents" version of a honeymoon, and it is a trend I am totally on board with. I love the idea of finding unique ways to honor this phase of your life and all that you have done—and are about to do. From a week relaxing at the beach to a weekend hunkered down in a cabin in the woods, it all sounds divine.

Think about how you can babymoon outside of the box. It doesn't have to be an elaborate vacation. Babymooning by yourself can be incredibly therapeutic, as can a weekend with your partner or best friends. You also don't have to go far—or go anywhere, for that matter. Maybe your perfect babymoon is a staycation at home with your favorite foods and most loved sitcom reruns on repeat. Or perhaps you sign up for that painting class at the local community college you've been eyeing for a while. Whatever you do, just consider taking some intentional time to focus on and celebrate you because you are pretty worthy of celebration.

everyone commits to a fair schedule and that the other parents have caregiving styles that work with yours (such as how much screen time is allowed, junk food, and so on).

Babysitter or Nanny   Babysitters or nannies are hired caregivers. They may work occasionally (date nights only), full time, or anything in between. You will also have the option to choose between someone who comes to your home or someone who watches your child in their home.

Recommendations from friends are a great place to start. There are also websites that specialize in finding care. No matter how you find the person, always be sure to request a background check, speak with references, and meet with them in person to ensure they are a safe and comfortable match.

Nanny Shares   A variation of hiring a babysitter or nanny is to co-hire them with a friend, neighbor, or family member. For example, perhaps you only need care 3 days a week, and a neighbor needs care the other 2 days. You can hire a full-time nanny and split the time between the two families.

Or the nanny can care for both of your children at the same time for a slightly reduced rate per family.

This can be a great option, but do make sure that you are familiar and aligned with the other family involved. Things could get messy if misunderstandings arise.

Au Pair   Au pairs are young adults who travel to foreign countries for a year or so to live with a host family and provide care for the children. In exchange, they receive room and board and a reduced salary. You can hire them through an au pair agency that has been sanctioned by the US State Department.

Au pairs can offer an exceptional level of convenience and security, as they live in your home (snow days won't be a problem), and you get to know them well. They become part of the family. You will need to consider how you feel about always having someone in your home. And think about what might happen if things do not work out well (for instance, it might be

BABY'S IN UTERO ACTIVITY CAN REVEAL THEIR PERSONALITY

By now you are likely feeling a whole lot of movement throughout the day as your little one prepares to make their debut. Maybe you get gentle rolls and big stretches, or just when you decide to call it a night, you get bounced with kangaroo kicks (which are more fun to watch on the outside than experience on the inside—ribs!). Either way, you can't help but wonder just what this little creature might be like.

Well, researchers have found there is a significant correlation between what your kiddo is doing on the inside and what they likely will be up to on the outside. So, if you think you have a little kickball player or an interpretive dancer in there, it might be a good idea to get used to the idea now. And this goes for temperament, too. That tumbler is as likely to meet the world with feistiness as the roller is to take it all in with calm. You are getting to know your little one even before they arrive. It's never too early to think about how you might support them in their own special way.

awkward living with someone you are in the process of firing). If you decide to go this route, it's important to write down all your childcare expectations and home rules before you hire the au pair. Being on the same page from the beginning is an especially important foundation for this kind of childcare arrangement.

Parent Helpers   A parent helper is often a younger person, like a teenager, who helps take care of your child while you are home. This can work well if you work from home or if you want help entertaining a toddler while you take care of your newborn.

Daycare/Preschool   Daycares are facilities where groups of children are cared for by licensed workers. In preschool settings, many teachers also have early childhood education. In these scenarios, kids have the benefit of socializing with other children and learning how to interact with teachers from a young age.

Being around many children can expose your child to more germs, which means they may get sick more often—at first. Eventually, they build up their immunity and thus get sick less in the long run! When they do get sick, though, it's likely that you or your partner will have to take the day off from work to stay home with them, which can be a stressor.

Just like when you hire a babysitter or nanny, make sure you investigate the daycare: Read reviews and make sure they are licensed properly and that all employees have background checks. It's also essential to ensure that they can care for your child in the way you want. For example, not all daycares allow cloth diapers and personalized nap schedules or administer vitamins and medications. Also check on the ratio of caregivers to children and the age range of children in one room.

Lastly, don't be afraid to trust your senses (and your instincts). Does it sound happy there? Does it smell clean and look bright? If something doesn't feel right, it's okay to move on to the next place.

Ultimately, finding childcare is about finding an extension of yourself, someone to help you care for your little bean while you continue to make life happen around you. If your initial choice doesn't turn out to be the best fit, keep looking. Having a reliable source of childcare that helps you and your child feel 100 percent comfortable and supported is essential to your family's well-being.

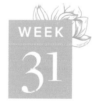

WEEK 31   Your baby is the size of a coconut when curled up, about 16.2 inches long when stretched. Your baby's eyebrows and eyelashes are fully developed, and the hair on

---

A DATE WITH DESTINY

Here you are, well into your third trimester, which might bring your due date into high relief. Will baby be born on that day? Before? After? A good thing to keep in mind is that for first-time moms, only 4 percent of births occur on the actual predicted date. The normal window for birth is 2 weeks on either side of the due date, since it is just an estimate, but the average time for a first baby to be born is 40 weeks plus 3 to 5 days. In other words, most first-time mamas go past their due date.

their head continues to grow. Their skeleton is nearly the size it will be at full term. The baby also has nearly fully developed lungs and intestines. Their remaining focus is to add fat and muscle over the next few weeks.

gather

- ○ Pregnancy support belt if your back is hurting
- ○ A birth ball (see "Birth Ball" on page 289 for guidance on finding the right size)
- ○ Yoga block or small inflatable ball (for inner thigh squeezes)
- ○ Glycine and omega-3 fatty acid–rich foods
- ○ A list of available childcare resources in your area

todo

- ○ Reflect: How will you foster your child's growth into the person they will become?
- ○ Schedule your next prenatal appointments and consider Tdap vaccines for you and those who will care for the baby.
- ○ Talk to your provider about their recommended way of assessing your baby's movement, and start counting!
- ○ Consider whom you'd like to be present during your birth.
- ○ Practice inner thigh squeezes.
- ○ Anticipate and write down what your child-care needs might be after the baby arrives and begin sorting through your options.
- ○ Plan a babymoon.
- ○ Schedule a hospital tour, if applicable (see "Questions to Ask Your Potential Birthing Place" on page 86).

- ○ Read chapter 22, "Pain and Coping Techniques"; chapter 23, "Interventions"; chapter 24, "Cesarean Births"; chapter 29, "Breastfeeding"; and chapter 30, "Pumping and Bottle-Feeding."

remember

You are growing a being who will become an adult with a unique and significant influence on the universe.

Month 8

WEEKS 32–35

I walk toward
and through
my fear.

note
FROM DIANA

This month, we are going to talk about fear. Birth is one of the most primal things we do, and fear is the most primal emotion we have: It only makes sense that it comes up in labor and birth.

Let's start by looking back to our hunter-gatherer ancestors.

Thousands of years ago, when a woman was giving birth, she was at the mercy of the elements. Say she looked up and saw a bear. Her brain would set off the "threat detected" alarm, which would trigger the stress hormones to start rushing through her body, causing what we know as the fight-or-flight instinct. This acute stress response, also called hyperarousal, sets off a cascade of physical reactions in the body: muscle tension, elevated blood pressure, racing heart, and rapid breathing, to name a few. The body also starts to turn glucose and fat into immediately usable energy.

All of these very intentional responses happen for a reason: survival. We instinctively know when we feel safe or scared, and our body reacts accordingly, including when we are in labor.

Researcher Judith A. Lothian wrote in a study about the importance of privacy in birth: "For animals giving birth in the wild, fear of predators in early labor triggers catecholamine release and labor stops, giving the animal time to move out of danger before labor begins again."

The animal focuses on finding safety, and when she does, and her body calms down again, labor will resume.

Yet here's the modern reality of this situation: Evolution does not happen quickly. The ancestral *Homo sapiens*' acute stress response is very much alive and well in us today.

What has evolved is "the bear." Instead of a massive beast with snarling teeth, the bear has become a traffic jam that makes us late for work, an aggressive email, or even a reminder letter when we forget to pay our cell phone bill—and of course, the intense anticipation of soon giving birth.

Our brains cannot tell the difference between the threat of a bear or the threat of a traffic jam. It all just feels like danger, and our bodies respond.

How does this relate to birth? The fear of birth can be cultivated slowly and subtly, but its impact is profound. We live in a society that tends to downplay the powerful and beautiful aspects of birth while playing up the scary and painful parts. We see TV shows and movies with dramatic birth scenes. We tend to hear more of the troublesome birth stories than the good ones. Plus, we are not exposed to birth in the same way humans used to be, even one hundred years ago. Your birth may be the first one that you experience, but in generations past, most women would have witnessed at least a few births by the time they had their own. This modern disconnection from the act of birth can add up to deeply seated unease.

You don't need a research study to tell you (but they went ahead and did one anyway) that women who hear negative birth stories from others are more likely to be afraid.

There is a scientifically demonstrated phenomenon called the "white coat syndrome" in which people (up to 40 percent of us) experience an acute stress response when we are near medical providers or in medical settings. (Oh, and hey, it's more common in women than in men.)

Lastly, as we discuss in the last step of the birth plan chapter (see "Is there anything else the team needs to know?" on page 329), we all have our stuff that can impact how we experience significant events such as labor and birth.

And so, darling mama, if you are scared, this is for you.

Do not be ashamed of your fear. Your fear is there to protect you from the bear.

You are normal. Nearly every woman I have worked with as a midwife has had some level of nervousness or fear about birth (including me, the midwife). Studies have found that almost 80 percent of women experience some degree of fear regarding birth. Whether it's of a precise detail or the process in general, or even of what comes after (aka parenthood), it is very natural to feel uneasy about something (or a lot of things).

You are not alone in your fear. And your fear is not your fault.

I want to convey to you, warrior mama, that research has found some specific ways to counter the fear of childbirth:

- Getting confident around your understanding of how reproduction and birth work
- Seeing a birth in real life—or online! (Though certainly you know yourself best. Some women find seeing a birth intensifies their fears.)
- Learning from friends about pregnancy and birth*
- Getting therapy

*My professional caveat is to choose whom you speak with wisely. If you have a friend who tends toward the dramatic, consider whether her stories would be helpful or frightening.

xo,

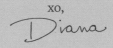

P.S. It is essential to note that while it's common for women to be nervous about birth, there is a point where professional help should be sought out. About 3 to 8 percent of women experience tokophobia, the specific phobia of pregnancy and childbirth. If you find that your fear is all-consuming, keeping you from enjoying your pregnancy, or making it hard to function, check in with a mental health professional. This applies even if you don't think you have tokophobia but want to talk through your concerns with someone. Research shows that at least 85 to 90 percent of people who seek therapy start to feel better. There is no shame in asking for help: It's just another sign of how brave you are.

Psychologist Carolyn Wagner says that if you are feeling intense fear, therapy can help significantly. While you are waiting for an appointment, and in conjunction with therapy, remember "that anxiety exists in the future. It is all about *what I'm afraid might be coming down the line.* So, if you can stay in the present moment, anxiety will significantly reduce, if not disappear."

Wagner recommends the following mindfulness strategies to bring you back to the present moment when you find your mind has gotten caught up in your anticipatory fears:

- Focus on what is going on right here, right now. "I'm safe, my baby is safe, and we're going to sit here together and breathe for a few moments."

- Project LETS (Let's Erase the Stigma) shares a wonderful strategy called the 5-4-3-2-1 technique: Name 5 things you can see, 4 things you can feel, 3 things you can hear, 2 things you can smell, and 1 thing you can taste.

Wagner encourages women to talk through their fears with their provider to get some solid data and action plans in place. Are you afraid that you won't be able to manage the pain? Your ob-gyn or midwife can explain what pain management options are available. Your doula can talk you through other supportive measures you can take.

Perhaps you're afraid that something will happen to you or your baby during delivery. In that case, you may benefit from learning more about who will be in the delivery room, how you and the baby will be monitored, and what happens if there's an emergency issue.

"While we don't want you Googling every story of deliveries gone awry," Wagner says, "it is always good to get reliable information from your own provider who knows the particulars of your pregnancy and birth place." Above all, Wagner recommends that anxious moms get a doula when they are able to. "There's no substitute for having that kind of intense, experienced, personalized support."

The meditation described below is intended for you to try self-relaxation at home. It will relax you deeply, so please use precautions. Do not attempt when driving or operating machinery or during a time when you cannot safely relax.

This exercise will guide you through releasing the tension within your body. To start, read through these instructions a few times. Then try to practice this as often as you can so that it comes naturally to you when you are in labor. You can also ask your partner to read it to you aloud. (For an audio version of this meditation, read by me, go to mother.ly /becomingmama).

Another option is to ask your partner to join you for this relaxation. As I mention each body part, have your partner touch or massage that part of you. Over time, you will learn to relax with just their touch. It's okay if this makes you giggle at first; that's totally normal. You'll get more comfortable with time.

Release the Tension Pregnancy and Birth Meditation

Find a comfortable place and position. Close your eyes if you'd like. Once you are comfortable, take a few big cleansing breaths. Release the used air in your lungs and breathe in cool, nourishing oxygen. Feel your body and your belly move with your breathing. Spend a few moments connecting to your environment. Hear the sounds around you. Perhaps they are pleasant, or perhaps you find them irritating. Hear them, but don't focus your attention on them. Slowly tune them out. The noises are around you but not inside you, and though they are there, they are not affecting you. Your mind is quiet and peaceful. Focus again on your breathing—how when you take a deep breath, you can feel your body fill with lightness, calmness, and restorative energy.

When you exhale, you feel the tension and stress leaving you. Breathe in calm. Breathe out tension. Now focus on the part of you that is touching the earth. It may be your feet on the ground, your side as you lie on a bed, or your bottom as you sit in a chair. Think about how that part of your body feels. You may not be directly touching the ground outside, but you are grounded to the earth. Let yourself feel supported and embraced and grounded by the earth.

Take a few more deep breaths. Now focus on your toes. Wiggle them, notice any tension that you feel, and release it. Now the soles of your feet. Your feet that work all day supporting and balancing the weight of your growing, beautiful baby. Release the tension in your mama-feet. Move your feet in circles, and as you do, relax your ankles. Feel the relaxation travel up your calves, your knees, the fronts of your thighs, and the backs of your thighs. Your strong legs carry your baby with you all day, lifting and lowering the body that is growing this tiny human. And before you know it, those same legs will be crouching down so you can kiss sweet chubby cheeks, will be folded in front of you as your baby sits on your lap listening intently to the words you read, and will be walking quickly behind a nervous but

READ AHEAD

Once you have read about the stages of labor, coping skills, and interventions, it is time to start thinking about what it all means for you. Read chapter 25, "Birth Plans."

thrilled toddler as you prepare to catch them as they fall, again.

Take another deep breath and allow your bottom to relax. Feel the strong, capable muscles of your vagina release their tension and the ligaments of your pelvis and your hips relax with your breath. Your body has spent months preparing your pelvis for birth. Trust your body and release the tension. And now your belly. Your swelling belly, filled with the energy of two incredible beings: a new baby, growing, changing, preparing to come into the world and fill it with love and excitement; and the strong superwoman who is growing that baby. Both of you creating so much energy in your belly. Allow the muscles of your belly and your uterus to relax. Your uterus knows exactly what it is doing. Your baby knows exactly what they are doing. Surrender to their wisdom.

Allow your back to release its tension. Your back is working so hard. Allow your back to completely relax as you breathe in fresh, clean air. Your lower back. Now your middle back. The space between your shoulder blades. Your shoulders. Let it all melt, as you continue to feel grounded and supported by the earth.

Now your neck. If you want, gently move your head from side to side and ease the tension in your neck. Find a comfortable way to support your head, so your neck doesn't have to. Relax your neck. Relax your jaw. Your jaw is connected to so much of your body, and relaxing it helps to alleviate tension everywhere. Even relax your tongue. Then your nose and cheeks. Your eyes and eyelids. Your forehead. Your scalp. Allow your whole head to just relax. Your head has been busy, after all. Full of thoughts about your birth. Your changing body. Wondering what to name your baby. Daydreaming about their sweet face. Worrying about being a parent. Yes, you've been very busy because you are already an amazing mama. So, allow yourself this moment to breathe, relax, and let go. Trust your body. Trust yourself. *You've got this.*

When you're ready, start to return to the room. Wiggle your toes; gently start to move your limbs. Come back to the present moment. When you're ready, slowly let your eyes open.

bonding WITH YOUR BABY

Starting around week 25, not only can your baby hear, they can also respond to sounds they hear in the uterus. Their heart rate goes up, and they may even open their mouth in response to hearing your voice. It is likely that this contributes to the immense mother-baby connection you are very close to experiencing.

What's more, recent studies have also found that babies start to learn about language, specifically vowels, in the womb. How wild is that?

The talking that you do in your normal daily routine is already shaping the way your baby will communicate and learn. You can also sing and read to them and ask your partner and village to do the same. Your baby will love

hearing from you, and chances are you'll love it, too.

You know how your favorite playlist can make you feel relaxed and nostalgic and happy all at the same time? There's nothing quite as quick and powerful as music to change your mood. And even in the womb, little ones respond to the vibrations and later to the beats and melodies that you play for them. Research also shows that music can help build the foundation for your baby's language acquisition, so you can think of taking a moment to jam out to your favorite songs as "educational." And even sweeter than that, you can begin exposing your child to the sound of you and your partner singing, which will no doubt soothe and relax them—even more so when you sing them lullabies later on.

Psst: A 2018 study found that pregnant women who took naps for 90 minutes, 5 to 7 days per week during late pregnancy were less likely to give birth to low-birth-weight babies. That is science we can totally get on board with. Yawn!

Symptoms YOU MIGHT FEEL

- Back pain/ache
- Braxton-Hicks contractions
- Constipation
- Fatigue
- Frequent urination
- Getting full quickly
- Groin pain
- Heartburn or reflux
- Hemorrhoids
- Hot flashes
- Itching
- Leg cramps
- Shortness of breath
- Sleep challenges
- Snoring
- Stretch marks
- Swelling
- Varicose veins
- Vivid dreams

To learn more about the symptoms that are impacting you—and how to deal—turn to the "Symptom Checker" on page 429. Remember,

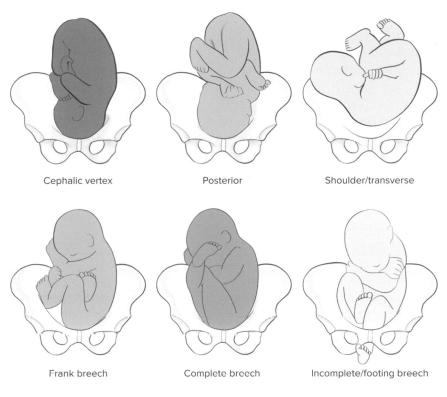

| Cephalic vertex | Posterior | Shoulder/transverse |
| Frank breech | Complete breech | Incomplete/footing breech |

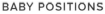

BABY POSITIONS

your provider is your first stop for any symptoms that concern you, so don't hesitate to reach out to them.

prenatal
VISIT THIS MONTH

Most women can expect to have two visits during their eighth month of pregnancy, which may include:

- Blood pressure check
- Weight check
- Urine sample
- Listening to the baby's heartbeat
- Belly measuring and fundal height check

- Follow-up on lab results from your last appointment

Your provider may recommend a repeat HIV screening during your third trimester. This is because transmitting the virus to an infant is easily prevented, and infection can occur after you've had your first HIV screening.

If you have been diagnosed with gestational diabetes, elevated blood pressure, or other complications, it is likely that your provider will start to monitor the baby more frequently this month in the form of ultrasounds and nonstress tests (NSTs). (See "Nonstress Tests" on page 457 for more info.)

Baby Positions

This month your midwife or doctor will start tuning in more to the position of your sweet babe. Up until now, it hasn't mattered if your baby is head down (cephalic), head up (breech), or head to the side (transverse). Your baby has had lots of room to flip around multiple times a day if they are channeling their inner gymnast.

But as you enter these final months of pregnancy, your baby starts to run out of room to flip. It's important to know what position your baby is in because it can impact delivery substantially.

Your provider will use their hands on the outside of your belly using a technique called Leopold's maneuver to determine where the head and butt are (cute!).

Here's what you need to know about breech and transverse babies: A breech baby has their bottom, knees, or feet pointing toward your vagina, essentially opposite of where they are supposed to be. A transverse baby is in a side-to-side, or horizontal, position. Being breech isn't actually a problem in and of itself, but there is a small increased risk of birth complications.

Breech babies were delivered vaginally all the time in the not-so-distant past, and there are providers who still attend vaginal breech births! If your baby remains breech, and you want a vaginal birth, you may be able to find a provider skilled and comfortable with vaginal breech births. Transverse babies who won't turn are not able to be born vaginally.

As you approach weeks 33 and 34, you'll want to start actively trying to flip your baby if they are breech or transverse, though it's never wrong to start encouraging optimal positioning earlier.

Here are some effective methods:

- **Watch your posture.** Good posture keeps your body more aligned, which can help with fetal positioning.

- **Plant your feet on the floor.** When you sit, try to keep both feet on the floor (avoid leg crossing). Also, see if you can sit with your legs angled so that your knees are level with or slightly below your hips.

- **Move your body.** Walking, yoga, and mild exercise can encourage your baby to be head down. By moving your body around and changing the space in your belly and pelvis, your baby may get the opportunity they need to flip. Start in a hands-and-knees position, or better yet, an elbows-and-knees position. Spend about 10 minutes in this position (as long as you are comfortable) twice per day. You can also lie on your back on a firm surface (such as the floor) and place some pillows under your hips to elevate them. Stay in this position for about 10 minutes (as long as you are comfortable) and repeat two times per day.

- **Get holistic.** Chiropractors, acupuncturists, and massage therapists use specific techniques to promote optimal positioning.

Anecdotally, the following tricks for turning a breech baby may work, and they don't cause harm:

- Shine a light on your belly above your pubic bone—the baby may get curious about the light and move to go check it out.

- Play music just above your pubic bone—baby might want to rock out and move toward the music so they can get a better listen.

Your provider may discuss the option of an external cephalic version (ECV). An ECV is a procedure usually done in the hospital (sometimes in the OR, though it is *not* a surgery). You'll lie on a bed, and the provider will put their hands on your belly and manually turn the baby from the outside. Risks are small, though sometimes an ECV can cause the baby's heart rate to drop, and if that happens, an emergency C-section may be necessary. Women also report that this can be an uncomfortable or even painful process.

Ultimately, you have to go with your gut. Some women want to pull out all the stops and do everything they can to flip their babies. Others take more of a "maybe there is a reason they're breech" approach and prefer not to do anything to encourage a position change. And many will choose to just try a few methods they are comfortable with to see what happens.

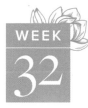

WEEK

32

Your baby is the size of a big cucumber, 16.7 inches long. Baby's starting to run out of room in the womb, so you may have begun noticing a change in their movements. It is important to note that they should be moving with the same frequency as before, it may just feel different now.

They also swallow almost a pint of amniotic fluid a day, and proceed to pee about the same

amount! You will likely gain about a half a pound per week for the rest of your pregnancy, so keep eating a healthy diet and taking your vitamins. (And by "healthy diet," we mean 90 percent good choices and 10 percent "Oreo ice cream delivery ASAP.")

nourish

Pump That Iron!

You're getting closer to meeting your sweet baby, mama! As you experience all the emotions leading up to your baby's birth, be sure to take care of your body with gentle nutrition, too. At this point in pregnancy, many moms begin to feel uncomfortable with eating or start to experience some unpleasant digestive issues (if they haven't already), including heartburn and constipation. These symptoms are the result of your growing baby taking up more space in your body, which begins to crowd your digestive system. Hang in there, mama. You're getting so close and won't be dealing with these side effects for much longer.

In the meantime, try eating smaller meals more frequently, stay upright after meals, and avoid foods that might trigger heartburn, like spices and foods that are acidic or high in fat. Be sure to drink adequate water and continue

---

FOOD PAIRING

Remember that pairing foods that are rich in vitamin C with iron-rich foods can help your body better absorb iron from food. Examples might be a citrus-based dressing on your spinach salad or fajitas with beef and bell peppers.

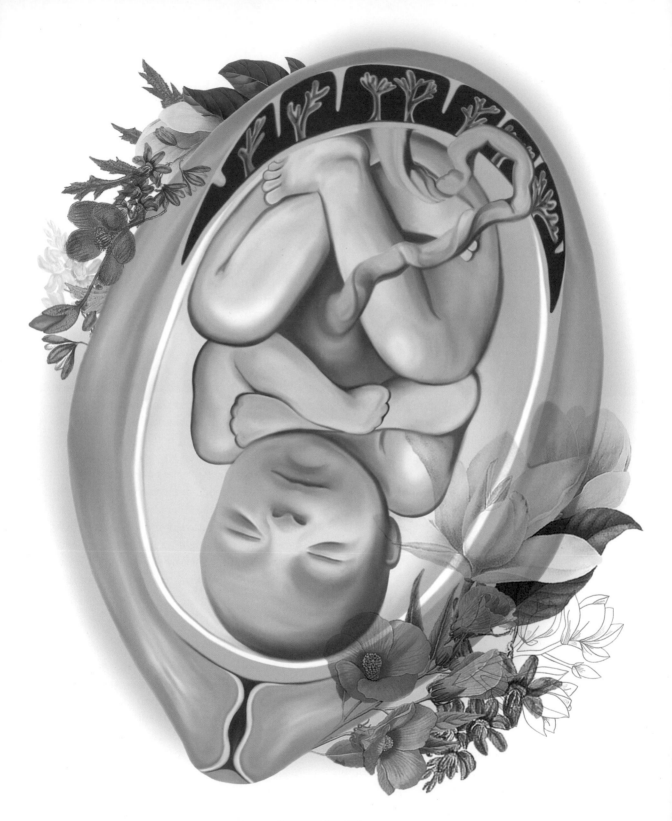

WEEKS 32–35

to aim for foods that are higher in fiber to keep you regular and help prevent constipation.

The third trimester is also a time when iron-deficiency anemia can occur. To help avoid this, aim for iron-rich foods, including lean red meat, dark leafy greens, legumes (such as chickpeas, lentils, and other beans), oily fish (like salmon), and fortified cereals.

Remember to stay consistent with prenatal vitamins as much as possible. Even though you're in the homestretch, your vitamins are still essential in covering your increased nutrient needs during pregnancy and post-partum. You'll want to continue taking your prenatal supplement after delivery and for as long as you're breastfeeding to help with recovery and healing.

move

Even though you are now feeling the bulk of baby and probably slowing down your gait, it's important to continue with a regular regimen of exercise if you have been active throughout the pregnancy. Walking, prenatal yoga, swimming, dancing, and strengthening exercises are great for keeping your energy up and maintaining your fitness level.

Diaphragmatic Breath Meditation

If you haven't done so yet (life is busy; I get it!), now is a great time to add in a daily meditation that helps you soften, destress, and enjoy the excitement of becoming a mother. Your practice doesn't have to consist of closed eyes, a quiet room, and sitting cross-legged. Integrate daily meditation into your life the way it works for you. Simply focusing on your breath and taking the time to quiet the mind while focusing in on baby can provide

a beautiful reset to your day. And going for a walk while clearing your head and breathing intentionally is another great way to press reset on your day.

Breathing and Fear

This is an opportune time to reflect on the value of diaphragmatic breathing (see page 119) and how it can ease the fear that comes up as birth draws near. Diaphragmatic breathing keeps you tapped into your parasympathetic nervous system (responsible for creating calmness through every cell in your body). Using your diaphragmatic breath to support you and your baby when fear shows up will prove to be a valuable practice both now and during birth.

Practice

Any time you begin to feel a sense of fear around your upcoming birth, stop and focus on deep, diaphragmatic breaths. Witness as this breath helps you feel better almost immediately. Remember that with each breath, the pelvic floor, deep abdominal muscles, and diaphragm all work in unison with one another.

As you do this breathing work, try repeating a calming mantra to yourself: "I am a strong, empowered woman. With every breath, I surround my baby with love and fill my body with the strength required to birth my little one."

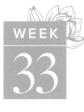

WEEK 33 Your baby is the size of a pineapple, about 17.2 inches long. *Psst: Did thinking about pineapples make you suddenly crave a piña colada? Curious about whether you can drink alcohol and breastfeed a baby?*

Check out "Drinking While Breastfeeding?" on page 402.

Deep breaths: Your baby is practicing breathing to get ready for life outside the womb! By the time of birth, they need to be able to take about 40 breaths per minute. You may feel like you are also taking some extra breaths, carrying around so much activity! It is okay to give in to the tiredness. It can only benefit you and your baby to increase your blood flow by lying down.

love
AND VILLAGE

With your mind full of thoughts about your birth, it can be easy to forget that at the end of all this, there will be a baby—your very own child that you get to raise.

Considering your parenting philosophies now can be helpful in easing some of the anxiety that this idea can provoke. Remember though that parenthood is fluid. You are allowed to—and will—reassess, make changes, and make mistakes throughout your journey. You, your child, and your partner, if you have one, will grow through this together.

Backed by decades of solid research, the predominant method of contemporary parenting advocated by therapists and psychologists involves establishing a strong emotional bond with your child, which helps them feel attached and, therefore, secure. Children who grow up with a strong sense of connection with their parents experience less stress, which can lead to lifelong benefits such as improved emotional regulation and increased independence as well as better physical health status.

So, what does this mean for you?

Attachment Parenting International (attachmentparenting.org) has laid out "Eight Principles of Parenting" to serve as a guide:

1 **Prepare for pregnancy, birth, and parenting.** Check!

2 **Feed with love and respect.** This means responding to your baby's hunger cues and instilling a positive attitude about healthy eating habits as they get older.

3 **Respond with sensitivity.** Pay attention to your child's emotional needs and respond with love and compassion.

4 **Use nurturing touch.** You know all that cuddling you are excited to do with your baby? Turns out it is excellent for their development.

5 **Ensure safe sleep, physically and emotionally.** Refer to "Safe Sleep and SIDS" on page 372 for more.

6 **Provide consistent and loving care.** Establish the trust that you will care for your child when they need you.

7 **Practice positive discipline.** Teach your child right from wrong in a way that feels like gentle guidance, not authoritarian commanding.

8 **Seek balance in your personal and family life.** Take care of yourself so that you can better take care of your child.

CHOOSING A HEALTH-CARE PROVIDER FOR YOUR BABY

Finding the right match in your baby's health-care provider is important. I always tell parents that while you want your child to grow to like their provider, it is also key that *you* like them. You'll be spending a lot of time with this person (especially in the first months of your baby's life), and they will be helping to guide you with some big decisions. It is awesome when you know that they share similar philosophies and that you can trust their advice.

Many offices offer appointments to meet with potential providers before your baby arrives, which is a great way to ask questions and set your mind at ease. I also love asking local parents for their recommendations.

Keep in mind that in addition to pediatricians (medical doctors who specialize in children), there are pediatric nurse practitioners and family practice doctors who offer wonderful care as well.

Here are questions to ask when you are meeting a provider for your baby:

- What are your philosophies (consider breastfeeding, vaccinations, circumcision, sleep training, nutrition, and so on)?

- Do you work with other providers? If so, will we still mostly see you, or will we rotate through all the providers? Can we meet them?

- What are your office hours? Do you have evening or weekend hours?

- Do you offer same-day sick visits?

- What happens if I have a concern in the middle of the night?

- What insurance do you accept?

- What other providers do you partner with or refer to beyond this practice (physical therapists, chiropractors, nutritionists, osteopaths, and so on)?

Other things to consider include the distance from your home (and possibly workplace or daycare) to the office and the overall vibe you get from the office staff.

It makes sense and sounds doable, right? Of course, no parent will be perfect all the time, and there will be moments when you yell or completely fail at your balancing act or let your kids stay up too late and eat too much sugar. But it's always good to have a baseline set of principles as a gentle reminder or to help get you back on track.

Over the next week, spend some time with this list. Talk about it with your partner and those who will be involved in your child's upbringing.

WEEK 34

Your baby is the size of a large cantaloupe when curled up, about 17.7 inches long when stretched out. Baby has gained a strong sucking reflex at this point and would likely be able to feed normally outside the womb.

They have likely turned head down by now, so you may be feeling serious pressure in your pelvis. Take heart: While baby does have a big head, the twenty-two separate bones that make up the skull are not yet fused. This will allow the head to be moldable and flexible when the baby is making their trip through the birth canal (see the image of a newborn skull on page 274).

PACKING YOUR BAG

This very well could be the most momentous trip you've ever had to pack for. And like a good vacation, some of your comfort and happiness will depend on how thoughtful you've been beforehand about what to bring.

Here are our tried-and-true suggestions for a starter list to make sure you have thought of everything.

Things to ask your birthplace about:

- Many hospitals and birth centers will provide diapers, wipes, onesies or T-shirts, a suction bulb, and blankets for the baby's stay.
- Some have birth balls and peanut balls available.
- Most provide mom with mesh underwear (ask for extras to take home!).

For a home birth, your midwife will provide you with a list of the additional specific items you'll need.

Let's get ready to go, mama. You're about to embark on the most exciting trip of your life!

Clothing
- ○ Hair ties
- ○ Flip-flops for the shower
- ○ Two changes of clothes to wear in the hospital or birth center
- ○ Nightgown and robe (you may want to use these instead of the traditional hospital gown)
- ○ Comfortable underwear
- ○ Glasses or contacts
- ○ Nursing bra
- ○ Nursing top
- ○ Clothes to go home in (maternity size)

Toiletries
Your hospital or birth center may provide some, but sometimes it's nicer to have your own.
- ○ Toothbrush/paste
- ○ Mouthwash
- ○ Lotion
- ○ Deodorant

- ○ Shampoo/conditioner
- ○ Lip balm
- ○ Hairbrush/comb
- ○ Soap
- ○ Earplugs
- ○ Breast pads
- ○ Nipple ointment
- ○ Makeup, if you want
- ○ Hairdryer, if you want

General Items

- ○ Birth preferences/birth plan
- ○ Bag
- ○ Picture ID
- ○ Insurance card
- ○ Quarters and cash (for vending machine)
- ○ Phone/camera
- ○ Chargers (with extra-long cords to reach the bed)
- ○ Contact info for anyone you and your partner may need to notify about the birth (family members, placenta encapsulation specialist, HR department, insurance company)
- ○ Snacks (freezer pops, crackers, applesauce, Jell-O)
- ○ Pillow(s)
- ○ Gatorade/coconut water/juice
- ○ Extra plastic bag for taking home dirty clothes
- ○ Magazine/book
- ○ Notebooks/pen
- ○ Gum/mints

Birthing Resources

- ○ Birth ball
- ○ Peanut ball
- ○ Rebozo (a specialized shawl used for traction and massage in labor)

- ○ Music playlists (on phone or otherwise)
- ○ Essential oils
- ○ Visual element (beautiful photo)
- ○ Mantras
- ○ Cord blood banking kit, if applicable

For Partner

- ○ Toothbrush/paste
- ○ Mouthwash
- ○ Deodorant
- ○ Two changes of clothes
- ○ Bathing suit (if tub or shower present; so you can get in with birthing mama)
- ○ Flip-flops and sneakers
- ○ Magazine/book

For Baby

- ○ One adorable newborn outfit
- ○ Receiving blanket (if you prefer your own)
- ○ Car seat (note that most hospitals will not release the baby until they see that you have a proper car seat for them installed in your car, when applicable.) Car seat installation can be checked by fire and police professionals at a local station. (See "Car Seat Installation Frustration" on page 206 for more details on car seats.)

Creating a Mama Ritual

As we talked about in chapter 11, work doesn't "just" mean a job that gives you money; it's about how you spend your days. And part of how you spend your days must be taking care of you.

It is incredible how quickly self-care can slip through the cracks when a baby arrives. All of our attention and energy is focused on

CAR SEAT INSTALLATION FRUSTRATION

One of the rites of passage of new parents is setting out to quickly install a car seat in the rear of a vehicle with the best of intentions, only to find (an hour later?) that the contraption is neither intuitive nor user-friendly upon first encounter. These things are designed to keep kids safe, not to make parents' lives easier! It's all for a good reason, and you will learn this skill over time. But is it any wonder that a whopping 59 percent of car seats are installed incorrectly? This is a huge deal because when car seats are properly installed, they can reduce the risk of injury in a car crash by as much as 82 percent.

But there is good news: You can have your car seat installation inspected for free by a certified technician. This is often done at special events, at local hospitals, or at police and fire stations (you usually have to make an appointment). I strongly encourage you to take advantage of this before your baby comes, and throughout their life, especially when they move from one type of seat to another. I have done it a few times, and each time they have made corrections for me (and they have been very friendly and nonjudgmental).

Your best bet is to do an Internet search for "car seat installation inspection near me" to find a location that works best for you.

our child, and we fall to the bottom of our priority list.

You are about to become a superhero (yes, motherhood is actually a league of superheroes: Welcome!), but you won't stop being a human, with human needs. It's easy to ignore those needs for a while, but it can get away from you quickly. One day becomes a week, and before you know it, you haven't done anything for yourself in months.

You may have heard the term "mom guilt." I will tell you that it can hit hard post-baby. Suddenly, the simple act of taking a shower feels selfish: "I should be spending time with my baby." We start to forego the things that give us joy because somehow doing them means that we are "bad moms." Mama, this couldn't be further from the truth.

On every airline's safety speech, they always tell you that, in the event of an emergency, you should put your mask on before your child's. That call to action exists for a particular reason: You are the most essential part of this operation. Your child can't thrive unless you do.

Listen. It's taken me three children to fully embrace this idea. I want you to embrace it sooner.

And motherhood as a whole needs your help. We need you to join us in changing the narrative for women and mothers. Self-care is not a luxury! It is a necessity!

So, this month, your assignment is to create a mama ritual. Something that is just for you, that only exists to serve you. It doesn't have to be elaborate or long, just a nonnegotiable, tiny (or not so tiny) piece of the day that you intentionally carve out for you to be your only focus.

Hold your mama ritual sacred. And start now. Make it a habit before your baby comes.

I find that spending time in nature offers me a total reset, whether it's a walk around my neighborhood, a hike in a nearby preserve, or simply playing outside with my kids. Something about being close to the trees and earth reminds me to trust the process a bit more, and I always feel more relaxed and grounded after.

Here are some of our mamas' favorite rituals:

"I wake up before everyone, do a workout, shower, and have coffee." AMBER

"I used to be an avid gamer before kids. Now I don't have much time for that hobby, and I miss it. So, a lot of nights after I put my son to bed, I will try to take an hour to play a video game before I go to sleep." LISSA

"A 6 minute yoga routine is the perfect length for me to change my mood and keep my flexibility intact through all of these pregnancy-birth-postpartum body changes." JESSICA

"Going to bed so early it might be considered a child's bedtime. Even, and sometimes especially, when I have a million things to do, the best thing I can actually do is let my mind and body rest." LIZ

"Each morning upon waking, my husband and I sit together and meditate. Our goal is 20 minutes, but sometimes we only have 5 minutes. No matter the amount of time, this practice helps me start each day with a fresh perspective (and it sets the tone for my well-being as a priority)." JAIME

"I love taking baths. I take all the kids' toys out of the tub, light some candles, add some bath salts (or my kids' bubble bath), and just soak." JANE

"When my son was a baby, I did training classes with my dogs. Once a week I had an evening with just my dog and a class full of people who didn't talk about babies at all. It was great (plus it helped make sure the dogs didn't feel pushed out by the baby because they were getting lots of attention). We're not in any classes right now, but dog walking sans child is my self-care." HEATHER

"Walking with a friend or making time for a regular girls' dinner with my friends always leaves my soul happy! Oh, and running errands solo when my kiddos were really young was so great. It truly felt like me-time to walk slowly through the Target aisles with a warm coffee." JILL

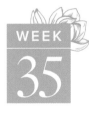

WEEK 35

Your baby is the size of a honeydew melon when curled up, about 18.2 inches long when stretched out.

Your little one now sleeps with their eyes closed, snoozes in a regular pattern throughout the day, and has coordinated reflexes.

Your body has been producing the hormone relaxin ever since you peed on that stick, but now it is working its magic, starting to relax the bones and ligaments that support your pelvis while beginning to soften the cervix. It likely also plays a role in relaxing the uterus so that it can stretch to accommodate baby's growth.

gather

- ○ A few nursing bras (see "Nursing Bras" on page 400 for more details)
- ○ Everything you plan to pack in your bag (same for your partner)
- ○ Items you might need for your mama ritual

to do

- ○ Reflect: Practice the "Release the Tension" meditation.
- ○ Schedule your prenatal appointments.
- ○ Schedule a car seat installation inspection (for each car if you have more than one).
- ○ Consider visiting a chiropractor, acupuncturist, or massage therapist.
- ○ Practice diaphragmatic breathing in response to fear.
- ○ Meet with potential baby providers (check out questions to ask on page 203).
- ○ Establish your mama ritual.
- ○ Pack!
- ○ Take a nap.

remember

Trust your body. Trust yourself. *You've got this.*

Month 9

I trust my body.

Oh, mama.

This is (potentially) my last note to you before you give birth.

(Don't worry; if you go past your due date, I won't leave you hanging. The next chapter is just for you.)

This month we are going to talk postpartum—a bit about what to expect and how to prep for it, so you can maximize your enjoyment of this soon-to-be precious time in your life.

Before we do though, let's take a few moments to reflect on how amazing you are. Seriously, look back at yourself over the last 8-plus months.

Are you in awe?

You have grown a human being (maybe several human beings!) from the size of a cell to the size of a pumpkin. That is superhuman.

You have experienced symptoms you never knew were possible and watched your body change in ways you always sort of knew about but never really believed could happen to you.

You have reflected, gotten excited, worried, and then gotten excited again about what this journey has meant to you and what your future holds as a mother. You've probably also had moments that I can't even imagine because they were unique to your individual experience.

Some of it's been great, and some of it's been challenging. But you've done it.

And you will continue to do it.

Because that is motherhood.

It won't always go smoothly. You will have glorious successes, and you will make mistakes. There will be moments of pure bliss followed (seconds later) by moments of "What did I get myself into?"

Motherhood is not perfect. But know this: You are the perfect mother for your baby. When you act out of love and good intention, you are doing it right. And your baby will adore you.

Enjoy these last weeks of pregnancy (at least a little; I know it's hard). Your sweet child will be here before you know it.

You should be so proud of yourself.

xo,

Diana

You have done all the planning and prepping you can do, and now it is time to give control over to nature. In other words, it is time to trust your body.

I don't mean this in a "sit back and let your body take over, and everything will be perfect" way, because sometimes our bodies and minds *do* need some help. Whether it's an epidural, Pitocin, or a C-section, sometimes interventions are necessary.

What I mean is, trust your body to tell you, and your providers, what it needs.

If what you need is to be left in your zone and do your thing with minimal interventions, your body will tell you that. You'll feel like you can cope with the contractions. If your baby is stable and happy, their heart rate will reflect that. When your provider assesses you, they'll see the signs that everything is progressing as it should.

If your body and your mind need help coping with the pain, you'll know. Pain medications and epidurals have a place in birth, for sure, and if you feel like you need them, ask.

And your body will let you and your provider know if an intervention is needed. If you're not dilating, if your blood pressure is high, if the baby is less than happy, your body and your baby will communicate these things, and everyone will adjust accordingly.

No matter how your story unfolds, you and your body will be the guiding light.

Take a few deep breaths and tell your body that you trust her. Think about all that she has done and marvel in her wonder. Thank her for her power and her work and watch her do her magic.

bonding
WITH YOUR BABY

Often during pregnancy, we get wrapped up in the planning. It's easy to do because there is so much to consider! But somewhere in the last weeks, it tends to dawn on you: Whoa, I am having a baby.

Write a letter to your baby. It can be sweet or silly, light or profound: Anything goes! And if you're feeling stuck, use the following letter featured on Motherly and adapt it for your purposes.

Psst: There's also an audio meditation version of this one on mother.ly/becomingmama.

Dear Baby,

I cannot wait to meet you. Experiencing you growing each and every day has been such an amazing journey. I am so eager for you to be born, so I can see your sweet face, smell your sweet baby smell, and hold you in my arms.

Getting to be your mom is the biggest honor of my life. I haven't met you yet, but I know it. I am already so proud of you and so excited to watch you grow into the person that you will become.

I'll admit, I'm a little nervous to become your parent. I'm doing everything I can to prepare for you, but it's a big job, and I know I won't get everything right. [Insert sentence about your personal visions of the life you want with your family.] I'll make some mistakes. I'll doubt myself plenty. But please know this: Everything I do comes from a place of deep, all-consuming love for you. Please don't ever doubt that.

I will love you completely—just the way you are.

So, take the time you need to grow. I'll be here: your rock, your warmth, your guardian, your mom. When you are ready to come out, I will make sure that your days are filled with silliness, adventures, and above all, love.

Love, Mom

Symptoms
YOU MIGHT FEEL

- Back pain/ache
- Braxton-Hicks contractions
- Constipation
- Fatigue
- Frequent urination
- Getting full quickly
- Groin pain
- Heartburn
- Hemorrhoids
- Hot flashes
- Itching
- Leg cramps
- Shortness of breath
- Sleep challenges
- Snoring
- Stretch marks
- Swelling
- Varicose veins
- Vivid dreams
- Water breaking

To learn more about the symptoms that are impacting you—and how to deal—turn to the "Symptom Checker" on page 429. Remember, your provider is your first stop for any symptoms that concern you, so don't hesitate to reach out to them.

prenatal
VISIT THIS MONTH

Most women will start to have appointments every week at this stage. Your provider will want to keep a close watch on how you are feeling, your blood pressure, how your baby is doing, and if there are any signs of labor. Here is what you can anticipate for these visits:

- Blood pressure check
- Weight check
- Urine sample
- Listening to the baby's heartbeat
- Belly measuring and fundal height check
- Assessment of baby's position
- Follow-up on lab results from your last appointment

Group B Strep

Between weeks 35 and 37, providers will recommend a screening for group B strep (GBS). GBS is bacteria that is present in some women's and men's bodies (in their reproductive, urinary, and gastrointestinal tracts). It is not a sexually transmitted infection or hygiene issue. We don't actually know why some women have this bacteria and others don't.

During normal life and pregnancy, GBS can cause urinary tract infections, but otherwise it is not thought to be a problem. However, if these bacteria are present in the vagina, and the baby comes in contact with them during birth, they can make the baby sick with a serious infection. This can lead to pneumonia, sepsis, and even meningitis—an infection of the fluid in the brain and spinal cord.

Between 1 and 2 percent of babies born to women with untreated GBS will be infected, and unfortunately, they can be severely at risk. In a previous era, GBS infections had a 50 percent mortality rate, which is why there are strict guidelines in place to screen and treat GBS. The guidelines have resulted in a dramatic reduction in the rate of infant infection since the 1990s.

Providers often recommend that women who test positive for the bacteria receive antibiotics during labor to prevent transmission to the baby. The drug of choice is penicillin, but if you are allergic, additional tests will be done to the bacteria to find another antibiotic that will work.

Some women may also have additional risk factors for having a baby with GBS, and they may be encouraged to receive treatment without a screening. For example, if you have already given birth to a baby who was infected with GBS, your provider will likely automatically start treatment, as your risks may be higher. Of note, GBS infection rates are higher for preterm or low-birth-weight babies.

To perform the screening, a cotton swab is inserted into your vagina and then into your anus (about a centimeter in) and then sent to the lab. Research has found that doing the test on yourself can be just as accurate as when a provider does it for you, so be sure to ask if that interests you! DNA-based tests that can give results within about 2 hours may be available as well.

Women who are having planned C-sections do not need to be treated for GBS but are usually tested. If your water breaks or you go into labor before your scheduled Cesarean birth, it may become necessary to start treatment.

The GBS Controversy The information regarding GBS screening is not foolproof. Your status can change after you have your screening, which may mean that some women are unnecessarily treated, and some cases are not detected. Providing antibiotics can affect the body's microbiome at a time when babies need to be exposed to healthy microbes to jump-start their immune systems. There's also the risk of widespread antibiotic use creating bacteria that are resistant to antibiotics.

BIG BABIES

If these last weeks of pregnancy find you worried about having a too-big baby, you are not alone. Many women are nervous about that, especially because our culture seems to love commenting on the size of women's bellies:

"Are you sure it's not twins?"

"You are ready to *pop!*"

Cool, thanks.

The truth is you can probably relax about this one.

A macrosomic baby, or big baby, is a baby that weighs more than 9 pounds, 15 ounces (though some providers use 8 pounds, 13 ounces as the criterion). Macrosomia is not that common: Only 1 out of 10 babies is macrosomic (and only 2 percent of all babies are 10 pounds or larger). There are some factors that can make you more at risk of having a large baby: having a BMI above 30, having gestational diabetes, or being older than 35. Now we need to take this seriously, of course. The concern with macrosomic babies is that there could be an increased risk of birth complications, such as cephalopelvic disproportion (see page 478) and shoulder dystocia (see page 480).

But I meet so many women who are terrified of birth because of this big-baby idea, and I don't want that for you, mama. To the extent that you can, try not to let this worry consume you. Your provider is assessing your baby's growth at each prenatal visit (with their hands or an ultrasound). If they are concerned, they will let you know, and then you can have a detailed conversation about what the best option is for your birth. Until then, remind yourself that your baby is perfect for your body.

READ AHEAD

Before you know it, this baby is going to be born, and you will officially be in your fourth trimester, otherwise known as the postpartum period. You can read all about it in chapter 26, "Self-Nurturing and the Fourth Trimester"; chapter 27, "Postpartum Physical Recovery"; and chapter 31, "Postpartum Love and Village and Returning to Work."

There are women who choose to use natural methods to prevent and treat GBS. This includes taking garlic, yogurt, tea tree oil, and more. Unfortunately, at this time the research around these methods is fairly limited, so we don't know for certain that they will work.

Sarah Bjorkman, MD, an ob-gyn, affirms that while this is very scary, neonatal infection with GBS is very rare, and more importantly, it can be prevented. "In the 1990s, before we started routine screening and treatment for GBS, it was the number one cause of early-onset sepsis," she said. "However, this is no longer the case as rates have dropped by more than 80 percent with screening and treatment. This is amazing! Antibiotics work, great evidence supports their use, and it could save their baby's life. ACOG, AAP, ACNM, and the CDC all recommend GBS prophylaxis/treatment, and so do I."

Ultrasounds

It is possible that your doctor or midwife will recommend an ultrasound during this time to confirm that your baby is head down if they are unable to tell by clinical exam.

If baby is breech, head over to page 198 for tips and info.

Ultrasounds are sometimes used to estimate your baby's size. Providers may use this information to make recommendations about induction of labor, but this measurement can be inaccurate. In fact, overestimation of fetal weight on ultrasound is significantly more common that underestimation. Now this is not to say that estimates should be ignored. But decisions about mode of delivery (spontaneous vaginal versus induction versus C-section) must not be made lightly, and they should involve an understanding of this research as well as the big picture.

Nonstress Tests

Nonstress tests are noninvasive tests that assess your baby's heart rate over a period of time to determine how happy and healthy baby is in there. More on this on page 457.

Vaginal Exams

Some providers may recommend a vaginal exam at your prenatal appointment to see if your cervix is starting to dilate. During an exam, they will wear a sterile glove and, using lubrication, insert two fingers into your vagina and reach back to feel your cervix. (Remember, if you are not a fan, go back to page 102 where I share some tips on making this procedure easier).

Vaginal exams are subjective in that there is no universal tool we use to see how open the cervix is. Tiny cervix rulers are not a thing. With a lot of experience, providers learn to assess the cervix by feel.

A quick note about vaginal exams: They *may* not be completely necessary at this point. It is entirely possible to be 0 centimeters dilated at your prenatal appointment in the afternoon and then in full-blown labor in the evening. It is also possible to be dilated a few centimeters and not go into labor for weeks—especially if you are having your second or third baby.

Another important point to consider is that an increased number of vaginal exams may up your risk of infections, such as chorioamnionitis (see page 479).

My professional practice involving vaginal exams—and many other tests for that matter—is this: I ask myself whether the information we gather from this exam or test is going to influence the plan of care. If the answer is "yes," it's probably an exam worth doing. If, however, it won't change things, and we are just curious, it is best to leave it alone.

In short, if you are interested and want a vaginal exam before you are in labor, discuss it with your provider. But if not, don't be afraid to ask questions about why your provider wants to do them and to decline if they not necessary.

Testing for Sexually Transmitted Infections

Many providers recommend additional testing for sexually transmitted infections, STIs, at this point, as birth is a time when the infection could be passed to the baby. For more info on STIs, see "Sexually Transmitted Infections During Pregnancy" on page 470.

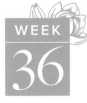

WEEK 36

Your baby is the size of a head of romaine lettuce, about 18.7 inches long when stretched out.

POSTPARTUM FOOD PLAN

Map out a postpartum food plan for yourself and your family and village. Meal kit deliveries can also be a lifesaver for the days and weeks after your baby is born. Consider subscribing to a meal delivery service or grocery delivery, even temporarily, to help ensure you have the needed food to nourish your body appropriately in the busy postpartum days ahead. Or better yet, see if you can put one on your registry!

Your baby's physical development is mostly complete, and the next 3 to 4 weeks are spent gaining weight (about an ounce a day), while your body is preparing to give birth.

You may be experiencing Braxton-Hicks contractions (see "Braxton-Hicks Contractions" on page 432), which not only help the uterus practice contracting for birth, but also provide stimulation for baby's developing senses.

Your expanding breasts are also kicking into action, making the colostrum for baby's first meals.

Meal Planning

You are getting so close to meeting your little one, mama! While these last few weeks leading up to birth can feel unnerving, it's a great time to make final preparations before baby's arrival.

If you haven't already, take some time to pack some healthy, nonperishable snacks in your hospital bag for you and your birth partner. You'll likely feel hungry at odd hours in the days after your baby is born, and you want to be sure you have extra, nutritious food on hand to keep your body fueled and satisfied. Some ideas include:

- Trail mix
- Dried fruit
- Jerky
- Granola bars
- Multigrain crackers
- Nut butter packets
- Dry cereals

Replenishing fluids is also essential for postdelivery, and you may want extra water or electrolyte drinks.

Lastly, consider preparing or stocking up on some extra meals that you can keep in the freezer for you and your family to enjoy after the baby arrives. This will help ensure that you have some nourishing foods on hand when you're less available for meal prep. Less time cooking means more time to snuggle with that new and precious baby!

EASY BAKED PESTO CHICKEN

Ingredients

1 lb. chicken tenders
3.5 oz. container of store-bought pesto
3 Roma tomatoes, sliced
8 oz. fresh mozzarella cheese, evenly sliced
Salt, pepper, and Italian seasoning
2 Tbs. Parmesan cheese

Directions

1 Preheat oven to 400 degrees F.

2 Place chicken tenders in a single layer in a large baking dish.

3 Spoon pesto evenly and thoroughly over chicken tenders in baking dish. Top pesto layer with a layer of sliced Roma tomatoes. Add mozzarella cheese over sliced tomatoes. Season with salt, pepper, and Italian seasoning. Top with a final layer of parmesan cheese.

4 Bake for about 40 minutes or until cooked through. Remove from oven and enjoy!

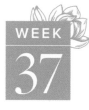

WEEK 37

Your baby is the size of Swiss chard, about 19.1 inches long. Baby's fine, downy hair (lanugo) is starting to shed, and fat continues to accumulate around your baby's wrists and neck.

You've reached another huge milestone: The baby is now full term! Your due date is still 3 weeks away, which means baby is technically "early full term." But if you go into labor today (which you could), there is a very, very good chance that your baby will thrive. Throughout this week and next, your baby's lungs and brain will fully mature.

move

Labor Prep Circuits

With birth drawing near, it's time to concentrate on labor prep. Training for birth both mentally and physically is a great way to enter your birth experience feeling more prepared and empowered about what you're about to experience. These labor prep circuits focus on strength, endurance, and

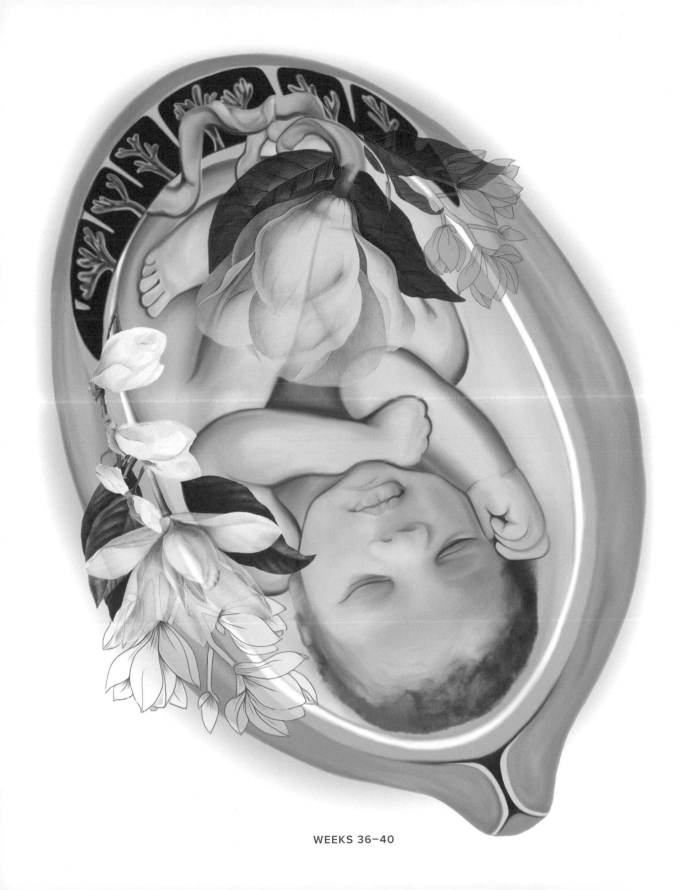

WEEKS 36–40

breath in a similar pattern to the contractions of labor.

Practice

Perform circuit-style workouts or "contraction stages" with four to five exercises lasting 1 to 2 minutes each. After performing one round of exercises, rest and come to a comfortable position to focus on diaphragmatic breathing. Use this rest period to calm and reenergize yourself for the next "contraction stage." As always, check with your provider to make sure these specific exercises are safe for you.

Psst: If you work out often and find that you'd like to add more challenge to this circuit, you'll find an added recommendation with each step.

POSTPARTUM NURTURING TECHNIQUES

Cultures around the world have beautiful ways of nurturing women during this vulnerable time.

In India, women might observe a 40- to 60-day period when they remain home in order to stave off potential infections. They receive herbal baths and daily massages to help rebuild their strength.

In Japan, women may practice *ansei*, which means "peace and quiet with pampering." They may spend the first 3 weeks in their parents' home, staying in bed with baby as others take care of their needs.

In Mexico, women might have *la cuarentina* ("the quarantine"), where they spend 40 days recovering from birth. They are encouraged to rest and eat well, and female relatives take over all the daily tasks.

You can perform these alone or with light weights (no more than 5 to 10 pounds).

Here are the steps in a labor prep circuit:

1 Squats (see page 148). Perform for 1 minute. (Add a bicep curl, with or without weights, for more challenge.)

2 Alternating reverse lunges (see page 167). Perform for 1 minute. (Add a shoulder press, with or without weights, for more challenge.) To do a shoulder press, take your arms out to the side and bend your elbows so that your hands are level with your ears (in a "goalpost" position). Slowly lift your arms up and bring your hands toward each other over your head. Then, lower your arms back down to ear level.

3 Inner thigh squeezes (see page 181). Perform for 1 minute. (Add front shoulder raises, with or without weights, for more challenge.) To do a front raise, start with your arms straight down by your sides. Slowly raise them in front of you, keeping them straight, until your hands are at shoulder level. Slowly bring them back down to your sides.

4 Alternating side lunges (see page 167). Perform for 1 minute.

Tips for Success

Remember to check with your provider before trying these exercises. These circuits are designed to mentally prepare you for getting through a contraction. They are based on the fact that labor isn't one long pain. It's 30 to 90 seconds of contractions followed by an even longer break. You just need to get through these intense contraction periods.

You can set your own time goal for each exercise. If your goal is to go for 35 seconds without stopping, try to stick to that time (no worries if you just can't make it!).

Try giving yourself a pep talk to make it through (just like you will in labor). Try these suggestions:

- Repeat to yourself: "Yes, I can."
- Remind yourself: "I can do anything for *x* number of seconds!"
- Breathe and soften into the intensity, knowing that your mental body is often ready to quit before your physical body needs to.

But don't overdo it! Mama, this is just to get you used to the idea that contractions come and go and that you can ride them through to the end. But if something doesn't feel right, stop immediately.

Many women I've worked with have found this exercise to be a helpful preparation for birth. You can even practice breathing during the same lengths of time so that you get used to what 30 to 90 seconds feels like. You can do it!

Planning for Postpartum

You and your village are ready for birth and baby, and now it's time to make sure that you have everything you need to heal and begin your life as mama.

The first few months of motherhood are sacred. For starters, you have become a mother, one of the most profound transitions a person can make. You will also be recovering from the intense physical experience of being pregnant and giving birth.

We have a "bounce back" mentality in our society that is, quite frankly, very unhelpful. For starters, there is very little bouncing in those first weeks. More importantly, the concept creates this idea that you were somehow better before and that you should get *back* to that state of being instead of embracing the *you* that just brought life into the world.

The post-pregnancy you is still *you*. You just have different needs. Honor them. Be gentle with yourself and accept the support of your village.

Talk to your partner and your village and decide some ways to create a haven in your home and what tasks you can delegate. They want to help you, truly, but sometimes they just don't know how. Don't be afraid to ask for what you need.

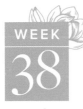

WEEK 38 Your baby is the size of a leek, about 19.6 inches long. By now, the circumference of your baby's head and abdomen are measuring the same.

For many mamas, this will be the last week of pregnancy. Multiples are more likely to come early, as are babies born to mothers with African and Asian ancestry.

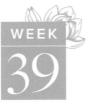

WEEK 39 Your baby is the size of a mini-watermelon, about 20 inches long. Their fingernails are perfectly formed and probably getting long; they may need clipping right after birth.

During this week, you may notice that the baby's head nestling into your pelvis means you have more breathing room, and your fundus has lowered a bit. But now the pressure is more on your bladder (as if you needed more trips to the bathroom)!

Not only is your baby ready to start life on the outside, they're prepared for their first meal. When your baby is born, their stomach is tiny, but that's okay! They have been developing fat stores to help them through the first few days of life while your milk is coming in.

work

Women often find that working gets significantly more taxing during this final stretch of pregnancy. We went straight to the source to find out how different moms handled these last weeks:

"I wanted to save most of my time for after the baby, but I also wanted a few days to myself, so I went out on leave about 10 days before I was due. This was perfect because my son was born exactly a week later."   MITZI

"I worked through but took off the week of my due date, and I was due on a Friday. I personally really needed that quiet and calm rest right before labor and birth. But if it makes any difference, I knew I would not be returning to work, so I didn't have to worry about saving my maternity leave."   ASHLEY

"I worked until birth with all three. First one, I was just trying to save up money. With my second and third, I really enjoyed my job, and it was better than being at home just waiting for baby. I'd rather save my leave for when baby was actually there."   SUMMER

"I had planned to work up until birth but got too tired and mentally checked out, so I stopped on my due date both times (both kiddos were over a week late). In some ways, it felt good to have downtime before birth, but it also made the last week to week and a half feel *so* long."   JENA

Listen to your body, and to the best of your ability, act accordingly. You'll know if you are able to keep working or if you have to slow down. There is not one right answer! And of course, you can always ask your provider for their insight.

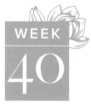

WEEK 40 Happy due date! That's 280 days! You did it! Your baby is the size of a pumpkin, possibly over 20 inches long. It will be exciting—after weeks and weeks of imagining your baby as a garden-growing plant—to discover that your baby is not a fruit at all! (But they will always be your little pumpkin.)

gather

Nothing. Take a break, mama. Consider setting up a meal train for after the baby arrives, but beyond that just relax, put your feet up, and wait.

to do

- ◯ Reflect: Trust your body.
- ◯ Schedule your last prenatal appointments!
- ◯ Work on meal planning.
- ◯ Practice your labor prep circuit.
- ◯ Read chapters 26, 27, and 31 about your fourth-trimester life.
- ◯ Take a nap.

remember

Trust your body to tell you and your provider what it needs.

Beyond 40 Weeks

There is magic
in waiting.

Oh, hey, me again. Not exactly what you were hoping for when we last "met."

If you are reading this, it is likely that you have enthusiastically and optimistically watched your due date approach, only to have it pass you by, potentially without even a hint that labor will start soon. It's like a bus that keeps on driving past the bus stop, leaving you late, uncomfortable, and still pregnant.

It can be so discouraging.

Everything and everyone is ready. Your bag is by the door. You've nested to your heart's content. You want to meet this baby already!

Not to mention, you feel so uncomfortable that it's nearly impossible to get a good night's sleep.

And if one more person texts to ask, "Is the baby here yet?" you might actually throw your phone out the window.

But you don't. You send a polite "he-he, not yet" text back. You take a deep breath, close your eyes, put your hands on your belly, and gently say, "Come, little one. I am ready for you."

Deep down, despite the difficulty of these days, you know that there is beauty in the waiting.

In the words of Colleen Temple, editor of *This Is Motherhood: A Motherly Collection of Reflections and Practices*, "Now is the time to appreciate the magic. Because this is a surreal, intense moment that you only get to feel so many times in your life."

If labor hasn't started yet, there may be a reason for it. We believe that, in addition to a number of maternal factors, babies send a signal of sorts when they are done cooking and ready to be born, so it's possible that your baby just wants to bake a bit longer.

Sometimes I wonder if our bodies subconsciously hold back when we feel as though we have some unfinished business to attend to (more on this in the reflection).

One thing is certain: You will not be pregnant forever.

The best thing to do? Enjoy some abundant self-care.

Nourish your body with decadent, nutrient-dense foods.

Speak lovingly to your body and to yourself.

And try to revel in the magic.

Your baby is coming, maybe even today. I promise you can do this. It will be so worth the wait.

xo,

Diana

Midwifery lore tells us that sometimes the powerful mind-body connection is what prevents labor from getting started. Perhaps you feel as though you have some unfinished business that must be taken care of before you can have your baby. Or maybe you have some anxiety or fear that is locking you into a holding pattern.

If you feel this could be true for you, take a few minutes to reflect on what may be happening.

- Is there a fear or anxiety that is consuming your attention?
- If so, can you name what it is?
- What might you be able to do to address this concern? Talk to your provider? A therapist? A trusted friend?
- Is there an unfinished project or task that is weighing on your mind?
- If so, can you knock it out before the baby comes, or is it too big/overwhelming/time-consuming?
- What parts of it could you delegate to help get it done?
- Does it really need to be done before the baby arrives?

If the project can be finished, go for it. But you are already working on quite the project—growing a human—so be gentle with yourself. The baby truly will not mind if their nursery is not painted yet: I promise! If the task is not going to get done, give yourself permission to let it go.

Symptoms
YOU MIGHT FEEL

- "All of them, okay? I have *all* of the symptoms."

To learn more about the symptoms that are impacting you—and how to deal—turn to the "Symptom Checker" on page 429. Remember, your provider is your first stop for any symptoms that concern you, so don't hesitate to reach out to them.

prenatal
VISIT THIS MONTH

You will still have the regular visits you have come to know and love:

- Blood pressure check
- Weight check
- Urine sample
- Listening to the baby's heartbeat
- Belly measuring and fundal height check
- Assessment of baby's position
- Follow-up on lab results from your last appointment

Now that you have gone past your due date, it's likely that your provider will want to add some additional testing. ACOG states that testing should start at 41 weeks, though there may be a reason your provider recommends starting sooner. The goal of these tests is to ensure that your baby is still happy and healthy inside and that your placenta is able to keep up with the demands of an advanced pregnancy.

Here's what you can expect:

- Nonstress test (NST; see page 457)
- Ultrasound, which can provide several pieces of information:
  - Ensuring that the baby is still head down (cephalic)
  - Estimating the size of the baby (remember, this can be quite inaccurate

at this stage in pregnancy; see "Big Babies" on page 213)

- ○ Checking the amount of amniotic fluid (see "Amniotic Fluid Index (AFI) and Maximum Vertical Pocket (MVP)" on page 454)
- Biophysical profile (BPP) (see page 454)

WAYS TO GET LABOR GOING AT HOME

Please check with your provider before trying any of the following methods. You may have specific circumstances that would make them unsafe for you and your baby. It's also important to note that it is hard to study these ideas, so very little has actually been proven to be safe and effective.

PREGNANCY TRADITION IN JUDAISM

Worry about pregnancy and its outcomes has motivated cultural traditions since the beginning of history. Sometimes these become superstitions. For example, many observant Jewish people never congratulate a woman upon learning that she's pregnant, but instead tell her *"b'sha'ah tovah!"* Translated as "in a good hour," this saying expresses the hope that the child is born at the right time. Some people may choose not to throw baby showers or buy the baby's gear before birth. These traditions seem to stem from the impulse to protect the parents. Yet Jewish tradition also offers an apt metaphor for the birthing process. In the story of the Exodus, the Jewish people travel through a narrow passage through the Red Sea before emerging into their promised land, not so different from the journey we all embark on during birth.

Sex

Although sex with a 40-week-pregnant belly may require some acrobatics, it may be worth a go. The theory behind this is that when you have an orgasm, oxytocin is released, which can stimulate contractions. If you have sex with a man, prostaglandins present in his semen can also help soften the cervix. The research jury is still out on this one; however, if the mood strikes (and your water hasn't broken), have fun.

Nipple Stimulation

Gently massaging your nipples can release oxytocin, which is responsible for initiating contractions. It therefore may effectively start labor—and make it happen faster. One small study found that it actually increased the odds of having a vaginal birth. It's important to note that since the studies have been small, we can't say for certain whether it is safe and effective (the concern is that it could generate too many contractions, which could cause fetal stress).

There are a variety of ways to do nipple stim, including with your breast pump, so check in with your provider to learn their preferred method if you are interested.

Walking

Walking can potentially help with labor because being upright and moving can help the baby get into a better position for birth. Make sure you stay hydrated, rest when you get tired, and bring your phone; you don't want to be far from home, alone, and suddenly in labor.

Spicy Foods

Legend has it that by activating the digestion system, eating spicy foods can trigger labor to start. This has not been proven but probably won't harm you either.

Herbs and Teas

A variety of herbs and teas are thought to potentially stimulate labor. These include:

- **Clary Sage Oil**   While it should not be used earlier in pregnancy, once you're at full term, clary sage can work its uterine magic. Herbal practitioners have used it for ages to induce contractions and improve the effectiveness of contractions in labor. However, it has never been clinically evaluated for this use, so you should always consult your practitioner before trying a new remedy.

- **Evening Primrose Oil**   There's no evidence to support that it works, but it also has not been found to be harmful.

- **Red Raspberry Leaf Tea**   There's no evidence to support that it works, but it also has not been found to be harmful.

Beware that a couple of commonly recommended herbs for stimulating labor are *not* proven safe:

- **Blue and Black Cohosh**   No evidence supports that they work, *and* they may be dangerous for the baby.
- **Comfrey Root**   No evidence supports that it works, *and* it may be dangerous for the baby.

Castor Oil

Castor oil is made from the bean of a castor plant. It has been used to induce labor since ancient Egypt! One method is to mix a small amount with orange juice to mask the taste—which it does not, even a little bit. Blech! The hope is that in stimulating the gastrointestinal tract, labor will also be stimulated.

A small study found that there is an increased chance of going into labor within the 24 hours following the ingestion of castor oil, but overall, we don't have strong enough research to say that it works. It also has not been proven that it does not work or that it is unsafe. Scientists did find that it generally causes nausea. Anecdotally, some women swear by it.

Castor oil notoriously makes people feel gross, with a fair amount of diarrhea being the norm. And if it does work, you are now in labor after having a long period of time having diarrhea.

My take: Talk to your provider and then determine your priorities. If you want to pull out all the stops to avoid a medical induction of labor, the potential symptoms may be worth it.

Acupuncture

Studies have found that acupuncture may help to soften the cervix, and one study found that it did make labor shorter. These studies also did not find any harm caused by acupuncture, either to the mom or baby.

Chiropractic

Some chiropractors use a labor induction technique late in pregnancy that combines chiropractic adjustments that stimulate the parasympathetic nervous system (your relaxation response) and release the ligaments around the uterus and pelvis.

STARTING LABOR ON YOUR OWN OR WAITING

As you can tell, we don't have much research to support the various methods of getting labor going on your own. However, many women have tried these techniques, and many of those women report great success! Talking with your provider will give you the best sense of which of these might be good and safe options for you to try—*if* you want to try them.

Some women feel that they want to try everything they possibly can to avoid a medical induction of labor. Cool.

Others find that these methods are uncomfortable and stressful, and they prefer to take more of a wait-and-see approach. Also cool!

No matter what you choose, continue to listen to your body. If you need a little medical help to start labor, see "Induction of Labor" on page 301.

nourish

Pre-Birth Energy Boosts

This waiting period is a great time to give yourself all the love you deserve. Choose to eat foods that are nourishing and satisfying to keep your body energized for the task ahead.

Listen to the cues your body is giving you as you anticipate labor. Some women may find that their appetite diminishes in the days leading up to birth. If this is the case, aim for simple, basic foods that are easy on your body while still giving you the boost of energy you need. This might be something like fresh fruit (again, cut up at home), whole-grain crackers, toast, or dry cereal. Stay hydrated by sipping on fluids, and rest as needed.

There are often questions about whether certain foods can help induce labor naturally, and while nothing has been proven, it certainly doesn't hurt to try. Some of these suggested foods include pineapple, curried or spicy foods (as mentioned above), and eggplant. While you're probably willing to try anything to get that baby in your arms sooner, there isn't a miracle meal guaranteed to bring on labor. The best thing is to continue to nourish your body with foods that sound appealing and hang in there, mama.

Although it feels like you are going to be pregnant forever, the end is in sight (and so close). Mama, the baby will come.

EARLY LABOR SNACKS

When you have officially transitioned into early labor (yay!), be sure to aim for easily digestible snacks (like the ones listed on page 216) because these will break down quickly into energy for your body during the birthing process.

When Pregnancy Is Hard

I'm not
doing it wrong.
Sometimes,
it's just hard.

Pregnancy and motherhood are piled high with "shoulds." You *should* be so excited. This *should* be the most magical experience of your life. You *should* savor this time because you'll miss it one day.

We spend a lifetime absorbing ideas about what this phase of our lives *should* look like. It can be so defeating when it turns out differently.

Maybe you have terrible symptoms that have lasted way, way longer than they "should."

Maybe you've been diagnosed with a complication that places severe restrictions on your daily activities.

Maybe you've received upsetting information about your pregnancy or baby.

Maybe your depression or anxiety is reaching new heights (or depths).

Maybe family members or co-workers are not supporting you the way you would like.

Maybe you are pregnant without a partner and feeling very alone in all of this.

Maybe every time you turn on the news you cry and feel scared to bring a baby into this world.

And maybe everything is "fine," but you really just don't like being pregnant.

Mama, you're not doing it wrong. Pregnancy can just be hard.

I am, as you now know, obsessed with pregnancy and birth. And you know what? Sometimes it just stinks. It's not fair, and you don't need to try to convince yourself that it is. We cannot control our feelings—physical or emotional—any more than we can change the wind.

And that's okay.

If the world is *shoulding* all over you, and you feel awful because of it, know this: You are doing exactly what you need to be doing right now.

If you feel like hurting yourself or someone else, call 911 or go to the emergency room. If you are scared or alone, or if you just need a shoulder to cry on, please get help from your provider or a mental health expert, a therapist, or someone in your life who can support you.

xo,

Diana

The Motherly community felt really strongly about letting you know that you are not alone in this struggle. Here is what they wanted to say to you:

"The physical symptoms of both my pregnancies were hard, but more than that, I was completely unprepared for its impact on my mental health. I experienced depression and anxiety for the duration of both my pregnancies. It almost sank my marriage both times. And I felt like I was doing something wrong. That I was a failure as a woman for not being able to handle it all better. I didn't ask for help when I needed it because I was embarrassed by what I saw as weakness. As difficult as pregnancy was for me, being a parent is the greatest gift of my life. Maybe the paradox of raising children is that the experience that brought me such misery led to immeasurable joy."   KATE

"I had hyperemesis gravidarum (severe nausea and vomiting) with three of my four pregnancies, and it was the hardest thing I've ever gone through. I found the lack of empathy from my providers particularly baffling. I want other mamas to know that it really *is* as hard as it feels. It's okay for a pregnant woman to dramatically 'lower' her expectations of herself during this time (survival is enough), and to request help in every possible way from her village. She won't feel this way forever, but survival mentality (and a recognition that it really is as hard as it feels) was key. I slept for almost 2 months straight in order to get through it. Medication helped, too."   ELIZABETH

"For most of my second pregnancy, we thought my daughter had Turner syndrome. While physically the pregnancy was a breeze (easier than my first, even though I had a 2-year-old running around at home and was working full-time), emotionally I was a wreck. I cried a lot, prayed a lot, and had a very hard time focusing and being excited about my baby. Basically, I felt like I was robbed of what should have been one of the most joyful times in life. Instead of feeling that joy, I felt a lot of fear and anxiety."
KATIE

"I wouldn't label my pregnancy as difficult. I didn't have anything like gestational diabetes or preeclampsia or anything, but it was not the sexy and magical experience I had expected either. It started with all-day sickness and debilitating fatigue, which got promoted to swelling and carpal tunnel, plus a few others. My biggest piece of advice is to share and ask for help. The more I spoke about my challenges, the more I found other women had similar experiences. It seems this storybook notion of pregnancy is not as common as we might believe, largely due to women suffering in silence."   LIZ

INCORPORATING MINDFULNESS INTO YOUR PREGNANCY

I wrote in the very beginning of this book about the wonderful benefits of mindfulness for your well-being. But sometimes we all need reminders, and this is a great time to nudge.

Remember how research is now suggesting that mindfulness can help with difficult aspects of our lives? When you cultivate moment-to-moment awareness of your thoughts and environment, you can keep your stress and negative emotions at bay, even during pregnancy. Pregnant women who have completed mindfulness trainings say that the practice allows them to struggle less and accept the situations they find themselves in more easily. They frequently pause throughout the day to stop and breathe, and they act less out of anger and more out of conscious intent.

Mindfulness doesn't have to involve meditation, and it doesn't have to take any extra time. It's more about staying present, noticing everything that happens, and not rushing to judge it. When you deliberately pay attention—while eating breakfast, while getting dressed, while walking to the bus— you can see that there are fluctuations in your mood or your energy levels. And you can reliably note that the sensations in your body and the thoughts you entertain are *always* changing. By calmly letting all these feelings and observations go, while staying rooted in the now, you can counter the more negative emotions.

The key thing about mindfulness, though, is that you have to practice it, just like any other skill. Just reading about it won't provide any benefits, unfortunately. So, look for other books, apps, and online tools to get started with your practice. Some hospitals and birth centers also have in-person childbirth education classes that teach mindfulness training, with sliding-fee scales.

Mindfulness will allow you to focus on the parts of your life that are working well and will diminish the attention you pay to the tough parts. Starting a mindfulness practice in pregnancy is actually the perfect time because you've already got a teacher! (*Psst: It's your baby!*) When you allow your baby to prompt you into paying attention, this is a pattern that will serve you well as a mom. Feel a kick? Focus on the baby for a few breaths. Envelop them in love and just be with your baby.

remember

I want you to know that while pregnancy is an important time, it is not the *only* time. It is just the beginning. Of course, you need to make good choices and be as healthy as possible. That your journey has gotten off to a rough start does not mean that it will always be like this. I know so many women who really do not enjoy pregnancy, yet they adore motherhood. This is a season, and it will pass. Your baby knows you love them (even if you complain about pregnancy), and ultimately that is what matters.

PART III

Giving Birth

DEAR MAMA,

Envisioning, founding, and nurturing Motherly has been one of the greatest honors of our lives. Seeing our dream become a reality is more breathtaking than we can describe.

But the real honor of it all comes from going deep into motherhood with the mamas who are in it—like you. Never is this more apparent than in the moment of birth (and adoption and gestational carriers/carrying, of course).

Just the idea of giving birth to another human being can be incredibly overwhelming—not to mention the fact that it often doesn't happen at a planned date or time! No matter how much you try to prepare, how many times you've given birth, or the number of Hollywood depictions you've seen, each birth experience is completely unique, intense, and awe-inspiring in its own way—and absolutely nothing can compare.

Mama, you are ready. You have prepared (even if you skipped over some chapters, even if you don't have your hospital bag packed yet—we totally get it). You have taken care of yourself (and therefore, your baby) and have imagined the emotions you'll experience when you see your baby's sweet face for the very first time. (Best. Feeling. Ever.) You may have even considered all the ways your life will change. And now, it's time.

Each contraction or each step of your C-section is another progression in your journey to becoming mama. You cannot anticipate everything that will happen (welcome to motherhood), but know this: being present in each moment along the way is all you need to do. These new experiences and milestones—from feeling the first "real" contraction or seeing your baby lifted over the C-section drape, to your first sleepless night with your little one—they are teaching you and forming you into a mother. You don't need to know exactly what will happen as you bring your baby into the world. You don't even need to know what you're doing. (Spoiler alert: none of us do, at first.) You just need to show up and be your glorious, powerful self.

As your baby's birth day draws near, remember this: Your baby is incredibly important, but mama, you are still at the center of this experience. So as your pregnancy culminates into one of the most epic accomplishments of your life, remember that your wants and needs matter. Advocate for yourself, surround yourself with a support squad, and believe in the inspiring woman you are within.

You have done the work, and now, it is time. We are cheering for you (can you hear us now!?) and cannot wait for you to fully understand just how powerful you are. You've got this.

xo,

Jill + Liz

Going into Labor

I've got this.

I want to mention an idea that might be on your mind right now. It's the oh-so-disappointing occasion of "false labor." False labor is when your Braxton-Hicks contractions are intense enough to make you (and your provider) think that labor has begun. However, these contractions are not dilating or effacing your cervix, which means you're not in "real" labor.

Before we begin, I am not a fan of the word "false." I prefer to call it "practice labor."

Toward the end of your pregnancy, it is possible that you will experience contractions that make you think—and feel—like you are in labor.

They may be uncomfortable and frequent enough that you head to your birthing place, thinking that surely labor has begun. But when you arrive, you are told that those contractions you had were not "real" contractions, and it was just a case of "practice labor." And mama, it can feel so discouraging.

One way to tell the difference between practice and real labor is that real labor contractions will not stop if you lie down or switch positions, while practice labor might. If you're not sure, try changing up your position. And remember, you can always call your provider for guidance.

A few things to keep in mind with "practice labor":

- What you feel is most certainly real; you are not making it up. It's just that the contractions you are having are not the type that cause your cervix to start to change, as they will when you are in real labor.
- Again, instead of thinking of it as "false labor," try to think of this as practice. You and your baby are doing a practice run of what will happen when you are actually in labor.
- This is a good sign that labor may be happening soon. So, try to practice extra self-care. Take a relaxing shower, have a delicious meal, take a nap, and stay hydrated.
- "Practice labor" often happens when women are dehydrated. The uterus gets irritable and starts having more Braxton-Hicks contractions. Make sure you are drinking at least ten glasses, 80 ounces, of water and fluid per day.

And hang in there. You're going to be meeting your baby very soon.

xo,

Diana

DUE DATES

Let's start by revisiting due dates—in other words, educated guess dates. The estimated due date (EDD) is calculated to be 280 days after the first day of your last menstrual period (LMP). This is the 40-week mark (which you have been working toward so beautifully). However, there are some other milestones to be aware of:

- At 37 weeks, your pregnancy is considered early term.
- At 39 weeks, your pregnancy is full term.
- At 41 weeks, your pregnancy is late term. You have gone past your due date.
- At 42 weeks, your pregnancy is postterm. Your pregnancy is now considered prolonged.

Only 4 percent of women have their babies on their due date. If this is your second time giving birth, you are more likely to give birth closer to your due date.

Most women will go past their due date. In fact, studies have found that 40 weeks and 3 days or 40 weeks and 5 days may be a more appropriate estimate.

You may be more likely to go past your due date if:

- Your first pregnancy went past your due date
- You have a sister who went past her due date

The bottom line is, you are *totally* allowed to be frustrated if your due date comes and goes without a baby. I may have sobbed both times this happened to me. I just hit that point where I was *so ready* to be done being pregnant and to have my baby in my arms. The important thing to remember is that passing your due date is normal, and even expected. So, brew yourself some tea, read chapter 15, "Beyond 40 Weeks," and hang in there. Your baby will come. I promise.

SIGNS THAT LABOR MAY BE APPROACHING

Remember that you do not have to figure out on your own if you're in labor. Your provider has a way for you to reach them at any time, so they can help guide you through this: when to leave for your birthing place, if applicable, and what to do to best take care of yourself and your baby in the meantime.

Nesting

Although it may sound like an old wives' tale, nesting is scientifically validated. A study found that as due dates approached, women tended to focus on preparing their environments for the arrival of a baby and were more selective about with whom they spent time.

You may find that sometime in your third trimester, or maybe even earlier, you get a sudden burst of energy that has you cleaning, organizing, and well, prepping your nest. Unfortunately, there is not an exact science to the timing of it. Nesting can happen days or weeks before the big day arrives. But it can be a great reminder that labor will come.

"I woke up super-early one morning (not by choice) around 34 weeks and had the sudden urge to clean out my entire fridge. Cleaned it top to bottom! And the day before I went to the hospital, I reorganized my entire pantry." BRITTANY

"I took a toothbrush to the grout in our shower one day about 3 weeks before my little one was born. I had *never* done that before! I felt so ridiculous but couldn't stop myself!" JENA

"Not so much on the cleaning the whole house side, but more of making sure the crib was set up, the clothes were washed and hung, and our hospital bags were packed months before I was due. I knew that at any moment it could be time to go, so I wanted to be extra prepared. And I'm not like that usually, so I know it was the mother inside me preparing." JULI

Psst: If the nesting bug does not hit you, don't worry. Just enjoy the time to relax.

Whatever you do, remember to stay safe: no inhaling nasty cleaning chemicals or climbing to the top of a ladder to dust the ceiling fans, please. And try not to expend all your energy. You may be going into labor very soon, and you'll need that fervor for birth.

Lightening

At some point toward the end of your pregnancy, your baby may drop lower in your pelvis. This is called lightening because many women feel much lighter after this happens (hooray!), though if you notice when it's occurring, sometimes it's uncomfortable momentarily. Afterward, your baby and uterus will be putting less pressure against your diaphragm, which means easier breathing for you. The downside is that you may have to pee even more (like that's possible, right?) with more pressure on your bladder.

Losing Your Mucus Plug

During pregnancy, a plug of mucus forms inside the top side of your cervix. It protects your baby by blocking bacteria that may travel up your cervix and into your uterus. As your cervix begins to soften for labor, your mucus plug may drop out. Don't worry. It doesn't hurt.

The mucus plug looks just like what you'd find on a tissue after blowing your nose when you have a cold, plus perhaps a few streaks of blood in it. This is sometimes called bloody show. If there is a teaspoon or more of blood, call your doctor or midwife right away.

As with the other signs listed above, there's no clear-cut answer for how long after you lose your mucus plug labor will start. Some women lose it weeks before labor, while others lose it once they've already started contracting. You might not even notice that it came out. The good news is that the process is moving in the right direction.

Diarrhea

Prostaglandins are hormones that help soften the cervix for labor, which is quite helpful. The nuisance side of prostaglandins is that they can cause diarrhea, which you may experience in the hours leading up to labor.

If you do have diarrhea, staying hydrated is vital. Be sure to drink at least ten cups, or 80 ounces, of fluid every 24 hours, and call your provider if you can't seem to retain the fluid.

Backache

Your back may ache in early labor. Sometimes early labor contractions (more on those in a minute) can be felt starting in the lower back and radiating or wrapping forward toward your lower belly. Think of these as a hug—much like the ones your toddler will be embracing you with before you know it.

Asking your partner or a friend to rub your back—with hands or a foam roller—can provide relief. Consider sitting on your birth ball and doing hip circles to help open up your pelvis and to encourage your baby to move into a good position for birth. Applying heat in the form of a warm compress, a hot water bottle, or a stream of water from the shower can also really help. Keep the temperature warm, not hot, to avoid overheating.

Water Breaking

You've likely heard the term "water breaking," which refers to when the thin membranes of the amniotic sac open and the amniotic fluid comes out. This is also called membrane rupture or water releasing. The words "breaking" and "rupture" sound scary, but rest assured, it is entirely normal, and it does not hurt because there are no nerves in your membranes.

The point at which your water will break during labor is a mystery! For about 10 percent of women with full-term pregnancies, it will happen before labor starts. This is called prelabor rupture of membranes (PROM). Of note, over 75 percent of women with PROM will go into labor within 24 hours of their water breaking, which is why we don't always swoop in to induce right away. If your water breaks before your pregnancy is full term, it is called preterm prelabor rupture of membranes (PPROM) (see page 467). In either case, your water may break when you are sitting on the toilet, lying in bed, or—my biggest worry when I was pregnant and living in New York City—on the subway. (And don't worry if it does! Your fellow commuters will have a story to tell for the rest of their lives, and they'll love you for it.)

Of the 90 percent of women who don't experience PROM, 89.9999 percent will have their water break while they are in labor. It may occur with a contraction, between contractions, or while pushing, or it may be done by your midwife or doctor in a procedure called artificial rupture of membranes (for more info on this, see "Artificial Rupture of Membranes (AROM)" on page 303).

So, what about the other 0.0001 percent? Their babies win cool-entry awards by being born "en caul," or entirely inside their amniotic sacs, which is exceedingly rare. Once the baby and the sac have been delivered, the provider makes a little opening in the sac and takes the baby out. (By the way, the very first baby I caught by myself was en caul—to date still one of the coolest experiences ever.)

When your water breaks, you'll either notice a big gush of fluid (which looks and feels a lot like peeing on yourself), or a slow and steady trickle. The trickle may be harder to detect because it can be subtle, especially because there is a lot of vaginal moisture happening at the end of pregnancy. If you are unsure, place a pad in your underwear. Lie down for 10 minutes and then stand up. If you have a small gush of fluid, it's likely your amniotic fluid.

And if you're still not sure, that's completely okay and quite common! Your provider can help you figure it out over the phone, or you can visit them for a quick and painless swab test to see if it is in fact amniotic fluid leaking out.

When your water breaks, there are a few things you'll need to report to your care provider. You can remember by thinking about the acronym TACO. (And why not have a taco while you're at it? Spicy foods are rumored to bring on labor, remember?)

T   Time. What time did your water break?

A   Amount. How much amniotic fluid came out (a gush or a trickle)?

C   Color. Healthy amniotic fluid is clear. If it looks bloody, green, or brown (like pea soup), call your provider right away.

O Odor. Amniotic fluid has a sort of earthy smell to it. If it smells sour or nauseating, call your provider.

So, now that we're all kind of craving tacos, and kind of grossed out by them, let's move on to what to do when your water breaks.

After Your Water Breaks at Home

As a general rule of thumb, it is a good idea to call your provider and let them know when your water breaks. They will be able to advise you based on your situation and the protocols of your birthplace and practice.

While there is a good chance that you will go into labor on your own, your provider may advise an induction. Recommendations vary on the amount of time a woman should have broken membranes (that is, her water has broken) before her baby is born because there is a concern for infection. Your practitioner may advise you to come in for an induction right away, or they may want you to wait up to 24 hours before starting an induction of labor, depending on their protocols. If you are GBS positive, you will likely need to start antibiotics as soon possible (see "Group B Strep" on page 212 for more details), and you will also probably have your labor induced.

After your water has released, avoid sex and don't put anything in the vagina, as these could increase the risk of infection.

Some providers are okay with having you take a bath after the water has broken, so if this is something you want to do, definitely ask!

Umbilical Cord Prolapse

One more important note on your water breaking: You need to be aware of the possible complication of a prolapsed cord. Very rarely (in about 0.16 to 0.18 percent of pregnancies), when the water breaks, a piece of the umbilical cord moves below the baby's head and sometimes emerges from the vagina. If you feel or see something in your vagina, call 911. While you wait for the paramedics to arrive, get in a hands-and-knees position and then lower down even farther so that your shoulders are on the floor and your bottom is sticking up. This will help keep pressure off the umbilical cord until help arrives.

CONTRACTIONS

Oh yeah, those.

First, let's go over what a contraction is: A contraction is essentially the tightening of the uterine muscle that works to dilate the cervix and move the baby down and out. You can think of the uterus contracting much like when you flex your arm and your muscle contracts. The difference is that we can't "tell" our uterus to contract in the same way we can "tell" our bicep to contract.

Contractions are like waves. They start small, build to a climax, and then gradually lessen. As your uterus gets tighter, the sensations get stronger, building to a crest, and then your uterus releases, as do the sensations.

Of note, there are many people who choose not to use the word "contraction"; they may prefer "surge" or "wave" or "pressures," for example. Before writing this book, I polled the Motherly community to see what they preferred: "Contractions" won by a landslide.

But you, of course, may refer to them however you like! Ultimately, it is about remembering how incredible your body is. Contractions are your body's continuous surges of power (and love) that are going to bring the baby that you have been growing

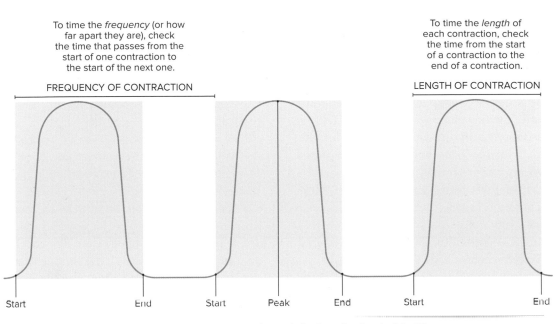

To time the *frequency* (or how far apart they are), check the time that passes from the start of one contraction to the start of the next one.

To time the *length* of each contraction, check the time from the start of a contraction to the end of a contraction.

FREQUENCY OF CONTRACTION

LENGTH OF CONTRACTION

Start   End   Start   Peak   End   Start   End

When we monitor contractions on an electronic fetal monitor, they look just like waves.

TIMING CONTRACTIONS

into the world. It is beyond wild to think about, and *you* are beyond amazing.

Although many mamas will have experienced Braxton-Hicks contractions for several weeks or even months leading up to their due date, "real deal" contractions feel different. For many women, early labor contractions feel much like mild menstrual cramps. They are low down in the groin area, and while uncomfortable, they are not all-consuming. In fact, a lot of women think it's "just gas" for a while.

The situation will gradually intensify until you have an exhilarating epiphany: "I think I'm in labor."

Of course, it is not always like this. I was fresh out of midwifery school and ready for my textbook labor when I was pregnant with my first baby. I went to sleep at 1:00 a.m. after a barbecue. (For the record, I do

not recommend this bedtime for someone approaching their due date. Do as I say, not as I do!) I woke up an hour later in booming labor with strong contractions every 2 minutes.

There is a wide range of normal when it comes to birthing your baby.

WHEN SHOULD I GO TO THE HOSPITAL OR BIRTH CENTER?

This is perhaps the most frequently asked question I get from women who are approaching their due date, and unfortunately, my answer is annoyingly vague: "It depends."

For women without complications who are hoping to have low-intervention births, we often recommend staying home through early labor. You will likely be more comfortable at home, and it will decrease your chances of interventions.

Psst: If you have a doula, this might be a great time to call them and ask them to head over to help you cope with labor at home.

If you stay home through early labor, most providers will encourage you to head in to your birthing place when your contractions are about 4 minutes apart, last for 1 minute, and this has been happening for an hour. When you are home, pay particular attention to your baby's movement (see "Kick Counts" on page 178) and call your provider with any concerns or changes. Certainly ask your provider what they recommend here, though.

If your water has broken, you may or may not be able to stay home for a while, depending on your GBS status (see "Group B Strep" on page 212) and your provider's guidelines.

If you have a high-risk pregnancy or complications, your provider will likely advise that you come in for monitoring.

Now, you will not have to make this decision alone. Your provider will help you over the phone. It is not uncommon for a woman in early labor to check in multiple times over the course of several hours for guidance. Your provider will ask you questions and guide you through what the best plan is for you.

PRETERM LABOR AND PREMATURE BABIES

Preterm labor means that you have gone into labor—with regular contractions and your cervix dilating—after the 20th week and before the 37th week of pregnancy. Sometimes these contractions can be stopped through medication (called tocolytics), and pregnancy can continue normally, with added precautions.

Signs of preterm labor may include:

- Consistent or repetitive uterus/belly tightening (painful or not)
- Lower back pain
- Downward pelvic pressure
- Water breaking (see "Water Breaking," on page 239)

If you have any concern that you could be in preterm labor, let your provider know immediately.

To diagnose or rule out preterm labor, your provider will monitor you for contractions and may recommend an ultrasound to check your cervical length, to see if it is shorter than expected for where you are in your pregnancy. They may also insert a small swab into your vagina to detect the presence of fetal fibronectin. This is a protein normally found on the bag of water that may be present in the vagina when labor is impending.

Preterm labor can lead to premature birth (when a baby is born before 37 weeks). If inevitable preterm birth has been diagnosed, your provider may start a type of medication called corticosteroids, which will help the baby's lungs mature more before they are born. You may also receive antibiotics to prevent infection.

About 1 in 10 babies is born prematurely in the US, but the vast majority of these are born after week 34, when they have more than a 98 percent survival rate. For babies born as early as 26 weeks, the survival rate is 80 percent.

Medical advances are continually improving, and premature babies are having better and better outcomes.

The earlier a premature birth happens, the greater the health risks for your baby, including a lower birth weight, difficulties with respiration, underdeveloped organs, and problems with vision. As premature babies get older, they may have more risk of developing learning disabilities and behavioral issues.

If you are before 37 weeks and notice a tightening of your uterus, whether painful or not, at regular intervals, call your provider—especially if you experience this more than five times in an hour. Many factors can lead to babies emerging early. These include:

- Mothers who are age 14 to 18 or over 35
- Women with gestational diabetes, preeclampsia, or an abnormal or damaged cervix
- Vaginal infections, viral infections
- Shock, trauma, and hard, physical labor
- Multiple gestation pregnancy
- Placental abnormalities

Studies have shown that non-Hispanic black babies are three times more likely to be born before 28 weeks than non-Hispanic white babies. Lesbian and bisexual women have a significantly higher risk of having a preterm baby than heterosexual women, likely stemming from prejudicial treatment and discrimination.

Babies born earlier than 37 weeks may require extra support, which will often happen in a neonatal intensive care unit (NICU; see page 477).

Some issues that early babies may struggle with are:

- Low weight

- No or little subcutaneous fat and underdeveloped thermoregulation, so they may not be able to maintain normal body temperature themselves

- Underdeveloped lungs, which may require supplemental oxygen

- Underdeveloped sucking and swallowing reflex, which requires them to be fed intravenously

Recent advances in treatments for premature babies means that there has been a steady improvement in expectations for babies born early. They have the chance to survive and thrive—even those born weighing less than a pound. Many premature babies graduate from their days in the NICU, meet developmental milestones, and have happy and healthy lives. Your baby's medical team will work closely with you and prepare you for what to expect each step of the way.

You might also want to read about breastfeeding in the NICU on page 403.

If your baby does come early, there is one more thing to remember, mama. An important one: you. Your baby is likely the star of the show right now, but remember that not only did you just give birth, you are likely under a great deal of stress, sleep deprivation, and worry. While you do the work of caring for your baby, please remember the importance of caring for yourself. Ask for help. Cry. Complain. And do things that make you feel good.

It's all okay. *You've got this.*

remember

Your labor story is starting, mama. Take this one step at a time. Breathe. Trust. Love. *You've (totally) got this.*

First Stage of Labor: Dilating and Effacing

This is
the moment
I discover
my power.

Labor is a momentous end to the process that began at conception. It's the grand finale to a biological tour de force.

Labor has four stages. The first stage is when you will go all the way from not being in labor at all to being fully dilated and ready to push! The second stage is pushing and the emerging of the baby. The third stage is delivery of the placenta. And the fourth stage is the hour following the birth of the placenta, in which the uterus begins its healing process and you begin life as a mama.

THE POWERFUL WORK OF YOUR CERVIX

To review what we learned about the cervix in chapter 2, over the course of the first stage of labor, your cervix will:

- Soften
- Efface (shorten/thin) from 0 to 100 percent
- Dilate (open) from 0 to 10 centimeters

Review the diagram "The Cervix in Labor" on page 29 for a refresher on what this process looks like.

During the first stage of labor your baby will also move lower down into your pelvis. All of this awesomeness is happening in response to your contractions.

ANTICIPATING THE TIMING

The first stage is almost always the longest of the three main stages of labor. If this is your first baby, the average length of the first stage of labor is around 12 to 20 hours. (If it's your second baby or beyond, this tends to be shorter.) It is not uncommon for labors to be much longer than this, and occasionally they are much shorter.

Studies have found that the length of time for labor varies based on certain factors. It decreases with increasing maternal age. It can vary depending on the mother's ethnicity. For example, a study found that black women tend to have a shorter pushing stage. Women with a higher body mass index have been found to have a longer initial phase of labor.

In the middle of the twentieth century, a doctor named Emanuel Friedman studied the course of labor to determine how long labor "should" take. His research led to a famous and widely used chart known as Friedman's Curve. This curve shows that women having their first babies should dilate no slower than 1.2 centimeters per hour between 4 to 9 centimeters (during active labor). Slower labors, according to Friedman, were an indication that something was wrong, which meant that intervention, like Cesarean section, was necessary.

The problem: His study included 500 Caucasian women from the same hospital in the US. And 70 percent of these women were between the ages of 20 and 30, while 95 percent were sedated using "twilight sleep."

Friedman's study was not exactly generalizable. The bigger problem is that we've been using the findings of his research for more than 50 years.

The good news is that there have been more accurate studies that point to an essential finding: You have more time.

Recent research suggests that for low-risk women having their first babies, labor can still be considered normal if you are dilating at 0.6 centimeters per hour or faster during active labor, as long as everything is progressing well, and baby and mama are fine and showing no signs of stress. That is substantially more time (in fact, it's twice as much!). In 2010, Jun Zhang and colleagues reported exciting new findings that it can be very normal for a woman to dilate quite slowly before she gets to 6 centimeters—and then it tends to really take off.

Why this matters: There are so many factors that contribute to how labor unfolds, and it must be looked at from the big picture. Friedman's Curve does not allow for the normal variation that occurs in birth. There are times when intervention is needed, of course. But research-based care is trending toward a more individualized approach to helping you bring your baby into the world. Now y*ou and your baby* are the most important variables.

Now on to what happens during the first stage of labor, which can be divided into three phases: early, active, and transition.

(Remember that your water can break at any time before or during labor. For a refresher, see "Water Breaking," on page 239.)

EARLY LABOR

Early labor is usually the longest phase of the first stage of labor. It can last roughly from 8 to 12 hours for a first-time mom and 0 to 8 hours for a repeat mom, though it's important to remember that this can vary widely.

During early labor, your cervix will soften, efface, and dilate to about 6 centimeters.

Contractions in early labor may start off infrequent (about every 30 minutes) and gradually become more frequent (about every 5 minutes). They will last about 30 to 45 seconds each and are generally uncomfortable but tolerable.

Most women find that they can talk through an early labor contraction. They feel these

TWILIGHT SLEEP

Way back in the early twentieth century, German doctors invented the procedure of injecting laboring mothers with morphine (a pain reliever) and scopolamine (a neurological agent). Known as twilight sleep, this combination of drugs reduced pain for the mothers a little and blocked their memory of the birth. Some women liked this, but it also led to problems. They couldn't immediately bond with their babies, and many of them had psychotic episodes while they were drugged, leading to the general procedure of strapping them down in their hospital beds to prevent them from causing harm to themselves or others. They also often needed to have operative deliveries with forceps because they were not alert enough to push. Thankfully, this practice was replaced after the 1960s with more humane methods of pain relief.

contractions, of course, but they are able to focus on other things.

Early labor contractions often start low down in your pelvis and feel a lot like menstrual cramps. It can sometimes take a bit for women to have the "Oh wait, maybe I am in labor!" thought, because the cramping can be so minimal. A lot of women think it's gas at first.

As early labor progresses, contractions will get more intense and more frequent. You may start to feel them in your lower back and find that they wrap around your belly toward your front. Eventually, you will feel them in your whole belly (your whole uterus).

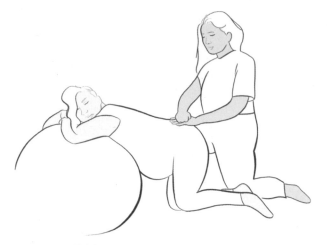

BACK LABOR SACRUM PRESS

This first phase of labor is exciting and even energizing. Things are happening, but it's bearable. You'll have a lot of adrenaline pumping through you, which may give you butterflies in your tummy. After all, you are about to meet the love of your life!

Steps to Take in Early Labor
Call your provider (**according to the plan you established with them**). It may not be time to head to your birthing place yet or to have your midwife come to you, but it's always good to check in. Your provider will ask you questions about what's going on and help you determine what the best course of action is (which varies from woman to woman). If you get the green light to stay home longer, and your provider has not recommended any restrictions, you can follow the rest of these steps. This is also a good time to contact your doula if you have one.

Have a light meal and stay hydrated. Remember that you are about to run a marathon, and you need good, sustainable energy. Registered Dietician Nutritionist Crystal Karges suggests multigrain crackers with nut butter, trail mix, and dried fruit to help keep you nourished.

Go for a walk with your partner or labor support person. Walking during early labor has a lot of benefits; it can encourage your baby to get into a good position to make labor easier, it can bring on more contractions while also helping you tolerate them better, and it's a nice distraction. Don't be afraid to lean on your partner and sway during the contractions. Your neighbors will love it! (Always keep your phone close by.)

Take a warm shower. Anecdotally, baths can slow things down in early labor, but showers are fantastic. They are relaxing and therapeutic, help with pain management, and will help lull you into the next step.

Take a nap. Again, the marathon is about to start. You may have a lot of energy and excitement during early labor, but see if you can lie down and close your eyes. Even if you can only drift off for a few minutes at a time, catnaps help restore energy. And don't worry; napping won't prevent labor from continuing.

Call your provider again if your water breaks, if contractions pick up, if the baby is not moving normally, or if you have bleeding or any other concerns.

BACK LABOR

Sometimes labor brings a significant amount of back pain, called back labor. This usually happens when the baby is positioned posteriorly, which means that their face is pointing toward your front and the heavy back of their head is against your tailbone. Ouch! Babies can be born in this position (they are called stargazers or sunny-side up), but it can make for a more difficult labor.

If you have back labor, one of the best things to do is move. Walk, lunge, dance, sway on a birth ball, and hang out in a hands-and-knees position: anything you can do to open up the space in your pelvis so that your baby can rotate. Ask your labor partner to press against your sacrum (see diagram on the previous page). Warm compresses also feel great in these scenarios.

ACTIVE LABOR

During the first stage of labor, early labor transforms into active labor. Active labor lasts an average of 7.7 hours for first-time moms and 5.6 hours for repeat moms. Generally speaking, your cervix will dilate from 6 centimeters to 10 centimeters.

Active labor contractions are more frequent, usually coming every 3 to 5 minutes and lasting about 60 seconds each.

Whereas in early labor, when you can likely do other things during contractions, contractions in active labor require all your attention. You will likely find yourself breathing harder through these contractions and unable to focus on anything else.

A NOTE FOR PARTNERS ON ACTIVE LABOR

Your role during active labor is to help mama stay in the intuitive part of the brain (refer back to "A Note for Partners on Staying in the Zone" on page 184), be prepared to guide her through the coping skills you know she likes (and to adjust as necessary should her preferences change), and be ready to act as her advocate—calling her provider, driving her to the birthplace, and so on.

Women often describe the sensations of active labor as waves of abdominal tightening and amped-up menstrual cramps. You may also feel your contractions in your thighs, bottom, and hips.

Many women will decide to head to their birthplace during active labor. The general rule of thumb is "4-1-1": Contractions are 4 minutes apart, they last 1 minute each, and they have been going on for 1 hour. (Be sure to call your provider to determine the best plan for you.)

It is now time for you to whip out all your coping skills from chapter 22. You'll likely want to use them during the contractions, and use the time between the contractions for resting and regular breathing.

TRANSITION

Transition is part of active labor, but it gets its own name because it can be quite momentous.

It is usually the shortest phase of the first stage of labor. It lasts about 30 minutes to 2 hours. This is the most intense part of labor, and we'll talk about what it feels like in a minute. But, first, here a couple of mantras to use during transition:

"It is so intense because it is almost over."

"I'm in transition. Transition is short."

Your profoundly smart body knows that your baby is now very close to being born. The baby is nice and low in your pelvis; your cervix is thin and almost entirely open. The intensity of transition mirrors the intensity of your situation: You are about to become a mama.

Transition contractions are frequent, coming about every 2 to 3 minutes and lasting upward of 90 seconds each. Many women describe these surges as whole-body experiences.

In addition to powerful contractions, you may also experience nausea and vomiting (maybe from the slowed digestion that

happens during labor, the hormones, or just the overwhelm of it all).

Psst: Your birthing place should provide you with a toothbrush and toothpaste, but you might want to bring your own (see "Packing Your Bag" on page 204 for things to pack in your hospital bag). You will appreciate the ability to brush your teeth if you do throw up. Also lip balm and hair ties for the same reason.

Transition can bring about the most dramatic emotional response of labor (aside from meeting your wee babe, of course). If you were modest and wanted to be covered up earlier in labor, you may find that you stop caring now. You may choose to be naked because you are hot or just annoyed by your clothes.

You may also start to doubt yourself. Women say things like "I can't do this," and even "Help me," or "Get the baby out."

Can I tell you a secret that might make you a little mad?

This is my favorite part of labor.

This is the moment where women discover their power. The moment where you think you *can't* but then realize that you *are*.

You are breathtakingly, awe-inspiringly fierce.

Even if you cry, even if you ask for help, even if you have an epidural: Those things don't diminish your fire.

I cannot be at your birth, take you in my arms, look you deep in your eyes, and make you believe me, so these words will have to do.

Mama, you are the essence of strength. You may think you can't. I know you can.

A quick note about the end of the first stage of labor: It is possible that you'll get the urge to push before you are fully dilated. This happens because the baby's head is low (which is a good thing) and pressing against your rectum and pelvis, triggering your push reflex. If this happens, your team will likely ask you not to push yet, which is really challenging.

So, here's what you are going to do: Pull your birth partner close to you and lock eyes with them. Instead of pushing, focus on the exhale of your breath, breathing out through pursed lips. You may find that your breath is a bit shallow for these contractions. That is okay, as long as you resume normal deep breathing when the contraction ends. Your partner will mimic your breath to help keep you focused.

Again, these will be extremely challenging contractions to get through, but you will get through them all!

Now you have reached the end of the first stage of your labor. You have done the miraculous work of going from being a normal person walking around to a fully dilated birthing warrior who is only a stage of labor away from meeting her baby!

Second Stage of Labor: Pushing

Come on out,
little one.
I'm ready for you.

You have done the extraordinary work of the first stage of labor. Your cervix is now completely effaced and dilated. It is time to push your baby out!

The second stage of labor starts when you are fully dilated and ends when your baby is born. First-time moms push for an average of 20 minutes to 3 hours, while repeat moms tend to push for less than 1 hour.

Here is what some mamas had to say about their experience pushing:

"It was definitely the time where I felt like I could do something and had some control. During contractions, it just feels like you are riding the wave of it, but with pushing, I could participate. It was empowering in the sense that it felt like I had the power now to bring my babe into the world." EMILY

"Pushing was awesome. I felt like the queen of the world and the most amazing human who had ever lived. Turns out I'm very goal-oriented." KATE

BIRTHING IN FRONT OF AN AUDIENCE

Historically, members of European royalty gave birth in front of audiences—large ones. The baby being born was of utmost importance to the nation and the world, so births were considered political events. Many witnesses needed to be present to ensure that babies were not secretly switched behind closed doors. It is said that 200 people attended Marie Antoinette's first delivery! (*Yikes!*)

"It wasn't the best part, but it wasn't the worst part either. It felt like a huge relief to be able to push and make progress, but it was *so much* harder than I anticipated. It just wears you out so fast. It was so great knowing that it was finally time to push and birth my baby!" AMBER

"Pushing was somehow so much harder than I thought it would be! I had heard so much about how women felt like it was a relief, and I didn't feel that way at all. It was my least favorite part! I will say, though, it was incredible how I mentally felt so different during the pushing phase. So much more present in between contractions." IVY

During this stage, you will work with your contractions to move your baby down and out. It is interesting to note that, technically, you don't *have* to push. Your contractions alone are powerful enough to do the work of birthing your baby. It would just take much longer. And eventually, you wouldn't be able to resist the urge, and your body would start to push involuntarily.

As your baby moves down your pelvis, we can measure their station—where the baby's head is in your pelvis. You may hear your providers mentioning these numbers during labor. At minus 4 station, the top of your baby's head is still high up in your pelvis; at 0, it is at the very bottom of the pelvis, and at plus 4, your baby is crowning, which means we can see their head. In other words, *oh, my goodness*, but more on that soon.

An important thing to keep in mind is that when you are pushing, babies generally take two steps forward and then one step back. They move forward with the push but then

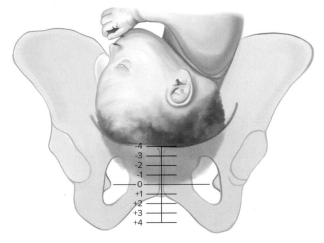

BABY STATIONS

slide back a bit in between pushes. All of your hard work will add up though, and progress will happen with most contractions.

SO, WHAT DOES IT FEEL LIKE?

The urge to push usually feels like you're about to have a bowel movement—a really big one. Yep, as your baby's head moves down, it applies pressure to your rectum, so it feels just like it does when you have to poop.

You will still feel the contractions, but many women find at least some relief from the pain because they are so focused on the act of pushing.

As the baby drops down, the urge to push will grow stronger. If you have an epidural, you should eventually feel the need to push. Epidurals take away the pain of contractions, but they usually do not eliminate the pressure that comes with pushing.

HOW TO PUSH

There's no glamorous way to say it, mama. Pushing your baby out is just like pooping. Imagine sitting on the toilet and bearing down

into your pelvis and bottom. It's the same thing in labor. Except, you know, you get a baby.

All right, let's pause there for a moment. The answer to the question in your mind right now: Yes, many, many women do poop while they are pushing.

As your baby's head presses on the rectum, and as you mimic the motion of having a bowel movement, some stool may come out.

Mama, hear my words: it's okay. It means that you are doing a great job of pushing and that your baby is getting closer and closer to entering the world.

Beyond that, I promise you that no one in the room will be bothered in the least. You will

---

A NOTE FOR PARTNERS ON HELPING BETWEEN PUSHES

You can help between pushes by offering her ice chips or sips of fluid (if allowed) and placing a washcloth with fresh, cool water on her forehead or the back of her neck.

be so focused on your work that you probably won't notice. Your partner will be so wrapped up in what's going on that they probably won't notice either. And the nurse and provider will just quickly wipe it away and continue cheering you on without missing a beat—no muss, no fuss. Never once have I ever had a post-birth conversation where a woman's bowel movement was discussed. It's just so normal.

So, if you can, try not to worry about that possibility anymore. From this point on, you've got bigger and better things to focus on. If anything, it's practice for when your baby becomes a toddler and barges in on you every single time you are going to the bathroom—and then wants to sit on your lap!

Back to pushing.

During the second stage, you will push when you have contractions and rest in between.

A NOTE ON EPIDURALS DURING SECOND STAGE

If you have an epidural, you may not have the urge to push right away. Some providers recommend the practice of laboring down, or waiting to push until gravity and your contractions bring the baby lower down and you have more of an urge to push. Of note, recent research shows that immediate pushing (i.e., not laboring down) decreases the risk of some complications, such as postpartum hemorrhage and chorioamnionitis, without making it less likely that you'll have a vaginal birth. Talk with your provider about what they recommend as the best plan for you.

You will discover your preferred method of pushing, with your provider's guidance.

Sometimes providers will recommend that you give about three big pushes with each contraction. You will start to feel the contraction build, or if you have an epidural, someone will tell you a contraction is beginning to be picked up on the monitor. You will take a deep breath in and then bear down into your bottom for about 8 seconds. You will then exhale, take another big breath in, bear down, exhale, and then repeat one more time.

My preferred method of pushing (when possible) is to skip the big, long pushes and opt for short, grunting pushes that last for a few seconds at a time. This type of pushing means that you are not holding your breath for long periods of time, and it often feels gentler on the body while still effectively moving your baby down.

Some providers count while you are pushing as a way to help you focus and to cheer you on. If this is helpful to you, awesome! If not, don't be afraid to ask to try uncoached pushing for a bit.

As the contraction fades away, you can stop pushing, catch your breath, and rest. During the rest, many women find they like to chew on an ice chip, close their eyes, and focus on their breathing. Pushing is hard work, so you will likely feel hot and sweaty.

Pushing Tip

You may be inclined to hold your breath while you are pushing, but this may not be supportive for the core and pelvic floor. Exercise specialist Brooke Cates advises that a more efficient way of pushing is to keep breathing in and out while you gently engage your core and relax the pelvic floor at the

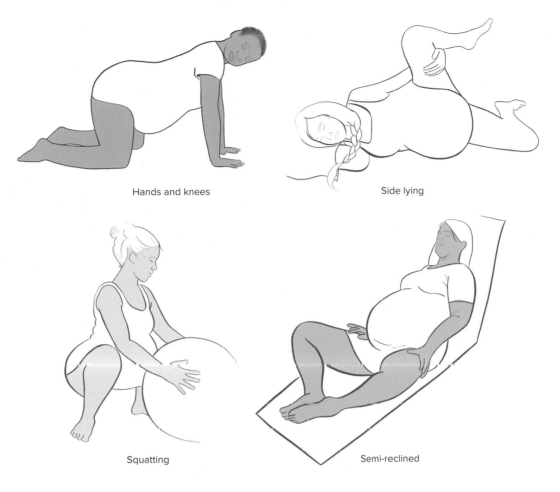

Hands and knees

Side lying

Squatting

Semi-reclined

POSITIONS FOR PUSHING

same time. This way you get the squeezing assistance of your corset muscle as the baby descends deeper into the pelvis. You're also allowing the pelvic floor muscles to soften for baby to emerge more easily.

POSITIONS FOR PUSHING

Spoiler alert: We truly don't know which pushing positions are best, so you get to decide.

Pushing in an upright position (sitting, squatting, kneeling) may lead to fewer operative deliveries using a vacuum or forceps (see "Operative Vaginal Deliveries" on page 306) and fewer fetal heart rate problems, but more tearing (see "Tearing" on page 261) and postpartum hemorrhage (see "Postpartum Hemorrhage: Warning Signs" on page 350).

Researchers have concluded that they could not advocate for one method as the best. Therefore, women should push in the positions that work best for them. Different positions can be helpful with different scenarios, and your provider will help guide you should they become necessary.

But ultimately, it is up to you. Don't be afraid to try out a few positions to see what works and feels best.

This is a good place to note that our "birth preferences" (covered in chapter 25, "Birth Plans") don't always match what happens or what we feel we need during labor. Know that at this physical and emotional peak of labor, you may have an instinct to get in an unexpected position (such as crouching) or that your plan to birth in water suddenly seems unappealing. Changes are super-common, so aim to flow through your needs without judgment.

For example, I assumed that I was going to push on my side, but when it came time, I found that I didn't feel powerful enough in that position. I experimented with all the positions for a few contractions and finally found (much to my surprise) that I did best semi-reclined.

When I am attending a woman in labor, I like to suggest trying a position for about 20 minutes. If the baby comes down and the woman feels good, we keep it going. But if the baby doesn't seem to budge much, or mama doesn't love it, we try something else.

Hospital labor beds have the ability to support many different laboring and pushing positions. They can lie completely flat or help you sit straight up, like in a chair. They have foot rests (aka stirrups), and many hospitals also have attachments available to give you more options.

The bottom half of the bed (the half closest to your feet) can also detach; this is called "breaking the bed." Some providers like to detach it to be able to comfortably reach your perineum, but others will not do so routinely. It may also be detached in the event of an emergency.

Birth centers often have regular beds for giving birth in. And at home, well, your bed, couch, kitchen floor, or anywhere else you see fit can serve as the perfect birthing spot.

Recumbent

This position is also known as lying flat on your back, with your feet in the footrests or propped on the bed. This position is not very common, since it pretty much defies gravity. It can be useful to get a baby under the top of the pubic bones, but that is not a problem most women need to worry about.

Semi-reclined (or Semi–Fowler's Position)

This is the most commonly used position in hospitals. In this position, you lie in bed with your back supported at about a 45-degree angle, with your legs up and about hip-width apart. Your provider may ask you to put your feet in the footrests, or you may be able to leave them on the bed.

You can put a hand behind each thigh and pull your legs toward you while you curl your body around your baby and bear down.

Hands and Knees

Many providers believe that if women were left to their own devices, this is the position that most women who have unmedicated births would assume. There is something very mama-bear powerful about it.

In this position, you'll push while on your hands and knees. You can do this on the floor (with a sheet or chucks absorbent pads underneath you) or in a bed.

If you have an epidural, you probably won't be able to get into this position on your own. But with some help maneuvering into position in bed, you may be able to support your weight and push. Just be sure to raise the side rails, so you don't fall out.

As a modification to hands and knees, you can kneel on the floor and rest your upper half against the bed or birth ball, or you can kneel in bed facing the head of the bed, with your upper half supported by the raised head of the bed or birth ball.

Squatting

Squatting can allow gravity to help move baby into an optimal position. Some hospitals and birth centers have bars that attach to the hospital

BIRTH ARCHAEOLOGY

Based on drawings and sculptures, archaeologists believe that women historically gave birth in upright positions, often squatting or sitting on birthing stools. Rumor has it that Louis XIV, the king of France, is responsible for changing this trend in the late seventeenth and early eighteenth centuries. He wanted to be able to see his wives and mistresses give birth, and this was more easily accomplished when they were lying on their backs. This was also around the time that forceps (a salad-tong-like device used to pull the baby out of the birth canal) were invented, and the recumbent position was best for their use.

bed that you can hold on to. There are also birthing stools that support you as you squat.

Side Lying

In this position, you will lie on your side and lift or scissor one leg while pulling back on your thigh with your hand as you push.

This position can be great if you want to lie in bed for pushing, but it is also used when baby is showing signs of stress. By lying on your left side, baby gets more oxygen. This puts less pressure on the inferior vena cava, a big vein that travels up your right side to bring blood to the heart.

Everything Else

If you and the baby are happy, and your provider can do what they need to do to catch baby safely, birth can happen in pretty much any position imaginable!

Perineal massage during pregnancy can help reduce the risk of tearing. You can do this yourself, though most women find it is hard to reach and instead have a partner do it for them. Two clean, lubricated fingers are inserted into the vagina, and then the perineum is massaged and released by moving the fingers in a U-shaped motion.

In a (very fast) birth I attended, as the woman sat up to get her epidural, she got a strong urge to push. So, she scooted her bottom off the side of the bed, and I got down on the floor and caught her baby.

Once a woman was going to the bathroom when she got the urge to push, so she moved her bottom forward, and I caught her baby on the toilet (he did not fall in).

Babies can be born in showers, hallways, and yes, even cars (but I promise that this is very, very rare).

WATER BIRTH

This is different from laboring in a tub in that the baby is actually born into the water. This is possible because until the baby takes their first breath, they still receive their oxygen from the umbilical cord. Water birth is fairly uncommon in the US but is on the rise around the world. In 2015, 9 percent of women in the United Kingdom gave birth in water!

Women often choose water birth because it feels like a peaceful way to transition the baby into the world and because water has tremendous therapeutic effects for easing pain and anxiety.

At this point, studies have shown that water birth appears to be a safe and reasonable option for low-risk women, in the presence of trained midwives or doctors. The American Association of Birth Centers, American College of Nurse-Midwives, Midwives Alliance of North America, and National Association of Certified Professional Midwives agree that after providing accurate information about water births, clinicians should support women in their decision to have a water birth.

However, the American College of Obstetricians and Gynecologists (ACOG) states that there is not yet enough evidence to say with conviction that water birth is safe, and they recommend that babies be born "on land."

There are also variations in state laws regarding water births and the practitioners who attend them. If you are considering a water birth, check with your provider to see if this option is available at their practice and the location where you'll be delivering. If not, and you want to explore this option further, your best bet is to discuss your options with an experienced midwife.

CROWNING

Just before your baby's head emerges from the birth canal, their head will crown. It is called crowning because your baby is emerging headfirst—or crown first. The perineum also can be said to look like a crown around your baby's head. This is an exhilarating moment. People in the room will be able to tell you if the baby has hair, and most importantly, you will be so very close to being done with labor and finally meeting your baby.

Women commonly refer to crowning as the "ring of fire" because the skin of the perineum stretches, causing a burning sensation. I won't lie: This is an uncomfortable experience for most women. Even if you have an epidural, you may still feel the ring of fire.

As your baby crowns, your midwife or doctor may tell you to hold back on any big pushes and give quick little pushes instead (about a second long, without too much force behind them). This is to slow down the baby's descent and reduce the risk of vaginal and perineal tearing (laceration).

Now we pause to talk through tearing.

TEARING

First of all, can we just agree that the word "tearing" is *ugh*? Who wouldn't be at least a little nervous hearing that word, especially as it relates to your vagina? (Better word below!) For a lot of women I work with, the idea of tearing is the thing that brings them the most anxiety. (It was my number one fear going into my first birth.) So, let's address it now.

Sometimes as your baby's head is being born, it needs a bit more room, so the tissue of your vagina or perineum will *release* (better, right?).

There are different degrees of tearing, which you can read more about on page 481.

Prevention of tearing may be possible. Some midwives and doctors will apply warm compresses to your perineum as you are pushing, which may help decrease the risk of serious tearing. Women often report that this feels comforting as well. Your provider may also massage your perineum while you are pushing. They'll insert two lubricated fingers into your vagina and use a U-shape motion at the bottom of your vagina.

BIRTH TRADITION IN ISLAM

At the time of birth, Muslim parents may whisper a prayer called the *Adhan* to the baby, a tradition that dates back to the prophet Muhammad.

GLIMPSING THE CROWN

As the baby is crowning, you can ask for a mirror if you would like to see this once-in-a-lifetime moment. You can also reach down and touch your baby's head. I did this with all three of my babies, and it took my breath away each time.

Another way to reduce tearing is to "blow" your baby out. As your baby is crowning, instead of pushing or bearing down forcefully, focus your energy on your breath: Put your lips together and blow. You'll still end up sending force downward (and your contractions will also continue to move the baby), but it will happen slower and more gently, which often means less tearing.

Still a bit uneasy about the idea? I get it. Here are four things I want you to know:

1 **Vaginas are smart.** They tear (or release, or give) exactly where the baby needs them to, providing just enough room for your baby to be born.

2 **Tearing is often better than an episiotomy.** Tears are often smaller than episiotomies, heal better and faster, and are less painful.

3 You will likely not feel yourself tear. There is so much going on in those last moments of your birth—physically and emotionally—that there is a good chance that you won't be aware of any tearing that does happen.

4 Vaginas heal quickly. Most tears are repaired with sutures (that dissolve on their own) and heal within a few weeks. For tips on recovery see "Vaginal Healing" on page 351.

EPISIOTOMIES

Episiotomies are surgical cuts made at the opening of the vagina (toward the bottom, into the perineum) at the time of birth to allow more room for the baby to pass through, or more room for delivery maneuvers by the provider.

The very good news is that although these used to be done all the time, research has found that there is not a benefit—and actually some harm—in routine episiotomies. Therefore, most providers only use them occasionally, when absolutely necessary. If you are concerned, this is definitely something you can ask your provider about and express your desire about not receiving one unless needed.

NOW FOR THE SHOWSTOPPER!

With each contraction and little push, your baby's head will move farther and farther until the entire head is out. Your provider will reach a finger in to check for a cord around the neck. They will then help guide out your baby's top shoulder, then bottom shoulder, abdomen, and legs.

And your baby, in all their supreme cuteness, will be born.

Once your baby's shoulders are born, you or your partner can often help deliver the rest of the baby's body. If this interests you, let your provider know ahead of time. I was lucky to be able to pull all three of my babies out. Each time was without a doubt the most amazing moment of my life.

THE MOMENT

As I try to craft this section, my firstborn is asleep next to me—wearing a tutu, arms around her teddy bear, breathing softly—and I am finding it impossible to convey in words the magnitude of the moment in which you meet your baby.

Your baby, who is here because of the culmination of your life's story up to this moment.

Your baby, who is already so unique, and will grow every day into an incredibly special person.

Your baby, who will leave you speechless.

And so instead of searching for words,

NUCHAL CORD

Did you know that about 25 percent of babies are born with the cord around their neck (called a nuchal cord)? In almost all of these cases, it is not a concern at all. The provider simply slips the cord in the other direction or does a cool somersault maneuver with the baby to get them out. In the unlikely case that the nuchal cord is causing problems, the baby will show variations in their heart rate pattern that may prompt the team to suggest an intervention, such as a Cesarean section.

I suggest that you meet your baby using your senses.

Look at their tiny body and count your baby's fingers and toes.

Hear your baby's cry for the first time.

Touch their slippery skin and kiss their birth-shaped head.

Inhale the earthy smell of the new life that you have created.

Embrace your new family.

And revel in the fact that you did this.

You are mama. And this is your baby.

Third Stage of Labor: Giving Birth to the Placenta

I am grateful
for everything
my placenta
did for us.

The third stage of labor begins as soon as your baby is born and ends after your placenta is born. It tends to be the shortest stage, lasting about 5 to 30 minutes.

While this stage is a short one, its importance is enormous. Your placenta has been with you for 9 months with the sole purpose of supporting and nourishing your baby, but its work is now complete. You will be thinking about one thousand other things, but if you can, after you deliver your placenta, take a brief moment to marvel at this extraordinary organ you made (see "Your Amazing Placenta" on page 166).

CUTTING THE CORD AND DELAYED CORD CLAMPING

In both vaginal and Cesarean births, the baby remains connected to the placenta via the umbilical cord until the cord is cut. We used to clamp and cut the cord immediately after birth, but research has found that there is actually a distinct advantage to waiting—a process known as delayed cord clamping.

THIRD-STAGE COMPLICATIONS

Some rare complications can occur during this stage of labor, and if you want to learn more about them, refer to the pages given here:

- Postpartum hemorrhage occurs in 2 to 5 percent of births (page 350).
- Retained placenta occurs in 0.6 to 3 percent of births (page 475).
- Uterine inversion occurs in 0.002 to 0.033 percent of births (page 481).

The placenta continues to deliver blood to the baby after the baby is born, and the cord actually pulses!

We have found that by allowing the baby to get that extra blood, babies start their lives with higher hemoglobin levels (the part of blood that carries oxygen) and less anemia. There is an increased risk of jaundice with delayed cord clamping, but it appears that the benefits still outweigh the costs. ACOG recommends delaying cord clamping for at least 30 to 60 seconds for full-term and preterm births, when possible.

When it's time to cut the cord, you can request for your partner or a member of your labor support team to do the honors. Don't worry; there are no nerves in it, so it doesn't hurt baby.

PUSHING OUT YOUR PLACENTA

Your uterus will continue to contract to help detach and deliver the placenta. Your provider will help guide the placenta out. You will need to give a little push or two, but after pushing out your baby (who is relatively big and of course has bones), delivering the placenta can feel like no big deal. I always imagine that giving birth to a jellyfish would feel a lot like giving birth to a placenta.

There are three ways that doctors and midwives may choose to manage the third stage of labor: expectantly, actively, or a mix of both.

Expectant management means that your provider stands attentively by and waits for the placenta to detach itself.

Active management involves a few things. They might first administer a drug to contract the uterus (like Pitocin, either in the IV or an injection)—sometimes as early as when just the baby's shoulder has emerged. When it's time to deliver the placenta, they may gently apply traction to the umbilical cord to guide the placenta out.

Some providers will also opt for a mix of these options. For example, they allow the placenta to detach on its own but will give a dose of Pitocin to help the uterus contract after the placenta has been born.

More research is needed in this area, but as far as we can tell, it appears that active management leads to a decrease in blood loss for women who are at risk of postpartum hemorrhage but does not have obvious benefits for low-risk women.

As of 2017, the World Health Organization; the American College of Obstetricians and Gynecologists; the American Academy of Family Physicians; and the Association of Women's Health, Obstetric and Neonatal Nurses all recommend active management. The American College of Nurse-Midwives recommends informing women of their options and helping them to make the decision that is best for them individually.

After you have delivered your placenta, your provider will likely massage your belly, which also massages your uterus. I'm not going to lie: This can be painful. The point of this un-massage-like massage is to help your uterus contract and clamp down so that you lose less blood, so it's important. It only lasts for about 30 seconds, so try to take a few deep breaths and focus on your sweet baby. You can do this.

You have choices when it comes to what happens to your placenta. To review them, see "What do you want to do with your placenta?" on page 326.

No matter what your plans are, see if you can take a few moments to look at your placenta and thank it. It grew alongside your baby, supporting them, keeping them growing (and keeping them company). Its function may be done now, but its importance in your family's story is immeasurable.

Fourth Stage of Labor:
The First Hours of Motherhood

My baby is instantly and adoringly attached to me.

The grand finale of labor happens after your baby and placenta are born and encompasses the first hours of your baby's life—and your life as their mother.

A lot goes on in those precious hours. Here is what happens during the fourth stage of labor.

YOUR BABY MEETS YOU

As I said earlier, words fall desperately short of describing what this experience is like for a new mama, and it's pretty amazing for a new baby too. Your baby knows you intimately, but for the first time, they will set eyes on their beautiful mother. Now they are in your embrace, smelling you, feeling you, and absorbing your love. Your baby is instantly and adoringly attached to you.

Birth is quite the milestone for your baby. They have spent the better portion of a year in your warm womb, and now they are here, amid all the struggles and joys that this world entails. Their surroundings are suddenly comparatively cold, loud, and bright—a system shock for sure. Your baby will take their first breath, which sets off an amazing cascade of physical changes (see "Your Baby's Heart" on page 275).

You get the award for *the hardest worker* during your labor and birth, of course, but remember that baby did a lot of work too and will go through their own recovery. When babies are first born, they often have a period of quiet alertness in which they are intently taking in the new sights and sounds around them. After about an hour, their energy level increases. They may start to kick their legs or even fuss. They want milk! This is because they are now hungry, so it is a great time to start breastfeeding if that is your plan. Once their belly is full, they will likely drift off into a very deep sleep, which can last for a few hours.

YOU START TO HEAL

You've only just given birth, but your body will start the process of healing right away.

Part of this healing may include closing any tears that occurred during birth. Your provider will gently inspect your vagina and perineum to see what may need to be repaired with stitches, also called sutures. If you do not have an epidural, they can give you a numbing medication called lidocaine before starting. It is injected into your vaginal tissue, similar to when you get numbing injections at the dentist.

Most tears are easy to repair, and the process happens quickly, often while you are busy cuddling your baby. If a more extensive repair is needed, your provider will communicate the plan with you (for more info on that, see "Vaginal and Perineal Lacerations (Tearing)" on page 481). Do be sure to let them know how you are feeling during the suturing process. If it hurts or you feel light-headed, there are things they can do to help you.

The stitches dissolve on their own—no need to have them removed.

If you had an epidural, the anesthesiologist will be called to your room to remove the catheter from your back. The worst part of this is peeling the tape off your back. Pulling the epidural catheter out feels like a tickle. If you had a urinary catheter, that will also be removed.

Psst: To learn about what happens after a C-section, see "Cesarean Section Healing" on page 352.

YOU MAY FEEL WEIRD

Immediately after giving birth, many women experience intense shivering. It can feel unnerving because often you don't feel cold; you just feel shaky. This happens for a variety of reasons: hormonal changes that occur after birth, IV fluids you've received (which can be cold), fluid shifts inside your body, and the adrenaline response to *OMG, I just had a baby!*

Your nurse can give you a warm blanket, which can feel soothing. And don't worry; the feeling usually doesn't last long.

It is also common to feel nervous at this time. In addition to unusual physical sensations, you've just gone through a massive transition and may be feeling worried about what's to come. Do not hesitate to check in with your nurse and provider, ask questions, and of course let them know about anything that is concerning you.

YOU GET TO REFRESH

After any suturing is done, your nurse and provider will help you get comfortable. They'll (very gently) wash away any blood or other substances and give you a fresh gown and sheets. This is also when you get inducted into official #momlife status: You get your first pair of mesh undies, a new mom's first fashion statement.

Inside the mesh underwear, you will get a big ol' pad (and possibly an ice pack that feels *oh, so good*). You can also ask the nurse for some witch hazel pads or spray to help soothe your sore areas.

If you give birth at home, your midwife will let you know when it's safe to shower. Most birth centers and hospitals will ask you to wait a few hours (and if you had an epidural, you'll have to wait longer until you are no longer numb). Definitely ask for help with this from your nurse or birth partner. Whether or not you had pain medication, you are likely to feel wobbly and weak on your feet, and falling in the shower is probably not on your agenda for the day.

Of note, this may be the first time you stand up after giving birth, and as such, a few blood clots may come out of your vagina. As you lie down, the blood pools and clots, and then it falls out when gravity takes effect. Clots are usually normal; however, if you have multiple clots or any that are the size of a golf ball or larger (immediately after birth or in the following days), notify your nurse or provider right away.

YOU CAN COMMENCE SKIN-TO-SKIN

The newborn phase can be trying (and we'll talk about it a bit more soon). But listen: Skin-to-skin with your baby is one of life's greatest joys. They are so warm and soft, and they smell so good (yes, even right after birth), and it's just the best.

To do skin-to-skin, you'll put your naked baby (except for possibly a hat and diaper) on your bare chest and then drape a sheet or light blanket over the pair of you.

In addition to the sheer loveliness of skin-to-skin, also called kangaroo care, there are many awesome benefits of skin-to-skin with your baby:

- Supports a more stable body temperature for baby
- Regulates heart and breathing rates for baby

> ### A NOTE FOR PARTNERS ON SKIN-TO-SKIN
>
> If mom needs some time before she holds the baby, you can absolutely ask to do skin-to-skin. There is a ton to be gained (by everyone involved), so go for it, and enjoy!

- Promotes weight gain for baby
- Increases the success rate of breastfeeding
- Decreases the severity of newborn illnesses, if present
- Reduces infant stress
- Leads to less crying
- Improves bonding between baby and mama
- Increases confidence among parents

And get this: It can increase the survival rate of very small babies. Oh yeah, and your baby is so soft and squishy and warm. In other words, it's *the best*!

A Few Notes on Skin-to-Skin

Some women feel ready for skin-to-skin with their baby right away, while others need a minute—or many minutes. And that is okay. You have just had one of the most intense experiences of your life, and if you need some time to simply *be* before holding your baby, that is completely allowed. You can try saying to your nurse, "I need a little bit of time. Can I let you know when I'm ready to hold my baby?"

If you want to do skin-to-skin but can't right away (for example, you need extra medical support after delivery, and holding the baby would be unsafe), try not to worry. Its benefits will still exist when the time comes. Skin-to-skin never gets old: Even toddlers and older children can benefit from it. (To this day, there are times when my toddlers are having rough moments that we do a version of skin-to-skin, and it still helps us both feel better.)

YOU CAN START TO NURSE

If you are planning to breastfeed your baby, the time has arrived! Lactation consultants recommend initiating breastfeeding within

the baby's first hour of life, when possible. See chapter 29, "Breastfeeding."

As more and more hospitals strive to be certified as "Baby Friendly,"* there is an increased emphasis on having the newborn remain in the same room with their mother (this is referred to as "rooming in"). In fact, some hospitals are doing away with the nurseries entirely (although NICUs remain for high levels of care). This has changed the way mothers and babies are cared for—from being considered as two separate beings to more of a joined entity known as a mother-baby dyad.

The theory behind rooming in is that it increases bonding and improves rates of breastfeeding.

If you are having a home or birth center birth, the decision has already been made to have baby with you. But if you are having a hospital birth, do you want your baby to room in or be sent to a nursery, if possible? I would encourage you to think about what you want—what you truly want—without fear of judgment.

I absolutely loved having my babies in the room with me. I still get emotional when I think of the first night with my daughter, just the two of us in the room. She lay in her bassinet and gave a little cry, and I jolted out of bed (the first of many, many times as a mom) to tend to her and thought, for the first time ever, "Oh, my gosh, I am her mama." It was so powerful.

But here's the thing: I am around birth and babies all the time, so her existence wasn't a total shock for me. I also did not have a traumatic birth, an experience I needed time alone to heal from. There are many reasons you might be considering asking the nurses to care for your baby overnight. If you had a long, difficult labor, you may need to restore your strength with a good night's rest. You just might not be ready, and that is okay. Ask for what you need. You deserve it.

*Baby Friendly hospitals adhere to rigorous standards that support breastfeeding and mother-baby bonding. For more, visit babyfriendlyusa.org.

YOU WILL BE CARED FOR AND LOOKED OVER

During this period of time, you will receive a lot of attention from your nurse and provider. They will make sure that you are comfortable and will keep a watchful eye on your bleeding, vital signs, and overall well-being.

You should be able to eat and drink normally now (except in a few special circumstances where precaution is needed). Are you already drooling thinking about that postpartum sushi, deli-meat, and soft-cheese buffet extravaganza? Seriously, you may want to think ahead to what you imagine you'll be craving after going through birth. Hospital food is still hospital food, so sending your friend or partner on a burrito or Greek salad run might be just what your new mama self needs—and deserves!

Within a few hours of giving birth, you'll be escorted to the bathroom to pee. A nurse will likely come with you to help you keep your balance. Remember, they have helped many women do this before you, so try not to worry about feeling self-conscious.

You Can Advocate for Yourself

You know yourself best, so do not be afraid to speak up if something is not right. Here are a few symptoms to look out for:

- Heavy bleeding: filling a pad in an hour or two
- Passing blood clots the size of a golf ball or bigger
- Fever
- Headache
- Blurry vision
- Difficulty breathing
- Leg pain or swelling
- Numbness
- Light-headedness and dizziness
- Anything else that feels off, really, anything!

YOUR NEWBORN WILL BE ASSESSED AND MONITORED

During your baby's first hours of life, a few assessments will be done by your provider, the nurse, and perhaps the baby's provider. More and more, these tests can be done at your bedside (or even while your baby is snoozing comfortably on your chest). Baby will be super-happy to have your love and warmth during these tests, and you'll get to have a thorough inspection of your little bean. Be sure to ask if this is important to you.

The Apgar Score

This is an assessment that happens two to three times in the baby's first minutes of life: at 1 minute, 5 minutes, and if needed, again at 10 minutes. The score was created by Dr. Virginia Apgar, a pioneering obstetrical anesthesiologist who used her own last name as a mnemonic device. APGAR stands for:

- **A**ppearance (is the baby's skin normal, or gray, purple, or blue?)*
- **P**ulse (we want their heart rate to be above 100)
- **G**rimace (does their facial expression respond to stimulation?)

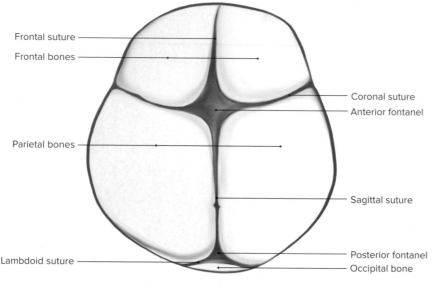

Frontal suture

Frontal bones

Coronal suture

Anterior fontanel

Parietal bones

Sagittal suture

Lambdoid suture

Posterior fontanel

Occipital bone

NEWBORN SKULL

- **A**ctivity (are they moving with appropriate strength?)
- **R**espiration (are they breathing normally?)

Each of the categories is worth 2 points, so a perfect score is 10, though we are happy to see numbers above 7. If the Apgar score is lower than that (especially at the 5-minute mark),

the baby may require a bit of support. This does not necessarily mean that something is wrong. Some babies just take a bit longer to adjust to the world.

*Almost all babies are born slightly purple or blue. The moment they take their first breath on the outside, their body starts to receive its oxygen through the lungs (instead of via the umbilical cord), and it often takes a bit for them to even out in color. In fact, their hands and feet can take up to 24 hours to reach their normal color. For this reason, babies rarely receive a "perfect 10" score.

Heart and Lungs

The provider and nurse will listen to your baby's heart and lungs periodically. Note that it is normal for newborns to have a bit of a heart murmur (a sound in between heartbeats) for the first day as their heart adjusts to its new way of pumping. Your provider will let you know if additional assessments are needed.

DO YOU HAVE A SOFT SPOT?

Ever heard the term "soft spots" when talking about a baby's head? Those are their fontanels! Parents often worry about hurting their baby's soft spots, but normal touching and care should be just fine. Oh, and heads up (pun intended): When your baby cries, sometimes their anterior fontanel will bulge. And if a baby is dehydrated, you may notice a significant dip in the anterior fontanel.

Standard Checks

Your baby's body will be assessed. The team will check the back and spine, genitals, anus, and belly by looking and gently feeling.

Hips and Limbs

Providers will assess your baby for a problem known as hip dysplasia. Hip dysplasia means that the leg bone fits more loosely into the pelvic bone, which means it isn't as stable. It is sometimes referred to as "loose hip." As many as 15 percent of newborns will have a very mild case of hip dysplasia that will heal on its own, but only 2 to 3 out of 1,000 babies will have a more serious case that warrants treatment. Treatment often involves wearing a brace. If the problem persists, surgery may be needed as your baby gets older. The outlook for a normal, healthy life is very good with hip dysplasias.

Your baby's arms and legs will also be assessed to ensure they can all move appropriately.

Head and Fontanels

Fact: Newborn babies' heads are weird. They're adorable, fascinating even, but weird. In adults, the bone plates of the skull are fused together, but in infants, they are not. This is so the bones can shift and overlap to fit more easily through the birth canal. Many babies are therefore born with "cone heads," which will reshape over time. The unfused lines between your baby's bone plates are called sutures. There are also two spaces called fontanels. The posterior (back) fontanel closes first (in a few months), while the anterior (front) fontanel takes longer (about 14 months, but this can vary).

YOUR BABY'S HEART

When your baby is in utero, they get their oxygen from the placenta via the umbilical cord. The heart does not pump nearly as much blood through the lungs in utero as it does after the baby is born. This means that some big changes need to happen when your baby is born to start routing more blood to the lungs.

When your baby takes their first breath, the air sacs inside their lungs begin to fill with air (instead of the fluid that has been there throughout pregnancy). Changes in your baby's blood pressure and the pressure in their lungs causes a shunt in the heart, called the ductus arteriosus, to close. This acts like a door. During pregnancy, it is open and allows blood to flow between the pulmonary artery and the aorta. At this time, pressure in the heart changes, which causes another shunt, called the foramen ovale, to close as well.

Baby's oxygen now comes only from their lungs!

GET HIP!

As your baby grows, it is important to support healthy hip development. If you plan to wear your baby (*yay for babywearing!*), proper technique is essential. See "Babywearing" on page 382 for some tips. The same goes for using a proper swaddling technique so baby's hips are not swaddled too tightly. Ask your nurse to help teach you how to swaddle your baby correctly.

NEWBORN MEDICATIONS AND TESTS

There are three medications/vaccinations that are routinely given to newborns, which are described below. They are all recommended by the leading health organizations; however, it is important to know that you may have the right to decline them, depending on where you live. You can speak to your provider for more guidance as it pertains to your specific situation. If you decide that you don't want your baby to receive the eye ointment, for example, make sure it is clearly stated in a birth plan and that you verbally mention it to your nurse in labor. It often gets done so quickly, and you will be focused on other things, so your preference may get inadvertently overlooked.

Eye Medication

Babies are routinely given an antibacterial eye ointment, called erythromycin, within minutes of birth to prevent eye infections, called ophthalmia neonatorum or neonatal conjunctivitis. The primary cause of these eye infections are the sexually transmitted infections chlamydia and gonorrhea. If the baby is exposed to these types of bacteria during birth, and they do not receive eye treatment, it can lead to blindness. Other non-sexually transmitted bacteria may cause neonatal conjunctivitis as well but are not known to lead to blindness.

Interestingly, studies have looked into using breast milk to treat eye infections (yes, by placing a drop of breast milk into the baby's eye)! The results have not been consistent though.

The vast majority of pediatricians recommend that all babies receive this medication. However, there are people who disagree.

There is growing concern for antibiotic resistance, and some are uncomfortable with giving medications that may not be necessary—and not even guaranteed to work. There is also controversy around how definitively one can say for certain that they do not have sexually transmitted infections (STIs). On the one hand, if a woman is having sex with someone, there is always a chance. But what if she is not having sex and has already tested negative for STIs? The issue is complicated, to say the least.

Hepatitis B Vaccine

Hepatitis B is a serious liver disease that can be short lasting or chronic. In babies, most cases are chronic (90 percent), and of those babies, 1 out of 4 will die.

Unfortunately, hepatitis B can remain undetected, which means that a mother can pass it on to her baby before or during birth. The CDC therefore recommends that a newborn's very first vaccination is the hepatitis B vaccine, given at or near birth. The baby will then receive two more vaccinations within the next 6 months to complete the series.

However, if they are confident that mama is not infected with hepatitis B, some families choose to delay this vaccine until adolescence, as it is mainly transmitted through sexual contact or drug use.

Vitamin K

Babies are born with low levels of vitamin K, a vitamin that contributes to the blood's ability to clot. This puts babies at risk for a rare but serious disorder called vitamin K deficiency bleeding (VKDB), in which they can experience bleeding in their digestive tracts and brains. Without preventive measures, 0.25 to

1.7 percent of babies are diagnosed with this very serious neurological disorder. Newborns are therefore routinely given an injection (usually in the thigh) of vitamin K shortly after birth. The injection gives babies enough vitamin K until they are able to get it from their diet, when they start eating solid food at around 6 months.

In the 1990s, a study came out that reported that this vitamin K injection led to an increased risk of childhood cancer, so parents began to decline it. However, numerous studies have followed refuting these original findings. The AAP recommends routine administration of vitamin K to newborns, but as with all of these decisions, you may be able to decline. There is also an oral vitamin K option that you can discuss with your provider.

Vital Signs

During your baby's first day or so of life, nurses will likely check their vital signs often, especially if you are in a hospital setting. The normal range of values is:

- Temperature: 97 to 100 degrees Fahrenheit
- Breathing rate: 30 to 60 breaths per minute
- Heart rate: 120 to 160 beats per minute

Jaundice

During pregnancy, the mother's liver does the work of removing the bilirubin from the baby's body, but upon being born, the baby's liver takes over—a job that it is sometimes not quite ready for. If this is the case, and bilirubin builds up in the baby, they can develop a condition known as jaundice, which usually appears on the second or third days of the baby's life. Jaundice is quite common: About 50 percent of full-term babies (and 80 percent of preterm babies) will have it! Jaundice is often detected during a routine blood test done in the hospital or at a pediatric visit or by using a light detector placed on the baby's head. You may also notice that your jaundiced baby has yellowing skin and sclera (the white parts of the eyes), is fussy, refuses the breast or bottle, and is extra sleepy or has trouble sleeping.

Jaundice can be treated by placing the baby under a special type of light or in filtered, direct sunlight (keeping baby near a window with sunlight streaming in), for phototherapy. Through a process called photooxidation, the light helps the body turn bilirubin into a form that is more easily processed and excreted from the body. Your baby may be placed in a bassinet under these special lights, or they can be wrapped in a blanket that has the lights in it (often referred to as a biliblanket), and sometimes you can even go home with this blanket or can rent one on your own. You will also be encouraged to feed your baby often, as this will increase their pooping frequency, and bilirubin is passed in feces.

Oftentimes when a baby has jaundice, pediatricians will advise giving the baby formula or donor milk. In the early days of breastfeeding, there is not much volume of milk produced (which is normal), and the medical team will be anxious to see that bilirubin number go down, something that happens faster when a baby eats more. Hence the bottles. If you are already formula feeding or feel comfortable with this plan, then that's great. Carry on!

If you find that you are disappointed by this because you wanted to exclusively breastfeed, consider talking to the doctor about your concerns. Studies have looked at the rate the bilirubin levels went down in bottle-fed and breastfed jaundiced babies. While bottle-feeding did bring the bilirubin levels down faster, the babies in the breastfed group did not experience any long-term consequences. In other words, as long as the bilirubin is dropping, it is okay if it does so slowly.

Your baby's provider will continue to monitor the baby's bilirubin levels until they reach a healthy level. If the jaundice persists after you return home from the hospital, it's likely that you'll need to bring the baby in for frequent blood tests to confirm that the levels are going down.

Untreated jaundice can lead to a dangerous condition known as kernicterus, a form of brain disease with lifelong consequences. It is very rare in the US and other Western countries, and children who develop it usually have other underlying conditions.

Other Possible Tests

Depending on the protocols of your provider and baby's provider, there are a number of tests or screenings that may be done in your baby's first week of life.

Frequent Weight Checks   It is normal for babies to lose up to 10 percent of their weight after birth. Periodic weight checks will make sure to catch it if it drops more than it should and to ensure that they are gaining it back at the right rate.

Blood Sugar   Your baby may have their blood sugar level checked (via a little prick on the heel) to ensure that it is stable. This is most common for the babies of moms with gestational diabetes, but it may happen for others as well.

Hearing Test   Babies will have their hearing screened during their first days of life to assess if there are any signs of a problem.

Heart Test   In order to ensure that baby's heart and lungs are healthy, a nurse will place a device called a pulse oximeter on the baby's right hand and one foot to assess how much oxygen is in your baby's blood.

Newborn Screen   Your child's provider will recommend a blood test called a newborn screen that looks for a wide range of illnesses. Generally, these illnesses are difficult to diagnose and can cause medical problems if not treated early. But there's good news: there are definitive treatment options available should your baby be diagnosed. The March of Dimes lists a number of conditions that can be tested for in the newborn screen (though which tests are done may differ by state), including the following:

- Phenylketonuria (PKU)
- Congenital hypothyroidism
- Galactosemia
- Sickle cell disease
- Biotinidase deficiency
- Congenital adrenal hyperplasia (CAH)
- Maple syrup urine disease (MSUD)
- Tyrosinemia
- Cystic fibrosis (CF)
- Medium-chain acyl-CoA dehydrogenase (MCAD) deficiency
- Severe combined immunodeficiency (SCID)
- Toxoplasmosis

GOING HOME

At some point after your baby is born, there comes a moment that may be the most surreal of all. Your provider or nurse walks in and says, "Okay, it's time for you to go home," (or "It's time for us to leave," in the case of a home birth).

I remember this so clearly with each of my babies. Each time, I just stared back blankly, not really computing what was happening. "So, I just . . . like . . . go home? And take the baby? Are you coming with me? Are you sure?"

It turns out, they were sure, even though I most definitely was not. The person telling you that it is time is in on a secret that you aren't in on (yet): Mama, you are ready.

Ready does not mean that you know all the answers. Ready does not mean you don't need help. Ready certainly does not mean that journey will be perfect.

In the case of motherhood, ready means love. You are ready to try things, make mistakes, and try again. You are ready to seek out support when you need it—or maybe even just before you need it. You are ready to embrace the wildly imperfect adventure.

You are ready to be mama.

Pain and Coping Techniques

Pain is a
formidable force.
But so am I.

All right, almost mama. It is time to dive into the topic of pain.

Pain is one of the most commonly cited fears about childbirth and an aspect of labor that women talk about frequently. You've probably thought about—and worried about—the potential pain of your upcoming birth. It's also true that we mamas have been giving birth for millennia and that more than two hundred babies will be born during the minute it takes you to read this paragraph (*what?*). It's facts like this that contribute to my deeply held knowledge that women are the most powerful beings on earth. We can hear all about how "painful" birth is, and yet time and time again, choose to walk bravely toward and through it to bring our children into the world.

We'll talk about this again, but it's really important to know that women experience their birth in many different ways. While listening to the stories of others is helpful, know that your story will be distinctly yours. What is on your mind right now about birth, how to feel your contractions, what you decide to use for coping skills: yours, yours, yours.

You've done really hard things before—I know you can do this, too.

Mama, if you're nervous about the pain, it's okay. For the record, midwives get nervous about their own birth pain, too. But I need to tell you that part of my deeply held knowledge is that you can do this. Yes, *you*.

So, let's demystify the sensations of labor and birth in an honest way so that you feel prepared and empowered to rock your birth.

xo,

Diana

THE PURPOSE OF PAIN

First, let's address the what and why of pain. Pain is protective. It communicates to the brain that something potentially harmful is happening to the body and that action is required to make it better.

Imagine you've started to wash your hands, and the water that comes out of the faucet is scalding hot. When your skin or tissues experience the pain of the hot water, they release signals for your nerves to alert the brain that pain is occurring. The pain signal travels through your nerve pathways (an amazingly complex web of connections throughout your entire body) to your spinal cord and finally to your brain. When the message reaches the brain, the brain sends a command back to the body instructing it what to do: "Pull hands out of hot water." This happens almost instantaneously and without our consciously thinking about it—and thank goodness! We would all be walking around with a lot more scars if it didn't.

Pain can also stimulate fear and the fight-or-flight instinct that follows—again, for good evolutionary reasons: "A bear just scratched me. That hurt. I need to run away."

In other words, "Aaaaagghhhhhhhhhhhhh!"

In chapter 13, we talked about how the body turns *perceived* threats into fear, even when the "threat" isn't necessarily a danger to our survival (such as arriving late for a meeting). The same thing can happen with pain. The important thing to remember here, though, is that not all pain is a signal that something is wrong.

The primary example of this is birth.

We are not "supposed" to burn our fingers in scalding water, and so it hurts.

We are not "supposed" to fall and sprain an ankle, and so it hurts.

P-A-I-N

We don't like to read the word "pain." As a general rule, we don't like to hear about it, think about it, or experience it. Our existence as a species has depended on developing an extreme aversion to pain. So, the word itself can be a trigger. If you find that you've got sensitivities around pain, know that (a) this is normal, and (b) you have choices to make. Other words can be substituted. Try "discomfort," "sensation," or "intensity." These are words that allow you to recover some resiliency in your response to what you are feeling.

When we polled Motherly readers during the creation of this book, they expressed a strong preference for the word "pain" to describe labor sensations, which is why we've chosen to use this particular language, but we encourage you to use the words that best suit your needs.

We are, however, "supposed" to give birth, in the sense that we have the capacity, and it's a natural body function.

WHY DOES BIRTH HURT?

This age-old question is indeed age-old, and as of yet, we still don't really know. But we have had plenty of ideas.

The obstetrical dilemma, a theory developed by anthropologist Sherwood Washburn in 1960, proposes that pain during birth stems from a combination of humans' unique ability to walk on two legs and our level of intelligence. Bipedal walking requires a narrower pelvis than walking on all fours, but intelligence requires a bigger brain (and thus a bigger head). A narrow pelvis plus a big head equals pain at birth.

This theory also addresses why human babies need so much attention compared to other mammals who can, for example, walk within minutes of being born. Washburn believed that we give birth to our babies relatively prematurely to prevent their brains from getting too big and, therefore, becoming undeliverable.

The obstetrical dilemma is being reevaluated, though, as some believe it is too simplistic and not entirely correct. Researchers have found that having a small or narrow pelvis is not necessary for biomechanical efficiency.

There's another possibility for childbirth pain: farming. When some of our ancestors started to rely more heavily on farming than hunting and gathering (about ten thousand years ago), their diets, and therefore bodies, changed. They began to eat more carbs and less protein, which likely made the adults shorter with narrower pelvises, while the fetuses grew chunkier—a less-than-ideal pairing. Anecdotal reports from history and anthropology reveal that if our early ancestors had not adopted grain-based diets, and continued to eat wild foods, we may have evolved to have easier, shorter labors and faster recovery from childbirth than we do today.

There's also some new thinking about how our modern culture shapes our bodies and biomechanics in a way that curtails full movement and flexibility in the core and pelvis. Prolonged periods of slouching and hunching in front of screens (guilty as charged) deprives us of strength and flexibility in our core and large muscle groups. In nonindustrial countries, people tend to develop stronger cores and flexible pelvises from squatting and sitting on the floor and engaging in much more movement in daily life. A supple pelvis and flexible hips can make birthing much easier.

And then, of course, there are the mechanics of what happens in birth. The uterus contracts, the cervix dilates, the vagina stretches, and a baby maneuvers out. The body is doing a ton of work, nerves are being activated, and well, that might just kinda hurt.

Okay, so now that we've looked at the causes of pain, it's time to explore what real women experience during labor. (We'll do the same thing for C-sections in chapter 24, "Cesarean Births.")

Here is how some Motherly mamas described the sensations of birth:

"I had an unmedicated, planned water birth at home, with 60 to 90 second contractions every 3 minutes for 18 hours straight, all in my back. There were painful moments

LABOR PAIN IS DIFFERENT FROM OTHER PAIN

You may have had a very painful injury or condition before. The pain of this did not let up (unless you took medication), and you did not know when it would end. Labor pain is different from this, though, because it is not constant. Contractions last 45 to 90 seconds, and in between them you can rest and prepare for the next one. This helps many mamas stay focused until the end because they know they will always be getting a break. And every contraction brings you closer to meeting your baby.

(like when I decided to walk down a flight of stairs halfway through my labor). But otherwise, I felt prepared for the sensations of labor and birth. I think that the same contractions can be interpreted as pain or just discomfort/pressure depending on so many factors. I find that I tolerate 'productive pain' (labor, tattooing) much more easily than I do 'unproductive pain' (migraines, dislocated/fractured bones), so much so that the former doesn't even feel like pain to me. Maybe it's the way my body releases endorphins, or maybe it's mind over matter, but that's my experience."   ELSPETH

"I had a 32-hour unmedicated home birth. I feel like I wasn't prepared for how painful it would be because people try to shy away from scaring new moms. But I think it's important to be honest as well. I would 100 percent do an unmedicated birth again, but it was *not* 'pressure' or 'sensation' or my body 'gradually opening up like a flower.'"   AMANDA

"For me, it was a pain unlike any other I've felt. But I was confident in myself and the work I'd done to prepare, and I think that helped me get through it. Having birth partners (my husband and doula) helping me through contractions and adjusting to different positions made it much more bearable."   LAUREN

"I knew from my previous births that I was going to want to get an epidural. I waited until things started to get intense, and then I asked for it. I was able to doze off during my labor, and I think that I was calmer during the whole process because I wasn't in pain. I did feel a lot of sensations during pushing, but since he was my third, it didn't last long."   WINNIE

"I did not experience much that I'd call pain. I called the contractions 'surges' to myself and in early labor, they were merely interesting. As labor progressed, they became more and more intense and I had to concentrate on my breathing and my visualizations to get through them. The only sensation that was painful was the moment of crowning—the ring of fire is REAL. I also had a leg cramp and a back spasm from holding a squat. Overall, everything except the very last hour of my labor was no worse than my very worst menstrual cramps."   LISS

EXPERIENCING PAIN

As mentioned in chapter 17, contractions are like waves: They start small, build to a climax, and then gradually lessen.

While the feelings of labor will vary for everyone, it is common for women to describe contractions as abdominal tightening with a downward pressure, much like a revved-up menstrual cramp that you experience throughout your torso. You may also experience discomfort or tightening in your lower back, hips, and thighs. Remember, the uterus is a big muscle, connected to ligaments and tissues (see the diagram on page 26), so it contracts, and the surrounding structures feel the impact as well.

And now for my heart-to-heart with you. Here are five things I want you to know, as a midwife and a mom of three:

1 **However you feel about pain is okay.**
  It's okay if you are nervous, and it's okay if you're not. We all have different backgrounds and experiences that determine our emotional responses to discomfort, and none of it is right or wrong.

The only caveat I will add is that if you feel like your fear of pain is keeping you from enjoying your pregnancy, or causing a significant amount of stress, consider seeking help from a mental health expert who can help you develop some coping skills. You can get referrals to qualified mental health specialists who take your insurance from your primary care provider.

Psst: Sometimes talking to your provider early on about your feelings around pain and coping methods that will be available to you will help relieve your concerns.

2 **People have different tolerance levels of pain.** This can vary by the individual and by cultural context. One study found that when women interpret pain as productive and purposeful, their experience of labor sensations are more positive, and they feel that they can push through it. Yet when they associate pain with negative and threatening situations and emotions, they are more likely to ask for help and doubt their own ability to cope.

3 **Pain can be cultural.** People from different cultures have grown up with different messages about pain, especially when it comes to childbirth. Wendy Christiaens and colleagues write that in the Netherlands, "pain is perceived as an ally in the birth process. Pain serves a biological purpose and is seen as constructive." Conversely, you may have grown up in a culture where pain has very negative connotations, a belief that is embedded deeply in you now.

In some cultures, there is an expectation that women remain stoic and relatively quiet during labor, while other cultures encourage expressiveness around pain. Your mental priming and social context have a big influence on how you experience birth.

Spend some time reflecting on how you grew up thinking about pain and consider talking to your provider about it. Your medical team has the responsibility of providing you with culturally sensitive care, and this is a big part of it.

4 **Women experience labor in many ways.** I am not going to sit here and tell you that giving birth does not hurt because for many women it does. I experienced each of my own labors as painful.

But I really and truly promise you that not everyone does. I have attended unmedicated births where women told me, in the middle of a contraction, that it felt more like pressure than pain. I have seen women laugh and smile and . . . wait for it . . . even orgasm during birth.

On the other hand, some women are more prone to experience labor as very painful. Rarely, intense pain is a signal that something is amiss and needs to be tended to right away. You can learn more about these rare complications on the pages given here:

- Placental abruption (page 474)
- Uterine rupture (page 481)

5 **Coping methods work, and you are in charge of the ones you use.** In the next few sections, we're going to discuss the many coping methods available to you. My advice is to read about them all, so you are

familiar with the full range of options to choose from.

This is a time to unapologetically focus on your own needs. What is true for you? What is your heart telling you it needs? The answers to these questions matter. There is a lot of noise out there about pain and birth, but ultimately your thoughts and feelings are the ones that matter. Tune in to *you*. The rest will follow.

With these concepts in mind, here is what I want you to know: *You've got this.*

I have not had the honor of meeting you in person. There is a lot about you that I don't know. But I do know this: You possess an innate, deeply rooted strength that will come out in force when you bring your baby into the world.

The specifics don't matter. Whether it is at home or in an OR, whether you choose hypnobirthing or an epidural (or both!), whether you smile or cry (or both!), there is nothing fiercer on this earth than a woman giving birth.

NONMEDICAL COPING METHODS

Every woman experiences birth differently, but there is one fundamental feeling that is at its core for everyone: intensity. Whether in physical sensation or emotional experience, in good ways or bad or a combination of all of it, birth is, well, profoundly intense.

And that is why we need coping skills. Think of this section as your bag of tricks: techniques and ideas that will help you handle what comes your way as your story unfolds.

Coping skills are for everyone, from home birth to planned epidural. Even if you know you want to get an epidural as soon as you possibly can, delays can happen—a rush-hour traffic jam, the anesthesia doctor is with another patient, or your baby comes quickly. And even with an epidural, many of these skills can still be used to help you cope mentally and emotionally.

No matter what your birth plans are, I suggest that you read through all of these methods and practice them as often as you can. Remember that something may not appeal to you now, but it may end up being your *favorite thing ever* when the big day arrives.

Before we dive into the bag of tricks, you must know that you always have the option to *not* cope in labor. The word "cope," I think, has some degree of expectation in it, that you are somehow expected to "hold it together" during your entire birth. And that's simply not the case.

Will coping skills help you? Absolutely. Does science show that these skills can make a real difference in your birth experience? Yes!

Are you allowed to let your guard down and *not* cope for a bit if you need to? Yes, 100 percent. If you need to cry, rage, complain, or all of the above, it is completely okay.

I have studied these skills thoroughly and taught them to thousands of women, and I *didn't cope* for many moments during each of my three births.

A NOTE FOR PARTNERS ON WATER THERAPY

If you are having a birth center or hospital birth, consider packing a bathing suit to wear in case you get in the tub or shower with the laboring mama. She will be allowed to be naked, but you may not be.

There is no expectation that you act in a certain way while you are in labor. Use these skills to make birth easier for you, but also give yourself grace if you need to fall apart a little, too.

It's always a good idea to check in with your provider about the various coping techniques to make sure they are safe for you and your baby.

The Power of Breath

Taking a deep breath during times of stress, pain, or emotional intensity is almost second nature to us, and for good reason. As Brooke Cates has taught throughout this book, deep breathing activates your parasympathetic nervous system, creating a relaxation response in your body. (Remember diaphragmatic breathing on page 119?) It can be so powerful during labor:

- Calming the body and mind for both mom and baby during and in between contractions
- Easing discomfort or pain during the birth process
- Creating a softer pelvic floor and abdomen during a time when tensing up can be automatic for a lot of women

Deep breathing can also help manage the stress of birth. Your body and your baby need oxygen to stay healthy and happy. Your uterus is a large muscle, and it needs oxygen to do its powerful work. So breathing is a great coping technique.

During a time when you don't have much control over what's happening within your body, you can control your breathing, and that can feel grounding for a lot of women. It also gives you something to focus on besides the discomfort. And studies have found that deep breathing can lessen the severity of pain.

When doing deep breathing work during labor, try to breathe as normally as possible between the contractions and leave the focused breathing until you feel the surge start to build.

After each contraction leaves, take a big, cleansing breath and send that contraction away. You never have to have that contraction again. It's done its work, and now it is over.

Middle-School Dance

I know you thought that the awkwardness of the middle-school dance was behind you, but I'm sorry to say it's back (but this time it is way sweeter and just so happens to be my favorite labor coping trick).

Place your hands around your labor partner's shoulders and have them place their hands on your hips. Lean your head against their chest, stick your booty out, and sway.

Unlike in middle school though (unless you were way cooler than I was), make sure your hips are sassy: Move them all around as you dance to increase your comfort and to help baby find their way down and through your pelvis.

As long as you can stand up, you can do this position while connected to a continuous monitor and IV fluids.

When women use this technique, often they decide to walk or pace in between contractions, and then as the contraction starts to build, pull their partner close and start to dance.

Water Therapy

People are naturally drawn to water, and many find that it has a healing and therapeutic effect on them. This is very much the case during labor. Spending time in the water, either in a warm tub or shower, during your labor can be absolutely lovely.

A small study found that women who spent 20 minutes in the shower in labor seemed to experience less pain and reported a higher satisfaction with their birth experience. Similar outcomes have been found from spending time in the bath.

As I mentioned on page 240, ask your provider if it is okay to take a bath if your water has broken.

Birth Ball

Birth balls (or yoga or exercise balls) are awesome. In one study, women who sat on a birth ball in labor had shorter first stages, used fewer epidurals, and had fewer C-sections. And birth balls can facilitate a number of helpful positions during labor, most of which you can do even if you have continuous fetal monitoring and an IV.

Ways to use your birth ball:

- Sit on the ball with your feet on the ground and rock from side to side or swivel your hips in a figure eight or circular pattern. You can sit upright or lean forward and rest your head on a bed or on your partner's lap as you move your hips on the ball.

- Place a blanket or yoga mat on the ground to kneel on and drape your upper body over the birth ball. Rock your upper body or lower body back and forth. You can also push in this position.

As long as you can stand up, you can use the birth ball in these positions while connected to a continuous monitor. You may be able to bring the ball into the bed with you and drape yourself over it as you kneel on your knees in front of it.

Peanut Ball

The peanut ball is a variation of the birth ball that looks like a peanut. It is a great tool, especially for a woman in bed (either because she has an epidural, complications, or is just resting). It can help you to feel more comfortable and can help you rotate your body into different positions, which may help facilitate dilation and the baby's movement through your pelvis.

A small study in 2015 found that women with epidurals who used peanut balls had slightly shorter labors, pushed for less time, and were less likely to need Cesarean sections. There is promising potential in the peanut!

Use your peanut ball:

- In a sitting position, place the ball on the bed and put one leg over the center of it. After about 30 minutes (or when you feel uncomfortable), switch legs.

CHOOSING A BIRTH BALL

When choosing a birth ball, pay attention to the size. Most women up to 5 foot 8 inches tall can use a 65 centimeter ball, though taller women should get a 75 centimeter one. When you sit on the ball, your knees should be at the level of or lower than your hips, not higher. Some birthplaces stock them, and for others, you'll need to bring your own, so be sure to ask.

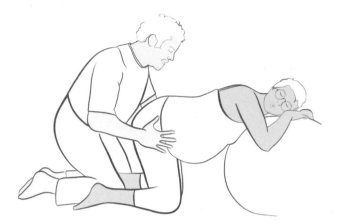

HIP SQUEEZE

- Lie on one side and drape the opposite leg over the peanut ball. After about 30 minutes (or when you feel uncomfortable), switch legs.

Hip Squeeze

In chapter 2 we talked about how the pelvis can move a bit like a clothespin (see "Bones" on page 23). Now we will learn how to take advantage of that during labor. Ask your labor partner to place their hands just under your hips and press inward. This can help to open the pelvis and often feels amazing during labor. You can use this while standing or while sitting on or draping over a birth ball.

A NOTE FOR PARTNERS ON BIRTH BALLS

While she is leaning on the ball, you can massage her lower back or do the hip squeeze (see above) or sacrum press (see diagram on page 248).

Rebozo

Rebozos are long, woven pieces of cloth that are used during pregnancy and birth in a variety of ways to support a mama and her baby. They originated in Mexico, and their popularity is spreading as more and more women find out about them. Rebozos are used to help women move in supported ways during pregnancy and labor, for comfort and for encouraging optimal fetal positioning.

If using a rebozo appeals to you, you may be able to find a doula with expertise or videos online that can offer guidance.

Hypnobirthing

Hypnobirthing is a birth education philosophy that teaches women to deeply relax in order to reduce—or even eliminate—fear and pain during labor. While many women who use hypnobirthing techniques plan to have unmedicated births, the technique can be applied to births with pain medications and even to Cesarean births.

A small study in Australia found that hypnobirthing helped women feel more relaxed and confident during their labors. Another study found that while hypnobirthing did not decrease the use of epidurals, women who used hypnosis during their labors reported less fear during their birth and through the first postpartum weeks.

If hypnobirthing appeals to you, you can find a local or online class to teach you how! My big piece of advice here is to practice—a lot. Hypnosis is not a skill that can be learned quickly, and the more you practice, the easier it will be to get into a relaxed state when you are in labor.

Aromatherapy

Aromatherapy is the use of essential oils to achieve various therapeutic benefits through the sense of smell. Its practice has been around for thousands of years, and Western medicine has started to take notice. Several small studies have found that aromatherapy may decrease a woman's experience of pain during labor, especially in early labor, without dangerous side effects.

Women who have hospital births sometimes appreciate the extra perk of a room that smells less "medical" (though you'll need to confirm that the hospital allows essential oils).

Essential oils and their potential effects for women in labor are:

- Frankincense (grounding)
- Geranium (calming)
- Jasmine (uplifting)
- Lavender (calming)
- Lemon or orange (energizing and nausea prevention)
- Peppermint (energizing and nausea prevention; anecdotally can cause a decrease in breast milk when used for nursing mothers)

ESSENTIAL OILS

If using essential oils in labor appeals to you, start now. Every time you take a relaxing bath or listen to a meditation, breathe in the scent of your essential oil of choice. When it comes time to use it in labor, your brain will remember the good vibes associated with that scent.

To use essential oils in labor, you can put drops into a water-based diffuser if your birthplace allows. If not, place a few drops on a cotton ball and place that on a surface nearby. People also make jewelry that is designed to have a drop of essential oil placed on it, so you can wear your aromatherapy.

It is important to note that essential oils are not regulated by the FDA, and most medical providers do not receive extensive training on them. To learn more about essential oils and to find a certified aromatherapist near you, visit naha.org.

Vocalization

Some women get inward and quiet in labor. Others are very vocal. Wherever you find yourself on this spectrum is, of course, fine. Studies have found that vocalizing can help decrease the pain of injuries and associated anxiety. And laboring women often later report that vocalizing gives them something to focus on, adds a sense of control, and provides emotional relief.

I want to share a quick personal story with you from my first labor. I was in the birth center, about 7 centimeters dilated, and *in it*—moving, swaying, and vocalizing deeply

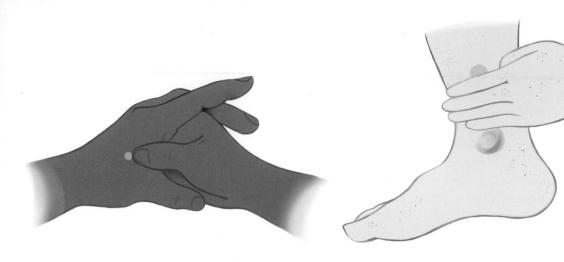

HUGO POINT (LI4)　　　　SANYINJIAO POINT (SP6)

and loudly. I have a very clear memory of suddenly thinking, "Wow, I sound like an animal. I need to calm down." I immediately felt self-conscious, stopped vocalizing, and lost my rhythm.

I still get sad when I think about that. Because the truth is that not only did no one care that I was making those sounds, they probably thought it was awesome. There is nothing more inspiring than walking into a labor room to find a woman who is owning her space—in body and in voice.

So, if you feel called to make noise, do so—loudly and proudly, mama.

When you do, try your best to use your deep, low, mama-bear growl voice (instead of a higher-pitched squeaking noise, which tends to make us tense up). That will help you move the baby in a more downward direction and remind you of the powerful force of nature that you are. You may also find that a calming "om" sound feels right, like in yoga.

Massage

Massage during labor can be just as wonderful as it is in everyday life. It can help with pain management, anxiety, and having a better sense of control and satisfaction with your experience.

Massage therapist and doula Kymberlie Berrien recommends the following: Sit on a birth ball, a stool, or the edge of a bed and lean forward slightly. Have your labor support partner use their fingertips to lightly stroke your back. They'll run their fingers down your spine, starting at your shoulders and going down and out over your hips. This can be done during or in between contractions.

Acupressure

The acupressure point known as the Hugo point, or LI4, is on the hands, between the pointer finger and thumb. A study found that women who had pressure applied to these points (on both hands) for 60 seconds on, then 60 seconds off for 30 minutes reported a decrease in labor pain and no dangerous side effects.

Similarly, the Sanyinjiao point, or SP6, on the lower inner leg (four fingers above the ankle bone) has been found to reduce labor pain when pressed and released over a period of 20 minutes.

Holding Hands

A small study found that when women held hands with their partners, they had a significant decrease in pain level. While the study looked at romantic partners, it is not hard to imagine that this would be the case in all trusted partnerships, to at least some degree.

Music

Many women find that music is a big part of their labor experience, especially if music helps to focus them or change their mood in daily life. Cue up a playlist (or several—maybe one upbeat and one more relaxing) and let the tunes flow.

Sterile Water Injections

Sterile water injections hover on the line between nonmedical and medical. They are essentially "just water" and can be administered in out-of-hospital births, but they do require the skills of a medical professional for administration.

To alleviate back pain in labor (see "Back Labor" on page 249), some providers may offer a series of sterile water injections into specific superficial areas of the back. The theory is that by doing something that causes pain to the body, the brain releases pain-fighting endorphins, which ultimately decrease the overall pain the woman is feeling. Some studies have found sterile water injections to be effective at relieving pain.

MEDICAL COPING METHODS

Maybe you're committed to using nonmedical coping methods, or maybe you know for a fact that you'll be asking for an epidural as soon as you arrive at the Labor and Delivery unit. Or like many mamas I work with, maybe you are waiting to see what labor is like before you make your decisions.

Knowing about all your options helps you be prepared for anything and stay focused on the one thing that makes it all worth it: your baby.

How Pain Medication Works

The nerves in your body are in constant communication with your brain. Pain medication works by dulling or blocking that communication.

Did you ever play "telephone" when you were a kid—the game where you pass a message around the circle by whispering it to the person next to you? Think of pain medication as the telephone game disruptor. The pain message is either diluted or blocked, so your brain does not respond with the same intensity it would otherwise.

There are two categories of pain medication used in labor: analgesics and anesthetics.

Analgesics

Analgesics are medications that decrease pain without making you numb or unable to move. Think of them as quieting the telephone game whisper. When Sally gets the message and tries to pass it on to the next person, she whispers it extra softly, making it harder—but not impossible—to hear.

Opioids, the primary type of analgesic used in labor, decrease the pain signal that is sent to the brain. It's still there; it's just decreased. Many women describe using an opioid in childbirth as "taking the edge off" the pain. Opioids are delivered through an IV and work very quickly. Yet as with all drugs, you could experience some side effects such as sleepiness, nausea, dizziness, and vomiting. The drugs may pass to the baby, making them less

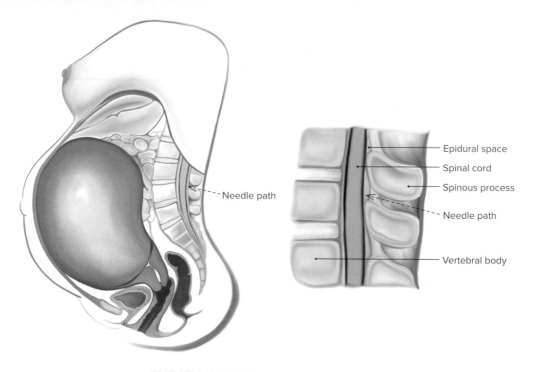

Labels on illustration: Needle path · Epidural space · Spinal cord · Spinous process · Needle path · Vertebral body

INJECTION INTO THE EPIDURAL SPACE

responsive and decreasing their respiratory rate, but they are generally harmless and have no long-term damage. This class of drugs includes morphine, butorphanol tartrate, nalbuphine, fentanyl, and meperidine. Also note that these drugs do not increase your risk of addiction to opioids if you have no history of opioid addiction. But if you do have a history of opioid addiction, you should avoid these drugs.

Another possible option, which is entering more and more birthing places (including birth centers) is nitrous oxide, which you may know better as "laughing gas." Delivered through a mask and at levels that the laboring mother controls, nitrous oxide does not affect labor or hormones, and it does not eliminate pain. Instead, it allows you to relax and focus less on the sensations. The dosage is controlled carefully, and it is one of the safest

comfort measures you can choose. If you feel nausea, dizziness, or any kind of discomfort, you remove the mask and resume breathing regularly. Research has found nitrous oxide to be safe for babies.

Anesthetics

Imagine if Sally (from the example above) received the telephone message and then just stopped talking. She decided that she was done playing, and the message would not move beyond her spot in the circle. Sally is an anesthetic.

Anesthetics work by blocking the transmission of pain signals in specifically targeted areas of the body. In other words, they make you feel numb.

There are several categories of anesthetics used in labor: local, regional, and general. The specific medications used may vary, so check with your provider about what they use, especially if you have concerns about allergies.

Local Anesthesia   This is much like the medication you get when you go to the dentist to get a cavity filled. A medication (usually lidocaine) is injected into the tissue of your vagina or perineum. While it doesn't decrease the pain of contractions or pushing, it might be used by your practitioner to numb a painful spot or to sew in stitches after the birth if you tear.

Pudendal blocks (another type of local anesthesia) are not common but still can be an option. They involve using a needle to inject medication that decreases the sensations of the pudendal nerve, which is located toward the side and back of the vagina. They are most often used just before the baby is being born if an intervention such as an episiotomy or forceps delivery becomes necessary.

Regional Anesthesia   Regional anesthesia numbs a large part of the body, but not all of it. Spinal blocks and epidurals are regional anesthetics.

A **spinal block** is most often used for a C-section. It is a single large dose of medicine administered via a long needle to the lower spine area, and it numbs everything from the waist down. You will not be "put to sleep" with a spinal. Women who have received a spinal block often don't have control over their lower body muscles, so it is not used when they still might need to push the baby out. With a one-time dose, it's usually not ideal for someone having a vaginal birth because the medication will wear off in a few hours, and you may still be in labor. It is a great option for Cesarean births, though, because we know how long

they last. Your surgery will be well behind you when the spinal effects start to decrease.

The **epidural** is the most frequently used (and talked about) form of pain relief during labor because while it numbs from the waist down, it still allows for muscle control, pushing, and mental alertness while in labor. It is also shown to be the pain relief method that mothers find most effective.

An epidural is different from a spinal in that when the needle is inserted into the space around the spine (called the epidural space), a catheter (like a tiny plastic straw), is inserted as well. The needle comes out, but the catheter stays in place for the duration of your epidural. (The anesthetic medicine flows into the spinal canal but outside the sac that protects your spinal fluid.) So, it doesn't matter if your baby is born an hour later or the next day: You receive medication continuously until you don't need it. Similar to a spinal block, an epidural will not put you to sleep.

There are also gradations of how strong the epidural can be and what types of medications are used to achieve the desired effect. For example, a "walking epidural" gives the laboring mama more connection to her contractions, though the name is a misnomer because you usually won't be walking around (though it does happen!).

If you have an epidural in place and then need a C-section, your anesthesiologist can often use the epidural and increase the dose so that you are numb enough for surgery.

Epidurals do have their potential downsides, however. With an epidural you will be hooked up to an IV, and your baby's heart rate and your contractions will be constantly monitored (if they aren't already). You will also likely have frequent blood pressure checks and possibly a monitor on your finger to assess your oxygen status. Most hospitals will restrict eating once an epidural is placed. Since you won't be able to get up to pee, your birth team may recommend an indwelling bladder catheter. This is a tube inserted through your urethra that removes your urine into a sealed container. Another option is to occasionally insert a straight catheter in to remove the urine—the benefit here is that nothing stays inside your urethra for a prolonged period of time.

A large study in 2019 found that women who have epidurals and who reach the pushing stage of labor may have a higher chance of having an instrumental delivery (with a vacuum or forceps; see "Operative Vaginal Deliveries" on page 306) but a lower chance of a Cesarean section. (It's important to note that the women in this study had a few things in common: it was their first baby; they were pregnant with only one baby, who was in a head-down position; and they reached full term. In other words, it doesn't necessarily apply to everyone.) And a 2018 study of 11,000 women found that for women who gave birth after 2005, epidurals do not seem to increase the risk of an operative delivery.

Some studies have found that epidurals can lengthen labor, while others have found that they do not. Historically, we have encouraged women to wait as long as they can before getting an epidural to lower the chances of longer labors and Cesarean sections. However, a recent large review of more than 15,000 women found that early epidurals do not seem to increase the rate of Cesarean births, instrumental deliveries, or adverse baby outcomes.

Side effects of an epidural may include nausea and itchiness. It does happen that some parts of the targeted area will never get numb, but in my professional experience, this is not common. In rare cases, patients experience headaches that can last for weeks as a result of epidurals (this is known as a spinal headache; see page 482).

If you're worried about the effect on your baby, recent studies have shown that epidural procedures don't seem to influence the Apgar scores (see page 273) for newborns. In rare instances, an epidural can make your blood pressure drop to dangerously low levels, which would impact your baby. This is why your blood pressure will be checked frequently.

Getting the epidural inserted can be a challenging moment, especially if you are experiencing difficult contractions. You need to stay very still to allow the anesthesiologist to apply a numbing agent and find the correct insertion spot for the catheter.

For many mamas, an epidural is just what they need to gather some energy to continue the laboring journey. Once the numbness has set in, you may feel relaxed enough to nap through your next period of dilation and wake up just before you need to push.

Don't worry, mama. I wouldn't leave you without telling you what getting an epidural feels like (from personal experience). It is a strong pinch, followed by a burn. So, here's the thing: In a scenario where you have not been contracting for a while, an epidural would be, in my opinion, uncomfortable. However, because you will (most likely) be in labor if you choose to get one, and having a hard time coping with the pain, the sensation of the epidural going in is almost welcome because you know what it means. And it is very brief.

It takes about 20 minutes for the pain relief to take full effect, but you will start to have decreased pain within a few minutes.

When you get an epidural, your provider will likely ask you to sit in bed with your legs dangling over the side, or you may lie on the bed on your left side in a curled position. A nurse or family member* may be positioned in front of you to provide emotional and physical support. You will be asked to stick your lower back out—a hard feat when you have a belly full of baby.

And don't worry; they will wait until you are not having a contraction to insert the needle.

*Some hospitals will ask that all support people step out of the room during the epidural to reduce the risk of infection and distraction. If this is the case, your nurse can stay with you and serve as your emotional support through the insertion.

General Anesthesia   General anesthesia is reserved for special cases, usually for the rare emergency Cesarean section where there is not enough time to insert a spinal or epidural. The risks of general anesthesia include aspiration (when vomit gets into your lungs), but this is very rare.

Women worry of course about the impact of the anesthesia on their babies. In most cases, the exposure time to the general anesthesia for the baby is very limited, so the potential for any long-term negative impacts is small. In an emergency Cesarean section, the medical team is able to deliver the baby extremely quickly.

With general anesthesia, you will be "asleep" for your Cesarean section and will meet your baby when you wake up. Good morning, indeed!

remember

As you approach your labor, it can be daunting to think about the pain that may come with it, especially since our society focuses on it so much and in such a negative light.

Yes, pain is a formidable force. But mama, so are you.

Use these coping skills to empower you through each contraction, one at a time. As each contraction ends, bask in the knowledge that you never have to have that contraction again. It has done its work, and now it is time to rest again. And every time you send another contraction away, you are one step closer to meeting your baby.

Interventions

I am present.
I am calm.
I can do this.

FROM DIANA

Most mamas I work with hope to spontaneously go into labor and progress through each stage on their own steam. They all want it to go well, and many of them even have a plan for the birth of their dreams.

Yet so many factors are at play with birth, and it's impossible to script the whole performance. It's more like improv. And sometimes that means that unscripted parts will play a starring role.

What am I talking about? Interventions. Tools and medicines that can help start your labor, keep it progressing, or make it safer and more comfortable for you and your baby.

Many of these have ancient histories, and some are relatively recent medical innovations. But all interventions have one thing in common: They're choices that you and your providers can discuss and modify for your comfort.

Pay attention to how your body feels as you read through these interventions. Is there one that makes you nervous? Consider bringing it up at your next prenatal appointment to relieve some of the worry. For example, you could say, "Last week I read about IVs in labor, and it made me feel concerned. Can we talk about them? Is it likely that I will have an IV, and is it possible to discuss alternatives? Can we talk through the research on why you think an IV may or may not be the right choice for me? Can you share the insertion process with me, so I know what to anticipate?"

Interventions are meant to be helpful, and it is a really great thing that they exist. But their existence does not mean that they are necessarily what you will need. Ask as many questions as you need to in order to feel comfortable.

Let's take a look at some of the interventions that may become a part of your story.

xo,

Diana

INDUCTION OF LABOR

Before we get into the specifics of inductions, I want to have a heart-to-heart with you (because I love heart-to-hearts, and this is a big one). Inductions often come with a strong emotional response. Some women feel almost desperate to avoid them, while others may get to a point where they want nothing as badly as to be induced. There is also a great deal of discussion and differing opinions surrounding induction from advocates, critics, researchers, and providers. It can feel overwhelming.

Mama, if you are finding yourself swimming in a sea of worry regarding an impending induction, please know that you are not alone. In fact, I have been there twice. I had a 41-week induction scheduled with my second baby, but he decided to come just a few hours before my hospital check-in time. And with my third baby, I was induced, again at 41 weeks. I was a bit of a mess during those times, concerned about the "right" thing to do and trying to balance my personal desires with my provider's recommendation (which was "It's up to you!").

If you are concerned about inductions (either avoiding one or getting one), bring your questions and emotions to your provider. They're all valid.

Inductions are not to be entered into lightly; they are serious business. However, know that if you do have an induction (or any intervention, for that matter), it is entirely possible to have a lovely, rewarding, beautiful birth.

The Nitty Gritty Details of Induction

Induction is when labor is started with the help of medications or other interventions (such as those we will address in this chapter), instead of by your natural hormonal process.

Past research has indicated that inductions may lead to more need for pain medication, longer labors, more interventions, and more Cesarean sections. Generally speaking, providers recommend allowing the body to go into labor on its own, a process known as physiologic birth.

That being said, inductions can become necessary. Reasons your provider may recommend an induction:

- You've gone beyond your due date. Some practitioners discourage mamas to go past week 41; others will stretch to week 42 (and still others feel comfortable going beyond 42 weeks, though this tends to be rare since there is concern for serious neonatal complications)

- There are concerns with your health (that could also impact the baby), such as preeclampsia (see "Preeclampsia" on page 466), cholestasis (see "Cholestasis" on page 459), or gestational diabetes (see "Gestational Diabetes Mellitis (GDM)" on page 460).

- Your age could be a factor. There appears to be a higher risk of stillbirth for women age 35 and older, so some providers advocate inducing to reduce the risk. (Protocols vary by provider. Some may recommend induction at 39 weeks while others may prefer 40 or 41 weeks.)

- There are fetus-related concerns, such as intrauterine growth restriction (see "Intrauterine Growth Restriction (IUGR)" on page 463), decreased placenta function (see "Placental Insufficiency" on page 475), or concern about the baby being too large (see "Big Babies" on page 213).

Elective inductions—done when there is no medical necessity—have generally been approached with caution. Many believe that if your body has not gone into labor, there may be a good reason (such as the baby not being ready yet). Unless there is a medical need to induce, many feel that we should just let birth happen naturally.

Other reasons to avoid an elective induction include the desire to avoid interventions like intravenous drips and continuous fetal monitoring, the ability to ambulate and shower during labor, and the effort to minimize the potential risks that come with inductions.

In 2018, a large, randomized study was published by the *American Journal of Obstetrics and Gynecology*. The purpose of the study was to determine if elective inductions at 39 weeks would lower the risk of serious complications and death for babies as opposed to waiting for spontaneous labor. The researchers were also interested to see if these inductions would reduce the rate of Cesarean sections. Only low-risk women who were giving birth for the first time were included in the study. The vast majority (94 percent) of the women in the study were cared for by physicians. The findings of the study did not conclude that there was a decrease in complications or death for babies, but it did find that there was a reduction in the Cesarean section rate from 22.2 to 18.6 percent.

Here's my take on this new finding: Welcoming a child into the world touches every aspect of your life. If the aim is to increase choices for women and offer holistic care, the recent findings from the trial are intriguing. Women may desire to have an elective induction for reasons that are incredibly important to them: presence of their partner, emotional well-being, and more. In accordance with research, her provider will help her make the best decision for her.

There is still a lot to learn. This study adds to our understanding but does not define it. I'd encourage you to have detailed conversations with your provider about elective inductions, this study, and what it all means for you.

Note that if medical induction is being discussed, depending on the scenario, you may be able to ask for a little more time to see if you can get your labor going in nonmedical ways. (See "Ways to Get Labor Going at Home" on page 226 for nonmedical induction methods.)

Ways Your Practitioner May Induce Labor

When it comes to choosing a method of induction, there are many variables to consider. Your provider will factor in your (and your baby's) current status and health history, how ready your cervix is (how "ripe" it is), the most recent research, hospital protocols, and your preferences.

Sweeping or Stripping the Membranes

This is done by your doctor or midwife, but it doesn't have to happen in a hospital. Your provider will place a finger into the cervix and sweep around the base of the amniotic sac. This will loosen the membranes from the bottom of the uterus and can often help your body produce prostaglandins, which can soften the cervix and initiate labor through contractions.

Truth time: This can potentially cause painful cramps and be quite uncomfortable (says the midwife who nearly kicked another midwife while having this done—not my proudest moment). Feel free to try this (the sweeping part, not the kicking part) and then decide whether it's for you and ask the provider to stop as necessary.

Artificial Rupture of Membranes (AROM)
At various times before (though this is rare) and during labor, the membranes can also be ruptured with a small tool called an AmniHook, releasing the amniotic fluid and bringing contractions or intensifying the ones that you already have. The reasoning behind doing this is that removing the cushion of waters that separates the baby's head and the cervix will allow the baby's head to come down, thus increasing the pressure on the cervix and hopefully causing it to efface and dilate faster. It also causes an increase in hormones and prostaglandins that help soften the cervix and kick-start labor.

Since the bag of water protects the baby and your uterus from coming into contact with bacteria, when it is broken, there is concern that an infection could develop, which is pretty serious (see "Chorioamnionitis (or Intra-amniotic Infection)" on page 479). So, after the membranes break, you have a window of time in which they consider it safe to labor and deliver without intervention (which varies depending on your providers' protocols). If you are still not in labor after this window of time, interventions will likely be discussed.

While providers may use AROM to speed the process up, a recent study showed that, in the case of spontaneous labor, rupturing the amniotic sac does not shorten the first stage of labor and may, in fact, increase the incidence of Cesarean births. So, in a labor that is progressing normally, there is usually no need to artificially rupture the sac. In induced and augmented labors, however, AROM may help prevent C-section. Remember that you can absolutely speak up and discuss the pros and cons of AROM with your provider.

Foley Bulb A Foley bulb is a mechanical way to induce labor using a cervical balloon attached to a catheter. Your provider inserts it through your cervix into your uterus when it is deflated and then fills it with sterile saline. The pressure from the balloon can help open the cervix and trigger the hormones of labor to do their work on the cervix as well. The Foley bulb will remain in place until your cervix dilates to about 3 centimeters (at which point, the Foley bulb will fall out) or until your provider removes it (for example, if it is determined that it is not working). Once the Foley bulb is out (and sometimes while it is still in), Pitocin can be started to encourage regular uterine contractions—more on this soon.

Foley bulbs are sometimes used in birth centers and home births, though they are more common in the hospital setting.

Women often say that the experience of having the Foley bulb inserted is rather uncomfortable, but once it's in, it is more of an annoyance than a discomfort.

Prostaglandin Medications Prostaglandin medications can assist the cervix in effacing—becoming soft and thin—to make way for baby's head. You'll be given either a pill (Cytotec) or a wafer-like cervical insert (Cervidil) that can work in a matter of hours or overnight to jumpstart labor.

WHAT CAN I EAT OR DRINK DURING LABOR?

Some hospitals restrict all food and drink, fearing that you may aspirate (inhale vomit) if you have to get general anesthesia later (see "General Anesthesia" on page 297). The theories that led to restricting food and liquid intake during labor date back to the 1940s but are alive and well today. However, current research suggests that it is safe to eat during labor and that it may even lead to a slightly shorter labor process! ACOG even states that "the oral intake of modest amounts of clear liquids may be allowed for patients with uncomplicated labor." This makes sense. If you were about to run a marathon, you would not do so without eating. Labor is a marathon, and getting hungry is natural.

I will say that most women I work with do not desire "meals" while they are in labor; they tend to want just snacks. (After the baby is out, well, that's when a double cheeseburger and milkshake will be your best friends. #sohungry)

The takeaway: Do not be afraid to talk with your care team about eating during labor. If you do decide to add liquids and foods to your labor plan, some of my favorites are coconut water, soup broth, fruit-flavored popsicles, crackers, and trail mix. Or choose something else that sounds delicious to you.

Pitocin   Oxytocin is the natural hormone in a woman's body that helps start labor, and Pitocin is its synthetic twin. When used for inductions, Pitocin is given through an IV. Contractions will eventually start, and they may be more frequent and intense than those with a naturally occurring labor.

The concern with Pitocin is that it can promote powerful contractions that the baby sometimes does not like (the baby will let us know they are unhappy by showing changes in their heart rate pattern on the monitor that your team will be watching closely). To reduce the risk of causing the baby stress, the Pitocin will be started at a low dose and increased very gradually until contractions are regular. Some women only need a tiny bit of Pitocin to get things going.

Women often describe Pitocin contractions as more intense than regular ones. Many women who get Pitocin also end up getting epidurals (though I have absolutely worked with women who did not). The skills in chapter 22, "Pain and Coping Techniques," will help you here—so much—either way!

Augmentations

Labor augmentation is induction's little sister—similar and related, but different. Sometimes labor starts on its own just fine but then stops progressing (the medical term for this is *stall* or *arrest*) and needs a boost. Usually augmentations are done with Pitocin or rupturing the amniotic sac.

You can always request to try a nonmedicinal approach first. For example, I have had many patients for whom some mid-labor nipple stimulation did wonders to reignite their labor. Walking (especially up stairs), squatting, and dancing can help as well.

OTHER BIRTH INTERVENTIONS

Intravenous (IV) Therapy

In a hospital birth, it is often customary to get hooked up to intravenous therapy (an IV fluid drip) upon arriving should you need antibiotics, fluids, or other medications. This does mean, however, that you are connected to IV tubing and a pole, which can restrict your movement. Instead, you can ask for a saline lock or heparin lock, which prepares a vein for an IV but allows you to move around without trailing the pole. In the event that they need to connect you to an IV, the hard part is already done.

Birth centers usually do not insert IVs, though they may if you will need medications, like antibiotics for GBS (see "Group B Strep" on page 212).

If you prefer not to have an IV, speak with your provider about it ahead of time.

Fetal Monitoring: Continuous Versus Intermittent

Your uterine contractions can have an effect on your baby's heart rate. When your muscles are tight, blood flow to baby slows down, which may decrease their heart's beats per minute. This is normally harmless and natural, but on rare occasions, it isn't.

If the baby's heart rate doesn't recover between contractions, it may be a sign that baby is not tolerating labor and can lead providers to want to intervene quickly to ensure a safe delivery. For this reason, we monitor the baby's heart rate throughout labor. There are several ways to do this.

Continuous electronic fetal monitoring (EFM) is the use of a machine that records the baby's heart rate and the frequency of uterine contractions. Two different types of sensors are placed on the mother's abdomen with belts. One sensor measures and records the baby's heart rate. The other sensor measures and records uterine contraction patterns. Be prepared for these sensors to fall off and require readjustment often.

The use of EFM varies greatly depending on your specific scenario as well as on the practitioner and birthing place. It's important to note that EFM can cause false alarms, and since it requires constant connectivity, mama can't always move around as much as she might like. Ironically, constant monitoring can actually lead to *more* oxygen deprivation for baby since moms may be laboring flat on their backs and compressing key blood vessels.

What's more, EFM has been found to increase the likelihood of Cesarean sections and operative deliveries (like forceps and vacuums), without improving outcomes for babies. In other words, the risk of an unnecessary intervention increases with EFM.

WHAT'S REALLY GOING ON WITH BABY'S HEART RATE?

Your baby's heartbeat is the single measure that matters most when assessing their health in utero. But know this: Most babies' heart rates will sound irregular at some point during labor. Your nurse and provider may suggest position changes (lying on your left side is often the best for the baby's heart rate) and other measures to keep everyone healthy and happy. Never hesitate to ask questions. And it's okay if you need to ask them a few times. You have a lot going on!

Now, sometimes EFM is necessary, and we are very glad that it exists. It can be lifesaving. I want to convey that being connected to a monitor the whole time does not mean that you can't have a lovely birth. Most of the coping skills from chapter 22 can be done while connected to an EFM. Don't be afraid to advocate for yourself; if no one asks if you'd like to get out of bed, go ahead and ring the call bell.

You have alternatives, especially if your pregnancy is low risk. There are now some EFM devices that are wireless, which means you can walk around during labor and generally assume any position you please.

The alternative to continuous EFM is intermittent fetal heart rate monitoring (or intermittent auscultation) via a Doppler wand or a special type of stethoscope. You might also try connecting to the EFM for a few minutes each hour, or just through a contraction, which can reassure practitioners that baby is fine. ACOG states that intermittent auscultation is appropriate for low-risk women, and ACNM goes further to say that it is the preferred method for low-risk women.

Something to keep in mind is that connecting women to an EFM is often done routinely in hospitals, but this does not mean you necessarily have to do it. You can speak with your provider and nurse (the more ahead of time, the better) and let them know you want intermittent monitoring or auscultation.

Internal Monitors

If your labor slows, your provider may suggest an intrauterine pressure catheter (IUPC). This can measure the strength, duration, and frequency of your contractions with increased accuracy, although it can occasionally also cause infections and fever for the mama.

Should the baby give off signs of distress, you might also have internal fetal heart rate monitoring. This is done by inserting a small electrode into the vagina and threading it up through the cervix onto the baby's scalp.

Operative Vaginal Deliveries

An operative vaginal birth (also called assisted vaginal birth) might be recommended near the end of the pushing stage to hasten the birth if there are concerns with the baby's heart rate or if your pushing efforts need some extra assistance. Despite the word "operative," these births don't always happen in the operating room; they can be done right in the delivery room. They involve tools (the vacuum or the forceps) and are used in about 3 percent of all births. Vacuums tend to be more common.

Vacuum Delivery A vacuum extractor is a device that uses a soft cup that is attached to a vacuum tube. The cup is placed on the baby's head while the practitioner or nurse pumps air out of the tube to create suction, which helps the provider guide the baby out.

Forceps Delivery Imagine some oversized metal salad tongs and you've got forceps. Each tong is slipped into the vagina and placed on either side of the baby's head. The provider then guides the baby's head out.

Your provider will continue to rely on your pushing efforts to help your baby be born with both vacuum and forceps births.

Possible risks of operative deliveries include:

- Perineal injury for the woman (more so with forceps than vacuums)

- Various scalp, head, and eye injuries for the baby (anywhere from 2 to 75 percent of babies can be affected, depending on the outcome being measured)

The short-term maternal risks from operative deliveries are thought to be less than the risks of C-sections, but there is more long-term risk for incontinence issues (due to injury while using the device).

The bottom line is that these tools sound scary, but they are great to have handy when needed. Most women don't need them, and most who do are fine! Know that you can ask any questions you need to in order to feel informed and comfortable with these procedures.

TRANSFER FROM HOME OR BIRTH CENTER TO HOSPITAL

If you've planned a home birth, no doubt your midwife will advise you about the possibility of needing to transfer to a hospital to deal with possible complications. Only about 10 percent of women who plan home births transfer to a hospital after labor has begun. This is usually for nonemergency reasons, like a slow progression. Good communication and coordination between your original provider and the one who may be joining your team or taking over your care is key and allows the family to trust and work cooperatively with the providers in the new setting. It's common practice for parents who are planning a home birth to tour and get familiar with their potential transfer hospital, which helps minimize potential anxiety.

If you are giving birth in a birth center, they likely have an agreement with a nearby (or on-site) hospital in the event that you need to be transferred.

remember

We may not love the idea of interventions, but we are very glad that they exist when they are needed. Remember that if your story unfolds in such a way that interventions are necessary, you can remain present in your body and in your birth and have a positive and empowered experience.

Cesarean Births

All birth is magic;
there is no
qualification.

note FROM DIANA

The words "Cesarean section" have the potential to stir emotions.

For some women, having a C-section is a relief, a safe way to deliver their baby. For others, it's a major disappointment. And still others are unsure, having more questions than opinions about the whole process.

Mama, where you fall on this spectrum is not for me to comment on. But there is one thing that I need to make abundantly clear: Having a Cesarean section *is* giving birth.

As I have shared on Motherly, "When a baby is born from your body, it is birth. Period. Saying that a C-section isn't *birth* because it didn't happen vaginally is like saying that soccer isn't a sport because it's not tennis. Cesarean sections and vaginal births are different, yes. But do you know what's not different? How hard a mother works to grow and birth her baby, how committed to her baby's health and safety she is, how proud she should be of herself when she's done, and how much she loves her baby."

Mama, however you feel about the possibility of a C-section is justified. You must promise me, though, that through it all, you will look on yourself with awe and celebration.

You are brilliant. *You've got this.*

xo,

Diana

TYPES OF CESAREAN SECTIONS

There are three categories of Cesarean sections: planned, nonemergency unplanned (the most common), and emergency unplanned (the least common).

Planned Cesarean Section

This is a scheduled C-section that has been decided on by you and your health-care team because it is likely that the outcome will be better than if you tried to have a vaginal birth.

Reasons for planned Cesareans might be:

- Breech* or transverse baby (see "Baby Positions" on page 198)
- Previous Cesarean section* or other uterine surgeries (see "Vaginal Birth After Cesarean (VBAC)" on page 316)
- Suspected large baby* (see "Big Babies" on page 213)
- Multiple babies* (see "Multiple Babies" on page 464)
- Placenta location or other problems (see "Placental Issues" on page 474)
- Active herpes lesions (see "Herpes" on page 472)
- High HIV viral load (see "HIV" on page 473)

*It is important to know that these are not automatic or guaranteed reasons to have a Cesarean section. Many women around the country and world have vaginal breech births, vaginal births after having a previous Cesarean, and give birth to big or multiple babies vaginally. The decision will depend on your preferences and your provider's concerns and protocols.

You have the right to ask questions and receive information about the benefits, risks, costs, and alternatives to any intervention suggested, including a Cesarean section. You also have the right to get a second or third opinion if the answers you hear don't feel right. You can seek out providers who match your desires. For example, there may be a doctor or midwife in your community with a lot of vaginal breech delivery experience who would be happy to work with you.

Elective Cesarean Sections   These also fall into the category of planned C-sections. This means that a woman has opted to have a Cesarean birth, despite not having a medical necessity to do so.

Elective Cesareans are controversial. Generally speaking, the birth community tends to advise against them. A C-section is major abdominal surgery, and with that comes risks. Many feel that there needs to be a strong health-based reason to warrant the decision to perform surgery when there is a lower risk solution—vaginal birth.

That said, this is your body, your baby, your birth. You've arrived at this place with a rich, deep story that you understand better than anyone else. You deserve to be listened to and respected. Have conversations early on in your pregnancy about your desires to see what options are available to you.

Nonemergency Unplanned Cesarean

This means that the woman started down the path of having a vaginal birth, but something came up during her labor that made a Cesarean birth appear to be a better option. Though these are unplanned, they are not emergencies. There is time to ask many questions and discuss the plan. Birth partners are usually able to dress in scrubs and go into the operating room, and "gentle Cesareans" can be an option (see "What Is a Gentle C-Section?" on page 314 for details).

Reasons for nonemergency unplanned C-sections might be:

- Labor does not progress (technical term: arrest of dilation).
- Baby does not move down during pushing (technical term: arrest of descent).
- Baby is not tolerating the stresses of labor, which can be determined by their heart rate.

Emergency Unplanned Cesarean

True emergencies are rare. They can occur when the woman or baby has a sudden and serious complication that necessitates immediate delivery.

Reasons for this might be:

- Severe or prolonged drop in baby's heart rate (see "Fetal Monitoring: Continuous Versus Intermittent" on page 305)
- Cord prolapse (see page 240)
- Placental abruption (see page 474)
- Uterine rupture (see page 481)

SO, WHAT HAPPENS IN A C-SECTION?

Let's start with nonemergency unplanned C-sections. Through various paths, you and your provider will arrive at the decision that a Cesarean section is the best way for your baby to be born.

After asking all the questions you have, you will sign a consent form, and the team will begin to help you get ready: You will get a lovely blue bonnet for your hair, and you may also be asked to remove all jewelry. Shaving pubic hair is not usually done anymore, as evidence to support its necessity is lacking. It may be clipped or trimmed, though.

You will be brought into the operating room (OR), usually via a wheelchair or in your hospital bed.

Partners are often asked to stay behind for a bit but will be escorted in before the birth starts. During this time, your partner will be given scrubs and a blue bonnet to match mama—gorgeous.

A note about ORs: They are cold, both literally and figuratively. They are cold in temperature because that helps them stay sanitary (though many hospitals do offer heated blankets to help you feel more comfortable). And they tend not to have much "warmth and personality." See if you can close your eyes, practice your relaxation exercises, and focus on maintaining your center and sense of calm.

In the OR, you will be assisted onto the table. If you do not have an epidural, the anesthesiologist will give you one or will give you a spinal block (see page 295). If you do have an epidural, they will adjust the dose higher. Before the Cesarean begins, the doctors will ensure that you are completely numb.

After you are numb, if you don't already have one, a urinary catheter may be placed to empty your bladder during your birth, though recent research has found that this practice may not be based on the best evidence. Studies have found that routine urinary catheters for C-sections may not be necessary for all women and that women may have fewer urinary tract infections and be able to walk sooner without them. You can definitely talk to your provider about your concerns.

Before your birth starts, a curtain will be put up just under your breasts so that you can stay focused on your breathing and positive thinking without being distracted by the team helping your baby to be born. Your partner will be invited to sit right next to you. They will be allowed to hold your hand, stroke your face, and talk to you throughout your birth.

The anesthesiologist will also be stationed by your head. Think of them as your Cesarean section master of ceremonies. If you have questions, concerns, or needs, let them know, and they will help you. For example, if you have nausea or heartburn (which we'll talk about more shortly), you can ask the anesthesiologist for medication.

THE BIRTH

Psst: We're about to get a little graphic here, so if details aren't for you, feel free to skip ahead to page 321.

Most women will have a horizontal incision just above the pubic bone, a few inches below your belly button. The incision is surprisingly small, usually about 5 inches long. Vertical incisions are sometimes used if the baby is premature or in a challenging position, if the baby needs to be born urgently, if the mother has a high BMI, or if the mother has had previous vertical incisions.

After the skin incision, the doctor will separate—not cut—the abdominal muscles. They will make an incision in the uterus and the amniotic sac. The baby will then be lifted out of the uterus, and in a scene that might be right out of *The Lion King*, the doctor will raise the baby over the curtain, so you can see them. Brace yourself for some powerful lioness-mama emotions.

The cord will be clamped and cut (delayed cord clamping is often an option here too, so be sure to ask for it if you want it), and the baby will be brought to a warm bassinet to be examined, dried, and wrapped in a blanket. When the baby is ready, as long as everything

READ AHEAD

If you know that you will be having a C-section, it is a great idea to read about postpartum healing now in "Cesarean Section Healing" on page 352.

is okay, the nurse will bring them over to you. Since you may not be able to use your arms yet, depending on your anesthesia, the nurse will hold the baby up to you so you can meet, or you can ask for your partner to hold the baby near you.

Sometimes the baby will be taken to the newborn nursery or NICU for evaluation and care. Your partner usually has the option to go with the baby, if you'd like. If, however, you would prefer that your partner stay with you for support as you complete your birth, that is fine! The baby will be well taken care of; it is okay to ask for the support you need. Another person may be able to accompany the baby as well. (Is your mom in the waiting room? I have a feeling she would be delighted to escort the baby!)

Your placenta will then be delivered through the incision in your belly. You have the same options with your placenta as in a vaginal birth (taking home, encapsulating, and so on), so be sure to make your wishes known to the team before the birth starts.

It takes about 15 to 20 minutes for your baby to be born via C-section. The second part of the procedure is all about closing the incisions and taking care of you, and this lasts about 30 to 45 minutes. It takes a longer time because the team goes slowly and methodically, stitching up layer by layer, to ensure the best healing process.

The outermost skin layer will be closed by sutures, staples, or glue, and then it's done. You did it! You will be taken to the recovery room where you will rest and be monitored for a few hours. During this time, you can nurse if you want to, spend time with your partner, and begin the process of healing from your birth.

Vaginal Seeding

During a vaginal birth, the baby is exposed to the healthy bacteria of the mother's vagina, which may help establish healthy microbes in the baby's gut. Since C-section babies do not have the same exposure, providers have developed a technique called vaginal seeding. In vaginal seeding, after the baby is born, the vagina is swabbed with a piece of gauze that is then rubbed on the baby's nose and eyes and placed in the baby's mouth. The theory is that this replicates the transfer of bacteria that happens in vaginal births.

At this point, we do not have enough research to routinely recommend this practice. Some hospitals are currently involved in studies around this, so if you are interested, definitely check with your provider.

If You Have a Planned Cesarean Birth

Your story will be very similar to what we just described. The main difference is that you may have an appointment the day before your birth to have some blood drawn in preparation for the procedure. On the day of your C-section, you will arrive at the hospital at the scheduled time, and a nurse will help you prep and take you into the OR.

Psst: The night before a planned Cesarean section is a great time to use your meditation skills. Talk about not being able to sleep!

If You Have an Unplanned Emergency Cesarean Birth

These can be intense. Once the decision has been made, there may be a rush of people into your room to help get you ready and into the operating room as soon as possible. You will still be able to ask questions, and you will be informed about what is going on, but be prepared to have it all happen quickly.

Once you are in the operating room, there is a chance that you will receive general

WHAT IS A GENTLE C-SECTION?

A gentle C-section intends to create peaceful energy during the birth, while mimicking the mechanics of a vaginal birth as much as possible.

The providers help guide the baby out slowly—head, shoulders, abdomen, and then legs—much like what happens in a vaginal birth—so that the baby has a chance to naturally remove fluid from the lungs as their body is gently squeezed on the way out. Skin-to-skin bonding is often done right in the OR, and sometimes breastfeeding can be initiated there, too.

A clear drape may be available to you if you are interested. With the clear drape, you can look down and watch your baby be born. (Don't worry; you won't be able to see much of the actual surgery because your belly will be in the way.)

A gentle C-section isn't always available, and of course it may not be what you want. It's just awesome to know that it exists, when possible, for women who do want it.

anesthesia (meaning you'll be asleep for the birth) if you don't already have a spinal or an epidural.

The actual surgery happens much like the one already described, but it happens faster. Your baby will possibly be handed over to a NICU team to ensure they are doing well and to give them any support they need.

When surgery is complete, general anesthesia will be removed (if you had it), and you will be given pain medication so that you'll be more comfortable as you wake up.

What Does Cesarean Birth Feel Like?

You should not experience pain during your Cesarean birth. You will, however, feel pressure on your belly as the baby is being born. It is also possible that you'll experience some nausea or heartburn. If you do, be sure to tell your anesthesiologist, who can give you an IV medication to help.

You may also have some intense shivering. This is due to the hormone surge, IV fluid, and the temperature of the OR. It can feel unpleasant. The nurses will give you a warmed blanket, which helps a lot. Know that this is temporary and normal.

Here is what Motherly community members who had Cesarean births want you to know:

"Know that you can still have a birth plan. My doctor knew what I wanted, but the hospital staff didn't. Don't be afraid to tell them what you want. I got it all! Saw my baby being born, had skin-to-skin the entire time they stitched me up, and started breastfeeding as soon as we got to the recovery room. You don't have to miss out on those special moments, but you have to ask for them specifically."

ANDREA

"I wish I had known that they happen even if you do everything 'right.' I thought C-sections could always be pinpointed to particular situations or health characteristics. Mine was completely random, and I was not prepared for that possibility, so I took it extremely hard during the C-section and postpartum. My advice: Be gentle and patient with yourself. You just had major surgery. It will take some time to heal, so take all the time you need."

PAMELA

"As someone who has had both a vaginal and C-section birth, both are still 'giving birth.'"

KATIE

And here is a note from ob-gyn Sarah Bjorkman, MD, to the mama who is feeling scared about a potential C-section:

I get it! A C-section is major abdominal surgery, and that is scary. But they are very common. (Did you know a C-section is the most common major surgery done in the hospital every day?) And they are safe. Giving birth is really hard. It takes a physical and mental toll on the body, no matter which route the baby joins us through. I know women who have had both vaginal births and C-sections and swear that their recovery from their C-section was easier. It is different for everyone.

Dr. Bjorkman recommends talking to your provider about concerns you have.

A NOTE FOR PARTNERS ON CESAREAN BIRTHS

Cesarean births can be difficult for partners and loved ones, too. If it happens quickly, all attention is on mom and baby, leaving the partner to "fend for themselves." In an emergency C-section, there may not be time for the partner to come back to the OR, and that can stink. You are alone in the room, after a whirlwind of activity, feeling unsure and scared.

Even in a nonemergency case, partners can have a difficult time coping. You might feel powerless or nervous to know that the person you love is having major surgery, or you may feel that your own needs are not being addressed because all eyes are on her.

It's tough, but I offer you this: Trust that she is in competent and skillful hands. C-sections are common, which means that doctors do them all the time.

Also, please know how important you are, despite feeling powerless. Your presence in the OR, or when she is recovering, matters more than I can describe. You are still very much a part of the birth story, and your support and love are significant.

"Sometimes the unknown is the worst part. Knowledge is power, and feeling like you have some control is so important," she said.

You can talk about:

- Your specific reasons for needing a C-section and whether a vaginal birth might still be an option for you
- What happens on the day of surgery
- Any fears about pain, recovery, breastfeeding, bonding, or previous trauma
- Risks
- Recovery, including pain management, sleep, and rest
- Goals for birth, like using a clear drape or baby having skin-to-skin with your partner immediately after birth

VAGINAL BIRTH AFTER CESAREAN (VBAC)

If you have had a previous Cesarean birth, you may have the option to have what is known as a TOLAC—trial of labor after Cesarean. This means that you try to have a vaginal birth. If you do, it is called a VBAC, or vaginal birth after Cesarean, and these are wildly cool.

In addition to the personal reasons you may want to have a VBAC, there are some medical benefits as well. First, when you have a VBAC, it eliminates some of the risks that come with major abdominal surgery. VBAC may be a good option for women who desire large families because it is generally not recommended to have more than three Cesarean births. If you are planning to have more children than that, VBACs may be a safer option. Lastly, recovering from a vaginal birth is usually easier than recovering from a C-section.

VBACs have historically been controversial. The primary concern is the increased risk of uterine rupture (see page 481). But a large review of studies found that the risk only increased by a small amount. In order to prevent one uterine rupture, we would need to do 370 C-sections.

About 60 to 80 percent of women who try a TOLAC will end up with a vaginal birth. This number varies depending on factors like your age and overall health, the reasons for the original Cesarean, and provider- and hospital-specific protocols.

ACOG's guidelines state that in consultation with their provider, women should be allowed to make the decision regarding a TOLAC or repeat C-section.

Here are seven things I want you to know about VBAC:

1 **Quiet the noise and listen to *you*.** You're probably surrounded by people giving you advice—well intentioned yes, but helpful? Not always. You don't have to take everything everyone says to heart. Have in-depth conversations with your doctor or midwife and really home in on what it is that *you* want and what feels right to *you*.

2 **Know the facts.** The American College of Obstetricians and Gynecologists and the American College of Nurse-Midwives (among many other organizations) support VBACs. You have the right to information and care that is based on evidence. Don't be afraid to ask questions and do your own research.

3 **Choose the right provider.** Remember that you are the customer here. If a VBAC is really important to you, and if your physical situation qualifies you to have one, make sure your doctor or midwife fully supports you and your decision. If they don't, you are allowed to ask for a second opinion, and find someone you feel comfortable with!

4 **Take a birth class.** Taking a birth class will empower you with knowledge and confidence to have the birth experience you want. Come hang out with me in Motherly's birth class (mother.ly /becomingmama)!

5 **Assemble an awesome support team.** Having consistent emotional support will increase your chances of having a VBAC. Talk to your partner about how important this is to you. And consider hiring a doula; they can make all the difference.

6 **Take care of yourself.** You want to approach your birth as healthy as possible to increase your chances of having a VBAC. Get regular prenatal care, eat really well, rest, and find ways to decrease your stress. Your body is a temple!

7 **Be gentle with yourself.** It is possible that your first birth experience left you feeling unsatisfied. You may also be feeling extra stressed now as you approach your birth. Give yourself permission to be gentle with yourself. Know that what's in the past is, well, in the past. Trust your body and be really, really proud of yourself. No matter what happens, you are absolutely a rock star.

A FEW ITEMS THAT MAY HELP AFTER A C-SECTION

Abdominal or Belly Binder   These are special types of compression garments worn around the belly. One of the oldest traditions, Bengkung belly binding, comes from Malaysia. Strips of fabric are ceremonially woven around a woman's abdomen after birth to offer support. Some women who have Cesarean sections report that belly binding helps decrease pain.

High-Rise Underwear   The waistband on bikini underwear usually lands exactly where your incision will be, so high-rise cuts will feel much more comfortable.

Comfy Pants   You'll want pants that won't rub your incision. Yoga pants with a wide and stretchy waistband work well, as do loose-fitting dresses.

MEDITATING DURING YOUR CESAREAN

Birth is birth is birth is birth. You are giving birth to your baby. Your work here is magic; there is no qualification. Look at what you have done! You have grown a human, and that human is now entering the world in all their glory. That is birth.

Mama, I want you to know that it is entirely possible to have a beautiful Cesarean birth.

Some women find it useful to have something to do or think about so that they can stay relaxed during a C-section. You might find solace knowing that you have a focus in case you need it for the procedure. Motherly's Cesarean Section Birth Class includes a C-section meditation, and we want to share it with you here as well. If a C-section is in your future, or you just want to be proactive, try this meditation. You can listen to it online at mother.ly/becomingmama or have someone read it to you. You can also use it while you are in the operating room, so add it to your packing list if desired.

A Cesarean Birth Meditation

This relaxation exercise will guide you through releasing tension in your body. Close your eyes if you'd like to. Once you are comfortable, take a few big, cleansing breaths. Release the used air in your lungs and breathe in cool, nourishing oxygen.

This is your birth. This is your baby's birth. You have worked so hard growing this baby, and you have done a beautiful job. And now, it is time for your baby to be born.

Feel your body and your belly move with your breathing. There may be noises and activity happening around you. These are the sounds of the people who are attending you as you give birth to your baby. You can hear them, but you can also choose to slowly tune them out. The noises are around you but not inside you, and though they are there, they are not affecting you. Your mind is quiet and peaceful. Focus again on your breathing, how when you take a deep breath, you can feel your body fill with lightness, calmness, and restorative energy. When you exhale, you feel the tension and stress leaving you. Breathe in calm; breathe out tension.

Now focus on the part of you that is touching the earth. As you lie where you are, you may not be directly touching the ground outside, but you are grounded to the earth and to Mother Nature. Let yourself feel supported and embraced and grounded by the earth.

Take a few more deep breaths. We're going to work on relaxing your body, little by little, part by part. It's okay if you've already received medication and aren't feeling each part of your body like you usually do. You can still visualize each part and be present in your body's awesomeness.

Focus on your toes. Notice any tension that you may feel and release it. Now the soles of your feet. Your feet that work all day supporting and balancing the weight of your growing, beautiful baby. Release the tension in your mama-feet. Relax your ankles. Feel the relaxation travel up your calves, your knees, the fronts of your thighs, and the backs of your thighs. Your strong legs carry your baby with you all day, lifting and lowering the body that is growing this tiny human. And before you know it, those same legs will be crouching down so you can kiss sweet chubby cheeks, will be folded in front of you as your baby sits on your lap listening intently to the words you read, and will be walking quickly behind a nervous but thrilled toddler as you prepare to catch them as they fall, again.

Take another deep breath and allow your bottom to relax. Feel the muscles of the ligaments of your pelvis and your hips relax with your breath. Trust your body, trust those around you, and release the tension. And now your belly. Your belly, filled with the energy of two (or maybe more) incredible beings: a new baby, growing, changing, preparing to come into the world and fill it with love and excitement; and the strong superwoman who has grown that baby. Both of you, creating so much energy in your belly. Allow the muscles of your belly and your uterus to relax.

Allow your back to release its tension. Your back has been working so hard. Allow your back to completely relax as you breathe in fresh, clean air. Your lower back. Now your middle back. The space between your shoulder blades. Your shoulders. Let it all melt, as you continue to feel grounded and supported by the earth.

Now your neck. If you want, gently move your head from side to side and ease the tension out of your neck. Your head is supported, so your neck doesn't have to work right now. Relax your neck. Relax your jaw. Your jaw is connected to so much of your body, and relaxing it helps to alleviate tension everywhere. Even relax your tongue. Then your nose and cheeks. Your eyes and eyelids. Your forehead. Your scalp. Allow your whole head to just relax. Your head has been busy, after all. Full of thoughts about your birth. Your changing body. Wondering what to name your baby. Daydreaming about their sweet face. Worrying about being a parent. Yes, you've been very busy because you are already an amazing mama. So, allow yourself this moment to breathe, relax, and let go. Trust your body. Trust yourself. *You've got this.*

Today is the day that you are giving birth to your baby. You are surrounding your baby with love and protection, just like a mama bear.

Your body is already beginning to heal itself. Your body knows what to do. Trust your body. Listen to your body as it heals. Take a few deep breaths as you prepare for the rest of your life. You are a mama now, and a pretty awesome one at that.

When you're ready, start to return to the room. Wiggle your toes, gently begin to move your limbs. Come back to the present moment. When you're ready, slowly let your eyes open.

remember

Reading about birth—especially Cesarean birth—can feel scary. It can be jarring to imagine being in labor, about to have a baby, and going through all the potential scenarios both good and bad.

But know that your birth is a story that will unfold over time.

When you were 12, if someone had shown you a photo of your future life as it is right now, you would never have believed it. It is next to impossible to fully imagine a reality that we've never experienced. But now, looking back at how your story has evolved, it all makes complete sense. One little step at a time, and you have ended up here.

Birth is almost always this way, too. It happens faster, but it is still a story that evolves over time.

The details will make sense as you progress through them.

You can be an active, empowered participant in decisions.

You will give birth with confidence and awareness.

Birth Plans

This is my birth.

Confession: I don't love the term "birth plan."

Here's why: Plans are rigid. When we sit down and write a plan, whether it's for our upcoming vacation, starting a business, or our birth, we are doing so based on predictions. I predict the weather will be good. I predict the economy is primed for this type of business. I predict that at 6 centimeters I will be ready for an epidural. While those predictions are based on evidence, they are not yet facts. When predictions do not become realities, especially when they involve something that matters deeply to us, we tend to feel like we failed.

- "It rained the whole time. The vacation was a bust."
- "The market changed. My business was a dumb idea."
- "I got my epidural earlier than I thought I would. I failed."

The idea that you could look back at your birth and feel that somehow you failed is simply not okay. At that point, no matter the direction your birth goes, you will have brought a human into this world. You are a goddess and should revere yourself as such.

I cannot get on board with a birth plan that will harm your self-perception.

What I can totally get on board with is you being an active member of your birth team. At this stage, I want you to think through the aspects of your labor and birth that are important to you and then to express those desires to a team who respects and listens to you.

This is achieved by establishing your birth preferences.

Your birth is a story that will unfold, and establishing birth preferences will allow you to be active in every decision and turning point that comes up.

Ultimately, I believe that what is important is not your birth experience—the specific details that add up to become your story—but how you experience your birth. If you feel heard, respected, and nurtured through the experience, you will be more likely to feel like that rock star you are when it's done, however it happens.

In this chapter, I'll take you through how to do that.

xo,

Diana

Before we get into the nitty-gritty of you writing your birth preferences, take a few minutes to be still. Get grounded in yourself and what you want. Remember, this is your birth.

Place your feet on the floor and take a few deep breaths. Close your eyes if you want to.

Now imagine that you are in your birthing room. Don't worry about the details yet; just focus on how you feel. Imagine that you are in labor, and everything around you is perfect.

- What is the energy like in the room? Is it calm and serene, or is it upbeat and energetic?

- How do you want to feel in this moment (supported, prepared, excited, calm, confident, loved)?

- What are you choosing to do with your body? Do you see yourself immersed in a bath, taking a shower, laboring in bed, or something else?

- What about this scene makes you feel safe?

- Who is in the room with you, and what support do they offer you?

There is no one way to achieve any of the feelings you just raised, except to be true to yourself, what you want, and what you need. You may feel safest at home, or you may feel safest in a hospital.

BIRTH PLAN TIPS

Most providers and nurses I know really do listen to or read your birth plan or preferences. They went into this work because they love birth, and it's important to them that you have a good experience. Before we go into *what* to include, here are some ideas about *how* to include your wishes.

Be Concise   If you write it out, try to keep your birth plan to one page. Your nurse may be busy when you arrive, and you want to ensure that they read it. Keeping it on the short side will help.

Choose Neutral Language   Consider the tone of your birth plan. Think about how the words you choose will be received by the team and try to stay neutral.

For example, instead of "DO NOT take the baby out of the room," try "I strongly prefer to have baby remain in the room at all times." It conveys the same meaning, but it won't put the reader on the defensive right off the bat.

Share Your Plan Ahead of Time   Bring your birth plan or preferences to a prenatal appointment during your third trimester and ask your provider to take a look. They can help assure you of anything you are worried about and answer any questions about hospital policies linked to your desires.

One more thing: Not every woman wants to write a birth plan, and that's okay. If you don't feel called to do it, don't force yourself. I would recommend reading through the following questions, though, just so that at some level you have considered what you might want under certain circumstances.

WRITING YOUR BIRTH PLAN

Here are the ten questions to consider when making your birth plan or birth preferences.

1. *Where do you want to give birth, and who will catch your baby?*

Midwives rarely use the word "deliver" when talking about attending a woman's birth. You are the one doing the work of delivering your baby into this world. My midwifery school director used to say that our role was to be the guardian of safety. So, who will be your guardian of safety?

If you need to refresh your memory on the birthing place and provider options available to you, look back at chapter 6, "Choosing a Birthplace and Provider."

There is a good chance you've already determined who you'll have catching, based on where and with whom you are currently receiving your prenatal care. However, this is an excellent time to reassess and make sure that your needs are being met.

If you feel respected and well cared for and are confident that your birth plans will be supported, then that is awesome, and you are good to go! If not, it may not be too late to switch to a different practice or location.

Often (though certainly not always) the scenario whereby women change practices mid-pregnancy has to do with a change in birth plan desires. For example, imagine that Luna started her prenatal care with the doctor she received her gynecology care from, but after attending a birth class, she decided that she would prefer to give birth in a birth center, so she transferred her care. Margo, on the other hand, started her pregnancy journey with a home-birth midwife because Margo's sister always raves about her home birth. But Margo realized that she felt safer knowing there was an operating room down the hall, so she transferred her care to a hospital.

There is no one way to do this, mama, except the way that feels right for you.

2. *Beyond your midwife or doctor and nurses, who would you like to have in the room with you?*

A doula? Your partner? Family members or friends? No one? For things to consider in making these choices, revisit chapter 12 to read "Love and Village" on page 183.

3. *What are your preferences around pain medications?*

Deciding whether you'd like pain medication during your birth is significant, and it's likely already on your mind. This is, of course, a very personal decision.

One aspect to consider is how—if at all—pain meds should be offered to you. (For more info on pain medication options, check out "Medical Coping Methods" on page 293.) For example, if you know that you want an epidural, do you want to get it as soon as possible, or would you rather wait until you are in advanced labor?

If you are undecided on your pain med plan, do you want someone to offer you an epidural once an hour and allow you the opportunity to consider and then say yes or no? Or would you prefer that no one mentions the word "epidural" unless you do?

Once you have decided what your preferences are, make sure you let someone on your birth team know so that they can help communicate your needs to the whole team.

4. *What is in your "bag of tricks" for coping with labor?*

In chapter 22, we went deep into nonmedical coping skills. Some of them will resonate with you, while others won't feel like the right fit. See if you can learn about and practice all of them.

When you are in labor, it is helpful to have a wide range of coping options. For example, perhaps you usually love massages, but when you go into labor, you suddenly find them annoying. Or maybe the idea of deep breathing feels boring right now, but in labor, you discover that it is the best thing to get you through a contraction.

Coping methods are essential for women who plan to get epidurals, too. First, you may be laboring at home for a while before heading to the hospital. There is also a chance that your epidural will be delayed (for example, if the anesthesiologist is with another patient, you may need to wait). And labor may progress quickly for you, in which case, you may not have time for an epidural. It is awesome to have some tricks up your sleeve for times like these.

Also, even with an epidural, you may have some symptoms that can be aided by comfort measures. You may experience pressure as the baby gets low (breathing exercises are great for getting through this rough patch). And you may feel nervous or even anxious at times (guided relaxation and visualization exercises are fantastic for helping you refocus).

Once you've homed in on the coping skills you prefer, make sure to practice them with your birth partner so that you can access them quickly when you need them most.

If you are writing out a birth plan, you might include a list of the coping skills you think you'd like to use in labor, as a sort of reminder sheet.

5. What preferences do you have for various interventions?

Depending on your birth setting, the use of certain interventions may or may not be routine, but that doesn't mean you don't get a say.

Here is a list of interventions that might come up during your late pregnancy and birth. Decide how you feel about them and whether you want to include them in your birth plan:

- **Inductions** Would you prefer a 41- or 42-week post–due date induction, if your practice offers a choice? (See "Induction of Labor" on page 301.)

- **Your Bag of Water, or Amniotic Sac** Would you prefer to let your water release (break, rupture) on its own over an "artificial" release done by your provider? (See "Artificial Rupture of Membranes (AROM)" on page 303.)

- **IV** Would you prefer not to be connected to an IV? If an IV is necessary, would you like to have a "saline lock" when not in use? (See "Intravenous (IV) Therapy" on page 305.)

- **Monitoring** Would you prefer continuous monitoring or intermittent monitoring or auscultation? (See "Fetal Monitoring: Continuous Versus Intermittent" on page 305.)

- **C-Section** Do you have specific desires if a C-section is needed? (See chapter 24, "Cesarean Births.")

6. How should your baby be cared for?

When it comes to caring for your baby in the hours after their birth, there are several decisions for you to make. It feels a bit overwhelming to think about all of this now, but if you can make your plan ahead of time, you'll have more time to enjoy the splendor of your new baby without being bogged down by all this stuff:

- Cord blood banking (page 163)
- Delayed cord clamping (page 266)
- Skin-to-skin (page 271)
- Breastfeeding (page 393)
- Eye medication (page 276)
- Vitamin K shot (page 276)
- Hepatitis B shot (page 276)
- Nursery or in-room care for baby (page 273)
- Circumcision (page 365)

7. What do you want to do with your placenta?

Your placenta is endlessly cool: an organ that exists for the sole purpose of nourishing and supporting your growing baby. After your baby is born, you will also deliver your placenta (see "Your Amazing Placenta" on page 166). It has done its job, and it's time for it to leave your body. Then you get to decide what happens to it.

In most Western medicine births, the placenta is discarded after birth, as it is considered medical waste. If this feels right for you, you'll get to look at it (if you want to), and then it will be taken away. Or it may be sent to the lab for testing (for example, if you developed a complication such as preeclampsia or an infection).

However, there are many people around the world—and a growing number in the US—who choose to keep or use the placenta for a variety of purposes. You have the ability to choose what you want to do with your placenta, though regulations in some

institutions or states may differ, so definitely ask. You may need to sign release forms, and having it outlined ahead of time will save a lot of stress and accidental oversight. Following are your options:

- **Take the Placenta Home** Many cultures around the world believe that the placenta holds deep meaning and importance. As such, the placenta is often taken home and celebrated. It can be stored in a ritual pot until it is ceremonially buried, interred in sacred ground, or planted in the earth to nourish a young tree. Various cultures have regarded the placenta as a soul container, a lifeless twin of the baby that was born, or a guardian angel. You may want to look into your family history and traditions to see if there was a belief or ritual associated with your ancestors' placentas.

- **Placentophagy (Ingesting the Placenta)** Humans are the only mammals—from mice to lions to chimpanzees—who don't routinely ingest the placenta after birth. There are a few theories about why this is done. First, it may hide signs of birth from predators. But it may also provide vital nutrients and replenishing proteins to the mammal mama who has just lost a lot of energy and blood and needs immediate sustenance. There is evidence that people from some cultures historically ingested the placenta. Traditional Chinese medicine views the placenta as an incredibly powerful source of healing, and practitioners have been drying and preparing it for hundreds of years.

  Placentophagy had all but disappeared in the industrialized world, but it was rediscovered and popularized by the home birth community in the 1980s. Since then, proponents of the practice claim that it can increase postpartum energy, improve lactation, decrease the risk of baby blues and postpartum depression, increase iron stores, decrease postpartum vaginal bleeding, and encourage quicker uterine healing. It is important to note that there are no big studies validating these effects, and some practitioners are concerned about the effect of ingesting the toxic metals that accumulate in placental tissue, along with the fact that the placenta is not sterile and could contain group B strep and other infections.

If you choose to keep your placenta and ingest it, one of the easiest ways is to have it encapsulated by someone local who offers this service. (This involves dehydrating the placenta, pulverizing it, and putting the powder into capsules.) Some women choose to ingest it raw or to have a salve or tincture made from it.

You can take the pills cautiously, watching for effects. Many women absolutely love how the placenta makes them feel, but if you don't, simply stop taking the pills. Some even share them with their partners or family members.

"I did have a great milk supply and not a ton of bleeding, so while I'm not positive that it was because of my placenta pills, I figure they must have helped at least a little! I knew someone trustworthy who did the encapsulation process and knew of other people who used her, so I didn't have to do a ton of research, which made it easier."
COLLEEN

"I was repulsed by the idea of ingesting placenta when it was suggested to me by my fiancé. But I kept an open mind and researched it. I ended up eating some raw and encapsulating the rest. As a bonus, my research led me to fall in love with this fascinating organ, sparking a spiritual relationship with the divine feminine as well."
VAL

If you would like to explore placenta encapsulation further, a local placenta encapsulation expert can address your questions. Keep in mind that safety is important here, especially when it comes to infection control. Be sure to ask about experience, training, and certifications.

- **Lotus Birth**   This is a practice that has ancient roots in many different cultures. In a lotus birth, the umbilical cord is not cut, so the baby remains connected to the placenta for varied amounts of time, sometimes until it detaches on its own, which can take up to 10 days. The placenta is washed after it is born and air-dried. Sometimes salt is applied to its surface to prevent spoiling. Cloth may then be wrapped around the placenta, and it is moved around with the baby in a basket or bin. Note: Most hospitals will not permit a lotus birth, but it can be arranged with a home birth. There are no medically proven benefits to the practice, but many people are motivated to keep baby attached to the placenta for spiritual and traditional reasons.

8. Do you have any specific requests for your birth?

Here are some examples of specific requests you might have:

- Do you want a mirror to watch while you are pushing?
- Would you like to touch your baby as they are crowning?
- Would you like to assist your baby out?
- Would you like your partner to help deliver the baby?
- Would you like your partner to cut the umbilical cord?

9. Are there any cultural or religious customs the team needs to be aware of?

Medical providers strive to respect cultural and religious needs whenever possible, but sometimes we forget to ask. Including your needs in your birth plan will draw attention to them to make sure that they are honored and observed.

SAMPLE BIRTH PLAN

NAME   Motherly Mama

AGE   28

PRONOUN   She

PARTNER'S NAME   Partner Papa

PRONOUN   He

OTHER SUPPORT PEOPLE PRESENT
Carin Foryou, doula

DUE DATE   April 10

OB'S NAME   Dr. Birthwell

PAIN MEDICATION   I would like to try to have an unmedicated birth but am open to getting an epidural if I decide I need one. I will request one if I need it. Please do not ask me.

COPING TECHNIQUES I WANT TO USE
Birth ball, shower, and music

INTERVENTIONS   I would like minimal interventions if possible, including intermittent monitor (as previously

discussed with my ob-gyn) and a saline lock. If I need a C-section, I would like a gentle C-section but not a clear drape.

BABY CARE REQUESTS
- Delayed cord clamping
- Immediate skin-to-skin
- Breastfeeding
- Baby in room with me
- Eye medication and vitamin K okay

PLACENTA   I plan to encapsulate my placenta. My doula will transport the placenta to my home after the birth.

BIRTH   If possible, I'd like my husband to help deliver the baby once the head and shoulders are out. He would like to cut the cord.

SPECIAL CONSIDERATION   I have a history of anxiety. Keeping the room calm and allowing me enough time to ask the questions I need to will help me a great deal.

Thank you for your time and attention!

For a birth plan worksheet, visit mother.ly/becomingmama.

For example:

- Do you prefer to be attended by only female providers and nurses when possible?
- Do you have special dietary needs?
- Will you and your family need time and a place to pray throughout the day?
- Is there a prayer that you will need to say just as the baby is born?
- Do you observe a sabbath, and how can the team support you during this time?
- Will you decline a blood transfusion for religious reasons?
- How do you feel about breastfeeding in front of others?
- Will you require a privacy screen if breastfeeding in an occupied room?

10. Is there anything else the team needs to know?

We all have our histories and experiences that make us who we are, but they can also burden us with painful memories or emotions. Birth can stir up some of the deep-seated parts of ourselves that we do not confront on a daily basis.

Consider if there is anything that might come up for you. Do you have a history of trauma that might impact how you cope with your birth?

As a reminder, pelvic exams and birth can be triggering for women who have experienced violence. Women who have lost a pregnancy or child can be profoundly affected by labor and delivery. Women with mood disorders or depression can spiral downward because of the stress of labor.

Your partner may have similar experiences as well that will come up for them.

Communicating these concerns to your team can help them support you better, in both preventing physical discomfort as well as helping you emotionally should you start to experience strong feelings.

Your birth plan is also an excellent place to communicate social needs. Are there any social situations/relationships the team needs to be aware of? What pronouns should the team use to address you and your partner (she, he, they, ze, or something else)?

This is not mandatory, of course. You do not have to share any more than you want to. The point is to make sure that you feel as safe, respected, and well cared for as possible. It is your team's desire and responsibility to care for you to the best of their ability, and communicating your needs and desires fully may help them do this better.

BIRTH PLAN WORDING

Here is a list of some concisely worded requests that you may want to include in your birth plan, depending on your preferences.

During labor:

- No offer of pain medication
- Pain medication offered if I ask
- Free movement, intermittent monitoring
- Water birth (if applicable for your birth location)
- Natural water rupture
- Limited cervical exams
- Music, low lights
- Food and water available and offered

After birth:

- Immediate skin-to-skin
- Delayed cord clamping

- Donate cord blood
- Bank cord blood
- Bathing baby delayed
- No vitamin K shot, eye ointment, or hepatitis B shot (my provider approves)
- All preventive health care for baby
- Placenta saved
- Breastfeeding encouraged
- No formula
- No pacifiers
- Nursery care
- Circumcision

remember

It can feel overwhelming to consider all the options for your birth, especially when you factor in the potential unpredictability of Mother Nature. Remember that your story is going to evolve over time, and you will be able to advocate for yourself every step of the way. Take some time thinking through each of the topics mentioned in this chapter, and then trust that when the time comes, you will be able to take it moment by moment and then, with the help of your birthing team, make the best choices for you and your baby.

This is your birth. Take some deep breaths and try to home in on what you want and need as you consider your preferences. And just think, one day not that long from now, you will have a birth story and a baby that comes from that story.

PART IV

The Fourth Trimester

DEAR MAMA,

Yes, you really just did that. You gave birth to a remarkable, beautiful, little human being. Congratulations mama, and welcome to your fourth trimester.

In many ways, the fourth trimester is a paradox. So much of what we as mothers experience during this period is similar, unifying us around the world and across time in solidarity. And yet, it is also during this period of time that so many new mothers feel lost and lonely, questioning their new identities and wondering if things will ever return to normal.

Mama, this new life can be absolutely overwhelming—and we have been there.

We, as planner Jill and one-day-at-a-timer Liz, were both confronted with the shock of new motherhood, but for very different reasons. Jill was shocked by how challenging breastfeeding was, and Liz was shocked by how unfamiliar her body felt. These adjustments were unexpected, and we'll be honest, really challenging.

But in time, your new normal will seem, well, normal. It might even feel like the life you dreamed of. (And if it doesn't, if it's harder than you realized, know that is so normal, too.)

In time, we also both found our own versions of motherhood that brought us peace and joy. For Jill, it came when she learned to accept being cared for by her husband and family as she took care of the baby. For Liz, it came with a new perspective on her life's mission, as motherhood ignited her conviction to carve a career with meaning—one that was worth sometimes being away from her child. (And she found it in co-founding Motherly.)

Mama, what will the fourth trimester mean for you?

We know that there will be hard times—Motherly's annual State of Motherhood survey tells us year after year that women do not receive the support they need during this vulnerable time. We, therefore, implore you to stand up for yourself and to ask for what you need loudly. And to know that you are truly not alone in this. There are so many mothers, women, and people who want to support you.

We also know that you are going to find your strength. And mama, there is no greater strength in the universe.

Be gentle with yourself. Dote on that baby. Take a nap (or ten).

Because mama, you've so got this.

xo,

Jill + Liz

Self-Nurturing and the Fourth Trimester

I am the trunk of my family's tree.

note FROM DIANA

You did it! You have crossed the threshold from woman to mother. You are still *you*, but now you are also a mama! I wish that we could sit down for tea together so that you could tell me your birth story. But even without knowing any details, I know that you were amazing.

We are going to spend a lot of time marveling at your wonder and reflecting on your importance in this part of the book.

You are the trunk of a beautiful family tree. Yes, you have a tiny, new budding twig to take care of. But always remember that *you* are still *you*: a woman with a history all of her own, a woman who has just shared her body with a growing life, a woman who has just given birth, a woman who is settling into her new role as a *mother*, a woman who now needs to heal from those massive feats of *giving* and *becoming*.

We spent a lot of time during your pregnancy discussing postpartum self-care. Now it is time to live it.

Hard to do, right? The constant pull of the to-do list and thoughts of "I should" swirling around in your head can be so much noise.

Please know that you deserve to revel in healing quiet and stillness, to bask in the rays of your own sunlight and the light of those who love you. I know that this is not a common experience for mothers these days, but that doesn't make you any less deserving of it.

You have your own birth story now. In this moment, the story is new and raw, but over time, it will settle in and become a part of you. Our birth stories make us strong, fierce, and vulnerable, all at the same time. However you feel about your birth is okay, and I am going to help you process the emotions that are coming up.

You also have a baby (or two? three?) now. How wild is that? A sweet child that seems to be at once a total mystery and an old soul whom you have known for ages. Meeting your baby is so many things at once—overwhelming in every sense of the word. But don't worry; I'm here to help walk you through it.

And you have this brand-new life. Your connections with your partner, village, work, and hobbies will evolve as you move through your journey as a parent. Sometimes it feels wonderful; other times it is confusing and awkward. That is all normal. Part of that will never go away. But I promise that the pieces will start to fall into place, and we're going to help you make sense of it.

Welcome to your postpartum guide.

It is organized a bit differently than your pregnancy chapters because women's postpartum experiences tend to vary even more than their pregnancy experiences do, which is part of the reason it can feel hard to find the support you crave.

Here you will find detailed sections on emotional wellness, birth recovery and healing, breast- and bottle-feeding, caring for and bonding with your baby, and finding ways to thrive through it all.

xo,

Diana

Birth is arguably the most intense experience we have in our lifetime. To bring life into the world through our bodies is to simultaneously access our deepest strengths and most raw vulnerabilities. After we have done this warrior work, we are immediately thrust into motherhood. We wrap ourselves around our babies, giving and nourishing and pouring our love into them, with little opportunity to process the torrent of emotions and sensations of the birth we just went through.

This part is so important.

Our ancestors gathered together to tell their stories, and in doing so found the peace and comfort that comes from shared experiences. But in our hectic lives, this rarely happens. Birth stories are told, but we are rushed through them, our concerns hushed, and our celebration reduced.

Mamas, tell your stories. Linger in the details, rejoice over your triumphs, cry over the disappointments, and revel in your magic. Your birth story tells how your baby came into being and how you became a mother.

So come, sit beside me, and tell me your birth story.

First, write it down. Record the times and sequence of events, people who were there, and any details you remember. It seems fresh now, but as the years pass, you may forget some of the specifics. You may find yourself coming back to this story as you celebrate your little one's birthdays and may even share it with them one day.

Next, reflect on and record the answers to the following questions. Jot down what comes to your mind first and know that you can come back and add more at any time.

- Describe a moment (or several) that made you feel proud.
- Is there an aspect of your birth for which you feel gratitude?
- What surprised you?
- What questions linger? Was there anything that you did not understand?
- What was it like to see your baby for the first time?
- Were there parts of your birth that felt scary?
- Did anyone stand out to you as being particularly supportive and helpful? Would it feel good to let them know?
- Was there an element of your birth that makes you uncomfortable to reflect on?
- Do you feel at peace with your birth? If not, can you tell what you need to get there?

It's important to feel safe and supported when talking about your birth. People mean well, but many tend to avoid talking about and listening to negative experiences, or maybe they don't let you dwell on the positive ones long enough. What is most therapeutic is to have empathetic listeners who don't judge you, gloss over your experience, or push your feelings aside.

If you're not finding these listeners in your daily life, you will want to find someone who can hear you and help you process your emotions about birth. A therapist, counselor, or psychologist is trained in how to do this, but you can also find support in a partner or friend.

And check out "To the Mama Who Had a Traumatic Birth" on page 345 to evaluate whether you feel your birth wasn't just difficult, but traumatic.

Sleep. Lack of sleep is probably the hardest part of being the parent of a newborn (we'll talk more about your baby's sleep on page 369). It can feel relentless. But know this, mama: This too shall pass. I promise. In the meantime, find pockets of sleep wherever you can. Research has found that even little cat-naps of 20 minutes can help restore energy.

Now, people are going to tell you to "sleep when the baby sleeps." This is a great concept, but the fact is that most moms have trouble following it. The time when the baby is napping is usually the only time you have to yourself, and it is so tempting to do "you stuff." That brings us to the next golden rule.

Be intentional with your time. Okay, the baby is asleep. You get to be the boss of your time. You can do whatever you want, but be intentional. So often we get into the habit of the "let me just." "Let me just do a load of dishes real quick" or "Let me just check Facebook real quick." And before we know it, the baby is awake, and we feel upset that we didn't get to do what we had really wanted to do.

Instead, try to do the most important thing first. If your goal is to take a nap, get right into bed. If your goal is to call your best friend, pick up the phone right away. If your goal is to check Facebook, that is completely fine! Just make sure you are doing it on your terms, intentionally.

Establish boundaries. This is a big one, and there are actually two parts to it: advice boundaries and space and time boundaries.

Remember all the (well-intentioned) people who had all kinds of advice for you during pregnancy? Now that the baby is here, they are back and probably more eager to help you than ever. They love you and want the best for you and the baby. But when you are trying to find your own way, their tips and opinions can be problematic in that they can make you question your instincts, values, and priorities.

Some moms can just tune it out. If this is you, great. If not, you could try saying, "I am so lucky to have your support. For right now, I am going to try things this way, but if it doesn't work, I will absolutely call you for advice."

The second boundary has to do with space and time, two commodities that become precious the moment you become a mom. People want to come to see you and fuss over the baby. They may even be staying in your home for a while to help. This is wonderful, of course, but it can be draining. Remember that even though they are being kind and helpful, you still have the right to (politely) set the rules. For visitors, ask them to come at a certain time that works for you, and when you are ready for the visit to be over, it is completely acceptable to say, "Thank you so much for coming. It was great to see you. I am exhausted, and the baby needs to eat, so we are going to retreat into the bedroom. Can't wait to see you again in a few weeks!" If you have houseguests for an extended period, be sure to carve out time for you to be alone with the baby.

I did not realize that I was an introvert until I became a mom. Until that point, I could "recharge" alone whenever I needed to, so I was always up for hanging or going out. Once my daughter came along, my opportunities to recharge alone decreased dramatically, and suddenly I found myself getting exhausted by social events. It took a while, but I have learned to schedule in "me time" so that I don't burn out.

Eat, drink, and be merry doing it. I've already mentioned my disdain for the idea of "bouncing back." Remember, you just grew life and gave birth. You are healing and growing and changing in thousands of ways. Dieting or "getting your pre-baby body back" does not need to be one of them. Eat healthy foods, absolutely. But try to release the idea of dieting for now. In these first weeks and months, the goal is healing and recovery. Nourish your body with amazing foods. Hydrate yourself with water and smoothies and tea. Be gentle with and talk lovingly to your powerful, wondrous body.

Cut your to-do list in half. (Then do it again.) If your body was making a to-do list during the first month of the postpartum period, here is what it would include:

- Shrink uterus hundreds of times over.
- Reestablish uterine lining while healing wound where placenta detached.
- Heal vaginal tears or Cesarean incision.
- Convert food and water into breast milk.
- Eliminate excess fluid.
- Begin the process of hormonal rebalancing.
- Respond to emotional swings.
- Attend to a tiny human's every single need around the clock.
- Function on minimal sleep.

I am tired just writing that. And you are *living* it!

Mama, the dishes in the sink, the unpainted nursery, and the blank thank-you cards and birth announcements can all wait. Your well-being cannot. If something on your to-do list does not directly impact the mental and physical well-being of yourself or someone who is dependent on you, put it off.

POSTPARTUM TRADITION IN BRAZIL
In Brazil, it is customary for new moms to give a small gift to everyone that comes to visit after the baby is born.

P.S. Etiquette expert Emily Post says you have 2 months after the baby is born to send thank-you notes for gifts. We give you permission to stretch it to 4 months.

Trust yourself. This is incredibly hard to do, but it is crucial. In the absence of the village-style living of the past, mothers suffer because we are simply not around babies and other mothers to the extent we used to be. For many women, the first baby they ever take care of or even hold is their own.

Even if you do have a lot of babies in your life, having one of your own is a completely different beast. You are, for the first time, the ultimate decision maker, the first line of defense. So much responsibility is on you.

And on top of it all, you are healing from the most physically demanding thing you've ever done.

No matter how much support you have, the fourth trimester is a vulnerable time. It is so easy for self-doubt to trickle—or flood—in. Even as a midwife and nurse, I questioned myself repeatedly when I was taking care of each of my three newborns.

You spent time during your pregnancy reflecting on your values, your parenting philosophies, and what type of mother you envisioned yourself being. Now it is time to set those reflections into action. It is okay if they have evolved, as long as it's on your terms. Tune out the noise and trust your intuition.

You are your baby's expert. You are your family's expert. You know what to do. Maybe you don't know how to take care of the umbilical cord stump (see "Umbilical Cord Care" on page 366) or how to freeze your breast milk (see "Breast Milk Storage" on page 409). It's okay; that will come. Your instincts and intention will guide the way, and the rest will fall into place.

Get the help you deserve. From everyone. The people in your life want to help you; they just don't know how. They will be delighted when you assign them a task.

Your mother-in-law's amazing lasagna? Ask her to make it and bring it over.

The high school kid who works at the grocery store? Ask him to help you wheel your cart out to your car.

The lactation consultant your sister used? Ask her to come over to just make sure the baby's latch is right.

The local moms' group you've been silently lurking in on Facebook? Ask them for their favorite local baby-friendly coffee shop, and see if any of them want to meet you there.

THE POSTPARTUM PARADOX

As I shared in chapter 14, many cultures around the world have long-established traditions of prioritizing postpartum care for new moms during the first vulnerable weeks. In addition to providing a nurturing environment to support the mother's process of healing, these practices convey an essential message to new mothers: "What you have done is challenging, and you are important and valued."

Unfortunately, this mentality is not communicated universally. A prime example of this is the lack of a nationwide paid maternity (and paternity) leave program in the US. In fact, an investigation done by the nonprofit magazine *In These Times* found that 1 out of 4 American moms return to the workforce within 2 weeks of giving birth.

Mama, if things seem really hard right now, it is because they are—really hard. The system is letting you down.

But because it is like this now does not mean it will be like this forever. There is much we can do to advance our situation and that of women around the world. Women are speaking up about their needs, calling attention to the inequities, and we are being heard.

In the meantime, mama, the task unfairly falls on you. Given what you know to be true for you and your life, see if you can find small ways to advocate for yourself. When someone offers you help, take it. And if no one offers help, ask for it. It won't be enough, but it will be something. The messaging around you does not speak the truth. You deserve so much. You are so important. You can do this.

Psst: This can be a time of profound transition and even upheaval in partner relationships. We are going to delve into this in chapter 31, "Postpartum Love and Village and Returning to Work," but if you need it now, jump to page 413.

Many hospitals and birth centers offer free breastfeeding groups with lactation consultants, so ask your provider to connect you.

In the absence of the village, we need to create our own. Don't be shy, mama. I bet you'll be blown away by the love that comes pouring in.

Be clear with expectations for the visit. The highest priority is that you don't feel like you have to entertain, clean, or assist your visitors in any way. The visit is about you, mama, and your precious baby, so let them know what time they can visit and how long they can stay, and make it clear that however much you want to help them feel comfortable, it will be up to them to find the water glasses, the snacks, and the door on their way out. Don't feel obliged to take care of anyone but you-know-who.

Request that everyone wash their hands right away. You and baby don't need any outside germs while baby is still developing their immune system.

Accept food and offers for help. Don't feel bashful about your guests' offers to help.

You don't need to fully answer every question, unless you want to. Perhaps you don't feel like going over all the details of the birth again and again, and you're fatigued describing your NICU experience. "It was intense" should suffice. Perhaps you had a rough night and don't feel like rehashing all the feedings and messes you cleaned up. "These first few weeks have been challenging, but I'm holding up" is a good response. Your guests should understand and not take anything personally.

If they do, practice this mantra: "What's mine is mine, and what's theirs is theirs." You can't take care of everyone's feelings and needs right now, and mature adults understand that.

nourish

Postpartum Nourishment
Your #momlife can make healthy eating challenging, to say the least. Your days are

---

POSTPARTUM DOULAS AND NEWBORN CARE SPECIALISTS

Postpartum doulas provide care for women and their families in the weeks immediately following birth. They nurture you as you heal, support you as you learn to breastfeed (or bottle-feed), and offer tons of education surrounding your physical and emotional well-being, as well as caring for your newborn. Some postpartum doulas offer services such as meal preparation and light household work.

While postpartum doulas are there to take care of the mother and the family as a unit, newborn care specialists (also known as baby nurses, night nurses, or night nannies) are there to mainly care for the baby. Some families choose to hire newborn care specialists to provide care overnight or for stretches during the day so that the mother can sleep or recover from birth.

If you are interested in one of these professionals, you might reach out to see if they have a registry plan: Sometimes you can ask friends and family to contribute to the fee as their baby gift to you!

consumed by taking care of a tiny human—as well as the exhaustion that comes along with that—so it can be easy to forget about nourishing yourself.

But mama, it is so important.

A nutrient-dense postpartum diet is critical to help replenish your energy and electrolytes and to support wound healing (such as tears or surgical incisions).

Not only does nourishment allow your body to heal physically from pregnancy and birth, research shows that it may also protect your emotional health. And though we need to learn more about it, it appears that good nutrition can decrease the risk of developing postpartum mood disorders. It can also support breastfeeding, which in turn supports your baby.

There are some key nutrients that are likely to be depleted after pregnancy and giving birth. These include:

- Iron
- Zinc
- Vitamin B12
- Vitamin B9 (folate/folic acid)
- Iodine
- Selenium
- Omega-3 fats like DHA
- Specific amino acids from proteins

So what's a tired but committed mama to do? First, consider the quality of the food you eat without aiming for perfection. Aim for whole foods that are minimally processed to support your diet. The fewer ingredients with names you can't pronounce on the label, the better.

To review, there are three main macronutrients to focus on during this time: carbohydrates, proteins, and healthy fats. If you are able to incorporate these into each meal and snack every day (and we'll show you how), you will officially be rocking your nourishment.

Carbohydrates   Healthy carbs are going to give you the sustained energy you need to care for your baby and heal your body. Specific foods to add to your daily diet include:

- Fruits and veggies
- Whole grains, such as oats, quinoa, brown rice, pasta, and cereals
- Beans
- Starchy vegetables, such as potatoes, squash, and peas

Protein and Iron-Rich Foods   These will help you rebuild your muscles and tissues as you heal, as they replenish blood store losses. When your body has what it needs to heal, you will have more energy and feel better in general. Protein will also support your milk supply if you are breastfeeding.

ON RESTRICTED EATING

Eating nutritious foods is essential, and mama, so is eating *enough* food. There is so much pressure on new moms to make their bodies look a certain way, and as a result, women are suffering. Studies have linked dieting in the postpartum period to the development of maternal eating disorders as well as difficulty with nursing.

Nourish your body and be gentle with yourself. And if the stress of dieting and eating is becoming intrusive in your daily life, seek help from your provider or a therapist, especially if you have had an eating disorder in the past.

Bonus: Protein can help you feel more satisfied after meals and keep your energy levels stable throughout the day! Specific food ideas include:

- Poultry and beef
- Seafood
- Eggs
- Whole-fat yogurt and cheese
- Nuts
- Beans
- Seeds

Healthy Fats These will help your body absorb the other nutrients you eat, as well as boost your energy and stabilize your hormones. Fat is also a major component of breast milk, supporting its ability to help your baby grow and develop. Foods with healthy fats include:

- Olive oil
- Hemp or chia seeds
- Avocados
- Coconut
- Eggs
- Fatty fish, such as salmon

Now that you know what you need, let's talk about how to make this happen: Make. It. Easy.

This is not the time for elaborate meal plans and recipes, unless that brings you joy (then, of course, go for it). Find easy ways to get power foods into your body with as little effort as possible. One of the easiest ways to do this is to combine foods from different groups into one snack or meal.

Pro tips for making this easy in nine (yummy) ways:

1 Make your own veggie plate (or better yet, ask someone else to make it) or buy a premade party platter of vegetables.

OVERNIGHT OATS

Ingredients
1/2 cup rolled oats
1/2 cup milk of choice (cow, almond, soy, or other)
1 tsp. cinnamon (or cocoa powder or dark chocolate)
1/2 tsp. pure vanilla extract
2 Tbs. chopped nuts/seeds (almonds, walnuts, chia seeds, flaxseed)
1 Tbs. sweetener of choice (honey, maple, agave syrup, or other)

Directions
Add ingredients to a glass jar, stir until combined, screw on the lid, and refrigerate overnight. Stir and enjoy cold, or heat in a pan or microwave-safe dish in the morning!

Include carrots, broccoli, celery, bell peppers, and anything else you love, and put a bowl of hummus or guacamole (or both!) in the center. As you are nursing (or Netflixing or just going about your day), you can grab a veggie, dip it, and enjoy. (Oh, and you can even add some flaxseed or chia seeds into the hummus for an omega-3 boost!)

2 Fruit salad is easy. After rinsing them off, cut up your fave fruits and place them in a bowl in the fridge. Berries and kiwis always work well, but of course, add anything else you like. You can simply pick from the bowl as you go through your day, or use it as a premade topping for cereal, yogurt,

oatmeal—and ice cream. (Add granola too for even more nutrients and yum factor.)

3 Speaking of oatmeal, you can batch-make overnight oats (see recipe on previous page). They make an awesome breakfast (and let's be honest, lunch, snack, and dinner, too).

4 Add nut butters to whole-grain breads and crackers.

5 Put avocado in your salads, sandwiches, tacos, and so on. A personal fave is avocado on toast with a drizzle of olive oil. Yum!

6 Stir chia seeds and nuts such as almonds, walnuts, and pecans into your oatmeal, cereal, or yogurt.

7 Make baked potatoes and top with fatty fish (such as salmon).

8 Add your favorite starchy vegetables (such as corn, sweet potatoes, squash, or peas) or beans to salads, soups, stews, or chili to increase the fiber/nutrient content.

9 Hard-boil eggs and keep them in your fridge for a snack or to add to sandwiches/salads.

Other ideas to consider for easy fourth-trimester nourishment:

- Ordering groceries online and having them delivered
- Using a meal-kit service
- Asking for help from loved ones for shopping and cooking
- Requesting that friends set up a meal train for you
- Setting up a stable routine where you share cooking responsibilities with others

Spending a short time on planning meals and snacks for yourself will help you be more intentional about how you are feeding yourself. And don't forget about hydration. It remains ever-important.

Food Restrictions

Many women worry about eating certain foods while breastfeeding. Unless a specific food allergy has been diagnosed in either you or baby, there is likely no need to restrict your diet. The food restrictions that are recommended during pregnancy no longer apply to breastfeeding.

Oh, hello, you gorgeous turkey sandwich, sushi roll, and soft cheese. How I've missed you!

If you do have food restrictions due to sensitivities or reactions identified in your baby, know that there are still many ways to get the nourishment you need. Working with a registered dietitian and lactation consultant can help you come up with a meal plan that meets your energy needs while also protecting your baby.

If You Need More Support

Do not hesitate to reach out for help; professional guidance can be a game changer.

If you aren't sure where to start, check with your health insurance to see if nutrition counseling is covered during your pregnancy or to ask for referrals to providers in your area. You can also check with your perinatal health-care provider for a referral to a dietitian who can help you with an individualized nutrition plan. Lastly, support groups or prenatal nutrition classes can be a lower-cost or free option for connecting with a nutritionist alongside other like-minded mamas. These groups are sometimes offered through clinics or birth centers in your community. Ask your provider if these resources are available to you during your care.

POSTPARTUM MENTAL HEALTH

Before we get into what postpartum mental health issues *are*, we need to discuss what postpartum mental health issues are *not*:

- They are *not* unusual. (Up to 25 percent of women experience postpartum depression, for example.)
- They are *not* a statement about your character.
- They are *not* a reflection of your "abilities" as a mother.
- They are *not* your fault.
- And they are *not* something to ignore.

We spend a lot of time considering all the ways our bodies change during pregnancy: The uterus grows, the pelvis widens, the blood volume increases. But did you know that the brain undergoes massive changes as well?

Neuroscientist Jodi L. Pawluski and colleagues wrote that "the maternal brain is a marvel of directed change, extending into behaviors both obvious (infant-directed) and less obvious (predation, cognition)." In other words, our brains change significantly in response to motherhood. During pregnancy, our brains lose grey matter (neurons) and develop new "neural architecture," all to support the new ways our brain must function as we care for our babies. One theory is that the loss of grey matter is an effort to declutter the brain of neurons it doesn't need, thus making it work more efficiently.

Though more research is needed, one thing seems clear: Pregnancy causes our brains to change in ways that can impact us greatly.

On top of the structural changes, we have intense fluctuations of hormones, and of course sleep deprivation, both of which have very real consequences for our emotional state.

We don't get mad at ourselves when we experience, say, lower back pain in pregnancy. We don't like it, but we know that it is not our fault. It is the function of a growing uterus, hormones, and a shifting pelvis. We don't judge ourselves for those changes because we understand they are beyond our control.

Mental health changes are no different.

Why then, are we so critical of ourselves when we experience them?

ROCK ON, MAMA!

It is a universal fact that music has the power to alter one's mood. So on that premise, researchers studied mothers with depressive symptoms to see what kind of music might help them feel better. They found that while classical music only helped half the mothers, rock music helped all the moms by either balancing the electrical patterns in their brains to buoy them up or by lowering their cortisol levels to calm them down. Either way, rock music had a positive effect on their moods and lowered their anxiety level. So, dig up that old leather jacket and crank the rock 'n' roll!

Like so many aspects of motherhood, a shift is underway. We are recognizing the stigma that exists in our society around mental health issues, and we are slowly but surely working to address it.

A big part of that is focusing on yourself—a brand-new mama. So, let's discuss what you may go through and what to be on the lookout for.

This cannot be emphasized enough: While we very much encourage you to advocate for yourself, you do not—and should not—attempt to diagnose yourself. If you have the slightest concern that something is wrong, please seek help from a mental health therapist. The symptoms of postpartum mental illness can be difficult to sort through and categorize. That is not your job here. Your job is to put yourself in front of a mental health therapist. They will take it from there.

If at any point you have thoughts of harming yourself or someone else, call 911 or go to an emergency room right away.

The Baby Blues

The baby blues are very normal; around 70 to 80 percent of new moms experience them. One moment you feel overjoyed and full of love, and a minute later, you are sobbing because you have no idea what you were thinking or how you are going to actually be this child's mother. (Yes, I have done this three times. I know this phase well.)

The baby blues generally last about 2 to 3 weeks and then taper off.

However, if they last longer than that, and the tear-triggering and downward spirals lead to feelings of despair, hopelessness, or unending bouts of negativity, you might be experiencing postpartum mental illness.

Postpartum Mental Illness

There are several types of illness that may occur:

- Postpartum depression
- Postpartum anxiety
- Postpartum obsessive-compulsive disorder
- Post-traumatic stress disorder
- Postpartum mania
- Postpartum psychosis

Oftentimes the symptoms of these illnesses overlap, and it can be difficult at first to arrive at a diagnosis (which is why consulting with a mental health therapist is so important). Symptoms can include:

- Feeling sad for long periods of time without an easy-to-pinpoint cause
- Lack of desire to do the things you used to love
- Difficulty getting out of bed
- Difficulty falling asleep
- Lack of motivation
- Feeling guilty often
- Anger or rage
- Worrying about things that seem odd or that you did not used to be worried about
- Repetitive thoughts or actions, such as the need to clean something over and over or ensure that a door is locked multiple times
- Fear of being left alone with your baby
- Reliving difficult aspects of your birth
- Not wanting to talk or think about your birth at all
- Inability to make decisions
- Periods of being extremely energized (lots of talking, moving, cleaning)

- Feeling invincible or that you have powers beyond human ability
- Hallucinations
- Intrusive and disturbing thoughts; violent thoughts
- Not being able to sit still
- Not feeling bonded to your baby

Examples of thoughts you may have include:

- "My baby doesn't love me."
- "I am not a good mom."
- "I want to run away."
- "I don't deserve to be happy."
- "Something bad is going to happen to my baby. I know it."
- "My family would be less burdened if I weren't around."

Mama, if anything resonated with you here, please reach out for help. Again, postpartum mental illness is complex. Any concerns or thoughts that just don't feel right warrant your attention.

Because here's the thing: Postpartum mental illness is treatable. Within a short window of time, you can get to a point where you are feeling significantly better. Whether it's talk therapy, medication, or a combination, there absolutely is hope. Please ask for help. For additional resources related to mental wellness, visit mother.ly/becomingmama.

TO THE MAMA WHO HAD A TRAUMATIC BIRTH

Birth has the potential to rock our worlds.

Sometimes our experiences leave us hurting, scared, and sad. Sometimes we feel cheated. Sometimes we just feel lost and confused.

While all birth is amazing, not all women feel amazing about their births.

Birth trauma is a very real thing, and we need to talk about it. Trauma is defined as "a deeply distressing or disturbing experience." A birth that leaves us feeling distressed or disturbed is a traumatic birth.

So, mama, if you are feeling unsettled, scared, or any other powerful and negative emotions about your birth, please know that your emotions are valid.

When we give birth, we do so from our core—not just the core of our bodies, but the core of ourselves. We are open and vulnerable during and after birth, and the energy that is around us is the energy we absorb. It becomes a part of the inner voice that guides us in motherhood.

Please remember that trauma is incredibly personal. What's traumatic for one woman may not be for another. One woman may be traumatized by a birth that happens very quickly, while another woman would call that her dream birth. One woman may be traumatized by needing to have a Cesarean, while another would feel relieved by it. A woman can have a perfect birth on paper but could have been deeply affected by a few careless words uttered to her in passing.

If you feel traumatized, it is trauma. Plain and simple. Don't let anyone make you feel like you are overreacting, and certainly don't ignore what your mind and body are telling you.

Please reach out for help because although the story has been set, the way you process it doesn't have to be. Mental health therapists can help you work through your experience in a way that is healthy and constructive.

remember

The truth is, no matter where you are on this journey, you will still be growing, changing, learning—and becoming mama. There's no one way you "should" feel about your new role, and there are as many different ways to mother as there are mamas. We all have negative thoughts and feelings about big life changes, so don't sweep those away and bury them because you think you shouldn't feel a certain way. What is most important is that you recognize that feelings change from moment to moment, from day to day, and from month to month. But if your feelings are consistently outside your normal range of highs and lows, you need to reach out for help. And that may be the biggest lesson of early mamahood: We can't do it alone!

Postpartum Physical Recovery

Moment to moment,
I am healing.

note
FROM DIANA

Getting reacquainted with your body after giving birth is a challenge that no one can prepare you for. When you are pregnant, you can wrap your mind around the changes that are happening: There are books to read (*hi!*), there are lots of prenatal appointments, and the experience somehow makes sense (though it is pretty weird). But when the baby is out and it is "just" you again, it can sometimes feel like you are a stranger in a new territory.

Your organs have quite literally shifted around your body and will take some time settling back into place. Your baby is born, but your uterus still makes you look several months pregnant. You have lines on your skin, pounds on your hips (and arms and legs), and your breasts, well, you've never quite seen your breasts like *this* before. The image you see in the mirror is not what you expected.

On top of it all, your stamina is (way) different and your body is healing from probably the most physically strenuous thing it has ever done.

Mama, you are not making this up. This is difficult. And this is a time for self-compassion.

Your body has gone through so much. She needs your kindness and gentleness in every way during this season. The time will come to return to the gym or those skinny jeans or whatever else you need (and that is completely fine). But for now, breathe and remind your body of how proud you are of all that she has done—and is doing.

xo,

Diana

BLEEDING AND YOUR HEALING UTERUS

Now that your uterus has completed the Herculean task of growing and giving birth to your baby, it needs to heal and recover. It takes about 6 weeks (this can vary) for your uterus to return to its prepregnancy size, though it does a significant amount of this shrinking in the first days of the fourth trimester. This process is called involution.

Postpartum bleeding is called lochia and happens whether you have a vaginal or Cesarean birth. Bleeding may last up to 6 weeks.

The bleeding and discharge happen for a few reasons. Blood remaining from birth and remnants of the pregnancy need to be expelled after the baby is born. Your uterus is also healing the site where your placenta was attached. It's much like a wound that needs time to get better.

Lochia changes as time passes. During the first 3 to 5 days after birth, it will be like a heavy period. The blood will be red or dark red with a moderate flow (called lochia rubra). You may see a few small pieces of the amniotic sac, vernix (the white waxy substance that covered your baby in the womb), or lanugo (your baby's downy body hair) in those first days. Lochia rubra generally smells like menstrual blood.

You may also have some blood clots, which can be normal. Blood clots form when blood is stagnant, or not moving. So, if you sleep for a period of time and then stand up, you may see or feel a clot or two come out. You may also have a gush of blood when you stand up because the blood has been pooling in your vagina while you were lying down.

I'll say this more than once, and I am emphasizing it here, because it is so important: If you are at all concerned about how much you are bleeding, *let your team know right away. This warrants a 2:00 a.m. call to your midwife or doctor.*

Danger signs include filling a pad with blood in an hour or two, passing multiple blood clots, or passing any one clot that is larger than the size of a golf ball.

Of important note: Native American women may be at an increased risk of experiencing a postpartum hemorrhage. And black women who have postpartum hemorrhages may have more serious cases.

Toward the end of the first week, the lochia rubra will transition into lochia serosa, which consists of a lighter flow and lighter color. It's usually light red or brownish-red instead of deep red. This lasts about 2 weeks, though this can vary. Some women will see this end at around 10 days, while others have this for up to 4 weeks.

After lochia serosa comes lochia alba. This is more like vaginal discharge than bleeding. It is yellowish-white in color and may last until around week 6.

If, especially during the first weeks, you notice a sudden uptick in bleeding, it can be a sign that you may need to be less active. Your body may not have been ready for that walk around the block yet. Take it as a signal that your body is asking you to rest more and call your provider with any concerns.

Managing Your Involution and Bleeding

Right after your birth and for the first days after (if you're still in the hospital), your midwife, doctor, or nurses will be checking and massaging your uterus. They will ask you to lie flat on your back. They'll place a hand on your belly to press down, feeling your uterus. They want to make sure it feels firm (and not floppy, flaccid, or "boggy," as it's termed) and also that it is decreasing in size. On the day you give birth, the top of the uterus should be approximately level with your belly button (when you are lying down), and we expect the uterus to be about a centimeter lower every day. The nurse or provider may also massage your uterus to help encourage it to clamp down. This is uncomfortable, but it should only last about 30 seconds.

For the first months of postpartum, pads or disposable underwear are the best way to manage bleeding. Tampons are not recommended. If you had a vaginal birth, your vagina is sensitive and healing, and tampons will impact that process. With either type of delivery, tampons can increase the risk of toxic shock syndrome. Try to choose pads or disposable underwear without fragrance, as your vulva may be extra-sensitive.

Make sure to pee frequently. When your bladder is full, it can push the uterus off to one side, which impacts the uterus's ability to heal and shrink. Stay hydrated and empty your bladder about every 2 hours while awake to prevent this from happening.

Cramping Versus Pain

Cramping during the first 3 to 5 days is normal—and actually a good thing! This is especially true for women who are breastfeeding. Every time your baby latches on or you pump, oxytocin is released. Yes, the same oxytocin that gave you labor contractions. The oxytocin tells your uterus to contract, this time to help reduce bleeding and to aid in healing. Ask your provider about taking a medication, like ibuprofen or acetaminophen, those first days to help with the pain (these are considered safe for breastfeeding).

If you feel that your pain is not related to breastfeeding and feels like more than just cramping, it may be a sign of a uterine infection, especially if you have had a Cesarean birth. You may experience pain in your lower abdomen, along with fever and chills. If that happens, call your provider right away.

Postpartum Hemorrhage: Warning Signs

Postpartum hemorrhage (PPH) is when a woman loses 1,000 milliliters or more of blood, or has blood loss with specific signs and symptoms, after giving birth. It is a leading cause of sickness and death for women around the world. A PPH can happen just after birth, but it can also happen days or even weeks later. This is called a late postpartum hemorrhage.

You know that I am not a fan of worrying you. But when it comes to postpartum bleeding, I drop my guard on that a bit because it's a big deal. It is essential to be aware of the risk because if you have a problem, it is likely that you are going to be the one to identify it first, not your medical team. This is a vital area to practice your self-advocacy. If you are concerned, call your provider, go to the emergency room, or call 911. Right away.

Signs to look out for:

- A sudden increase in bleeding or sudden return to bright-red bleeding when it's been brown or pink
- Foul-smelling vaginal discharge
- Filling a pad in 1 to 2 hours
- Chills
- Blurred vision
- Dizziness, light-headedness, or weakness
- Fast heartbeat

- Rapid breathing
- Clammy skin
- Confusion
- Nausea or vomiting
- Swelling in the vaginal area
- Fever

VAGINAL HEALING

Whether you tore or had an episiotomy or "just" stretched during delivery, your vagina now needs to recover.

If you had a Cesarean birth after pushing for some time, it is possible that you'll also experience some vaginal discomfort during these first days or weeks.

The good news: Vaginas are exceptional. They are designed to heal from birth and return to pretty much the same shape they were in.

So, how long will the pain last? With a huge caveat, the standard answer is up to 6 weeks (but often it's much shorter). Depending on how severe your injuries were, this time period can vary widely, though many women experience a great deal of relief by the end of the first week. From my experience, many women find that at about 2 to 3 weeks postpartum, they are not thinking about their perineum nearly as much as they were those first days.

Following are my two favorite remedies for perineal pain.

Sitz Bath   This is a plastic basin that goes on your toilet. It is filled with water and acts like a whirlpool for your bottom. Your hospital or birth center may send you home with one for free, or you can usually buy them at a local pharmacy or medical supply store. Several times per day for about 20 minutes, sit with your bottom immersed in the sitz bath. You can use room-temperature or warm (never hot) water. Or you can make a mixture of water, two tablespoons of witch hazel, and a few drops of lavender essential oil. You can also sit in your bathtub if you don't have a sitz bath, but it's very important to make sure the tub is clean so that your perineal area does not become infected. Ask your partner or a friend to disinfect the tub with the agent of your choice—vinegar, hydrogen peroxide, or bleach—and rinse extremely well before getting in.

Padsicles   You can make these ahead of time or as needed. Take a regular menstrual pad and line it with witch hazel (either poured from a bottle or presoaked towelettes). You can then add a tablespoon of aloe vera and a few drops of lavender essential oils if that's

VAGINAL BLEEDING WITH C-SECTIONS

Many women are surprised to learn that they will still have vaginal bleeding after a Cesarean section, even if they did not go through any contractions. The blood comes from your uterus, which is healing where the placenta detached, recovering from surgery, and healing from all those months of pregnancy. So, your bleeding will be much like the bleeding experienced after a vaginal birth (see "Bleeding and Your Healing Uterus" on page 349). It is vital for you to report too much bleeding, which is when you fill a pad with blood in just an hour or two.

your preference. Place the pad in your underwear, or if you don't need it right away, wrap it up and put it in the freezer until you do.

By the end of 6 weeks, stitches are usually dissolved, and the perineum, vagina, and surrounding parts appear to be back to normal. But here is the caveat: We do not currently pay enough attention to postpartum healing, and that is a problem.

Yes, most women (95 percent, in fact) who have a vaginal birth experience some degree of vaginal and perineal pain after delivery. This is expected. But if your pain has turned into suffering, attention may be needed, and you might need to advocate for it.

For a long time, we have been normalizing pelvic pain after birth. In doing so, many women have not received the help they need for experiences that extend beyond what is considered normal and expected. So, if you

have a lot of pain, trouble holding your urine, difficulty with sex, or any other concerns, ask for a referral to a pelvic floor physical therapist (more on that soon).

CESAREAN SECTION HEALING

After your Cesarean section, you'll likely stay in the hospital for about 3 nights. When your birth is complete, you'll be brought to a recovery room and monitored closely.

As the anesthesia wears off, you'll likely start to experience pain at the incision site, and you may also have nausea, itching, and heartburn. Communicate all of this to your nurses and provider, as there is medication available for all of it.

If you have a urinary catheter, it may be removed when you are able to walk to the bathroom, though providers are starting to remove them even sooner (or not place one at all).

A significant milestone after a Cesarean birth is passing gas: Yup, everyone around you wants you to fart! Abdominal surgeries slow down digestion and can (rarely) cause a serious intestinal blockage called a postoperative ileus (more on this on page 481). Passing gas is a sign that everything is in good working order. Studies have found that chewing sugar-free gum after a C-section can speed up movement of the digestive system, thus making you pass gas and even poop sooner, which can decrease your risk of complications. When you pack your hospital bag, throw in a few packs of your favorite gum!

You will not be able to eat immediately after your C-section (and you likely won't want to, either, due to some post-surgery nausea). But when you do get hungry, let your nurse know! When you get the green light to eat, start slowly to make sure it sits well.

REIKI FOR C-SECTION RECOVERY

Reiki is a form of complementary healing whereby the therapist channels energy throughout the body using light touch, and it can be great for new mothers. A study found that Reiki resulted in decreased pain for women who were recovering from Cesarean sections.

This form of healing is not covered by insurance, so it is important to know the rates of the practitioner you plan to work with and whether they can accommodate different income levels. You can also look into working with someone who is training, as they may be able to offer discounted rates.

You will be encouraged to get out of bed and walk within the first day—with plenty of help, don't worry. This will help to wake up your digestive system, as well as prevent blood clots and get you ready for going home. Many women I work with say that although those first walks are difficult (you may feel weak or have pain), they make a world of difference in the speed of recovery.

Pressing a small pillow lightly against your incision as you walk, cough, and sneeze can be helpful in decreasing the amount of pain.

As you recover from surgery, you can expect some pain, especially in the area of your lower abdomen. You will be given pain medication in the hospital, and possibly some to go home with. Do not be afraid to be very vocal about what you are feeling and to ask for medication when you need it—or even before. It can be easier to prevent pain than to make it go away once it sets in.

If everyone is healthy, most babies can be brought into the recovery room with you and stay with you throughout your time in the hospital. You will also be able to breastfeed almost right away. Your nurses will help you find positions that are comfortable with your incision, and I'd strongly encourage that you ask to see the hospital lactation consultant as well—the more help, the better! C-section mamas usually opt for the football hold (see page 396) or side-lying position (see page 396) in those first days and weeks of recovery, though I know some women who were able to do cradle and cross cradle using a soft nursing pillow.

The method used to close your incision (Steri-Strips, staples, or other) will vary, so your nurses and provider will give you detailed instructions about how to care for your wound and when to return to have the strips or staples removed. In general, you want to be gentle with the area: Wash it carefully, pat dry, and keep an eye out for openings, bleeding, redness, swelling, pus, or severe pain.

Once home, you may have trouble walking up and down stairs, and you likely won't be able to drive for a period of time. This is a great time to call on your village for help.

Other aspects of your recovery will be similar to the process that women who had vaginal births go through, so be sure to review the earlier sections in this chapter. Remember, you gave birth to your baby, and that makes you a warrior-mama, plain and simple.

ALL THE OTHER RECOVERY ISSUES

Peeing

Nothing can really prepare you for how many thoughts and questions you might have about another person's pee and poop when you have a baby. It turns out that your own elimination will be on your mind as well.

The first days after you give birth, your medical team will ask you many times about your urination. This is to ensure that your system remains healthy after labor or surgery, especially if you had a urinary catheter. Don't worry; complications are rare.

What is more common is discomfort when you pee. Women usually experience a burning sensation on their perineum, the skin just outside of the vagina. Whether the skin has been stitched or simply stretched, these abrasions or wounds burn when urine passes over them. But don't worry; there's a trick (or two) for that.

Stay Hydrated The possibility of burning may not inspire you to want to drink a lot, but by staying hydrated, your urine will be less concentrated and will, therefore, burn less. Try to drink at least ten 8-ounce glasses of water a day.

Use a Perineum Bottle Many hospitals and birth centers will send you home with a plastic bottle called a peri bottle. If not, they are available for purchase online, or you could use another plastic bottle that has been thoroughly cleaned and disinfected. Fill the bottle with tepid or room-temperature water, and as you are peeing, gently pour the water over your vulvar area. This dilutes the urine, washes it quickly from your skin, and makes it so that you don't have to wipe with toilet paper. It can also be used to keep your perineal area clean. Make sure you dry the area well, using a patting motion (not wiping).

Urinary Tract Infections

It's important—but sometimes difficult—to distinguish between the normal discomfort of peeing after birth and a urinary tract infection (UTI). UTIs can be more common during pregnancy and immediately after, due to the structural shifts within your body that have occurred, the presence of a catheter, and just a lot of attention to that area in general.

The primary difference between the "normal" pain and a UTI is that a UTI tends to hurt or burn more on the inside when you pee, as opposed to on the outer skin. That said, that's not a foolproof method for distinguishing them, so if you are at all concerned, call your provider.

Staying well hydrated is a great first step in prevention. Also, when you wipe, always do so from front to back.

Symptoms of a UTI include:

- Burning when you urinate
- Cloudy or bloody urine (which can be hard to see when you have postpartum bleeding)
- Foul-smelling urine
- Intense and frequent need to urinate, with only a little urine actually coming out
- Fever or chills
- Lower back pain

Incontinence

Incontinence, or losing your urine when you don't mean to, is common after giving birth.

Researchers have not yet found concrete evidence that this is a hereditary condition, but they have found that Caucasian and Hispanic women tend to have a higher risk of urinary incontinence.

Other contributing factors include weakened pelvic floor muscles, episiotomies, structural changes that occurred during pregnancy, and damaged bladder nerves.

Some women try to avoid losing their urine by not drinking as much fluid. Unfortunately, this doesn't usually work, and it can increase your risk of other problems like UTIs, dehydration, and decreased breast milk production.

If the incontinence lasts beyond the first postpartum weeks, report it to your provider.

Pooping

The very first bowel movement you have after delivery is notoriously scary. You've just given birth, you may have stitches (either in your perineum or your abdomen), you're sore, and quite frankly the idea of having to push something else out of a tender and vulnerable part of your body sounds like a terrible idea.

The bad news is that you do have to do it. The good news is that chances are it will be okay. And I'm here to walk you through. It is my midwifely duty (pun intended) to help you with this as well. Here's what to know.

Delayed First Poop   If you didn't eat while you were in labor, there may just not be anything in your system to digest yet. Your GI tract also slows down during birth, so it may take a bit for it to wake up. You also may have pooped during birth. Your bowel may have been stressed during labor as well. Lastly, the stress factor may contribute to some holding back, either consciously or subconsciously.

If you have stitches, know that they are designed to withstand pressure. Some women like to get their squat on with a toilet footstool, which supports elimination with a more natural squat position.

Some providers will prescribe stool softening medications for the first few days postpartum. It can also be bought over the counter. These can be a great help. Just be sure to also follow the other healthy-bowel tips here in addition to using the meds: The meds should be a temporary measure.

Foods That Can Help
- Water, water, juice, and more water (hydration is key to a healthy and pain-free bowel movement)
- Fruits like apples, prunes, figs, and berries
- Coffee
- Oatmeal, bran muffins
- Chia seeds

Taking Deep Breaths   Yes, I am offering a guided imagery exercise to help you poop: We've bonded enough by now for this.

When you have the urge to go, do what you can to make it a relaxing experience. Ask

PELVIC FLOOR PHYSICAL THERAPY

You may have heard that in some countries—like France, Holland, and Australia—women are entitled to pelvic floor therapy after birth through their national health-care service. New moms there don't suffer as much from incontinence or other pelvic floor issues that are so common in the US because their providers routinely prescribe physical therapy post-birth, known as perineal reeducation, which can cure incontinence in over 60 percent of women. Hopefully the US will follow this trend soon. In the meantime, you may need to ask for it. Your provider may have a pelvic floor physical therapist to refer you to (who may take insurance). There are also providers who do not take insurance.

The important thing to note here is that "Yeah, you had a baby. This is how it is now" is not an appropriate response. You deserve help and very likely do not have to just deal with this.

someone to watch the baby and find a time and place where you won't feel rushed.

Sit on the toilet, take some deep breaths, and relax your pelvis. Close your eyes and try to visualize the digested food leaving your body. It nourished you and gave you the energy to get through labor. Now it's done its job, and it will be on its way. It's just some old food remnants—nothing to be scared of.

Instead of forcefully pushing the bowel movement out, simply allow your bowels to relax and open. If the poop needs a little nudge, you'll know and can do so safely, but otherwise, just let your smart body and gravity do the work.

No rush. No pressure. Just poop.

Constipation   If you don't have a bowel movement within a few days, if it hurts to poop, or if the poop is hard or rabbit-pellet-like, call your provider. They can recommend a medication to help you.

Fecal Incontinence and Uncontrolled Gas

It doesn't seem quite fair that, after all you've been through, this is something you might need to now deal with, but it's the unfortunate truth for up to 25 percent of women, so let's talk about it.

"Anal incontinence" is the term that means not being able to stop feces or gas from passing. Reasons that it could happen include injuries during birth, operative deliveries (like with forceps), episiotomies, pushing for a long time, having a large baby, and general instability of the pelvic floor after pregnancy.

For some women, this may go away with time. But it can last for up to 12 months or longer without treatment, so please do not be embarrassed to seek help from your provider. Treatment may involve medication to bulk up your stool or physical therapy to restore your pelvic floor.

It's also important to note that women with anal incontinence are at high risk for depression and anxiety. Speaking to a mental health therapist and finding support groups can help you cope emotionally as you physically heal.

In the meantime, women find that wearing pads or disposable underwear can help them feel more confident about going out and about.

Hemorrhoids

Postpartum hemorrhoids are much like the ones you may experience during pregnancy, though the pushing and general strain on your pelvis during birth can make them worse. Whatever the reason, they are painful, but treatable. Try witch hazel pads. Sitz baths can also be soothing and healing, as can padsicles (see page 351). Of course, there are also over-the-counter hemorrhoidal creams. If all of these fail, discuss other treatment options with your provider.

Night Sweats

Postpartum night sweats can be quite annoying to the almost 30 percent of women who have them. Your precious few hours of sleep are hard enough to come by, and now you have to spend them sweating like you just ran a marathon.

Postpartum night sweats are caused by the lower levels of estrogen that your body is adjusting to now that your baby has been born, and by your body's effort to release the extra fluids from pregnancy and delivery.

Don't worry; they won't last forever. They tend to start to go away around week 2. In the meantime, continue to stay hydrated. I know this seems backward, but hydrated veins actually help your body release fluid. Wear cotton and other light, natural fabrics and avoid sweat-inducing foods like caffeine, spicy foods, and alcohol.

If your night sweats don't go away after a few weeks, talk to your provider about checking your thyroid.

Hair Loss

Many women enjoy the lustrous-hair effect of pregnancy, only to be disappointed when

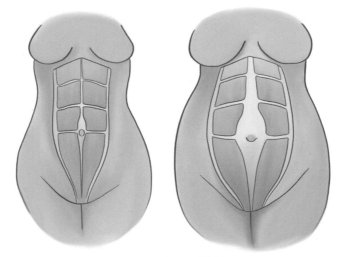

DIASTASIS RECTI

that lustrous hair starts to fall out postpartum. Most of the time, you are not actually losing more hair, your body is just shedding the hair it didn't shed during pregnancy. This tends to be most extreme around month 3 but can take about a year to stabilize.

In the meantime, treat yourself to a new haircut—mom bob, anyone? Use volumizing products to help boost up your roots to hide any thinning patches. Or just embrace it and wait for it to stop, which it will. You are gorgeous, mama.

If you are concerned about the hair loss, talk to your doctor or midwife about whether a thyroid test is in order.

Birth Control

You may want to start a form of birth control, either to prevent pregnancy or for other medical reasons. Choosing a birth control method is complicated. There is no perfect choice, and it all depends on you (and your partner). Unfortunately, all the contraception methods out there come with a downside—especially

for women. That said, there are a lot of options to choose from. Take your time, talk to your provider, and listen to your gut.

Following on pages 358–359 is a guide to help you begin to consider which hormonal or non-hormonal method might be for you. This is not meant to be comprehensive. There are a lot of details to know about each option, and only your provider can give you all the info you need to make the right choice for you.

Diastasis Recti

As your abdomen stretched to accommodate your growing uterus and belly, your abdominal muscles may have shifted to the sides to make more room. In doing so, they can separate in the middle, causing what is known as a diastasis recti. Research estimates that anywhere from 30 to 100 percent of pregnant women will experience this to some degree.

Your provider can tell you if you have this, or you may be able to feel it yourself. Lie flat on your back, lift your head up to contract your

HORMONAL BIRTH CONTROL METHODS

METHOD	EFFECTIVE WITH TYPICAL USE	DESCRIPTION	BREAST-FEEDING SAFE?	PROS	CONS	NOTES
Implant	99.9%	Matchstick-sized rod inserted into forearm that releases progesterone.	Yes	"Set it and forget it." Lasts 3–5 years (unless removed sooner).	May cause heavy periods or irregular bleeding.	Usually inserted during a quick office procedure.
Hormonal IUD	Mirena, Skyla, Liletta, Kyleena: >99%	Small, T-shaped device placed in your uterus. Works by thinning the lining of the uterus, changing the cervical mucus, and stops ovulation.	Yes	"Set it and forget it" (check placement monthly). Lasts 5+ years (unless removed sooner). May eventually ease period symptoms.	May experience spotting. 5% risk of falling out in the first year.	Can be placed immediately after birth, though failure rates are higher if done so.
Injection	96%	Injection of progesterone hormone received every 12 weeks.	Yes	Only have to think about once every 12 weeks.	Have to wait until the dose fades if you don't like the side effects. Long-term use can cause bone loss, weight gain, and other hormonal birth control symptoms.	Ask to pre-schedule appointments for the year, so you don't go too long between injections.
Minipill	93%	Pill taken by mouth daily that contains progesterone only, which prevents sperm from meeting egg.	Yes	May eventually stop your period.	Must remember to take every day. Not safe to take with a history of certain medical problems.	Should take it within the same 3-hour span each day for it to be effective.
Patch	93%	Skin patch that releases estrogen and progesterone, which stops ovulation; changed every 3 weeks.	Yes, after 6 weeks postpartum when milk supply is established	Can regulate periods and related symptoms.	Increases risk of blood clots, heart attacks, and strokes in some women.	Be sure to wear the patch on a spot that won't often be rubbed by clothing.
Pill	93%	Pill taken by mouth daily that contains estrogen and progesterone, which stops ovulation.	Yes, after 6 weeks postpartum when milk supply is established	Can regulate periods and related symptoms.	Must remember to take every day. Increases risk of blood clots, heart attacks, and strokes in some women.	May not be immediately effective, so discuss the need for a back-up method with your provider.
Ring	NuvaRing: 93%	Plastic, bendable ring inserted into the vagina (by you) that releases estrogen and progesterone, which stops ovulation. Removed after 3 weeks, so you can have a period.	Yes, after 6 weeks postpartum when milk supply is established	Can regulate periods and related symptoms.	Increases risk of blood clots, heart attacks, and strokes in some women.	You can talk to your provider about using the ring to skip a period.
Emergency contraception (Plan B)	75%–89%	Pill(s) taken after intercourse that prevent(s) fertilization from occurring.	Yes, though repetitive use may decrease milk supply	Can buy over the counter.	Lower efficacy rate. Can be difficult to find depending on where you live.	The sooner you take it after intercourse, the more effective it is. Consider keeping some on hand. Inserting an IUD within 5 days of intercourse is also a form of emergency contraception.

NON-HORMONAL BIRTH CONTROL METHODS

METHOD	EFFECTIVE WITH TYPICAL USE	DESCRIPTION	BREAST-FEEDING SAFE?	PROS	CONS	NOTES
Abstinence	100% with perfect adherence	Abstaining from vaginal sex with males.	Yes	100% effective.	May not be appealing to all.	Trigger warning: does not work in the event of nonconsensual sexual encounters.
Male sterilization (vasectomy)	99.9%	Procedure to block the tubes that carry sperm.	Yes	Permanent. More effective and less invasive than female sterilization.	Must wait for all sperm to leave the body before man is sterile.	Reversals are sometimes possible, though it's safest to assume it won't work.
Female sterilization	99.5%	Surgery that blocks fallopian tubes from allowing egg to travel down and become fertilized.	Yes	Permanent.	Permanent. Requires invasive minor surgery.	Essure is a metal coil that is placed in the tubes without surgery that has the same effect.
Copper IUD	ParaGard: 99.2%	Small, T-shaped device placed in your uterus, which works by keeping sperm and egg from meeting.	Yes	"Set it and forget it" (check placement monthly). Lasts up to 10+ years (unless removed sooner). Immediate return to fertility when removed.	May experience heavy periods for the first year. 5% risk of it falling out in the first year.	Can be placed immediately after birth, though failure rates are higher if done so.
Lactational amenorrhea method (LAM)	98% with perfect use	Breastfeeding-induced lack of ovulation.	Yes	Can be effective for the first 6 months. No need to buy anything or put anything into your body.	Only works if you are exclusively breastfeeding and never go longer than 4 hours between feedings during the day and 6 hours at night. Only effective if you are less than 6 months postpartum and have not gotten your period.	LAM is not effective if: baby is 6 months or older; breastfeeding frequency is less than described to left; bottles are introduced; or your period returns.
Male condom	87%	Sheath that goes over the penis to catch sperm.	Yes	Depending on material made from, can provide STI protection. Can buy over the counter.	Decreased sensation for men. Requires male cooperation.	Lambskin condoms do not protect against STIs.
Diaphragm and cervical cap	83%	Dome-shaped device inserted into the vagina (often used with spermicide) to prevent sperm from passing through cervix.	Yes	Female controlled.	Must be comfortable inserting your fingers into your vagina. Must remember to put it in.	Most women wait to start using until 6 weeks after birth. Must be refitted by provider after giving birth.
Female condom	79%	Sheath that is placed inside the vagina to catch sperm.	Yes	Provides STI protection. Can buy over the counter.	Must remember to put it in.	Can be inserted several hours before intercourse, if desired.
Spermicide	79%	Gel, cream, or foam inserted into vagina to kill sperm on contact.	Yes	Can buy over the counter.	Can cause burning and skin breakdown, which can make you more susceptible to contracting HIV over time.	Needs to be inserted within about 20 minutes before intercourse.
Withdrawal (pulling out)	78%	Male ejaculates outside of vagina.	Yes	Increased sensation for both parties (compared to male condom use).	Risk of some sperm leaving the penis before ejaculation.	Requires willpower.
Natural family planning (fertility awareness)	77%–98%	Timing sex based on your knowledge of your cycles and fertile time.	Yes	Feeling of empowerment for many women.	Can be tricky to learn at first.	Look for a local class to learn how to do natural family planning!
Sponge	If you've never given birth: 86% If you've given birth: 73%	A squishy sponge with spermicide in it that kills sperm on contact.	Yes	Can buy over the counter.	Must remember to put it in.	Can be inserted several hours before intercourse, if desired.

abdominals, and press your fingers into your belly a few inches above your belly button. You may be able to feel the separation.

Diastasis recti can resolve on its own, depending on how severe it is. Ensure that you maintain good posture and body mechanics as you are healing: Lift with your legs, not your back, and support your upper body as you get into and out of bed.

If it is still present 6 to 8 weeks after birth (which it often is), talk to your provider about the possible need for physical therapy or other support resources.

Getting Your Period

If you are not breastfeeding, you can expect your period to return about 40 days after giving birth because your ovulation hormones are not interrupted by the milk-producing hormones. If you are exclusively breastfeeding, enjoy the reprieve from bleeding, since it may take 27 to 38 weeks to resume menstruation. If you're both breastfeeding and bottle-feeding, your period's return can be hard to predict.

Anecdotally, some women report that birth changes their periods. They may be longer or shorter than before or have more or less blood. You may also find that they are irregular at first, especially if you are breastfeeding.

Remember that you ovulate before you see the blood of your period, which means it is possible to get pregnant just weeks after giving birth. Refer to the previous chart for birth control ideas if you are ready to resume sex and need birth control.

move

Most providers recommend waiting about 6 weeks after a vaginal birth and 8 weeks after a Cesarean birth to start exercising again. It is essential to ensure that you are physically ready to work out so that you don't get injured. Be sure to ask your provider if you can start exercising at your postpartum visit. But before then, let's talk about core rehab.

During pregnancy and then again during birth, our core and pelvic floor experience a good amount of pressure and stretching. It's important that we rehab our core in the early days of the postpartum period to support even the simplest daily movements. This rehabilitation will also help you better prepare for getting back into your exercise routine at 6 to 8 weeks postpartum (if desired), while helping to heal your core in the most supportive of ways. Get clearance from your provider, and then try the following.

Practice

In the first few days postpartum, reconnect to your diaphragmatic breathing (see page 119). This provides powerful healing to your core and any abdominal separation that may be present.

Begin reimplementing the belly pump (see page 132) and focus on feeling the sensations in the pelvic floor and corset muscles as you activate them. You can expect these muscles to feel weak at first, but you'll be surprised at how quickly they seem to find the familiar activation from before.

Refer to "Lift and Wrap in Everyday Life" on page 108, where we talk about implementing correct core recruitment in various daily movements. This can begin soon after you give birth to provide the most support possible to your body in the early days, especially now that you'll probably be carrying the 6- to 10-pound weight of your baby.

As you begin to feel stronger and more connected to your core in the first few weeks postpartum, it's important to continue to rehab your core via gentle core recruitment exercises before jumping back into a full-on exercise routine.

Pay attention to your body. If you notice an increase in bleeding, pain, or any other concerning signs, report the symptoms to your provider right away.

Tips for Success

- Most expecting women experience some level of naturally occurring abdominal separation (diastasis recti), and it's important to evaluate the depth, width, and length. If you're experiencing any discomfort, urine leaking, or bulging sensations in your pelvic floor, seek guidance from a pelvic floor physical therapist in your area. The sooner these things are addressed, the better.

- If any of the above symptoms are present, seek out a specialist before returning to your regular exercise routine to ensure that you've healed in the most supportive ways as you move forward in motherhood.

pause
AND REFLECT

Ah, mama. It is in this moment that you might be susceptible to all sorts of unforgiving self-talk. You may be idolizing women who appear to have it all together just moments after giving birth. But anything you read in glossy magazines or see on TV about the postpartum period is likely to be fiction.

If I could give a prescription to postpartum mamas, it would be to only engage with media that soothes you, if you engage at all. This is a quiet, healing time when focusing on your baby is a joy, and taking time to build up that rapport is all-encompassing. Don't distract yourself with what others are doing. You and baby are the stars of the show right now.

It's common to speed up and try to cram more in when we become stressed or overwhelmed. We try to push ourselves because we want to feel like we are accomplishing something, and we become tired and depleted. Stress causes us to be unkind, judgmental, and unempathetic toward ourselves. "I can't believe I can't do this," we say. "Look at her! She can do it! What's wrong with me?" Our breath becomes tight and shallow.

So, take a few moments to be still and connect. Are there any messages you have received that didn't nurture you or help you in the moment? Are there people whose examples you just can't follow? Imagine these thoughts falling like leaves into a burbling brook and washing away in the stream. Are there images of the "perfect you" that you think you'll never attain? Imagine ripping them up and giving yourself a hug instead. Stay with what is. You are a mom. You deserve the best. You are enough. No one else gets to live *your* life, so know that you are living it in the best way possible.

remember

Your body has given birth to a baby. Be nurturing and gentle with her.

Your Baby and Bonding

If you do it with love,
you are doing it right.

This chapter is about how to take care of your baby, and I promise we'll get there. But before we do, we need to address the most important aspect of your baby's transition into this world: *your* transition into this world.

In chapter 5, we first touched on the weight of all the questions—tiny and huge—that encompass the journey of pregnancy and parenthood. Things that we never even considered before suddenly take up so much space in our awareness.

From figuring out the intricacies of daily life with this new creature (it feels like a game of Jenga some days, doesn't it?) to massive shifts in the way you view, well, everything, it all contributes to the very real mental overload of motherhood.

And then there is the new-mama self-doubt. It starts as a tiny seedling, but it takes root, and like an out-of-control weed can grow until it becomes all-consuming. It seems all we can do is ask ourselves on repeat: *Was I enough today?*

Yes, mama. A thousand times, yes.

We see ourselves through lenses warped by all the "shoulds" we have absorbed since we were children. If I could impart one piece of knowledge to you, it would be this: The impossibly idealized notion of a "good mom" is not real.

Here's what is real: *you*. You, with all your quirks and "flaws," your questions and worries, your mistakes and do-overs—you are the real deal, and you are perfect for your baby.

Mama, if you could see what your baby sees, you wouldn't have one seedling of self-doubt left.

I'll tell you again what I told you in the beginning: The answers of motherhood will rarely come easily. We have access to so much information, and there can be so much noise out there, that it can be hard to know what the right thing to do is. So here is my advice, for now and for always: Ask for opinions, look for research, and then do your very best to tune it out and listen to your heart. We all make mistakes, we all change our minds, but if you make these decisions from a place of intuition and love, you're doing it right.

Just like your new babe is learning how to be a human in this world, you are learning how to be a mama, each and every day. Give yourself grace and patience on this path.

xo,

Diana

The first week is all about adjusting, for both you and your baby. Your baby is having more milestones than you can keep up with: first breath, first pee, first poop, first feeding, first nap, first snuggle, and so much more. By caring for them through it all, you are laying the foundations of trust, love, and safety.

It is incredibly important to take care of yourself as you care for your baby, so do not be afraid to delegate baby care to a partner or family member.

Psst: You are still going to be your baby's favorite for a while now. Taking an extra nap while grandma bonds with the baby will not impact your baby's love for you at all.

Sometimes, mamas miss these firsts, and I want you to know that it is okay. Perhaps you had a complication that required prolonged hospitalization, for example. It can be incredibly painful to miss any aspect of your baby's life, especially in the earliest days. There are two things to remember here:

- There will be so many firsts that you *will* see. And mama, they never lose their grandeur, ever.

- In many ways, you *were* there for the first. Maybe not physically, but in the thousands of ways that you grew and nurtured your baby leading up to the moment. Your effort and love are why your baby had the first that they did. Mama-power goes far beyond where you are located at any given moment.

Do what you can to release the feelings of guilt (because it was not your fault), and focus on all the ways that you *have* supported your child.

FALLING IN LOVE WITH BABY

Did you know that it takes some women time to fall in love with their babies? You may already be head over heels, or you may be waiting for it to click, and that's okay. Sometimes not bonding with your baby can be a sign of postpartum depression, so if your baby arrives and you're concerned, reach out to a therapist. But overall, remember that everyone's love story is different.

CIRCUMCISION

If you have a boy, one of the first decisions you'll need to make is whether you'd like him to be circumcised.

Circumcision is an elective procedure in which the foreskin (tissue that covers the head of the penis) is removed. It can be done by a provider in a hospital (usually on the day of discharge) or by a mohel, who is a ritual circumciser in the Jewish religion (traditionally on the baby's eighth day of life). Of note, mohels usually perform circumcisions in the home or at a religious center, and you do not have to be Jewish in order to hire one for your son's circumcision. There are several techniques for the surgery, so if you are curious on the specifics, your best bet is to check with the person who will be doing the circumcision. Note that many hospitals offer numbing creams and pacifiers dipped in sugar water to help ease the baby's discomfort.

The circumcision decision can be complicated—and controversial.

The official statement by the AAP is that "the health benefits of newborn male circumcision outweigh the risks, but the benefits are not great enough to recommend universal newborn circumcision. The final decision should still be left to parents to make in the context of their religious, ethical and cultural beliefs."

A report from 2016 stated that 71.2 percent of boys in the US are circumcised. It is interesting to note that the number varies widely around the world. It ranges from almost none (for example, 0.15 percent in Costa Rica) to almost all (99.9 percent in Morocco).

Here are some of the pros and cons people cite when making their decisions. If you are unsure, you can turn to your pediatrician for guidance.

Reasons some parents may choose to circumcise:

- Prevention of urinary tract infections, decreased risk of contracting HIV and some sexually transmitted infections, and decreased risk of penile cancer (per the AAP)
- Religious, cultural, or traditional beliefs
- Desire to have him look like his father, brother, or other family members
- Enabling him to "fit in" with peers, if most males in the community are circumcised

Reasons some parents may choose not to circumcise:

- Risk of pain, infection, and error (though complications are rare)
- Religious, cultural, or traditional beliefs
- Enabling him to "fit in" with peers, if most males in the community are not circumcised
- Concern about the ethics of performing an elective surgery on someone who cannot give consent

- Concern about potential nerve damage and decreased sexual sensitivity (though this is disputed by the AAP)

Circumcision Care If you decide to circumcise your baby, the hospital staff (or the mohel) will give you detailed instructions about how to care for your child's penis, depending on the procedure they choose to perform. Generally, you will apply petroleum jelly directly to the penis or to the gauze that covers the penis for the duration of the healing process, which is usually 7 to 10 days. Keep the area as clean as possible (gently washing away pee and poop that may get on the wound), and watch for signs of irritation and infection:

- Constant crying
- Spot of blood on diaper larger than a quarter
- Pus
- Swelling
- Redness
- Fever

UMBILICAL CORD CARE

The umbilical cord connected your baby to your placenta, providing all the nutrients and oxygen they needed as they grew. Now that they are born, it is time to thank the umbilical cord for all it did and send it on its way (or keep it somewhere sentimental).

After birth, the umbilical cord will look like a yellow, squishy cord, about the width of your thumb. Exactly how much is dangling from your baby's belly depends on where it was cut. You may bring baby home with a small clamp, or the clamp may be removed prior to discharge. Over the course of about 7 to 10 days, the cord will dry and shrivel and eventually fall off. When it falls off, it is not usually a momentous thing. You'll just check the diaper as usual and notice: *Hey! There's a raisin in here! Oh wait, that must be the umbilical cord.* You can choose to save it or throw it out—totally up to you.

After the cord falls off, there will be a small wound in the belly button, but that will heal quickly.

The main thing to know about umbilical cord care is to keep the area as dry and clean as possible to discourage yucky bacteria from growing where it does not belong. Also, avoid submerging your baby's body in a bath until the cord has fallen off.

In the meantime, sponge baths work well. If—let me rephrase—*when* pee or poop gets on the cord, it is fine to use some soap and water to clean it. As long as it stays mostly dry, it should heal well.

PEEING AND POOPING

Welcome to the world of being fascinated by and constantly discussing someone else's bodily functions! If they are consuming your thoughts, you are not alone. A baby's pees and poops can tell you a lot about their general health, so good for you for being so aware! Keeping a log of your baby's pees and poops, on an app on your phone or on a piece of paper, is incredibly helpful (see the chart we've provided below).

As a general rule of thumb:

- On the first day of life, baby should pee once.
- On the second day of life, baby should pee twice.

YOUR BABY'S FEED, PEE, AND POOP CHART

DATE	TIME	FEED	PEE	POOP

- On the third day of life, baby should pee three times.

(See, they're not that tricky.)

By the end of the first week, your baby should be peeing about six or more times per day. You'll soon learn your baby's normal rhythm, so if that varies, you can contact your baby's provider.

Your baby's very first poop is called meconium: It is dark and sticky, much like tar. This poop will slowly transition to newborn poop. In breastfed babies, it looks like mustard mixed with sesame seeds, and in formula-fed babies, it is less seedy and a bit browner.

Babies usually poop at least once per day, but they often poop much more frequently than that. If you're concerned about their output, talk to your baby's provider.

DIAPERS, DIAPERS, DIAPERS

Which Type of Diaper Will You Choose?

Your baby will go through nearly four thousand diapers in their lifetime, so choosing what those diapers are made of is an important decision! Here are some factors to consider:

MECONIUM CLEANUP

Meconium is sticky and hard to remove. When your baby has a clean bottom, you can apply a thin layer of petroleum jelly so that next time they poop, it will be much easier to wipe it away. As soon as they transition to newborn poop, it becomes much easier to clean.

Benefits of cloth diapers:

- They use fewer environmental resources.
- There is less or no chemical exposure for baby's skin.
- After the initial investment, they are less expensive than disposable over your child's lifetime.
- Many parents say that after learning how to use them, they're not hard or burdensome.
- They come in cute styles and designs.

Drawbacks of cloth diapers:

- Your child is immediately uncomfortable when wet or soiled, so more changes are necessary.
- They can be inconvenient because you have to carry around soiled diapers when you do diaper changes away from home.
- They must be carefully managed so as not to smell or create a biohazard.

Benefits of disposable diapers:

- They're convenient.
- There is less initial investment.
- They are easier to learn to use.
- They are less bulky.
- They come in cute styles and designs.

Drawbacks of disposable diapers:

- They may accustom the child to not needing frequent changes because they are comfortable even when soiled, potentially making toilet training harder.
- They use more environmental resources.
- They are more expensive than cloth in the long run.

Compostable diaper services carry nearly all the same benefits of disposable diapers, but they are also good for the environment. Prices for compostable services in urban areas are comparable to those for cloth diaper services.

You can also experiment. Some parents use cloth at home and disposable when they are out and about. There are tons of different cloth diaper styles out there, so if you are curious, head to your local baby shop, where someone will be able to walk you through your options. There are also many different diaper services that will deliver fresh diapers each week and take your soiled ones to clean.

Diaper Rash

Diaper rash is an irritating rash that develops on your baby's bottom. It often develops when their sensitive skin has prolonged contact with pee or poop in the diaper, though sometimes it can happen if the baby is exposed to a new product, starts solid foods or a new medication, or has another type of infection. Breastfed babies may sometimes get a bit of diaper rash if *you* eat certain foods: strawberries and oranges being some of the common culprits. And sometimes it just happens. Please hear this: Almost all babies get diaper rash at some point, and it doesn't necessarily mean that you've done something "wrong."

If your baby develops diaper rash, you can use an over-the-counter diaper cream (that is free of dyes and scents) or coconut oil (if they are not allergic). If it doesn't clear up, or seems to be getting worse, reach out to your baby's provider, as occasionally they need stronger treatment.

The best way to prevent diaper rash is to change your baby's diaper frequently and to expose their bottoms to air. Perhaps every time you change their diaper, you can let their bottom air out for an extra minute or two before putting the new one on. Baby powder is not recommended because the particles are very fine and can be inhaled by the baby.

While we're on the topic of changing diapers, remember to always wipe babies from front to back so that you're not pulling bacteria from their bottom toward their urethra (where pee comes out). Some parents choose not to use wipes with chemicals on them. You can simply use a washcloth with water (that you wash after each use) or buy a commercial brand wipe that only uses water. You may want to cover their genitals with a cloth while you are changing them to avoid getting peed on!

SLEEP

Ah, infant sleep, or lack thereof. This is a topic that gets a ton of attention—and for good reason. Your baby's sleep has a tremendous impact on your sleep, which in turn impacts your life, ability to function, and emotional and physical well-being. In short, it's a big deal.

My wish for parents regarding sleep is this (and I know it is way easier said than done): Do what you can to encourage good sleeping habits, but don't get consumed or stressed by it.

A story: My firstborn was a dream baby. She slept well, ate well, rarely cried, the whole deal. My middle one, on the other hand, had a tough time. (Note: I have stopped saying "he was a tough baby." One of my favorite parenting quotes from a friend is "My baby is not *giving me* a hard time, they are *having* a hard time." It made a big difference in my mental framework on the really hard days.) He cried all the time and woke up every half hour for 8 months. To this day when I take naps, I tell my husband it's because I still have to make up for that lost sleep.

The exhaustion of that period was like nothing I have ever experienced. But the thing that made it unbearable was my guilt. I remember so clearly thinking that I had done something wrong, that I somehow broke him, that it was my fault that my baby didn't know how to sleep. Unfortunately, many of the messages I received from the resources I turned to did not help alleviate my concern. I could cry now just thinking about the frustration and heaviness I felt during this time.

Then one day I found (like a beacon of light) a short article written by Dr. William Sears in which he described my son to a T, and I realized two things. First, my son was a "high needs" baby. He was not, in fact, a "tough" baby; he was a normal baby with intense needs. And second, his sleeping was a reflection of his temperament, not of my parenting.

This shift in attitude was everything for me. He still did not sleep through the night after I discovered this (or even close), but the relief I felt from learning that my baby, and my parenting, were okay made the challenges so much easier to deal with.

So now I share with you, mama, that the newborn sleep struggle is real. It is okay to be frustrated if it is not going well, and it is more than okay to ask for help and support from your village or professionals. Please just don't blame yourself. If a "bad" habit forms, it probably developed out of necessity.

Ten Sleep Habits to Establish from the Start

Sleep consultant Rachel Gorton offers the following advice:

1 **Use light and darkness to your advantage.** In the first few months of life, your baby won't quite be able to tell the difference between day and night. So, exposing your baby to light first thing in the morning and throughout the day will help them make this distinction and help drive their circadian rhythm. Natural sunlight will also keep your baby alert and stimulated throughout the day, which is important for development.

Darkness is equally important. Your baby's room should be dark for all naps and bedtime, signaling to their body that it is time to sleep. In the evening, you can start dimming the lights in the house about 2 hours before bedtime to prepare your baby for the transition to sleep.

2 **Develop a routine.** Even when your baby is a newborn, you can start thinking about a routine that will help them learn when sleep is coming. Although a newborn's sleeping patterns can be erratic and unpredictable, a bedtime routine is still beneficial at any age.

When your child is younger, the routine will likely include more rocking and helping to settle, whereas an older baby might fall asleep more independently.

Some ideas of what to include in a routine are bath, books, rocking, swaddling, infant massage, and singing. Of course, you can decide what works best for your family and your baby.

3 **Eliminate exposure to blue lights and electronics before bed.** This is true at *any* age, because lights from screens can easily suppress melatonin, our sleep hormone,

and it happens fairly quickly. This is why it is best to turn off the TV and any other electronics near your baby at least 2 hours before bedtime.

4 **Keep your baby's sleep environment consistent.** When your baby is first born, it might seem like they will fall asleep anywhere and everywhere, and it will be tempting to let them do so. While napping on the go is somewhat inevitable for the first couple months, I always encourage sleep to happen in your baby's own sleep environment when possible.

Whether that is in a bassinet in your room or a crib in baby's room, teaching them to sleep in the same environment consistently will help avoid difficult transitions later and encourage longer sleep stretches without distraction. It is also safest to have your baby nap on a firm surface (such as in a bassinet or crib), rather than allowing them to take naps in areas that weren't designed for sleep. Your baby will, of course, fall asleep in all kinds of places in the beginning—strollers, carriers, swings, and more. When this happens, it is recommended that you move the baby to a place designed for sleeping (like a crib or bassinet) as soon as possible.

5 **Encourage healthy sleep "tools."** Many parents worry that the use of a pacifier or other sleep objects creates a habit that is difficult to break later. But I highly encourage the use of sleep objects as long as they don't become the only thing that will get your child to sleep.

A pacifier, white noise machine, or swaddle/sleep sack are all great sleep-promoting objects. Many babies will naturally transition out of using one or more of these items as they get older, and if they don't, you can help them do so using various methods.

6 **Honor sleepy signs and cues.** Most babies will show clear signs that they are ready for sleep as early as 6 weeks. You can start following appropriate awake windows for your baby's age immediately, which will help avoid overtiredness, but sometimes listening to your baby is all you need to do.

Babies tend to have small sleep windows, meaning that there is a brief period during which falling asleep will be easiest. Once the window passes, it may be harder for them to fall asleep because they get overtired. When your baby is yawning, becoming fussy, and overall seems less alert, these are all signs that they are ready for sleep soon, and it is important to put them down quickly to avoid missing that sleep window.

7 **Make sure your baby's environment promotes sleep from the start.** When possible, the area that your baby is sleeping in—whether they have their own room or are sleeping in yours—should have few distractions, which include toys, lights, artwork, and colors. It is best to have minimal objects in the room and neutral colors to eliminate overstimulation, when possible. Room temperature is also key because you don't want your baby waking because they are too cold or too hot. The recommended room temperature for your baby is between 68 and 72 degrees Fahrenheit.

8 **Learn how to respond to your baby's different sounds and movements.** As new mamas, we are very in tune with every sound and stir our baby makes, and it can be hard to ignore any slight movement or peep. But remember that it is normal for your baby to go in and out of sleep cycles, and as they do this, they will likely make many noises that sound like fussing or grunting.

Because this will happen consistently, there is no need to rush to comfort them each time you hear them. It is important to help them establish some independence by giving them the opportunity to fall back asleep on their own. If your baby starts to cry or become upset, that is a different story and I do encourage tending to them if that is the case.

Psst: Did you know that it is normal for babies to have nonrhythmic breathing? They may breathe quickly for a few breaths, followed by a few deep breaths, then a several-second pause, and it is completely normal! Of course, if you are worried, you can always call your baby's provider. And see "Trouble Breathing" on page 378 for more on emergency breathing signs that you should get attention for right away.

9 **Cycle through soothing methods with your baby.** One of the most common sleep challenges I see with older babies is that they have developed a reliance on just one way to fall asleep and stay asleep. While some of these habits might be unavoidable in the beginning, you can be mindful of this by cycling through different methods of soothing with your baby instead of reverting to one way to get them to sleep.

Basically, you want to teach your child that there are many ways to fall asleep. So, this might mean one night you rock them until they're sleepy, and the next night you soothe them without picking them up. I encourage parents to use Dr. Harvey Karp's 5 S's from *The Happiest Baby on the Block*, which can be used all at once or intermittently:

- Shushing
- Sucking (such as pacifier use)
- Swaddling
- Side or stomach position (*only* while soothing, *not* for sleep)
- Swing (*only* while soothing, *not* for sleep)

10 **Bond with your baby at bedtime.** Studies have shown that an emotionally secure child is more likely to sleep well than a child who is anxious or unsettled. And while your newborn is not going to be experiencing anxiety or stress the way we do, it is a great practice to use bedtime as a time to bond with your child.

This is something you can carry on as your child becomes older, helping them to relax and become ready for sleep by spending that one-on-one time connecting and being close, so they can fall into dreamland without a worry in the world.

Safe Sleep and SIDS

Fair warning: This is the scary part of the chapter, but we would be remiss in our commitment to providing you with holistic information if we didn't cover it, mama. Sleep and the prevention of sudden infant death syndrome (SIDS) go hand in hand, so let's discuss what it is and how to prevent it.

SIDS is when a baby dies inexplicably during the first year of life, most often while they are asleep. This may be caused by a brain or breathing problem, environmental or unsafe sleeping factors, or for reasons completely unknown. SIDS is part of a larger group of infant deaths known as sudden unexpected infant death (SUID), which also includes strangulation or suffocation.

It is unbearable to think about, I know.

SUID is rare; in 2016, there were 91.4 cases per 100,000 babies. That means 0.09 percent of babies. The risk for SIDS begins to drop after 4 months (though again, it can happen up to the first birthday).

There are many steps we as parents can take toward greatly reducing the risk:

Put baby "back to sleep." You and I were likely put to bed on our sides or tummies. The thinking at the time was that if we threw up in the middle of the night, we'd be less likely to choke. But research has overwhelmingly demonstrated that when babies sleep on their backs, they are significantly less likely to die from SIDS.

Babies should sleep on a surface designed for sleep. As mentioned earlier, babies should not sleep in car seats, swings, or other devices not intended for sleep. These items may position them in such a way that their airway becomes obstructed, and they do not have the ability to reposition themselves.

Put nothing in the crib with baby. If your baby will sleep in a crib, the crib must have only a well-fitting and firm mattress (without a gap between it and the bars) with a fitted sheet. No bumpers, toys, pillows, blankets, pacifier clips or strings, or anything else can be in there with them. The concern is that if one of these items obstructs the baby's ability to breathe, the baby will not be capable of moving themselves or the item away.

There should be no smoking near the baby or in the baby's home. Even smoke on your clothes can have a harmful effect.

Keep the home cool. When in doubt, a cooler temp is safer than a warmer one. Again, the ideal indoor temperature is 68 to 72 degrees Fahrenheit.

Keep the air circulating near baby's bed. Having a source of moving air can be beneficial. You don't have to put a fan directly blowing on the baby (and probably shouldn't), but a fan off to the side is great.

Breastfeed. Babies who receive breast milk during the first 2 months of life have nearly a 50 percent decreased risk of dying from SIDS, and it doesn't have to be exclusive breastfeeding. It works even if they are also getting supplemented with formula. The longer they receive breast milk, the more benefit there is.

Avoid additional products. AAP's position is that parents should not use home monitors or commercial devices in baby's crib, including wedges or positioners, marketed to reduce the risk of SIDS. Wedges and positioners can actually lead to suffocation, and the FDA states that they have "*never* cleared an infant sleep positioner that claims to prevent or reduce the risk of SIDS. And, there is no scientifically sound evidence to support medical claims about sleep positioners." Consult your baby's provider if you have questions about how this applies to your baby.

Pacifiers can help. The use of pacifiers decreases the risk of SIDS. Just make sure the pacifier is not attached to a clip or string, as this could pose a threat. Additionally, ensure that you check pacifiers routinely, as they may get loose or damaged.

Check the environment. Make sure there are no cords, chargers, or other objects that could be pulled into the crib.

So, Where Should Baby Sleep?
First, the lingo:

- Co-sleeping: sharing a sleeping space (a room) with your child
- Bed sharing: sharing a sleeping surface (a bed) with your child

If you bed share, you co-sleep. But if you co-sleep, you do not automatically bed share.

It is also essential that we understand that bed sharing happens around the world and has since the dawn of babies.

The AAP recommends that the safest place for a baby to sleep is on their own sleep surface, in the parents' room, for the first 6 to 12 months of life to reduce the risk of SIDS.

Now, when we are as tired as we can be during early parenthood, we simply do not have the ability to control our bodies in the same way as when we are well rested. Regardless of your intentions, it is quite possible that you will fall asleep with your baby at some point. One study found that 25 percent of mothers reported falling asleep with their

babies in dangerous locations (like armchairs and couches). So, my very strong belief is that all parents should know how to make bed sharing safer so that if it happens, they know how to do it in a way that minimizes accidents.

The AAP has recently revised their sleep guidelines to state that if there is a chance that you will fall asleep (for example, while you are nursing) the safest place to do this is in your bed. When you wake up, they advise placing the baby back on their own sleep surface. But the most important piece of this is that bed sharing should happen in a bed—never on a couch or chair because very scary accidents can happen.

Other recommendations for safe bed sharing, as outlined by Dr. James McKenna of the University of Notre Dame Mother-Baby Behavioral Sleep Laboratory:

- Follow the same guidelines regarding safe sleep detailed on page 372.

- No pillows or blankets around the baby.

- Bed sharing should only happen if you are breastfeeding, not bottle-feeding.

- If you share your bed with a partner, both partners should agree to bed sharing and be aware that the baby is in the bed.

- Ensure that there are no places where the baby can get wedged (such as between a mattress and headboard).

- No bed sharing with other children or pets.

- No bed sharing with anyone under the influence of alcohol, sedatives, medications, or with conditions that do not allow them to wake up easily.

- Long hair should be tied back.

- No cords (chargers, blind cords, and so on) in or near the bed.

If there is a chance you may fall asleep with your baby, do a scan of the surroundings to ensure that it is safe. As always, your baby's provider is the best person to talk to for guidance.

THE PERIOD OF PURPLE CRYING AND COLIC

All infants cry. They also all cry a lot during certain periods. This is normal behavior. Some babies have excessive crying, without any identifiable cause, and this is also considered normal, although if you have any concerns about your infant's crying, talk to your health-care provider right away. The truth is that crying can become a huge challenge for parents to deal with, especially when the infant cannot be consoled for long periods of time.

"The Period of PURPLE Crying" is a relatively new term, coined by Canadian developmental pediatrician Ronald Barr, to describe a period of time when infants cry a lot. It has nothing to do with them turning purple. The letters in PURPLE stand for:

Peak of crying
Unexpected
Resists soothing
Pain-like face
Long lasting
Evening

This type of crying usually starts around week 2 and lasts for a few months. The child simply cannot be soothed during this period, though parents will try everything to relieve them. It may last up to 5 hours and begin during the late afternoon or evening. In the absence of illness or injury, purple crying is normal—but very difficult for parents. For more, visit dontshake.org.

Colic is defined as crying for 3 or more hours per day, 3 or more days per week, for 3 or more weeks. There are many theories as to the cause of colic, which is more common for premature babies. It may be due to tummy troubles or even baby migraines.

If you have a baby who cries a lot, talk to their health-care provider. They can help determine if the cause is medical or developmental. Beyond that, carefully read the following section on shaken baby syndrome (because this is one of the prime scenarios when it can happen) and do whatever you can to take care of yourself.

SHAKEN BABY SYNDROME

It's scary, but we need to address this. Shaken baby syndrome occurs when a baby is shaken back and forth so forcefully that their brain is injured. It can lead to very serious consequences, including death. Moment of truth: Almost every parent I work with during pregnancy grimaces when we talk about this and comments that they don't understand how anyone could shake a baby. Almost every one of them comes back a few months later and says, "I haven't shaken my baby, but I think I understand now how it can happen."

New parenthood can be exhausting in a way that we've never experienced, and extreme exhaustion does things to our brains and bodies that we don't expect. Add to that the profound stress of being a new parent and having a baby who just . . . won't . . . stop . . . crying, and we start to see how someone might find themselves in a situation of extreme frustration. It can—and does—happen, to moms and partners alike.

If, or rather when, you feel overcome by this type of extreme frustration, stop. Whatever you are doing, no matter how hard the baby is screaming, just stop, put the baby down in a safe place, and walk away (staying in the home with them). You will feel guilty to walk away from your crying infant, but really this is the most valiant thing you can do—recognizing that you are having a moment of vulnerability and responding in a way that keeps everyone safe. Take some deep breaths, call your partner or a friend to take over for a bit, or cry it out yourself. If you feel like you can't stop yourself from harming the baby or yourself, call 911. It is the most loving thing you could do.

And take care of yourself. This is one of those key instances of putting your oxygen mask on first. If you are as well rested and nourished as possible, you will be able to think a bit more clearly during the moments of stress.

Remember that when we find ourselves feeling weak, we often find our deepest reserves of strength. This is one of those times.

Psst: For more on baby crying, see "The Period of PURPLE Crying and Colic" on page 375.

LEAVING THE HOUSE

Trips out of the house, even a quick walk up the block, can do wonders for new mamas and babies alike. Some women find that those first weeks can be isolating, so making a point to get out into the "real world" can be

a great reminder that life goes on around you. And you never know when you might meet a new friend!

Those first trips out of the house can feel like a comedy of errors. You'll pack and unpack the diaper bag six times, and just when you think you're ready to walk out the door, your baby will have a total poop blowout. You'll take a deep breath, get them all cleaned up . . . and then it will be time for a feeding.

Remember to keep your sense of humor and don't blame anyone. Even if your afternoon out gets shortened to a 20-minute walk around the block, it will still be worth it.

Pediatrician Niki Saxena says that if your baby is healthy, with no medical issues, it is generally safe to take them to places where they won't come into contact with lots of germs. This includes large well-ventilated spaces like parks. When possible, Dr. Saxena recommends waiting to take your baby on a plane or to more crowded places (like visiting your place of work, for example) until the baby is at least 1 month old, and preferably after their 2-month-old vaccinations. "If an infant less than 28 days old develops a fever (defined as a temperature of 100.4 degrees Fahrenheit or higher), the current medical standard of care requires admission to the hospital for an infection workup, and why take the chance?"

If your baby has ongoing medical issues, speak with your pediatrician about trips outside of the home.

WHEN TO CALL YOUR BABY'S PROVIDER

Can I tell you a quick story? I called 911 once because my son was having a nightmare. Yup, uh-huh, me, with over a decade of medical experience. He was breathing a little weirdly

YOUR 1-MONTH-OLD BABY

Tracking your baby's development can be an exciting part of parenthood, and a stressful one as well. Remember that all the milestone guides out there are estimates. Just as with adults, babies have their own temperaments and abilities. Try to avoid comparing your baby to others you know. Trust your baby's provider and your instincts. If you and your provider do have concerns regarding your baby's development, your baby will be referred for an evaluation. And if an issue is found, know that treatment and support are available and often very effective.

YOUR 1-MONTH-OLD'S DEVELOPMENT

It is amazing to consider how much your baby has changed over the course of a few weeks! Here are some of the most exciting milestones, and how you can help foster their development:

Thinking/Vision Your baby can see about 8 to 12 inches in front of their face. One of the best ways to bond with your baby early on is to spend lots of time holding them close. When your baby is close to you, they can smell you, hear your voice, and see your face—all things they adore doing. Babywearing is fabulous for this (see page 382).

Engaging They will react to familiar sounds. Sing to your baby! (Don't worry; they'll love your voice.)

Communicating Their only way of communication is crying. Experts agree that it is not possible to spoil a baby, so go ahead and pick your baby up when they need you. As we discussed in chapter 13, the prevailing child-raising philosophy today is attachment parenting, which suggests that we respond to our babies when they cry.

Moving They can move their head from side to side. While they are awake, dangle toys in front of them so that they can practice looking as they learn to move their head. They won't be able to track the items just yet, but that's coming!

Ready for a super-cool science moment? A study was done where mothers who spoke different languages wore recording devices as they cared for their babies. The results showed that although the words they said were different, the sounds they made were the same. (Mama wisdom for the win!) No matter how new to babies we are, we inherently know how to do this job. This means that you can trust your instincts. Talk to your baby in the way that feels right, and before you know it, you'll have full-on conversations, though you may have no idea what those adorable coos mean.

and acting lethargic, so I freaked out and called. The unnecessary ambulance ride that ensued was over the top, yes, and we were extra tired the next day from the middle-of-the-night commotion. But my son was thrilled when three "firefighters" (paramedics, actually) walked into the house, and now I have a funny, albeit embarrassing, story to tell.

Part of being a mom is possessing an inexplicable amount of love for another human being that makes us do some pretty wild things. I was scared and couldn't think clearly, so I called for help. To this day, I do not regret it, and I would urge you to do the same.

If something doesn't feel right, call your baby's provider and ask, even in the middle of the night. Many hospitals also have 24-hour nurse call lines that can help you if you are unsure. If it's very concerning, take them to urgent care or the emergency room, or call 911. It is okay if you are wrong, but often you won't be. A parent's intuition is second to none, and it is okay to listen to it when it alarms.

Here are some specific symptoms to look for:

Trouble Breathing   Grunting, shallow breathing, nostril flaring, skin turning pale or blue, and sucking the skin in around their ribs are all indications of respiratory distress. *This is a 911 call!*

Inconsolable Crying   Especially if this is an unusual behavior for your child.

Fever   A fever in a newborn should be treated as an emergency. You can check their temperature under their armpit, though a rectal temperature is the gold standard. (However, thermometer technology is advancing, so there may be additional options available. Ask your baby's provider which method they recommend.) When taking a rectal temperature, insert the thermometer about a half an inch inside their rectum (no more) and wait for the temp to register. If their rectal temp is 100.4 degrees Fahrenheit or higher, call your pediatrician or take them to the hospital.

Pee and Poop Changes   If you notice a decrease in the number of pees and poops your baby has in a day, call. If they are straining to poop, and the poop is hard (rabbit-pellet-like), or the pee or poop is bloody and looks unusual, call. If your baby goes longer than 8 hours without peeing, you should always give their provider a call.

Vomiting   It is normal for babies to spit up. But, if they vomit, especially if the vomit travels (projectile), call.

Lethargy   If baby seems extra tired, unarousable, or floppy, call 911 right away. Another sign that a baby is lethargic is if they miss two feedings in a row (because they are too tired to eat). If this happens, give their provider a call.

Umbilical Cord or Circumcision Site Concerns   If there is bleeding, pus or drainage, a foul smell, redness around the area, or excessive pain, call.

Thrush   See "Thrush (Candida or Yeast Infection)" on page 400.

BABYPROOFING

The good news is that newborns give you a grace period in that they are stationary and

YOUR 2-MONTH-OLD BABY

This is such a fun age for a newborn! They are still so tiny, but we can start to see little glimpses of personality peek through, and mama, it is the best.

YOUR 2-MONTH-OLD'S DEVELOPMENT

Thinking/Vision   Your baby can focus on and track objects and faces with their eyes. Read to your sweet baby. They may not understand the plotline just yet, but the sound of your voice and the pictures in the book will still do wonders for their learning. In fact, evidence suggests that babies who are read to develop more advanced vocabularies and have improved reading skills as older children.

Engaging   They may start to smile. (Brace yourself, this is a pretty powerful moment!) Most often, babies smile at familiar faces, especially when those faces are smiling at them. You know how when you look at a baby you instinctively raise your eyebrows and smile? That's on purpose! In following your instincts, you are giving your baby the very first lessons in social interactions. Bonus: They get to have those lessons with their favorite person. You!

Communicating   They will start to coo. When your baby coos, coo or talk back. You can mimic the sounds they make or tell them about the movie you saw last night. Anything goes when they are hearing your loving voice.

Moving   Their movements will start to become smoother. Continue tummy time to help them build up their strength and even get down on the floor with them, so they can be inspired to look up at your beautiful face (and your dry-shampooed messy bun).

Giving your baby a very light massage using specialized stroking motions can not only help them feel good, but it also has been found to improve the parent-baby bond and increase parental confidence. You can find instructional videos online, and there are certified professionals who can teach you as well.

don't require immediate babyproofing. They do, however, tend to start rolling and moving before we are ready for it, so it's never a bad idea to start prepping.

The specifics of how you make your home safe for your baby are dependent on the layout, of course. One of the most important things to do is to mount any furniture to the wall that has the potential to fall on a child. Bookshelves, armoires, TVs and stands, and dressers are the usual culprits, but you'll have to take a look to see what else needs to be secured. The statistics on this are staggering: According to anchorit.gov, someone in the US is injured by tipped-over furniture every 17 minutes, and two-thirds of those injured are toddlers.

Unfortunately, "It took three grown adults to move that bookcase in here, so there is no way a toddler could tip it over" doesn't fly here. Kids are smart and crafty and can often find a way to get themselves into trouble.

Some other areas of your home to babyproof:

- Doorknobs and handles
- Stairs
- Stove and oven knobs
- Medicine cabinets

- Cleaning products
- Cords and wires
- Blinds and pull strings
- Plugs and outlets
- Fireplaces
- Sharp furniture corners
- Glass tabletops
- Toilet bowls
- Pet feeding areas
- Large equipment (treadmills, musical instruments, and so on)
- Toys and other small objects that can fit in mouths
- Windows (to prevent falls)
- Hot water heater (set at 120 degrees Fahrenheit or lower)

You should also buy (or test existing) carbon monoxide and smoke alarms, and you should have your home assessed for lead paint if you live in an older (pre-1978) home.

Remember: Never leave a baby unattended on an elevated surface such as a table or bed.

SETTING UP YOUR BABY'S "OFFICIAL" LIFE

There are some official items that require your attention when you have a baby:

Health Insurance   Your baby will not be automatically added to your health insurance. Most plans require that you call them within 30 days of your child's birth to get them on your plan and covered. For more info on acquiring health insurance if you don't have it, see "Health Insurance" on page 152.

Birth Certificate   When your baby is born, your health-care team will usually give you the paperwork to request a birth certificate.

NEWBORN CARE IN NIGERIA

In Nigerian tradition, a baby's first bath may be given by the baby's grandmother or other female relatives other than the mother, in an effort to remind the mother that she has a community of women to support her through motherhood.

YOUR 3-MONTH-OLD BABY

Can I tell you something? Each time one of my babies turned 3 months old, I got a little sad. Why? Because it meant that technically, they were not newborns anymore. Of course, I was filled with so much gratitude for every day I got to spend with them, but it was at the 3-month mark that it first occurred to me that this little baby was growing up.

Spoiler alert: I am now almost a decade in, and they are all very much still my babies. They do grow up, but they also still need us so very much—with the added benefit of letting us sleep through the night (most of the time).

And mama, it just keeps getting better. My eldest just asked me to go on a "sushi and makeup-store date" (which is my perfect afternoon exactly) and my little guys crack me up daily with their antics.

Enjoy these precious moments, but do not be afraid of what's to come. You should know by now that you will positively rock it.

YOUR 3-MONTH-OLD'S DEVELOPMENT

Thinking/Vision   Their vision is improving, and they can see things farther away (even across the room!). It can be fun to take walks and point out interesting things to look at. Don't worry; your living room counts if it's freezing or raining outside.

Engaging   They enjoy playing now and will respond to facial expressions and sounds. Continue reading to them as often as you can, and add in your own commentary to the story. "Look, this is a sheep! Sheep say bah."

Communicating   Coos become more babbling in nature, and your baby may try to imitate sounds. These are just the beginnings of conversations. Respond to them with interest, smile, and talk back.

Moving   Your baby has more control over their hands: They can swat at and grasp some objects. Dangle baby-safe toys and objects in front of them to encourage them to reach out and grab (improving their hand-eye coordination). They will be fascinated by touching different textures, too.

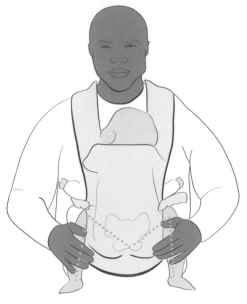

BABYWEARING SAFETY

If not, you can visit your state's Department of Health website to find the application and instructions for completion.

Social Security Card   When you complete your child's birth certificate form, there will be a box to check if you would also like them to receive a Social Security number and card. You can also go to a local Social Security Administration office to complete the process in person. Be sure to check ssa.gov ahead of time to see which documents you are required to bring with you.

Will or Trust   See "Wills and Trusts" on page 153 for info on this important step.

Qualified Tuition Plan (529 Plan)   These plans allow you to begin to save money with tax advantages for future education expenses. Visit sec.gov for more info.

Beneficiaries   If you have any investment or retirement accounts, contact the organizations to discuss naming your child as a beneficiary.

BABYWEARING

Babywearing is ancient. It can make breastfeeding easier and ensures that your baby is tended to, while also giving you a lot more freedom to move about your home and out of it, hands-free! Babies tend to love it, so it is a wonderful way to soothe them.

Plus, it is super-cozy and sweet! Seriously, those little beans are just so warm and soft.

There are all kinds of wraps and carriers out there. Honesty moment: It can feel a bit overwhelming at first. I would suggest talking to people in your village about what they have used and even borrowing their carriers and experimenting to find which one suits you best. Baby shops can assist you as well.

Proper positioning is essential when you wear your baby. Here are a few rules to follow:

- Baby should be positioned high enough on your body that you can easily kiss the top of their head.

- Baby's face should be to the side with nothing in front of their nose or mouth, so they can easily breathe.

- Proper leg and hip alignment is important for prevention of hip dysplasia (see "Hips and Limbs" on page 275). The International Hip Dysplasia Institute provides the following guideline for wearing newborns: "Thighs spread around the mother's torso and the hips bent so the knees are slightly higher than the buttocks with the thighs supported."

As noted, there are a number of different carriers and techniques to try, especially as your baby gets older. Ask for help from a local babywearing group or a babywearing consultant near you.

TUMMY TIME

When babies are born, they don't have much neck and back strength. To help them develop their muscles and postural skills, you can introduce some exercises: Think baby planks!

When baby is awake (and always with you in attendance), place them on their belly on a firm surface. A blanket on the floor works well. Avoid putting them somewhere high, like a changing table, couch, or bed, because they will be able to roll before you know it! The baby will instinctively start to push down with their arms and try to raise their little head.

If your baby was born at full term and healthy, you can usually start tummy time right away. Start with about three sessions a day—just a few minutes each. Babies tend to fuss during tummy time in the beginning because it is hard work. (This is me at the gym, so I can't blame them.) Once they get stressed, it is okay to pick them up and take a break. A little tummy time goes a long way.

THE FIRST BATH

There is something universally terrifying about the first time you give your baby a bath. I say this not to scare you, but so that when it happens to you, you don't feel like there is something wrong with you. It just feels so . . . real! Not to mention, they are wiggly and slippery, and the process is new. Don't worry; I promise that you will get the hang of it quickly.

Babies do not need to be bathed often because they do not get dirty like older kids or grown-ups. A few times per week is fine! This will also help prevent their sensitive skin from drying out. You can also forego the immersion bath and stick to sponge baths in the beginning.

First things first: *Never leave a baby unattended near water*. They can drown in an inch of water.

If possible, give the first bath with a partner. It helps to have some emotional support, someone to grab missing supplies, and someone to take pictures!

Supplies you'll need:

- Bathtub, sink, or basin
- Washcloths

- Baby soap/shampoo (anything mild, with no alcohol or fragrance, is great)
- Dry towel for after
- Clean diaper

The ideal temperature for bath water is just about 100 degrees Fahrenheit, and the ideal temperature in the room is 68 to 72 degrees Fahrenheit.

Place the baby in the water and make sure their head is supported. While most newborns hate those first sponge baths, they tend to adore baths where they can sit in the water; it feels like home. Newborns really don't need much washing or scrubbing, but if you choose to, use a very mild soap without chemicals or additives.

The bath can be brief or leisurely, just not so long that the water gets cold. And it's worth noting that some newborns have a habit of peeing or pooping during bath time, so be prepared for a "rinse, clean, repeat" moment if this happens to you. After a bath is a perfect time for some skin-to-skin to help calm them down and warm them up, and you get to inhale all that fresh, clean baby smell.

Cradle Cap

Some babies develop cradle cap, which is a bit like baby dandruff—white or yellow flakes and patches on the scalp. It doesn't seem to bother babies, but parents usually want to treat it. If you do, there are commercial shampoos available. I will say that my personal favorite remedy is to take a bit of coconut oil (if they are not allergic), rub it onto their scalp, let it sit for a few minutes, and then exfoliate with a soft-bristled brush. Just be careful: Coconut oil can make bathtubs and floors very slippery!

Hey there, you two (or three or four). The busy, sometimes chaotic world is spiraling around out there, but you have found your way into this quiet moment, just the two of you. Find respite from the noise in the soft ebb and flow of each other's breath.

Find solace in the inner peace you feel when you are together.

Breathe each other in deeply. As you do, inhale each other's scent. You are each in the presence of your favorite person on earth. Just their scent grounds you and centers you in a way you never imagined possible, so breathe each other in.

Touch each other's skin. It's perfect, right? In one touch, you find grace and strength, beauty and awe. Marvel in that perfection.

Take a moment to look at each other. Truly look at each other. If you find the feelings too strong, that's okay. Close your eyes and just be present with each other. You are looking at life. Everything beautiful and pure and right is there in front of your eyes. This is powerful stuff.

Baby, do you have any idea how much your mama loves you? And that even when she's not thinking about you, she is actually still thinking about you? She has loved you since the day *she* was born.

Mama, do you have any idea how much your baby loves you? During the first year of life, your baby does not even understand that you are two separate people. To your baby, you are happiness, peace, and life. Mama, to your baby, you are home.

Take as long as you want to enjoy this moment with each other and bask in these moments as often as possible. And know that the bond you two share is unlike anything else. Absolutely nothing comes between you two, so whether you have 5 minutes or the whole day to spend together, whether the day has been filled with simple pleasures or utter mess, you are entwined into each other's lives deeply and beautifully, forever.

remember

Pediatrician Niki Saxena says that if she could say one thing to all new parents, it would be this:

> Take a deep breath, put the phone down, and know that you can do this. Do not get so caught up in the worry that you forget the miracle that is your baby. Don't try to be the perfect parent: Your baby does not need you to be perfect. But your baby does need you to be present. Don't forget to take care of yourself and your partner, if you have one. Don't be hesitant about accepting help, and *sleep whenever you can!*

Breastfeeding

I am magic.

You know by now that if I had my way, we could talk about all of this in person, so I could give you hugs (if you want them; I'm a hugger), and I could look you in the eyes as I tell you the most important things. Mama, this is one of those moments, big time.

Breastfeeding is intense.

In a way, it is like giving birth: It involves a complete sharing of yourself, emotionally and physically. It can be one of the most beautiful, awe-inspiring experiences of your life, but it can also be one of the most draining and frustrating.

You did a great job taking care of yourself while you were pregnant, and it is paramount to keep that going through your nursing journey. In fact, your body may be working even harder now than it was during your pregnancy. Exclusively breastfeeding an infant requires the same amount of energy as walking 7 miles a day. (*Whew!*)

Be very gentle with yourself as you embark on nourishing your baby.

Mama, this next adventure is a big one. But I know you are going to rock it. Here are six things I need to tell you about breastfeeding:

1 **It is natural, but that doesn't mean it's easy.** Yes, of course, breastfeeding is natural in that it is something nature causes our bodies to do. But the word "natural" implies that breastfeeding *should* come naturally. It might, but it might also be tough. If it is difficult for you, that doesn't mean there is anything unnatural or wrong with you or your baby. Sometimes it's just hard.

2 **It can be awkward at first.** One of the very first midwives I worked with as a student used to say that breastfeeding is like ballroom dancing when both partners have watched it on TV, but neither has actually done it. In other words, it's awkward. I teach women to breastfeed every day, and yet with each one of my three children, I felt like I had to relearn how to nurse them. Each baby will have unique preferences and needs, and it can take a while to learn them. You are, after all, meeting your dance partner for the first time.

3 **It takes a while at first.** For those first days or weeks, it is okay if it takes you several minutes to set yourself up to breastfeed each time—getting the pillows just right, adjusting your top, having to look up diagrams of feeding positions. Chances are that you will get the hang of it, and before long you'll be a total breastfeeding boss . . . or you won't. And both are okay.

4 **It is ideal for babies; however . . .** There are days when I am fully convinced that breastfeeding is a form of magic. In short, it's amazing. As you'll see in the next pages, nursing your baby provides so many benefits.

However.

What your baby needs most on this planet, more than breastfeeding, is you. If breastfeeding is causing so much pain that you cry every time you nurse or making you so stressed or sad that you are developing postpartum depression or anxiety, you are allowed to reassess. You are allowed to think about your own well-being in this relationship and prioritize yourself if you need to.

There are many ways to get help for breastfeeding issues, and I strongly encourage you to do so. But you know what? Sometimes it just doesn't happen. And if this is the case, you are still a good mother. I promise.

5 **Perfect is the enemy of good enough.** Another way to say this in relation to breastfeeding is that every drop counts. As we'll discuss, organizations like the AAP recommend breastfeeding through the first year of your baby's life. But if, for whatever reason, that can't happen, it does not mean that the breast milk your baby does get is not meaningful. *Every single time* your baby nurses, they benefit from it.

As an example, a 2017 study found that babies who are breastfed for at least 2 months have a 50 percent reduction in sudden infant death syndrome (SIDS), even if they also receive formula during that time.

6 **Ask for help, even if it's going well.** Whether breastfeeding is challenging or a walk in the park, don't be afraid to ask for help. Most hospitals and birth centers have lactation consultants, and there are many who will come to your home. In fact, the Affordable Care Act now requires most insurance plans to cover breastfeeding support professionals. Some hospitals also offer free breastfeeding groups where a lactation consultant or counselor attends. (Hint: This is a great place to make new mom friends.) You can also find out if your local La Leche League has a support group near you. Or you can ask your baby's provider or your midwife or ob-gyn for help. You can also turn to trusted friends and family members. You do not have to face your struggles alone, even if all you need is someone to say, "Yeah, mama, you're doing great."

xo,

Diana

THE POWER OF BREASTFEEDING

Before we get into the specifics of breastfeeding, I just want you to marvel at yourself for a moment. We spent so much time during pregnancy reflecting on how incredible you are, and it is essential that you know that your magic is still alive and well now as you feed your child. The time you spend with your baby now is invaluable. You are laying the foundation upon which they will grow for the rest of their lives.

These first weeks can be oh, so hard. It's not glamorous, but mama, it is magic.

POSITIVE EFFECTS ASSOCIATED WITH BREASTFEEDING

Benefits of breastfeeding for mama:

- Promotes bonding with your baby
- Improved uterine involution and decreased bleeding after birth
- Reduced risk of ovarian and breast cancers
- Reduced risk of osteoporosis
- Quicker postpartum weight loss for some (you know by now that this one makes me twitch a little, but I'll leave it here nonetheless)
- Decreased risk of postpartum depression
- Portable
- Can provide contraception for some (see page 359)
- Less expensive

Breastfeeding doesn't cost much in terms of money. But as the writer Zuzana Boehmová said in a 2018 *Slate* article: "It's only free if your time is worthless." (And your time, indeed, is not worthless.) The truth is that breastfeeding does take a lot of time, and time is not a resource that all women are afforded equally.

Finding the time to breastfeed (or pump) is not easy, especially given our shortened (or nonexistent) maternity leaves, workplaces that may not accommodate breastfeeding and pumping women, and more. The decision to breastfeed is far more complex than "wanting to" or not, and the economic factors are very real. We have work to do here, mamas. A cultural shift that recognizes a mother's value is underway, and it's our job to do what we can to support each other as we grow through this.

Positive effects of breastfeeding for baby:

- Promotes bonding with mama
- Decreased risk of infection, such as respiratory illnesses and ear infections
- Decreased risk of sudden infant death syndrome
- Decreased risk of allergies
- Decreased risk of chronic illness, such as asthma, diabetes, and celiac disease
- Decreased risk of obesity
- Improved digestion, which means less constipation or diarrhea

HOW LONG SHOULD YOU BREASTFEED?

The American Academy of Pediatrics (AAP) recommends that babies be breastfed exclusively (which means that breast milk is the only nutrition they receive) for the first 6 months of life. At 6 months, additional foods can be introduced while breastfeeding continues to at least 12 months or beyond if desired by the mother. Babies do not need any other type of hydration when you are exclusively breastfeeding, so no need to give them water. They get everything they need from breast milk (with the exception of vitamin D, so talk to their pediatrician about supplements).

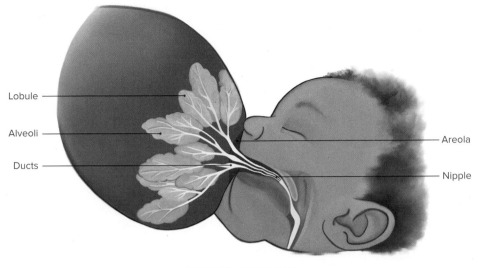

Lobule

Alveoli

Ducts

Areola

Nipple

BREAST ANATOMY

The recommended time frame is 6 months for a few reasons. First, many of the benefits listed above amplify in effect around the 4-month mark and again at the 6-month mark. Also, your baby's gut matures a lot in their first half year of life, meaning that at around 6 months old, their intestines are much better prepared for other, more grown-up foods.

THE AMAZING BREAST

So now that we know why breastfeeding is valuable (magical, even), let's chat through how the breast allows this to happen. Although to be honest, it's so amazing that we could probably just settle on "unicorn fairy dust" as an explanation and be done with it.

First, your awesome breasts' anatomy: Alveoli are grapelike pockets deep inside your breasts that make and store breast milk. They form a cluster called a lobe, of which you have about fifteen per breast. Ducts and ductules

act like highways to carry the milk from the lobes to the nipple and out to the baby.

The dark part of your breast is called your areola, and the nipple is the part that protrudes.

Montgomery tubercles are the tiny bumps on the areola. They provide lubrication for breastfeeding, and get this: That lubrication

BREASTFEEDING WITH A HISTORY OF TRAUMA

Women who have experienced trauma sometimes find that breastfeeding is triggering and distressing, but it can also be a pathway to healing. Please remember that you can speak up about your needs. Let providers (such as lactation consultants) know what you require to feel safe and comfortable.

smells like amniotic fluid, which makes your breasts even more enticing to your newborn baby. (See what I mean about unicorn fairy dust?)

Fun fact about your nipples! We likely envision milk coming out of one "hole" at the end of each nipple. But milk actually leaves the breast through small pore-like openings called milk duct orifices, and you can have up to twenty on each breast. When you take your first shower after your milk comes in, you may leak breast milk for the first time and see that your breasts act like sprinkler heads of milk!

When you are pregnant, your breasts actually go through a second puberty (say what, now?). You gain more ductules, and with the help of the hormone prolactin, you start to produce breast milk. You may find that your breasts leak during pregnancy, or they may not. This has no bearing on your ability to make milk after the baby comes.

When you give birth to your placenta, estrogen and progesterone levels drop, which makes prolactin increase even more. This signals to your body that it is time to start doing this breast milk thing.

On a related note, breastfeeding keeps estrogen levels low. Because of this, you may experience some uncomfortable symptoms like vaginal dryness. Try a water-based personal lubricant for daily discomfort and more enjoyable sex or talk to your provider about other options.

HOW BREASTFEEDING WORKS

When your baby latches on to your breast (takes your nipple into their mouth for nursing), your brain releases a hormone called oxytocin—yup, the same one that brings on labor contractions! Oxytocin stimulates the milk ejection reflex, which makes the milk squirt out of your breast.

At first, your baby will signal to your body that it is time for a feeding by doing a nibbling sort of suck—very tiny little sucks. Once the milk starts flowing, your baby will slow to a deeper, more rhythmic sucking. You may notice their little ears bobbing up and down as they suck and hear a slight "kah" sound as they swallow. I know, adorable.

Milk is made by a supply-and-demand system. The more your tiny boss demands, the more milk your body will supply. So, every time your baby latches on, they send a signal to your body that basically says, "I am here and hungry. Please keep it comin'!"

For this reason, most breastfeeding support people will encourage you to spend at least the first weeks feeding on demand—nursing every time your baby "asks." This is a lot, yes. But feeding on demand can help to establish your milk supply in those early weeks as your body is getting frequent "please make more milk" signals.

Certainly, this is simply not possible for many women, often because we have to go back to work. To the extent that you can, see if you can pump every 2 to 3 hours while away from the baby, and then nurse on demand

THREE BREASTFEEDING FUN FACTS

1 In most women, the right breast produces more milk than the left.
2 Mothers of boys tend to produce more milk than mothers of girls.
3 A mother's age and number of past babies does not impact her milk supply.

when you are together. (We'll cover pumping extensively in the next chapter, but if you want to read ahead, flip to "Pumping and Bottle-Feeding" on page 405).

Your baby will eat about eight to twelve times per day. Most babies will continue to nurse at night for the first year or more of their life.

There are also periods of time when your baby will feed even more than that. This is called cluster feeding. During these periods—that last about 3 to 5 days—your baby will want to eat seemingly all the time. It may be as frequent as every 60 to 90 minutes. And it is quite exhausting.

Knowing that it is normal can make it much more bearable. Cluster feeding may happen when your baby goes through a developmental or physical growth spurt or when they are exposed to an illness. In both cases, they know that they need more breast milk—because your baby is so smart, after all.

It may feel like you are not making enough milk, which can be stressful. It is also really hard to be feeding *that* frequently. Remember, as long as your baby is showing the signs that they are getting enough milk (see "How Do I Know That Baby Is Getting Enough Milk?" on page 394), they are probably fine, but don't hesitate to call their provider if you are worried. Your body will catch up to their demands soon. And this won't last forever.

BREAST MILK

The first milk that your baby will get after they are born is called colostrum. It is nicknamed "liquid gold," both because it is gold in color and because it is worth its weight in gold. It is just so darn good for your baby. Colostrum is calorie dense, very filling, and packed with immune-boosting antibodies. It also acts as a natural laxative to get your baby's GI tract moving.

If your baby ends up spending time in the NICU or needs to receive formula, you may still be able to give them colostrum for its benefits. Talk to the baby's provider about hand expressing some colostrum and then using a cotton swab to rub it around your baby's mouth.

After about 3 days, your milk will, as they say, "come in." This means that your colostrum has transitioned into breast milk, and chances are good that you'll know when it's happened. Your breasts will be larger and feel much fuller, and there is a good chance you will become engorged. Engorged breasts are full of milk. They can feel heavy and swollen, may be a bit bumpy, and may start to leak milk.

Mama, this is uncomfortable. Not exactly painful, but definitely not "normal" feeling.

The best thing to do with engorged breasts is to nurse your baby or use a breast pump, which many hospitals will rent out to patients if you don't have your own. International Board Certified Lactation Consultant (IBCLC) Sharen Medrano recommends trying manually expressing before using the pump because pumping "tends to take longer to get the milk out because it can't get as deep behind the areola or do the work that your hand can." Reminder: We'll get into pumping and all of the related information in the next chapter (see "Pumping and Bottle-Feeding" on page 405).

Medrano also advises that you alternate applying cold and warm compresses to your breasts when they are engorged, using mainly warm ones if you're having trouble getting the milk out.

You will quickly learn what kind of eater your baby is: delicate and slow or voracious and fast (mine were the latter: cute, hungry monsters), requiring both breasts at each feeding or satisfied after one. There is much variability here, and the only way to know is to wait and meet your baby and to see how your breasts respond.

So, say you learn that your baby gets full after about 20 minutes of nursing. Instead of automatically dividing that time between both breasts (10 minutes on the right and 10 minutes on the left), let them finish on one side before moving on to the next. Medrano also says that your baby will signal that they are done with one breast when their sucking and swallowing is no longer steady. When this happens, move them to the next breast.

If your baby eats first on the left and then tops off on the right, start the next feeding on the right side to ensure equal emptying.

It's a good idea to keep track of your baby's feeding sessions. Download an app or use a chart like the one on page 367.

How Do I Know When Baby Is Done Eating?

They will let you know. Babies, especially newborns, often fall asleep at the breast. When you pull them off your nipple, if they wake up and start searching again, you know they need more milk, but if they stay asleep, they are likely done. There is also the hand-clench test. If your baby comes off the breast with their hands clenched into fists, they are likely still hungry. But if their hands are open and relaxed, they are enjoying their post-nursing nap (and mama, maybe you should, too).

Hunger Cues

You will become your baby's expert very quickly, so you'll know better than anyone when they are hungry. Here are a few things to look for:

- Waking up. Newborns tend to wake up for one thing: milk.

- Lip smacking and tongue thrusting. Brace yourself for a cuteness overload with this one.

- Rooting. If there was a mantra to go along with this baby instinct, it would be "please be a nipple, please be a nipple!" Your baby's head will turn toward anything that touches their face in the hope that it might be a breast.

- Hand sucking. "Please be a nipple!"

- Getting angry. In other words, your baby is *hangry*.

If you can start a feeding at the beginning of this sequence of cues, it will save you the frustration of a hangry baby, but sometimes that is simply not possible. Just do the best you can!

How Do I Know That Baby Is Getting Enough Milk?

Great question! There are two main ways to tell:

1 **Checking their weight.** It is normal for babies to lose a bit of weight (up to 10 percent of their body weight) after they are born. You will have a few check-ins with the pediatrician those first weeks and

months to weigh the baby and ensure that their weight is continuing to increase.

2 **Pees and poops.** Keep a log of your baby's pees and poops, either by way of an app on your phone or an old-fashioned notebook and pen (see chart on page 367). If you learn that your baby normally pees about nine times a day, and then one day they pee only four times, it may be an indication that they are not getting enough milk. Likewise, if they are not pooping at least once every 24 hours, something might be up, at least in the very beginning (as babies get older, they may poop less). Your baby's provider will help you assess what is normal for your child. More (so much more) on pees and poops starting on page 367.

Latch and Positions

Latching can be tricky at first, but with practice (for you and for baby), it usually gets easier.

To start each feeding, bring the baby to your breast (not your breast to the baby; save your back, mama). Start by tickling your baby's mouth with your nipple to encourage them to open their mouth wide—the wider, the better. That ensures that your baby will take in as much of your areola as possible, which in turn ensures a deep latch. If the latch is shallow (that is, just on the tip of your nipple, break the baby's suction with the tip of your (clean) pinky finger and try again.

You will know you have a good latch when it doesn't hurt, and the baby is taking sips of milk (you will hear that "kah-kah" sound and see their ears bob up and down).

There are a number of positions you can breastfeed in; whichever one (or ones) you like best is great. See if you can try them all a few times, and then stick with the ones that work best for you and your baby. Following are the most common breastfeeding positions.

Laid Back You lie back or recline at a 45-degree angle, baby lies on you belly-to-belly, bobs their head until they find your nipple, latches, and eats.

Cradle Baby lies in your arm across your abdomen. Their head is supported from

LACTATION COOKIE BITES

Ingredients
1 cup whole rolled oats
1/2 cup shredded, unsweetened coconut
1/4 cup sesame seeds
1/2 cup ground flaxseed meal
1/4 cup honey (can substitute maple syrup)
3/4 cup almond butter
1 tsp. cinnamon
1/4 tsp. sea salt
Optional add-ins: chocolate chips, raisins, or dried cranberries

Directions
1 Mix all ingredients in a large bowl, and refrigerate for about 10–15 minutes or until mixture is firm.

2 Using damp hands, scoop out about 1 Tbs. of dough and shape into 1-inch balls. Set aside on a plate and repeat.

3 Enjoy as a snack or store in your fridge/freezer to eat later!

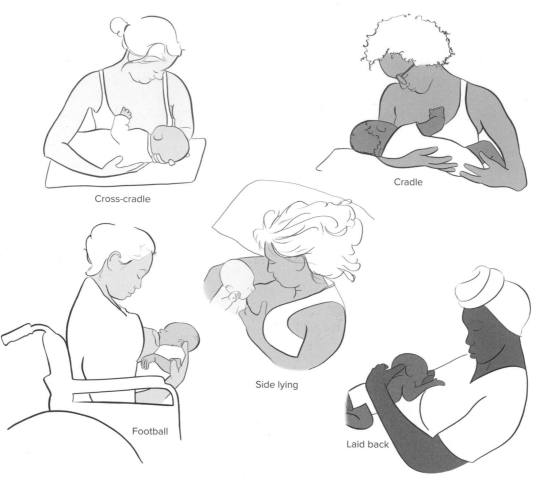

Cross-cradle

Cradle

Football

Side lying

Laid back

BREASTFEEDING POSITIONS

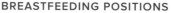

your arm that's on the same side as the breast they are nursing from.

Cross-Cradle Baby lies in your arm, across your abdomen. You support their body with the opposite arm from the breast they are nursing on.

Football Baby is at your side with their head toward your front and their legs pointing toward your back. They nurse on the side they are being held on.

Side Lying You lie on your side with baby also lying on their side, facing you. They nurse from the breast that's on the side you're lying on. (There is a good chance you'll fall asleep using this one, so please see "Safe Sleep and SIDS" on page 372 for safe sleeping guidelines.)

One thing to note is that breastfeeding is time consuming for the first several weeks and even beyond. You may find yourself with a baby at your breast for upward of 6 hours per day, and this is totally normal. Some days it may be less, some days more. But think of it as your main activity immediately postpartum. As baby's capacity to eat larger quantities grows, they will become more efficient feeders, and you will be able to fit feedings more smoothly into your routine.

Five Tips to Get Breastfeeding Off to a Great Start

International Board Certified Lactation Consultant Sharen Medrano offers these five tips:

1 Attend a breastfeeding support group or meeting while you are pregnant. They tend to be very welcoming (and free or inexpensive), and it is so helpful and empowering to actually watch a woman breastfeed in real life—to see how she moves and holds the baby. You can ask your provider about local groups or visit llli.org.

2 Ask for a breast assessment prenatally. Some women have breast issues that can make breastfeeding more challenging. These could be developmental or structural in nature. A breast exam may help reveal an issue, which means you can prepare and plan (instead of feeling shocked and stressed after the baby arrives). You can ask your provider to do the exam or reach out to a local IBCLC. This prenatal meeting may or may not be covered by insurance, so definitely ask.

3 Avoid bottles for the first few days, if possible. Babies are very smart and learn quickly that it's much easier to get milk from a bottle than a breast, which can lead to something called nipple confusion.

Nipple confusion can lead to babies rejecting the breast and preferring the bottle. By waiting to add bottles for a bit, they'll learn to latch first. It's interesting to note that we have long counseled women that pacifiers can also create nipple confusion, and they may! Studies have found, though, that nipple confusion may be more of an issue with bottles than it is with pacifiers.

4 If the baby does need to be fed pumped milk or formula, know that there are other ways to feed a baby besides a bottle! Medicine cups, shot glasses, syringes, and even spoons can be used to give milk to a baby. Just put the spoon (for example) right up to the baby's lips, offer slowly, and they'll start to eat. This will lead to a better transition to the breast when you move to nursing. Be sure to feed them slowly, though, giving small amounts at a time and allowing them to swallow completely before offering the next sip.

5 Hopefully, your experience will be wonderful, but some women do end up feeling intimidated or without the energy to advocate for what they want. Don't be afraid to ask lots of questions and tell your providers what matters to you.

TROUBLESHOOTING

You may experience some bumps along your breastfeeding path. Don't worry; these can often be overcome. And remember, you don't have to go it alone. The moment you suspect a problem, you can call your nurse or provider, baby's provider, or a lactation counselor or consultant.

Low Milk Supply

Since breastfeeding works on supply and demand, the best way to increase supply is to demand more—that is, nurse, nurse, nurse, nurse, nurse (or pump, pump, pump, pump, pump). When possible, rather than making each nursing session longer, see if you can add extra nursing sessions in. The act of latching and letdown can help trigger the production of more milk.

Remember also to focus on your nutrition and hydration to support the production of milk. While there are no studies that support the use of breast milk–making foods (known as galactagogues), it certainly couldn't hurt to try. Foods like oatmeal (and oatmeal cookies; see "Lactation Cookie Bites" on page 395) and apricots have anecdotally worked, as have herbs such as fenugreek, milk thistle, and goat's rue. Consult with your provider before trying the herbs though, as some women and babies have allergies to them.

Lastly, do not hesitate to speak with your provider or a lactation consultant regarding your low supply. They may have additional strategies to try and might recommend the addition of certain prescription medications that can help.

Oversupply

While it may seem at first like producing too much breast milk is good thing, women who experience it know it can be very difficult to deal with. Symptoms of oversupply often include breasts that are always full or engorged and a baby who is unhappy at the breast—fussy, gagging, or spitting up frequently.

The problem is that the symptoms of oversupply can also be connected to other breastfeeding issues, such as a baby with a lip or tongue tie (see page 399). Therefore, if you suspect that you have an oversupply, your best bet is to consult with a provider or lactation consultant to get an accurate diagnosis and appropriate treatment.

Reflux

Almost all babies have some degree of spit-up. For most, it just means lots of dirty bibs, but for some, keeping enough milk down is particularly difficult. Your baby may spit up frequently, may appear uncomfortable after feedings, and in more serious cases, may have slowed weight gain. Reflux is diagnosed by your baby's provider, who can help you develop a treatment plan; sometimes medications are necessary.

Latch Issues

Latch issues can stem from several areas, so seeking the aid of a lactation consultant early is usually the best thing to do, when possible. If it hurts when your baby latches, if baby seems stressed at the breast, if your nipples are cracked or bleeding, or if baby can't seem to maintain a latch, something might be up. It could be anything from needing to tweak your positioning a bit to a structural issue with your breast (for example, flat or inverted nipples) to a structural issue with your baby's mouth (like a tongue or lip tie).

I want to address the commonly heard breastfeeding mantra, "Breastfeeding shouldn't hurt. If it hurts, something's wrong." This is true—to an extent. Certainly, if when your baby latches it makes you get tears in your eyes (not the good kind), cry out in pain, or flinch from discomfort, something is likely wrong. At the first consideration of "hmm, I wonder if this is a problem," call for help.

But my concern with that phrase is that it discounts the widely shared experience of many brand-new mamas: Those first days of breastfeeding are not always awesome. A very sensitive part of your body that is probably not used to getting *this* much attention is suddenly being tugged, rubbed, and sucked for hours every day. It is bound to be at least a bit raw and uncomfortable.

It cannot be overstated that if you are worried, seek support. You do not want to ignore a potential problem that might only get worse. But if everything checks out, and "all" that is required is a period of adjustment, please know that this is normal. I have worked with many women who thought there was something wrong with them because they didn't enjoy breastfeeding their baby in those first days, often telling me, "I'm obviously not cut out for this."

Mama, you are.

Be patient, and it will get so much better. In the meantime, try the following:

- If you suspect that your nipples are just adjusting and need a little TLC, try expressing and rubbing a bit of breast milk into them, as breast milk has healing properties (*I know, right?*).

- Expose your breasts to air. Try for a few 20-minute sessions per day (though more definitely won't hurt).

- Use a baby-safe nipple ointment between feedings.

Lip and Tongue Ties

Sometimes a baby's mouth structure can make it difficult for them to get a proper latch, resulting from a too-tight frenulum (the membrane that connects the tongue to the bottom of the mouth or the one that connects the upper lip to the upper gum). You may notice these visually, or you may find out your baby has a tie because they are having issues latching. It is actually quite common (about 1 out of 7 babies) and rather easy to fix. An otolaryngologist (ear, nose, and throat doctor) will do an in-office procedure to release the tie, either using a laser or a scissor snip. (This is sometimes done in the hospital before discharge if you have a hospital birth.) Tongue and lip ties are not always a problem, though. My youngest had a pretty substantial lip tie and was my best nurser. If you do need to get it fixed, don't worry. The process is usually well tolerated and works wonders on fixing a latch problem. Most insurance plans will cover this procedure, but you may need to get a referral.

Mastitis

If bacteria enter the breast where there is unmoving milk, an infection called mastitis can occur, and mama, it stinks. In addition to the symptoms of a clogged duct, you will usually feel generally sick, much like you have the flu, with chills, body aches, and a fever. These symptoms warrant an immediate call to your provider (yes, even at 2:00 a.m.). They can sometimes even diagnose you over the phone.

Mastitis is treated using oral antibiotics, and it is almost always safe to continue breastfeeding (your provider will guide you here). It's actually the best thing to do, as it will help prevent the condition from worsening.

To prevent clogged ducts and mastitis, try not to skip a feeding or suddenly go much longer between feeds, as this can lead to a buildup of milk that can cause a problem. A study also found that stress and lack of sleep (both common for new mamas!) may make you more prone to mastitis because they can weaken your immune system. And sometimes it just happens despite your best efforts, so don't be hard on yourself if it does.

Plugged or Clogged Duct

Sometimes milk can get obstructed in one of the ducts (the highways that transport the milk from the lobes to the nipple). When this happens, it is usually on one side and can cause a painful, hard, warm, red lump.

To relieve it, try taking a warm shower or applying a warm compress and massaging it. And nurse your baby—*a lot*. While it may take some acrobatics, I have seen success when women position the baby so that their chin is pointing toward the clog because that is where they are most efficient at removing milk. You can also try "the dangle," where you place baby flat on their back on the floor and then position yourself on all fours over them, dangling the breast with the clog for them to nurse from. If these tricks don't work, call a lactation consultant or your provider.

Thrush (*Candida or Yeast Infection*)

Thrush can develop in your breasts, in the baby's mouth, or both. Babies naturally get a white tongue when they breastfeed. If you can scrape the white off with your fingernail, it's likely milk, but if you can't, it could be thrush. The baby may also develop a bumpy diaper rash.

You might know that you have thrush if your nipples burn, or when the baby latches,

you get a sharp, shooting pain in your breast. Thrush is usually treated with an antifungal medication for you (often a cream for your nipples) and the baby (often a gel that is applied in their mouth).

Some women choose to avoid prescription medications by using traditional remedies instead. Historically, gentian violet (a blue dye) was applied to the mouth and breast to treat thrush, but it can cause ulcers and should not be swallowed, so speak with your provider before trying this. Some women have had success applying a combination of vinegar and baking soda, yogurt, or probiotics to the breasts and baby's mouth, but these have not been studied well.

To prevent thrush, wash your hands well before breastfeeding. Try to minimize sugar in your diet, and up your intake of foods with healthy bacteria, such as yogurt, sauerkraut, and kombucha (which contains a small amount of alcohol, so discuss with your provider first). And just like mastitis, sometimes thrush is simply unavoidable.

Dysphoric Milk Ejection Reflex (**D-MER**)

Some women experience intense sadness just as their milk is letting down, possibly caused by an abrupt drop in the hormone dopamine. It can be very disconcerting to experience this, but hopefully you feel comforted knowing that this is a "real thing." Speak to your provider or a therapist about it, as treatment may be available.

BREASTFEEDING GEAR

Nursing Bras

Nursing bras can be a real game changer if you normally like to wear supportive bras. They provide support specially designed for your hard-at-work breasts, and they have ingenious little snaps and flaps that allow quick and comfortable access to your nipples. That said, they are not always a necessity, and plenty of women choose to wear camisoles, bralettes, sports bras in a larger size, or nothing at all.

If you do get a nursing bra, stores that offer bra fittings can be a huge help. Bra experts recommend getting sized for your nursing bras when you are about 8 months pregnant if possible, as your breast size at that point often reflects what it will be when you are nursing. You can also wait until about a month after your baby is born to get fitted. In the weeks immediately after you give birth, you may be engorged, and therefore measurements may be off. You can expect to gain several cup sizes and at least one band size from your prepregnancy bra size.

In the first month of breastfeeding—and sometimes beyond—try to stick to wireless options. Underwires can prevent milk from moving in your breasts, which could lead to plugged ducts. A lot of women love nursing tank tops during this time. Some women also find that they want to wear bras at night to be more comfortable. If you do, avoid underwire and make sure your breasts get some free time in the breeze. It is possible to develop yeast infections and heat rashes around your breasts if they don't get enough air.

You may choose to buy new bras or take hand-me-downs from friends: Both are great! If you buy, I'd suggest starting with one or two to make sure you like them, and that may be all you end up needing. If you get used ones, do keep in mind that they have likely been exposed to someone else's breast milk, so consider disinfecting them before wearing:

FEEDING TUBES

Special feeding tube systems can be used to give your baby milk at the breast. A container of milk (breast or formula) connects to a small tube, which you then tape to your chest, leading to the nipple. When your baby latches, they take your areola and the end of the tube in their mouth, and get milk from the feeding system, and possibly your breast at the same time.

Tube feeding may be recommended to encourage your milk supply to come in, if the baby is not getting enough milk from breastfeeding alone, or if you have a non-lactating partner who wants to feed the baby at their chest. Your baby's provider or a lactation consultant can help you get started with feeding tubes.

washing in hot water with a bit of 3 percent hydrogen peroxide. Drying them in sunlight can also be effective.

Breastfeeding Pillows

Helping your baby to nurse for hours a day doesn't have to cause muscle fatigue or soreness. There are specially shaped pillows that provide a "shelf" for the baby to lie on that sits right under your breasts. These breastfeeding pillows can be helpful for positioning your baby comfortably in the beginning (for you and for the baby). Later, when nursing takes less time, you won't need so much support, and you will likely have built up strength in your arms to support baby more easily.

OTHER BREASTFEEDING CONSIDERATIONS

Nursing in Public and Around Others

Ugh, people, right? Just kidding, sort of. I mean people are lovely, but sometimes they have a hard time knowing how to give a vulnerable breastfeeding mama the support she needs. Unhelpful comments that make us feel judged (or that are actually judging) have a way of quickly working their way into our psyches and making a lasting impression.

You get to decide what makes you feel comfortable. Some women breastfeed in public without covering, while others choose to use a blanket, shawl, or nursing cover. Still others find a place where they can be alone.

Know that the law is on your side. It is legal to breastfeed in public in all 50 states in the US. Beyond that, do what you can to ignore others, and trust that you are doing the best thing for you and your baby—whatever that means for *you*.

Drinking While Breastfeeding?

You may have heard that certain beers can increase your milk supply. This is true, sort of. Studies have found that sugar in the barley that beer is made from can increase the hormone prolactin, which is involved in triggering letdown, or the release of breast milk.

However, in general, research has found that alcohol can slightly decrease your breast milk production. And alcohol may also temporarily change the flavor and smell of your milk, which can impact how much your baby eats. Babies tend to nurse slightly more but take in less breast milk after their moms drink.

Only about 2 percent of the alcohol consumed gets into your breast milk. The alcohol amount in your breast milk peaks about 30 to 60 minutes after you drink (60 to 90 minutes if you drink while eating).

Here's the golden rule: If you feel the effects of the alcohol, alcohol is in your breast milk. When you are feeling sober, your breast milk is safe.

If you want to drink while breastfeeding, Dr. Jack Newman of La Leche League International says, "Reasonable alcohol intake should not be discouraged at all. . . . Very little alcohol comes out in the milk. The mother can drink some alcohol and continue breastfeeding as she normally does. Prohibiting alcohol is another way we make life unnecessarily restrictive for nursing mothers."

To get highly specific, the American Academy of Pediatrics states that the "ingestion of alcoholic beverages should be minimized and limited to an occasional intake." The maximum recommended for a mother weighing 60 kilograms (about 130 pounds) is 2 ounces of liquor, 8 ounces of wine, or 2 beers. They also state that "nursing should take place 2 hours or longer after the alcohol intake to minimize its concentration in the ingested milk."

Pumping and Dumping You may have heard about "pumping and dumping," which is when a breastfeeding woman pumps her milk after she drinks and then dumps it (throws it away). The good news is you almost never actually have to do this. Once the alcohol is out of your bloodstream, it's out of your breast milk. It doesn't linger in your breasts until they are emptied. Pumping also won't speed up the rate that the alcohol is processed by your body. Your liver is handling all that.

It's important to empty your breasts at regular intervals to maintain your milk supply (and for your comfort), so pumping and dumping can be great for this when you're drinking.

Say, for example, you are at a wedding, and your baby is home with grandpa. If you are used to nursing every 3 hours, you should try to pump every 3 hours when you are away from your baby. If the milk you pump has alcohol in it, dump it. If not, save it and add it to your freezer stash when you get home.

Cheers!

Breastfeeding a Baby in the NICU

If you have a baby in the NICU, breastfeeding can be a unique journey. Your baby may have specific nutritional needs as well as challenges related to their size, age, and physical abilities. The overarching stress and emotional intensity of the whole experience can weigh heavily on you. In short, this is hard, mama.

First, bathe yourself in gentleness. You are going to do the best you can do, every day. Your best is going to look different at any given moment, and that is okay. Your baby's needs and abilities are going to shift as well. "One day at a time" will be your motto for this phase of motherhood.

Here are a few tips for feeding your NICU baby:

- Don't be afraid to voice your desires. If breastfeeding is important to you, let the NICU team know. They are there to support you.

- Remember that every drop is gold. It may be that your baby is getting formula in addition to breast milk right now, and that is okay. Every time your baby gets breast milk, they benefit. And every time they fill their tiny tummies with nourishment, they will grow.

- Talk to your baby's team about swabbing your baby's mouth with your colostrum to help them develop more normal gut bacteria.

- Get a team feeding plan. There are many people involved in your baby's care right now. Making sure that nurses, doctors, aides, and any family members are on the same page regarding the baby's feeding will help a lot.

- Ask to see the lactation consultant—a lot. They will help you navigate the challenges that come up as your baby's story unfolds.

- Pump. Pumping often (about every 2 to 3 hours) will help to establish your milk supply, even if your baby isn't getting it all right now. You can freeze the milk for later or donate it. See chapter 30, "Pumping and Bottle-Feeding," for more.

remember

Breastfeeding can be a rewarding and amazing experience, but it can also be very challenging. Taking care of yourself is just as important now as it was when you were pregnant, so do everything within your power to nurture yourself through this.

Pumping and Bottle-Feeding

I am nourishing my baby, and my baby is thriving.

note FROM DIANA

There are so many possible reasons that you have arrived at this chapter, and more important, reasons why you plan to give your baby a bottle—or a lot of bottles.

Maybe you will be working outside the home. Maybe biology or circumstances have prevented you from being able to breastfeed to some extent or at all. Maybe you want to have the option to go out to dinner without the baby from time to time, or maybe you just don't want to nurse.

I could spend pages listing all the possible explanations for why you are here, but honestly, it doesn't matter.

There is one person who knows the whole story, and that is you. That means that there is one person who can make the best decision about feeding your baby—also you. I hope that you have support, both professional and personal, to help guide you through your options. But ultimately, you are the expert on your life, your family, and your baby.

The world is not always great at supporting moms, especially when it comes to matters of feeding. There is a lot of judgment out there, and at times it can be hard to stand tall in its wake. I sincerely hope that you don't feel any negativity, but if you do, remember that you arrived where you are for a reason that matters, and it is okay to trust yourself.

xo,

Diana

P.S. This chapter is your introduction to pumping and bottle-feeding. If you plan to bottle-feed without pumping, you can jump right to "Bottle-Feeding" on page 410.

PUMPING

For those who choose to use one, your breast pump is a tool meant to help you. There is not one definitive way to use it: You get to decide! Ask your village for their experiences. They will likely have many tips and tricks to share. But remember that ultimately your pumping picture is going to look different from theirs.

The ability to pump breast milk is an incredible gift. It is wonderful that we have a tool that can allow us to nourish our babies while doing #allthethings we need to do. But pumping is not always everybody's favorite activity.

Maybe you'll find it sterile and mechanical, or maybe it will be a good excuse for you to sit down and relax. It is also a fair amount of work, especially if you are carrying your equipment back and forth to work, washing all the pieces, and figuring out how much milk you need to thaw and when. It can be tedious. But breast pump technology is improving all the time, and it's wonderful to have a convenient way to provide breast milk while away from your baby, or to express breast milk when nursing is not an option.

Reasons you may decide to pump include:

- Having a supply of breast milk for when you are away from the baby (going back to work, dinner out with your friends, or an opportunity to sleep for an extra stretch at night)

- Increasing your milk supply

- Maintaining your milk supply while not nursing (for example, while drinking alcohol; refer to page 402 for guidelines on this)

- Relieving engorgement or a plugged duct

- Providing breast milk to your baby, who is unable to nurse

- Enabling your partner to feed the baby

- Preferring not to nurse but still wanting to provide your baby with breast milk

- Wanting to donate your breast milk

Prepping to Pump

What you'll need:

- Pump
- Accessories (may include tubing, flanges—the parts that go on your breasts—valves, and bottles or bags to pump into)
- Freezer-safe storage containers (bags, ice cube trays, freezable glass jars)
- Bag to carry pump and accessories
- Freezer bag or ice packs to transport breast milk
- Pumping bra/tank top

If you can, try to secure your pump during your pregnancy. Many insurance companies now cover the cost or send you one for free, so definitely start by calling them first!

In addition to the pump, you'll need the accessories for the pump, which usually include tubes, valves, bottles or bags for the milk to go into, and flanges. The specifics will depend on which pump brand and model you use. Most of the time when you get a new pump, it will come with a kit of accessories you need to get started.

Flanges are the trumpet-looking plastic parts that "latch" onto your breasts. Okay, let's be real. They look like burlesque dance accessories. It is important to have the correct size flange; not doing so can limit the amount of milk that comes out and can hurt. (*Ouch!*) Most pump brands have guidelines on their websites to show you which flange size in their lineup is correct for you, depending on the size of your nipples. So, get out your ruler and measure those areolas!

If you will be taking your pump with you outside of your home, you will likely want a bag to carry it and the other gear in. Many pumps come with a bag or even a handy backpack to travel with. You can also use that tote bag you have had in your closet for years. If your pumped milk will spend more than 4 hours at room temperature out of a refrigerator, you will also need a freezer bag or some ice packs to keep it from spoiling. Note that the sooner

you get your milk into a fridge, the longer it is likely to last. See "Breast Milk Storage" on page 409 for more information.

Another helpful item for mamas who pump regularly is a hands-free pumping bra (or an old sports bra with small holes cut into the center of each cup), which allows you to secure the flanges to your breasts and maintain suction without constantly holding them.

The other factor to consider is where you will pump. If you'll pump at home, think about a place where you can sit comfortably, with good back support. Yes, the couch in front of your TV is a perfectly good place. If you'll be pumping outside of the home, you might talk to your workplace about securing a private and comfortable spot or chat with co-workers who have pumped to see where they did it. If you are the first pumper among your team, consider yourself the pioneer. Do not be afraid to ask for what you need.

YOUR PROTECTIONS AT WORK

Section 7 of the Fair Labor Standards Act states that employers are required to provide "reasonable break time for an employee to express breast milk for her nursing child for 1 year after the child's birth each time such employee has need to express the milk." Employers are also required to "provide a place, other than a bathroom, that is shielded from view and free from intrusion from co-workers and the public, which may be used by an employee to express breast milk."

If you are concerned that your rights are being violated, contact your human resources department or an employment attorney.

Pumping Session

Start off your pumping session by wiping down the surface that you will set your pump on and washing your hands for 20 seconds. This will help keep bacteria off your pumping supplies, which will help your milk last longer.

Set up your pump. If it needs power, you can connect to an outlet or use a battery pack.

When you pump, you have the option to do both breasts at the same time or one breast at a time. What you choose will likely depend on why you are pumping and when you last fed your baby. For example, if you will be away from the baby for a period of time and are pumping to maintain your supply and bring milk home, you will probably choose to pump both breasts. If you are home with the baby and they have just nursed on the left side only, you may choose to then pump the right side to increase your supply or to add some milk to your freezer stash.

Be sure to consult your pump's instruction materials to confirm that you're operating the pump correctly and that the flanges are optimally positioned for you.

When you're done pumping, follow the manufacturer's instructions for cleaning the pump and accessories. If your baby is younger than 3 months old or has specific health concerns, your baby's provider may advise sterilizing the equipment between uses, so be sure to ask.

When to Pump

How often you pump will depend on why you are pumping, so there will be a lot of variation here. The most important thing to know, though, if you want to maintain your milk supply, is to try to pump as frequently as your baby eats. As we discussed on page 392, breast milk is made on a supply-and-demand system, so the more you pump, the more milk you will make.

If you will be exclusively pumping, or away from your baby for a period of time, pump as frequently as the baby eats—about every 2 to 3 hours. This will maintain your supply and help prevent clogs and engorgement.

If you are pumping once per day to increase your freezer stash, you might try to pump in the morning, as many moms find that they have the most milk early in the day.

Mamas who exclusively pump will generate anywhere from 19 to 30 ounces of milk per day (though this can vary a lot). If you pump eight times per day, you can expect anywhere from 2.5 to 3.75 ounces per pumping session (and again, your own amounts may be different).

BREAST MILK STORAGE

If you are going to give your pumped milk to your baby within the next 3 to 8 days, you can simply keep it in the fridge. If you plan to store it longer, you can freeze it. In cases where you plan to store the breast milk for later, it's recommended that you refrigerate or freeze the milk immediately after pumping to ensure maximum freshness down the road. Please see the following chart for Motherly's pumped milk guidelines.

PUMPED BREAST MILK STORAGE GUIDELINES

FRESHLY PUMPED MILK	TIME	NOTES
ROOM TEMPERATURE	4 hours	Keep covered.
COOLER BAG	24 hours	Keep ice packs in contact with milk. Avoid opening cooler.
REFRIGERATOR	3–8 days	Store in back of fridge. Clean hands, pump, and pumping surface will increase shelf life.
FREEZER INSIDE FRIDGE	2 weeks	Store in back, away from sides.
SEPARATE FREEZER	3–6 months	Store in back, away from sides.
DEEP FREEZER	6–12 months	Store in back, away from sides.

Thawing Frozen Milk

When you thaw your milk, you can either put it in the fridge overnight, run the bag or storage container under warm water, or place it in a bowl of warm water. Never microwave your breast milk, as it can create tiny hot pockets within the milk that could burn your baby's mouth, and you also run the risk of damaging the nutrients in the breast milk. Once milk has been thawed, it should be used *within 24 hours* and cannot be refrozen.

COMBINATION FEEDING

Many moms end up combo-feeding, meaning that they feed their baby by both nursing and bottle-feeding pumped milk or formula. This usually involves a period of experimenting and learning—mostly about your baby. After some trial and error, you will determine exactly how much milk your baby needs every day, their favorite bottle and nipple type, and what feeding schedule works best for your family. Although I know it sounds daunting now, you will get it. I promise.

Figuring out how much bottled milk to give your babe requires a bit of math. The average 1- to 3-month-old baby consumes 25 ounces of milk per day over eight to twelve feedings, so start with that and adjust as you get to know your baby.

So, say your baby eats ten times per day: Dividing 25 ounces by 10 feedings is 2.5 ounces per feeding, so each of the bottles would be about 2.5 ounces. When you nurse, there's no need to track how much they get (and no way to really do it either, except for a detailed weighing before and after!).

If you would like to maintain your milk supply, remember that you'll need to continue to empty your breasts at the same frequency that your baby eats, about every 3 hours. If the baby is getting a bottle for a feeding, consider pumping during that time.

BOTTLE-FEEDING

When introducing a bottle to your baby, there seems to be a golden window between 4 and 6 weeks. Earlier than 4 weeks can cause nipple confusion, which may make them prefer a bottle over the breast because drinking from a bottle is easier. It's worth noting that for cases when a bottle needs to be introduced earlier, some lactation consultants recommend using special newborn slow-flow nipples anytime you bottle-feed—even beyond the newborn phase—to restrict the flow of milk so that babies need to exert a similar level of effort for both bottle and breast (and so are less likely to develop a preference).

Introducing a bottle later than 6 weeks old risks having them refuse the bottle because they have grown very fond of nursing at the breast. If possible, ask your partner or a friend to feed your baby their first bottle. They are more likely to take it if they don't think mama is around to feed them.

I would suggest not investing in a huge supply of one brand of bottles just yet (register for a gift card instead). Each bottle and nipple has its own qualities, and your baby may have preferences or requirements that you won't find out about until you start bottle-feeding them.

Used bottles are generally considered safe to use. Sterilize them in boiling water or the dishwasher (if the bottle is dishwasher safe) to kill any germs. It is best to buy new nipples, though, as they can break down over time.

DONATED BREAST MILK

Some families decide to feed their babies donated breast milk. You can do this exclusively, or as a supplement to your breast milk or formula.

Donor milk banks have become more popular in recent years and can provide your baby with safe milk from another woman. Being able to have some breast milk can make a difference for many health factors. To locate a milk bank, visit the Human Milk Bank Association of North America online. And note that this option can, unfortunately, be quite expensive.

There are also ways to get free donated breast milk. An Internet or social media search may help you find some, as can word of mouth. You can also ask a friend or family member who is producing breast milk. Donated milk may come from women who have produced more milk than their baby needs or women who have lost a baby and choose to donate the breast milk they are still producing as a way to honor their journey.

Unofficial donations are not regulated in any way, so there are concerns regarding the possibility of contaminated milk (infections, drugs, and so on), as well as the safety of online transactions in general. Studies have found that unofficial donations tend to be more contaminated with bacteria than milk received from a bank, and AAP cautions against them for this reason. Still, many families choose this option, perhaps because they trust the person donating the milk and feel strongly that they want their baby to receive breast milk. Speak with your baby's provider for additional guidance.

FORMULA

If you need to go the formula route, do so with confidence. Formulas are getting better all the time and are highly regulated. I usually advise women to start simple. Did you get a sample of formula in the mail? Try it! If your baby tolerates it (which they most likely will), then perhaps your search has ended.

There are tons of options out there. Some moms choose organic formulas, as they want to be extra careful about pesticides. Some mamas are even sourcing formulas from European countries, since they don't include synthetic ingredients like those found in the US (note that this option can be quite expensive).

Do not go straight to soy formula, goat's milk formula, or anything highly specialized without consulting with your baby's provider first. These are great options for babies who need them, but they can be difficult to digest, so it's best to avoid them unless necessary. A few formulas contain high-fructose corn syrup, which can promote tooth decay, so you may choose to stay clear of those, or make sure to wipe down those adorable little gums (and eventually teeth) every day (with a washcloth and water).

Do your research and decide on the formula that is the best fit for your baby's needs and your family budget.

remember

As with all areas of parenting, feeding your baby can be highly complex. Ultimately, you must trust yourself and your decisions. Your baby will be fine because they have you. That is what matters most.

Postpartum Love and Village and Returning to Work

We are in this together.

note
FROM DIANA

There's no time like birth to remind us of our biology. When it comes down to it, we are governed overwhelmingly by the instincts and functions of our bodies. This means we have a finite amount of energy before we need to rest, and we are susceptible to the effects of stress.

Stress can be good, or it can be bad, particularly if it is prolonged, but we can't tell the difference between the two. All we feel is a cascade of physical responses that we tend to interpret negatively. This is why, even the most joyful times—weddings, moving into a new home, starting a new job we love, and yes, welcoming a baby—can leave us feeling anxious, tired, and depleted.

Enter parenthood, where, in addition to the happy stress, you are dealing with recovering from pregnancy and birth, shifting hormones, adjusting to a wonky sleep schedule, and, oh yeah, taking care of a totally dependent human 24/7.

This is hard, mama. So, if you are feeling some new pulls on your inner harmony, especially when it comes to relationships, village, and work, please know that this is completely and overwhelmingly to be expected.

As discussed, many cultures treat this postpartum time as a rest and recovery period for the new mother, allowing her to forget all about her other tasks and responsibilities and focus on baby. It's one of the most powerful traditions that we all would do well to incorporate.

But for those of us who don't have that social support or cultural heritage to lean into right now, there are still a million things you can do to be thoughtful and intentional about this super-formative time. This chapter offers a handful of strategies that I've seen work well for families just starting out.

xo,

Diana

Parenting Together

If you are parenting with a partner, you are in the midst of one of the most profound transitions you will go through together, especially when it comes to how you might be accustomed to relating to one another. Prior to having a baby, you were both individuals who primarily looked out for yourselves. Yes, you took care of and supported each other, but caring for an adult is very different from caring for an infant.

Research has found that within 3 years of a first baby, about two-thirds of married couples note a decline in the quality of their relationship. In 13 percent of married couples, this leads to divorce by the time the child is 5. But take heart. For couples heading into the new vista of child-rearing, there are steps you can take to keep your relationship as happy and healthy as possible.

Five tips for protecting your coupledom:

1 **Anticipate conflict and have a plan ready to go.** Chances are good that you will argue more than you are used to, for a little while (for all the reasons stated in my note). Know that it is normal, but that doesn't mean you have to settle for it. During a time when you are not upset, talk with your partner about how you will handle the disagreements to come.

2 **Consider couples therapy.** Just as every individual could benefit from seeing a therapist, every couple probably could as well. Even if things in your relationship seem great, consider seeking professional help. It's just like getting coaching for something you want to improve at. They can help you talk through things before they become issues in addition to working through the tough stuff that already exists.

3 **Practice forgiveness.** You are on the same team. Remember that you are both learning and allow space for the mess ups and confusion.

I came home from work one night, and my husband proudly reported that he had given our daughter her first haircut because it was in her eyes and bothering her. "I did it when she was in the bath!" he said. "Okay, great. Thanks! Where is the hair you cut off, so I can put it in her baby book?" (Which, for the record, I still have not made for any of my three kids.)

Cue blank stare. After a long, painful pause, he said, "Um, it went down the drain?"

Not going to lie: There were some serious tears on my part and a strong feeling of "*How could you?*" But after these emotions, it was up to me to realize that my husband had no way of knowing what my plan was for her hair and that he was really trying to help—and *did* help, even if it wasn't the way I would have done it. And how important is that lost lock of hair, anyway? (Hint: Especially unimportant for a nonexistent baby book.)

4 **Keep your sense of humor.** Sometimes, you just have to laugh. Like just now, as I was writing that haircut story.

Parenthood is serious business, but it is okay not to take every moment as a matter of life and death, especially when you can laugh together. When we went away on our first overnight with our newborn, she had so many poop explosions that we had to buy a new set of onesies. You know what? That was pretty funny.

When my husband was in a big photography contest that we all went to, and not one but all three of our kids had massive meltdowns while the judge was presenting awards in front of a large crowd—also funny.

It is not going to be perfect, but that is where the beauty comes from. Don't be afraid to laugh.

5 **Remember what brought you together.** Think back on when you met and those early days together. Before the baby, there were the two of you. This is part of your adventure together, but it's not the sum total of who you are together.

Sharing Household Duties

Talk with your partner about how you will share the responsibilities of caring for the baby and the rest of the household. This is going to look different for every family, so it might even be helpful to make a list of the duties.

They might include:

- Daytime feedings
- Nighttime feedings

- Washing bottles and pump parts
- Laundry
- Baby health-care appointments
- Baby announcements and thank-you notes
- Meal prep
- Dishes
- Housecleaning
- Errands
- Pet care
- Older sibling care

Decide who will be responsible for what ahead of time so that it doesn't have to be a conversation or negotiation every time.

And know that this will change as time goes on. For example, if you have maternity leave, and your partner does not have much leave, it may make sense for you to be the one to take your baby to their appointments in these first months. But when you head back to your job, maybe your partner will take over that task because your pediatrician's office is closer to their workplace.

Or perhaps your partner is handling most of the cooking right now, so you can get an extra nap in every day and heal from birth, but when you are feeling better, you plan to take over cooking because your partner will be back at work and gets home late.

Things will continue to shift as life unfolds, and that's okay. Make sure to have conversations about your needs as they come up and to respect your partner's needs as well.

Making Time for Yourself

You know the saying that you cannot pour from an empty cup? They may have been talking directly to new mamas.

Taking care of yourself is so essential, for you and for your partner. And it is something that is so easily overlooked or skipped. Prioritize time to do things that you love. If you have time to go swimming, and your partner has time to read quietly (or whatever it is that lights you both up), you will have more love and energy and happiness to share with each other.

Making Time as a Couple

After you've taken care of *you* time, be sure to add in couple time. Fair warning: This is going to look different than it used to.

Remember that this is a season, and it will pass. Romance will take more effort, which can take some of the fun and spontaneity out of it. But this season also has the potential to open your heart in ways you never imagined possible.

Use a pen (not a pencil) to add some date nights (or mornings) to the calendar. Communicate. Then communicate some more. And trust that the love that brought you together will get you through this time.

Here are some of the Motherly mamas' favorite post-baby date ideas:

"Sometimes we wait to eat our dinner until after the boys are in bed, so we can enjoy wine and an actual conversation without the chaos."   ASHLEY

"We plan dates way in advance, like concerts or events. You set it up, and then you kind of forget about it, and it pops up, and that's exciting."   COLLEEN

"We try to do something active rather than just dinner, so we don't feel bad if one of us is too tired to have an engaging convo."

EMILY

"I actually really *missed* my husband so much after [my son] was born. I realized I had to make a conscious effort and set aside time to see him as him, and talk to him and connect, even if it was just on our couch or at the dinner table. We love to cook together and binge-watch shows together, but we also prioritized finding a date-night sitter so that we could go out."   KARELL

Sex after Giving Birth

One of the most common questions among new mamas is when they can start having sex again (this includes vaginal, anal, cunnilingus, and external stimulation). Many providers suggest waiting about 6 weeks after giving birth. This is because at the 6-week mark, the uterus has returned to its prepregnancy size, the cervix has recovered, and most tears have healed.

So, the short answer is about 6 weeks.

The longer answer is that it's complicated, mama, and *you* are the one who gets to decide what is right for you.

First, depending on your birth and body, you may be ready to have sex sooner, or you may need more time to physically heal. It can take longer to fully recover from pregnancy and giving birth, especially when it comes to your pelvic floor, up to a year or even longer for some women.

There is a huge emotional component to having sex after giving birth. Your body has gone through extraordinary changes. A human has just come out of you! If the idea of intimacy feels nerve-wracking or scary, you are not alone.

You may also have concerns about your new postpartum body and being naked in front of someone else. Your body went through an enormous metamorphosis and is still transforming each day, whereas it is likely your partner's body stayed the same. You may assume that your partner has incorporated some bias about how pregnancy changed you: your breasts, your belly, and your vagina. This is a time to courageously ask for what you need, and it's a moment to revel in all that you have built with your beautiful body: a new baby and a family. You might feel more relaxed and gain trust if you open up about these issues.

Try something like this: "Honey, I've been through so much and felt so powerful from creating new life, but I want you to know that I'm feeling insecure about my body after the baby. I want us to focus together on how awesome my body is. I need you to tell me that you appreciate my body right now, as it is."

Lastly, you are now a parent, and with that comes a tremendous shift to your daily reality. The lack of sleep and omnipresence of baby poop in your new life are not exactly sexy, not to mention the fact that many mamas find it hard to get into the mood after being physically touched by a tiny human all day. The drop in estrogen that you experienced after birth means there is a concrete reason you may not feel very aroused.

Mama, it is okay.

If you're healed and ready to get it on, go for it. But if instead of excitement, you feel panic, take some more time.

Here are a few midwife tips for making postpartum sex more enjoyable for you.

Starting Alone Your pelvis is the seat of your power and is responsible for your sense of security, safety, and grounding as well as your emotions and sexuality. Giving birth can stir up a lot in your pelvis (physically and

emotionally) and leave you feeling vulnerable. Before opening yourself to someone else, you might think about reconnecting with yourself. You can gently feel around with your fingertips to get the new lay of the land or touch yourself in a way that feels good. Remember, this is your body.

Going Slowly with No Expectations There is no rule that you have to go "all the way" the first time you have sex after giving birth—or the second or the fifth. Try not to pressure yourself to achieve a certain outcome, and instead focus on connecting to your partner. If that is "just" kissing and cuddling, it is fine! It might actually be kinda sexy.

Being in Charge Tell your partner that you are into the idea of having sex again but that you would like to be the initiator and power holder. You control the timing, speed, actions—everything.

Using Lots of Foreplay and Lubrication Giving birth and breastfeeding can make your vaginal mucosa drier, which can lead to painful sex. Spend lots of time with foreplay to get yourself in the mood, and do not skimp on the lubrication.

If you are having sex with a man, it is important to know that it is possible to get pregnant pretty quickly after giving birth. Often times women ovulate before they see the blood of their period, meaning that you may be fertile without knowing that your menstrual cycle has returned. Plus, irregular cycles may make it hard to predict when you are ovulating. So, before reengaging in sex, consider your desires for expanding your family and consider your birth control options accordingly. (See "Birth Control" on page 357.)

One thing to keep in mind is that persistent lack of sexual desire can be a sign of postpartum depression. So, if you are just not in the mood ever, don't ignore it. Check in with your provider or therapist.

SINGLE PARENTHOOD

Single parenthood is a challenge that many say is both hard and very rewarding. The buck stops with you, which is a *huge* responsibility, but you also get all the freedom to make decisions about your life with your child.

Being a single mom can release superpowers that you never knew you had. Pay extra attention to the support system you build for yourself, as it can make such a difference.

Building Your Support Team

Consider who you can call on to help with childcare and household tasks, whether paid or unpaid. You absolutely need a sick-day fallback hero—someone who will take over when you just can't do it—even if it's backup daycare at the gym or the kind neighbor next door.

Next, who are the people you can trust to give you good advice about all of the questions that come with parenting and work? These are the types of issues that you may feel better discussing first instead of acting on alone: It is always helpful to have a parenting sounding board for the tough questions.

And then there are the work advisors. Work, whether at home or somewhere else, is important for all of us and especially for single moms who are the sole breadwinners. Many single mamas don't have, or necessarily want, child support from family or their ex. Since having a steady income is essential for single mothers, it's really helpful for a member or members of your support team to understand your work life and career goals in addition to your parenting goals, whether it's a best friend, a business partner, or a close colleague at the office. Good communication and a healthy relationship with this person are key, just as they would be with a romantic partner. It's often helpful if this person is also a parent.

And just because you are a mom now (and extremely busy!) does not mean you should give up the search if you still desire a partner or co-parent in your life. Many single moms by choice (and chance) end up in wonderful and supportive relationships down the road.

RETURNING TO WORK

Many providers recommend that new moms wait about 6 to 12 weeks before returning to the workplace. The body is still healing, and it's physically much more comfortable to be at home. Plus, the first weeks provide bonding time, and if you're breastfeeding, this is when you will be spending hours and hours a day nourishing your babe. You may need even more time if you have any complications you're healing from or if your child needed special treatment or time in the NICU. Unfortunately, a lot of moms just can't take as much time off as they would like because of economic and workplace realities—an issue that Motherly is committed to addressing.

Try to get your health-care provider's okay before you go back. The risk is that you slow your healing process and add extreme exhaustion onto your already full (and fatigued) plate.

Arranging Childcare

Back in chapter 12, we covered many of your options for childcare. If things have shifted—your career or your desires—you might want to review your options (see "Finding Childcare" on page 186). For better or worse, childcare is often an evolving process as your needs (and the needs of your child) change. It is normal to reassess from time to time and make adjustments.

Creating a Baby Schedule

One of the biggest concerns moms have about going back to work outside the home is getting enough time with the baby. It can be really hard to suddenly not be able to spend every moment with them.

I won't lie to you. The adjustment is difficult. Most moms find that after a period of time,

it does get easier. One thing to try to do is to schedule in quality time with your baby every day. This will make the transition much easier.

Build in rituals such as a morning walk, bedtime routine, or something else that creates a special, intimate time for just you and the baby.

Setting Boundaries at Work

Before you become a mother, your boss's requests for overtime and your co-workers' invitations for after-work happy hours are fairly easy to handle. That all changes when you have a baby. If you want to and are able to continue to say yes to those things, of course, that is fine! But it is also well within your rights to establish a clear and firm set of boundaries. It can be helpful to determine what your boundaries are ahead of time: What time do you have to leave by? Are you able to pick up extra duties and projects at the last minute, or do you need at least a week of advance notice to secure childcare? Are there certain days of the week that you have more flexibility than others? Considering the answers to these questions ahead of time will make it less likely that you *accidentally* agree to something that you wish you had said no to.

Changing Your Mind About Working

Most of the time, we walk around thinking our decisions are final. That is certainly true in a lot of areas. My kids often ask me when I am going to wipe off my tattoos(!), so at my house we spend a lot of time talking about decisions that cannot be undone. But it's important to remember that matters of career do not always have to fall into this category. With over 70 percent of mothers employed in this

---

WHEN WORK MEANS STAYING HOME WITH THE BABY

As we've discussed, being a stay-at-home mom is bona fide work, so having a schedule with the baby can be incredibly helpful here as well. You can still get to the end of the day and think, "Wow, we were so busy that I didn't actually get any quality time with my kids today." So, rituals can be a really important idea for you as well. Beyond that, you might consider making sure to schedule one activity with your baby every day: A music class, a walk to the park, or a trip to the grocery store all count. Having one thing planned to help get you out of the house can be really valuable. Just remember to give yourself flexibility. If you have a busy day of activities planned but wake up to heavy rain or an extra-cranky baby, you have my full permission to stay home and snuggle instead.

country, this is not to say that if we want to quit our jobs, we can. For most working moms, their salary is not optional; it is necessary. It does mean, however, that we are allowed to pivot and make shifts as the stories of our lives unfold, without guilt or shame.

These shifts might look different for everyone:

- Maybe you always thought that you would continue to work full-time but suddenly fell in love with the idea of being a stay-at-home mom.

- Maybe you quit your job because you had always planned to be a stay-at-home mom but are now yearning to be back in the office setting.

- Maybe you find that you are in a situation where you need to make more money to cover expenses, so you are adding work hours into your day.

- Maybe you decide you want to quit full-time work in an office and start your own business so that you have more flexibility to balance work you love and spending time with your kids.

- Maybe you decide to make a lateral move at your company that allows you a little more flexibility with a slightly lower paycheck.

Or maybe you get an opportunity to write the book of your dreams, and you hustle to find more-than-full-time childcare so that you can make it happen, which makes you both sad and ecstatically happy at the same time (*just sayin'*).

remember

There is no wrong way to do this, mama. And chances are good that however you are doing this now will change, many times over. There is simply no way to prepare for all the ways motherhood will alter our lives, desires, needs, and goals.

I often joke that a significant part of my job entails writing the word "journey."

I have tried countless times to find other ways to describe motherhood, but no other word seems to do it justice.

Because the truth is that you will always be *becoming mama*. It will always be a journey. The events of your life that led up to your pregnancy; the way that your pregnancy and birth story unfolded; the first time you looked at your baby, and the infinite moments that come after; every celebration, setback, worry, smile, frustration, sleepless night, and moment of breathless wonder—it is all your journey.

Not long ago, you stood in front of a door, not knowing quite how you got there or what was on the other side. You placed your hands on the door, and despite the uncertainty and the doubt, despite not knowing what lay on the other side, you pushed.

You pushed through the nausea, the testing, the worry. You pushed through the fear and the discomfort. You pushed into your pelvis, or you pushed into the operating room. And you arrived on the other side.

But to arrive in motherhood means to realize that the path is not linear: It peaks and troughs, twists, loops back, and spirals in on itself. Because becoming mama was never going to be easy, but mama, it is so worth it. You are a true warrior—and I am not sure a greater journeyer has ever lived.

To walk beside you on this small part of your journey has been my absolute honor. Thank you for your trust, but more important, thank you for making motherhood better. Because in redefining your own pregnancy, birth, and postpartum journey, you have laid the groundwork so that every mother who follows can do the same.

You are a marvel. And for one last time I will remind you: *You've got this.*

xo,

Diana

Welcome to #TeamMotherly

Motherhood is better together, and that's why we're so excited to welcome you to #TeamMotherly, our supportive community providing advice and encouragement for your journey. Read more about the digital and physical resources Motherly offers to help you thrive every step along the way.

MOTHERLY DIGITAL

Becoming Mama Companion Podcast

A week-by-week listening guide to enjoy along your journey to becoming mama. Listen along as Diana provides encouragement for each week, from planning your pregnancy through postpartum, and hear encouraging stories from other mamas like you. You can access the *Becoming Mama Podcast* on Apple Podcast, Spotify, or wherever you listen to podcasts.

Email Newsletter

Sign up for Motherly's email newsletter at mother.ly/join as a digital companion to this book. This newsletter will offer you a week-by-week guide to new motherhood—personalized for exactly where you are on your journey from planning a pregnancy through the toddler years and beyond.

Becoming Mama Site

There may be times while reading this book that you want to delve deeper into a topic—we've got you covered. We invite you to check out mother.ly/becomingmama, where we've curated the best of Motherly to provide you with the additional support, resources, and inspiration you need on your journey.

The Motherly Podcast

While you are waiting for your little one to arrive, we invite you to check out *The Motherly Podcast* (hosted by Liz!), featuring empowering conversations with some of the world's most inspiring mothers. You can download and subscribe to *The Motherly Podcast* on Apple Podcasts, Spotify, or wherever you get your podcasts.

#TeamMotherly on Social

In so many ways, your motherhood journey has just begun. Join our #TeamMotherly community on Instagram @mother.ly and Facebook @motherlymedia for daily inspiration and support. It takes a village, mama, and we've got this, together.

Motherly IRL Events

Our signature events—Becoming Mama and our Postpartum Wellness Workshop—provide transformative in-person experiences for pregnant women and new mamas. Starting with NYC and LA, our event series is going nationwide and is soon coming to a city near you. Check mother.ly/events for the latest opportunity to experience Motherly in person.

This Is Motherhood *Book*

Our debut book, *This Is Motherhood: A Motherly Collection of Reflections + Practices*, delivers inspiration for each chapter of your motherhood journey. From accepting your post-partum body, to learning how to simplify, to writing your family manifesto, this book is our love letter to you. No matter how challenging or magical the season you're in, *This Is Motherhood* reminds you that you're not alone, mama. You can find *This Is Motherhood* at mother.ly/motherlycollection or wherever you purchase your books.

Shop Motherly

Motherly is your source for products that make your life as a woman, and as a mother, better—and more beautiful. Shop Motherly to get exactly what you need to set up your small-space nursery, go back to work from maternity leave in style, and find the perfect toy for every stage, all curated by the content experts you trust.

Psst: Love The Motherly Guide to Becoming Mama *artwork? Shop Motherly to make it yours.*

I trust my body.

Symptom Checker

Pregnancy is weird. I mean, it is beautiful, yes, but the things it can do to your body can be all-out bizarre. But don't worry, mama. We've got you.

Here you will find a guide to symptoms you may be experiencing and ways to help you cope. You can use this section however you like: Look up only the symptoms you are experiencing or read through it from start to finish.

Remember, your provider is your go-to resource for all symptoms. They can best determine if what you are feeling is normal or if it warrants medical attention.

Baby Hiccups

Feeling your baby hiccup inside you is one of the strangest and loveliest experiences of pregnancy. What causes hiccups remains a mystery, though it may help strengthen baby's diaphragm (the muscle under the lungs) to prepare for breathing.

Not all babies will hiccup, so no worries if yours does not (you may also not be feeling their hiccups). A hiccupping fetus will make you feel like you have a ball in your belly that is gently and rhythmically bouncing for a few minutes at a time.

After 28 weeks, if your baby has hiccups every day and more than four times a day, research indicates that the baby should be evaluated. This can be a sign that the umbilical cord is being compressed.

Back Pain/Ache

There are several causes behind this common symptom of pregnancy. Your growing uterus causes significant changes in the way your spine curves, which can lead to a lot of discomfort. Your back also needs to support your uterus and baby, in addition to larger-than-normal breasts, which is hard work. The hormone relaxin, which is prepping your body for birth, causes your ligaments and tendons to loosen, which means that your back muscles don't have the support they are used to. Lastly, our culture is usually not great at maintaining proper posture (written by a lady who is currently hunched over her computer, typing away). All these things can lead to a pretty achy back.

Psst: Be sure to read about pelvic girdle pain on page 465, as it can be a cause of back pain, too.

With the following tips, there is hope, however:

- Strengthening your back and core muscles through pregnancy-approved exercises can do wonders for reducing your pain. Don't forget to check the "Move" content of each chapter for core-strengthening tips.

- Sit on a birth ball. Birth balls are not just for birth. Many women find sitting on their ball and rocking from side to side to be phenomenal for stretching the lower back and relieving some pressure on the pelvis. (See "Birth Ball" on page 289 for how to choose the best birth ball.)

- Prenatal yoga is a great way to gently stretch and strengthen your back.

Once you have been cleared by your provider, you can attend a class or find a free video online (just make sure it's prenatal).

- Get a massage from a certified prenatal massage therapist (see "Massage Therapists" on page 94) or ask a partner or family member to follow these instructions recommended by massage therapist Kymberlie Berrien: "Find her sacrum, the flat triangular bone just above her bottom [see "Bones" on page 23 for a reminder]. Place your thumbs in the center of this bone, and then move them in circles, traveling from her spine outward."

- Check in with a chiropractor (see "Chiropractors" on page 93). A chiropractor with a prenatal specialty can do wonders for back pain (and help to prepare your body for birth).

- Reassess your chairs. Make sure that the chairs you sit on regularly provide enough lower back support.

- Consider how you sleep. Is your pillow super-supportive, or do you wake up with a knot in your neck? It might be time to treat yourself to a new pillow. Many women also find that propping themselves with pillows or using a body pillow as they sleep can offer relief.

- Pregnancy support belts can lift up your belly to reduce the strain it places on your lower back.

- Opt for comfy, flat shoes (avoid high heels). The flashy pumps can make a reappearance after the pregnancy, I promise (though maybe in a larger size).

- Warm baths, warm showers with the jet pointed at your back, or a warm compress can feel great. Just make sure it doesn't get too hot: nothing above 104 degrees Farenheit.

Rarely, lower back pain can be associated with a urinary tract infection (see "Urinary Tract Infections" on page 354). If you also feel tightening of your uterus, it could be a sign of labor (see "Preterm Labor and Premature Babies on page 242)." Reach out to your provider with any concerns.

Benign Pregnancy Tumor

Small, noncancerous blood vessel growths can sometimes develop on the gums and skin of pregnant women. These are called pregnancy tumors, or pyogenic granulomas. Hormonal changes cause your body to respond differently to injury. If something irritates the gums or skin, your body might overreact, growing one of these tumors (or a cluster of them in an area). It's important to keep in mind that despite the scary name, *this is not cancer*, and these little guys are generally harmless—though they can be painful, especially when they become large. They can also bleed easily, and the oral ones can make eating difficult.

For pregnancy tumors in the mouth, your dentist will help you with diagnosis and treatment. Seeing your dentist regularly throughout pregnancy can lead to faster diagnosis, and good oral hygiene will help keep these at bay. If you notice one on your skin, tell your doctor or midwife, who may refer you to a dermatologist.

The tumors can be removed by a dentist or doctor using surgical instruments or laser treatment. Follow-up care is important because they can grow back.

Bleeding Gums

To deal with bleeding gums, the first step is to make sure you are seeing your dentist regularly. It is safe to have dental cleanings and most other procedures while pregnant, and these can encourage a healthier pregnancy. (For more on dental care during pregnancy, see "Visit Your Dentist" on page 7.)

In addition to the increase in blood volume you experience in pregnancy, the increase in the hormone progesterone can make your gums more sensitive to bacteria and plaque, which can lead to gum disease, specifically pregnancy gingivitis. You may also develop a bump that can bleed on your gums. This could be a pregnancy tumor, but don't worry; it is benign despite its scary name. See the previous entry, "Benign Pregnancy Tumor."

If the gingivitis is severe enough, your dentist may recommend antibiotics to get it under control.

Be sure to brush your teeth at least twice daily (consider switching to a softer bristle toothbrush), floss daily, and use an alcohol-free mouthwash (some women like using a warm water and salt wash). You may notice an uptick in bleeding for a bit, but ultimately it will decrease as your gums get healthier.

Ensure that you are getting enough vitamin D (a few ideas: salmon, fortified juice and milk, and egg yolks) and vitamin C (a few ideas: citrus fruits, broccoli, and brussels sprouts). Research finds that people with adequate levels of these vitamins may have less gum disease. Probiotics can help too!

Bleeding Nose

Your increased blood supply in pregnancy means that all of your mucus membranes (like inside your nose) get more blood and are therefore more likely to bleed.

To prevent nosebleeds, make sure to drink plenty of water and keep the air around you moist with a humidifier (which needs to be cleaned regularly, with vinegar or bleach, FYI). You can also try an over-the-counter saline nasal spray. If you blow your nose, blow gently, and avoid picking.

If you get a nosebleed, lean forward and pinch your nose halfway down for a few minutes. You can also try applying ice to constrict the blood vessels. If the bleeding doesn't stop after several minutes, call your provider.

Bloating

We have progesterone to thank for this one. It relaxes the muscles in your intestines, which slows down digestion. This is on purpose: Slower digestion means your body has more time to absorb the nutrients present in your food. But it also means more gas and therefore bloating.

What you can do:

- Eat smaller, more frequent meals and eat them slowly to help minimize gas.

- Stay hydrated. Drinking about ten 8-ounce glasses of water per day will help prevent constipation, which would add to the yucky tummy feelings you're already experiencing.

- Fiber up. Fiber will also help prevent constipation and make digestion smoother. Some ideas: barley, oats, bananas, carrots, apples, bran, flaxseed, chia seeds, and squash.

Braxton-Hicks Contractions

Braxton-Hicks contractions are uterine contractions that happen when you are not in labor. They can start in your second trimester and last all the way until you go into labor. They tend not to be painful: Most moms describe a squeezing sensation and a hard belly, but no pain. If you are not feeling Braxton-Hicks contractions, don't worry; you are likely having them and just not noticing, which can be completely normal.

If you have repetitive Braxton-Hicks contractions (five or more in an hour), even if they are not painful, call your provider to make sure it's not preterm labor (see "Preterm Labor and Premature Babies" on page 242).

Breakouts (Pimples)

The uptick in hormones during pregnancy can lead to increased oil production in your skin and therefore breakouts. Thanks so much for that one, pregnant body.

But don't worry; they'll go away. In the meantime, be nice to your skin. Do not use medications or over-the-counter treatments without talking to your provider first because some are contraindicated for pregnancy and breastfeeding. Wash your face daily with mild soap and moisturize using an oil-free moisturizer. (Note: Some mamas report having drier skin during pregnancy. If this is you, you may need extra moisturizer during this time.)

Breast Soreness/Tenderness

You may be months away from the possibility of breastfeeding your baby, but the rising levels of progesterone, estrogen, hCG, and prolactin in your body are already contributing to some dramatic changes.

Increased blood volume and tissue swelling can make your breasts feel tender and heavier in early pregnancy. Lobes—the glands that produce breast milk—start to increase, and ducts, which act like milk-transporting highways in your breasts, are developing. All this activity can lead to some discomfort, for sure.

If you're into wearing a bra, bra-fitting experts usually suggest waiting until your second or third trimester to invest in nursing bras (see "Nursing Bras" on page 400), but a comfortable and well-fitting bra may help you with any first-trimester discomfort. For now, focus on a bra that provides good support and allows for some flexibility; underwire is fine for now if that's your jam. Beyond that, you may find that warm showers or compresses on your breasts feel good. And take heart: You'll likely get some breast relief in the second trimester. If you're a no-bra gal, or only wear a bralette, keep doing what works!

Carpal Tunnel

Carpal tunnel (wrist pain) is super-common and happens to up to 62 percent of women during pregnancy, and many also experience it postpartum. It may be caused by pregnancy- and birth-related swelling or overuse and positioning as you care for your baby. Note how you are positioning your arms as you hold your baby. Try not to maintain a bent wrist position for a long time or repeatedly.

Rest is usually recommended for treating carpal tunnel. You can try an elastic bandage or wrist brace for extra support (it can also remind you to be aware of your positioning and usage). Ice packs can help ease the pain, and after baby is born, you may take anti-inflammatory medications like ibuprofen. If the pain persists, talk with your provider about other possible interventions, like steroid injections and physical therapy.

Congestion

This not-so-fun side effect is also called pregnancy rhinitis and makes you feel a bit like you have a never-ending cold or seasonal allergies. It is caused by the enlarged blood vessels in your nose and the hormones of pregnancy.

The first thing to do is to make sure it is "just" pregnancy rhinitis. If you have a fever, cough, chills, facial pain, or any other symptoms, check in with your provider. Once you've ruled out an infection, try this:

- Drink lots of water to keep the mucus loose and flowing (hey, it's better than clogged).
- Try a saline mist nasal spray.
- Use a cool-water humidifier.
- Take warm (not too hot) showers and breathe in the steam.
- Try a neti pot with distilled water, which allows you to clear out your nasal passages.

I'm sorry to say that congestion often gets worse before it gets better, but you should find quick relief after the baby is born.

Constipation

Not everyone will experience constipation, but those who do know it is a real bear to deal with. Progesterone slows your digestion, which means that food can sit in your system longer and get clogged up.

Here is my advice: Don't "wait and see" with this one. A lot of symptoms get better over time, but constipation tends to get worse. So, if you notice it, act on it.

To prevent or ease constipation:

- Drink a lot of fluid, *at least* ten 8-ounce glasses per day.

- Increase your fiber: Aim for 25 to 35 milligrams per day. Some surprisingly delicious foods with fiber are raspberries, raisins, artichokes, lentils, kiwi, and popcorn. Yum!

- Probiotics, like those found in kefir and yogurt, can help make you more regular. You can also add a probiotic supplement to your daily routine (as always, please check with your provider first).

- Don't hold it. When you have the urge to go to the bathroom, go. Holding it can increase your odds of getting backed up.

- Go for a brisk walk or do some yoga. Daily exercise has been linked to improved bowel functions.

- Avoid straining. When you do poop, avoid pushing really hard or sitting on the toilet for a long amount of time, as this can cause hemorrhoids.

- Check in with your provider. They can recommend medications or supplements that can help.

Cramping

If you have found your way to the cramping section of the "Symptom Checker," there is a good chance that you are early in your pregnancy and scared that something is wrong. I get it, mama. I have been there, as have so many others (85 percent of women experience early pregnancy cramping). I know that solidarity may not help you, but I do want you to know that you are not alone. I cannot promise you that everything is okay, but I will tell you that there are a lot of possible causes of your cramping, most of them completely normal.

In their 2016 study, researcher Katherine Sapra and colleagues write that "lower abdominal cramping appears to be the norm rather than the exception during early pregnancy, and cramping is not associated with pregnancy loss per se."

In the first days of your pregnancy, the fertilized egg will burrow its way into your uterine lining. Some women experience a bit of cramping with this.

Once the embryo has implanted, it starts to grow, which means that your uterus does, too. All this activity may go totally unnoticed by you, or you may become aware of cramping. This cramping can continue as your pregnancy progresses, or you may experience it in waves.

Starting around the second trimester, cramping may actually be something called round ligament pain, a normal, albeit painful, stretching of the ligaments that support your uterus (see "Groin Pain" on page 438 for more info).

Cramping can also come from digestive issues, such as gas, constipation, food poisoning, or a stomach bug; having sex; and dehydration.

There is also the possibility of labor—preterm and full term—as many women start their labors with feelings of "crampiness." If you sense that the cramping brings a tightening in your belly, it could actually be a contraction (see "Signs That Labor May Be Approaching" on page 237 or "Preterm Labor and Premature Babies" on page 242 for more details).

So, what are the steps to take if you have cramping?

Drink a glass of water and rest. If you can, lie down on your left side. You can also take a warm bath or put a warm compress where it hurts (just not too hot). Unfortunately, NSAIDs (like ibuprofen) cannot be taken during pregnancy. You can talk to your provider about taking acetaminophen, however. Take deep breaths and try to encourage your body to relax. If the cramping subsides, take the rest of the day easy and gently. If it doesn't, if it comes with other symptoms, or if you have vaginal bleeding along with the cramping, don't hesitate to reach out to your provider, who can help you determine the cause.

I would be remiss if I didn't add that sometimes cramping can be a sign that something is wrong. Examples of this could be:

- Ectopic pregnancy (page 57)
- Miscarriage or fetal loss (page 52)
- Placental abruption (page 474)
- Urinary tract infection (page 354)

Drooling

In today's episode of *Nobody Told Me I'd Have THAT*: drooling. Otherwise known as ptyalism, excessive saliva, and therefore drooling, it is a normal side effect of pregnancy. Nausea and heartburn may be behind this odd symptom, as are hormonal changes.

Sometimes by addressing your nausea and heartburn, your saliva amounts will decrease, though not always. Brushing your teeth and using mouthwash a few times per day may provide you with relief, as can sucking on a piece of candy: This won't decrease the saliva, but it will make it taste better. Many women also carry around a water bottle to spit in. You may be inclined to decrease the amount of water you drink, but that likely won't help and will only make you dehydrated and more uncomfortable. Take heart: The drooling usually goes away as your pregnancy progresses.

Dry Skin

See "Itching" on page 441.

Fatigue

Insert "welcome to the next 18 years of your life" joke here. Just kidding. In fact, those jokes bug me a bit. Yes, those first months of motherhood are exhausting, for sure, but your child *will* learn to sleep, and you *will* get the sleep you need again. I promise.

It just may not be during your pregnancy.

There are several reasons that you may not feel super-rested these days. First, your body is diverting a lot of its energy to growing a human (and their placenta), supporting that growth with more blood, and helping your baby eliminate what they don't need. This is a lot of work. Progesterone can also make you sleepy. As your pregnancy progresses, it can be harder to find a comfortable position to sleep in. And once you do, you are likely to be awoken by the need to pee or a kick to the ribs from your baby. And if you've given up caffeine, that doesn't help the situation much either (the process of giving up caffeine is discussed on page 11, if you're interested).

The good news is that there are lots of little tricks you can try:

- Shift your mindset. This one is first on purpose. We live in a go-go-go culture that thrives on the ideal of being "productive."

Many of us are so used to pushing ourselves that it is virtually impossible to step on the brakes when something big comes along—like pregnancy. Remember that the work you are currently doing is the very definition of productivity. You are making a person (or several, maybe).

- Nap. As often as you can. Even if they are only 15 minutes long, naps can add a great deal of energy to your reserve. (Research says it's healthy for you and the baby, so enjoy your slumber guilt-free.)

- Make sure you are getting adequate sleep every day. All adults should get between 7 and 9 hours of sleep per night. Pregnant women need to add 1 to 2 hours to that.

- Try to get into the habit of eating small, frequent meals throughout your pregnancy. Your body is processing food differently now. You are sending extra glucose (a form of sugar) to your baby to help them develop, which can make it easier for you to feel tired, or even light-headed. Having a more constant supply of delicious energy may help you feel more awake.

- Talk to your provider. The tricky thing about a very general and common symptom like fatigue is that sometimes we can dismiss a real problem as normal. If you've tried the above measures and have not had any relief, talk to your provider about some deeper investigation to make sure nothing is wrong, such as anemia (see "Iron-Deficiency Anemia" on page 464) or a thyroid condition (see "Thyroid Issues" on page 468).

For more tips and information, also see "Insomnia" on page 440.

Fetal Movement

See "Kick Counts" on page 178.

Food Aversions

Many women find that the idea of their favorite foods suddenly makes them want to throw up, especially during the early weeks of pregnancy. Your hormones are definitely to blame here. There is also the thought that nausea is evolutionarily protective: In limiting the foods you want to eat, there is less of a chance that you'll eat something that could harm the pregnancy.

Honor your aversions. There is no need to force yourself to eat something that will make you feel gross. I would encourage you to retry things from time to time because your aversions may evolve (especially if it's an aversion to a healthy food that would provide you and the baby good nourishment).

Keep your provider up to date with the foods that you are unable to eat. They may be able to refer you to speak with a nutritionist who can help you come up with inventive ways to get the needed nutrients in, without making you feel ill.

Food Cravings

While I have never actually met a woman who craved "ice cream with pickles," food cravings in pregnancy are very real. Ask anyone who has had a baby, and they will likely be able to share their random, very specific (and sometimes funny) preferences. I wanted red meat—*all the time*. For the record, I'm a vegetarian.

Some other examples from Motherly mamas are:

- Peaches and oranges
- Spring rolls
- Stuffed grape leaves
- Freezing cold milk
- Cereal
- French fries with yellow mustard
- Melted cheese dip
- Waffles and lemonade
- Root beer

Some suspect that when we have a craving, it is the body's way of telling us it wants a certain type of nutrient—even when that nutrient doesn't actually exist in the food we are craving.

Food cravings are not usually harmful, so I say go for it—in moderation. Remember that the whole "eating for two" thing isn't accurate. It is generally recommended that you add about 200 to 300 extra calories to your diet per day in pregnancy and that those calories come from healthy sources. But that absolutely does not mean you can't indulge in your waffle or french fry need from time to time. Enjoy!

The really important caveat here is when you start to crave nonfood items like ice, dirt, paint, and other items. This is called pica and requires a discussion with your medical provider. For more on this, see "Pica" on page 465.

Frequent Urination

Constant trips to the bathroom are one of the hallmarks of pregnancy, and this often starts sooner than you'd expect! From early on in your first trimester, the increase in blood volume, as well as the influx of hormones, can up the number of times you need to pee. As pregnancy progresses and your baby (and therefore uterus) gets bigger, more pressure is applied to your bladder. And then, of course, there are your sweet baby's kicks (and, um, body slams) against your bladder.

Unfortunately, there is not a whole lot you can do to minimize your potty runs. While it is so tempting to drink less water, that will end up causing more harm than good as it can lead to dehydration and urinary tract infections (UTIs), which only make this symptom worse. So, stay hydrated and see if you can turn the frequent bathroom stops into mini-mindfulness breaks: Each time you wash your hands after you pee, close your eyes, take three deep breaths, and mentally send your baby a little hug.

Occasionally frequent urination is a sign that you have a UTI. If you also have burning when you pee, your urine is cloudy or smells bad, your lower back hurts, you have a fever, or only a tiny bit comes out, call your provider (for more on UTIs, see "Urinary Tract Infections" on page 354).

Gas

I'll spare you the flatulence jokes, although you are not far away from having a toddler, which means that your world is about to explode with them (pun intended). Most women experience at least some degree of gas during their pregnancies. Progesterone, and eventually your growing uterus, can cause your digestion to slow down, which can make you more prone to tummy troubles like gas. Some people are able to dismiss it as a funny little side effect, but for others, it has a pretty substantial impact on their lives. Gas can be uncomfortable, causing significant belly pain at times.

Here are a few things to try:

- Don't drink during meals. Get your hydration in throughout the day but avoid taking big gulps of liquid while you are eating.

- Eat small, frequent meals.

- Experiment with foods. Common gas-causers are broccoli and cauliflower, onions and garlic, cabbage, asparagus, dairy, high-fructose corn syrup, and of course, the musical fruit (aka beans, for those who do not yet have a toddler in their lives). See if cutting out a food for a few days makes you feel better, and you may be able to identify the culprit.

- Move your body. Sometimes all we need is a little repositioning to let the air flow through us. Try going for a walk or doing some gentle stretches.

- Talk to your provider about medication if these tricks don't work.

- Don't dismiss pain that won't go away. Sometimes pain that we think is gas is really something more: preterm labor (see "Preterm Labor and Premature Babies" on page 242), appendicitis, or heart issues, to name a few. If you are worried, never be afraid to reach out to your provider, even if it turns out to be nothing.

Getting Full Quickly

It is 11:00 a.m. when a co-worker mentions the amazing burrito they ate last night, and now it is all you can think about. You get through the daydreaming about dinner (which you order online from the parking lot at work), and at last you get home, and the glorious burrito is in front of you. But after about six bites, you are completely full. It is one of pregnancy's great annoyances.

We hear so much about how hungry pregnancy makes you, so it is often a surprise to find that you get full quickly from your meals. Your slowed digestion and the growing babe crowding your stomach can lead to this issue. Just listen to your body. Eat a few bites, take a break, and come back when you are hungry again. You can also try eating and drinking at separate times so that the liquid doesn't take up all the room in there.

Groin Pain

Sudden, sharp pain in your groin is often caused by round ligament pain.

As your uterus grows, the ligaments that support it are stretched, which can cause sudden, sharp pains in your groin area. You may especially feel them when you change positions (stand up or roll over in bed, for example) or cough, and you may also notice them when you've been on your feet for a period of time.

Although it's unpleasant, it is usually nothing to worry about. To avoid the pain, try to change positions slowly, stretch frequently, exercise routinely, and drink plenty of water. When you have the pain, try moving into a comfortable position slowly, like lying on your left side. If the pain does not go away or is severe, call your provider.

Hair Growth

The higher levels of the estrogen hormone can lead to hair (and nail) growth that makes you feel like you've just stepped out of the salon every day. Some women find that their hair texture even changes with pregnancy: Your curly locks may be a bit straighter, or your straight hair may develop a wave. "Why yes, I did wake up like this. Thanks for asking."

You may also notice more hair growth on other areas of your body: legs, armpits, pubic area, and random places like your breasts or chin. It is normal, and there is no way to prevent it. If you would like to remove the hair, just be sure to do so in a way that isn't harmful for baby (for example, no depilatories until you get the okay from your medical provider).

Headaches

Headaches during pregnancy are very common. (They were always my very first symptom of pregnancy.) They can be caused by a number of factors (as listed below), though I will say that in my professional experience, the most common causes are not enough food and water. Causes of headaches include:

- Hormones
- Increased blood volume
- Fatigue or tiredness
- Adjusting to caffeine reduction/ elimination
- Hunger
- Dehydration
- Posture changes
- Worry/stress
- Complications like preeclampsia and blood clots

The first thing to do when you have a headache is drink some fluid—water, coconut water, or juice if you can—and have a healthy snack that consists of carbs and protein. You could try an apple with peanut butter or an egg-salad sandwich.

If your headache doesn't go away, consider a nap and a shoulder massage (*yes!*). It is generally considered safe for pregnant women to take acetaminophen (Tylenol) during pregnancy, but never ibuprofen, so ask your provider if this is an option for you.

Women also find comfort from acupuncture, stretching and yoga, resting in the dark, cool compresses on the forehead, ginger, and eliminating common triggers like caffeine, chocolate, and processed foods.

If your headache is severe, does not go away, or is accompanied by blurry spots in your vision, abdominal pain, dizziness, difficulty breathing, nausea and vomiting, confusion, or other worrisome signs, seek medical attention right away.

A special note about migraines. If you have a history of migraines, you may find that you get some relief during pregnancy: Those hormones do have some upsides. Some women will get their first migraine during pregnancy, though, and it can be really hard because many medications are not safe to take during pregnancy.

Heart Rate Increase

The extra blood volume moving through your body leads to a faster heart rate. You will likely feel it when you've walked up a set of stairs or jogged to catch the bus or maybe when you're just sitting still.

Sometimes an elevated heart rate can be a sign that your body needs attention. For example, you can experience it with stress, dehydration, fever, or in response to a medication, or it can be due to an underlying medical condition. It is never wrong to consult with your provider about your worries. If you also feel light-headed, if you faint, or if it feels like your heart is skipping beats, call your provider right away or go to the hospital.

Heartburn or Reflux

The hormone progesterone causes your gastrointestinal tract to relax during pregnancy, and this includes a valve that acts like a door between your stomach and esophagus. This means that stomach acid can move upward, causing you a fair amount of discomfort. If you've had heartburn or reflux before, it may get worse with pregnancy, or you may have it now for the first time.

There are lots of little tricks to try, but always check in with your provider because medications may be necessary:

- Eat small, frequent meals.
- Stand or sit upright for 30 to 60 minutes after eating.
- Use antacid medications (but with guidance; too much can be dangerous).
- Decrease the amount of greasy, spicy, and citrusy foods (all the good stuff—sorry!).
- Decrease caffeine.

You can also try eating papayas, bananas, or yogurt to calm a burning tummy.

Hemorrhoids

The pressure of your growing uterus, increased blood flow, and straining to poop when you are constipated can all lead to a common pregnancy ailment: hemorrhoids. These occur when veins in your rectum and anus enlarge and stick out. They can bleed and be itchy or painful.

Hemorrhoids are usually nothing to worry about, aside from the discomfort. If you have concerns, you can always consult your provider to make sure, as rarely do they require medical intervention.

To prevent or improve hemorrhoids, address constipation so that you don't have to strain. Eat lots of fruits and veggies along with at least ten 8-ounce glasses of non-sugary, non-caffeinated fluid per day.

Once you have hemorrhoids, you may find relief by using witch hazel pads. You can buy these over the counter at most drug and health food stores. Fold them in half and place them—forgive me for my nonmedical terminology—between your butt cheeks. You can also try a sitz bath, which is a plastic basin filled with warm water and herbs that fits onto your toilet seat so that you can sit comfortably in it. Lastly, padsicles can feel great too (see page 351).

If these tricks don't provide you with relief, talk to your provider about stronger medications.

Hot Flashes

If you are insisting on sitting directly in front of the air conditioner, naked, in winter, you might be pregnant. There are a few reasons behind these hot flashes: more estrogen hormone, extra blood volume, and carrying around the weight of your growing baby. As long as you don't have a fever (100.4 degrees Fahrenheit or higher), it's usually nothing to worry about. Hot flashes can be uncomfortable though! Be sure to drink plenty of fluid to avoid dehydration. Wear layers so that it's easy to take something off, and try to wear cotton fabrics, since they are more breathable. Beyond that, just remember: The person growing the baby gets to control the thermostat. It's the law.

Insomnia

It seems quite unfair that you are exhausted and crave sleep all day, but when you finally get into bed, it doesn't come. Unfortunately, this is a common pregnancy symptom.

The first thing to do is see if you can figure out if a certain symptom is keeping you from getting sleep—back pain, vivid dreaming, nausea, heartburn—and try to address that. Your waking at night and having trouble getting back to sleep may be caused by your frequent trips to the bathroom. Try drinking most of your fluids before 2:00 p.m. and avoid drinking anything in the hour before bed.

The other part to consider is your sleep hygiene. Coming from a lady who routinely falls asleep checking her Instagram feed in bed, I fully acknowledge how hard it is to change habits, but these changes can make a huge difference:

- Avoid caffeine in the afternoon.

- Skipping breakfast and irregular eating has been linked to poor quality sleep, so make sure you're getting regular nourishment.

- Use your bed for only sleep and sex.

- Avoid technology for at least an hour before bedtime because the blue light disrupts the sleep hormone melatonin.

- Dim the lights and make everything feel "sleepy" in your home for an hour before bedtime.

- Develop a bedtime routine and try to keep it consistent. This could include a warm shower or bath, reading, and a warm cup of chamomile tea.

- Don't just lie in bed for hours waiting for sleep to come, or worse, worrying about not sleeping! Make a plan for what you will do during the sleepless time (catch up on knitting? read romance novels?). Sleepiness will resume faster if you take your mind off it.

- Do relaxation exercises before bed or during your restless hours. There are so many apps available these days, and you can also find free guided meditation audios online.

- Consult an herbalist, acupuncturist, massage therapist, or your physician for insomnia remedies that they recommend for pregnancy. Lots of women find relief with things like tart cherry juice, magnesium supplements, and other natural treatments.

- See related information in "Fatigue" on page 435.

Although insomnia is common, it should not be ignored. Unfortunately, insomnia can be connected to some complications, such as elevated blood pressure. Be sure to let your provider know about your insomnia, so they can assess your overall well-being.

Itching

You may experience slightly itchy skin due to the extra blood volume in your body and because your skin may be stretching to accommodate your growing breasts and uterus. You may also find that you are more sensitive to skin-care products and are itching in response to them. Use a mild, fragrance- and alcohol-free lotion on your skin and stay hydrated to help fight the itchies. Skin can also become drier during pregnancy, which can lead to itching. You may need to apply lotion more frequently for the next several months (and be sure to rub it in well).

Sometimes itching can be a sign of a complication, though. It could be PUPPP, an unharmful but hard-to-deal-with condition (see page 468), or cholestasis, which is dangerous (see page 459).

Leg Cramps

Leg cramps, also known as charley horses, can be wildly painful and unexpected. They often happen in your calves in the middle of the night. They can be scary (in that they wake you up suddenly), but they are usually not dangerous.

The best thing to do when you have one is to gently stretch out the area by flexing your toes toward your knees (the opposite of pointing them). The muscles will slowly relax, and relief will come.

If the area is hard, red, and warm as well as painful, avoid rubbing it, and call your provider to ensure that it is not a deep vein thrombosis (DVT; see page 459). It is important to note that black women have an increased risk of developing a DVT, so any symptoms of this nature should be reported to your provider immediately.

Drinking water during the day and ensuring that you get plenty of movement every day can help prevent leg cramps.

Lightning Crotch

Yes, this is what we actually call it, because as you may already know, that's exactly what it feels like—a sudden, sharp pain in your vagina. It usually happens toward the end of pregnancy in response to the baby moving or because of the increasing pressure being applied to your cervix by the baby's head. So, it is a good sign that things are moving in the right direction.

Unfortunately, there is not much you can do about it when it strikes, though you can try lying down on your left side to decrease some of the pressure.

Linea Nigra

Linea nigra is a vertical line that appears on your belly's skin that runs from your belly button to your pubic bone. This line is always there, but it gets dark and visible during pregnancy due to the changes in the cells that cause pigmentation. The line will fade slowly after pregnancy.

Mask of Pregnancy and Skin Darkening

Known as melasma, the mask of pregnancy develops on more than half of pregnant women's (glowing) faces. It usually appears as darkening skin on the cheek bones, upper lip, forehead, or chin. Melasma happens when the cells responsible for coloring your skin work harder (in response to the pregnancy hormones). It is not dangerous, but it can be surprising to have your skin appearance change.

In addition to changes on your face you may notice it on other areas, such as armpits, forearms, genitals, and areas that are exposed to the sun.

You may be able to minimize melasma by being extra careful in the sun: Wear sunscreen (even in the winter), avoid the sun at peak hours, and wear a wide-brimmed hat. Also, avoid waxing, as that can irritate skin and make the melasma more apparent. Melasma usually goes away slowly after you give birth. If it doesn't, and you are concerned, talk with a dermatologist about remedies (just make sure to let them know if you are breastfeeding, since some meds will be off limits). Insurance may not cover these meds, however, and they can be quite expensive.

Metallic Taste

You are not imagining that weird metallic taste in your mouth. It's called dysgeusia. The changes in your estrogen hormone levels are likely to blame here. Unfortunately, there is not a whole lot you can do to prevent it. Many women find that sucking on a citrus- or sour-flavored piece of candy can make the taste go away, as can foods with vinegar (like pickles), at least temporarily. Brushing your teeth and tongue can help too. Hang in there. This is an odd one for sure!

Nausea and Vomiting

This dynamic duo makes up the most infamous of the pregnancy symptoms. About 70 percent of women experience at least some degree of nausea and vomiting, and it can be quite unpleasant. Nausea tends to start around week 5 of pregnancy, peak in severity during week 9, and get better between weeks 12 and 14, though there are certainly women who experience nausea for their entire pregnancy (and, ugh, it's the worst).

Many scientists believe that nausea and vomiting help protect you and your growing baby. The first trimester, when nausea is usually at its worst, is also when the baby is starting the delicate process of developing all their major organs. Nausea greatly reduces the variety of food a woman is able to eat, meaning that there is less risk of harmful substances being ingested and negatively impacting that organ development.

Anthropologist Kari Moca writes that morning sickness may exist to help the embryo develop. When you are nauseated and vomiting (and therefore eating less), your body burns fat stores. This generates more ketones in your body, which in this context are awesome brain-developing fuel for your baby.

So, what can you do about it? Most women find that they have to try different techniques to figure out what their nausea-reducing recipe is. Below are some ideas.

But one thing first: Pregnancy nausea is a big deal. It is common, and therefore we tend to dismiss it as a rite of passage, but when you are going through it, it can be truly miserable. It is okay to complain about how you feel; it doesn't make you ungrateful to be pregnant. It's also okay to ask for help, both in your daily life and from your provider. There are times when women require medical attention for their nausea and vomiting. If you go 24 hours without being able to keep food or water down, or if you feel light-headed or just really ill, call your provider or head to an emergency room.

Things you can try:

- **Acupressure Wrist Bands**   In most pharmacies, you can find elastic wristbands with plastic knobs that apply pressure to a specific area in your wrist. While they are marketed for decreasing seasickness, research has found that they can be very effective at decreasing pregnancy-related nausea.

- **Acupuncture**   Acupuncture has not had a ton of evidence to support that it works for morning sickness. However, many women swear by it, so it may be worth considering. You can also ask about acupressure.

- **Eating Often**   Many times women find that they get nauseated just as they are also getting hungry. To avoid this, keep crackers (or something else that you enjoy that is easy to eat) with you at all times, in your bag, your bathroom, your bedside—everywhere. Try to graze on the snacks all day (and in the middle of the night when you get up to pee) to keep that yucky tummy at bay.

- **Ginger**   Ginger comes in many forms and can help with nausea. You can add ginger to your food or find capsules, candy, or (real) ginger ale (beware the high sugar content). And don't forget Crystal Karges's ginger tea recipe on page 119.

- **Mint**   Peppermint candies and mint tea can be awesome for nausea. Smelling mint can also be lovely: You can get a few mint leaves and grind them up to release the smell, smell a bag of mint tea, or add a few drops of mint essential oil to a diffuser if you have one.

- **Tart Food**   You may find that tart food (like a lemon or lemon-flavored candies) makes you feel better. (I used to suck on lemon slices.) But make sure you are keeping up with your dental care. Citrus fruits are not great for the enamel of your teeth. Simply smelling lemons can help as well.

- **Vitamin B6 (Pyridoxine)**   This vitamin has helped women lessen their nausea. It can be purchased over the counter, but it's best to talk with your provider about it first because it is already in your prenatal vitamin. (You can also get a prescription for it.) Vitamin B6 can be found in milk, sunflower seeds, salmon, eggs, sweet potato, bananas, beans, and many cereals.

- **Prescription Medications**   There are a number of prescription medications available to help, so be sure to talk with your provider about them if you are interested.

When you leave the house, pack yourself a little kit of items to help you cope: bags to throw up in, gum or mints, snacks, a fresh shirt (and maybe pants, too), and wipes.

This is an area where it might be beneficial to check in with some trusted members of your village. Much of coping with nausea is trial and error, and someone you know may have discovered something that works for you, too.

Hyperemesis gravidarum (HG) is a severe form of nausea and vomiting. For more info on this, see "Hyperemesis Gravidarum (Excessive Nausea and Vomiting)" on page 463.

Nipple and Areola Darkening and Enlarging

The areola is the dark part of the center of your breast, where your nipple is, and it may get darker during pregnancy, which feels strange but is totally normal. Some theorize that the reason for nipple darkening is to help promote breastfeeding: Babies see best when there is contrast, so by making the nipples dark, your body is creating a target to help the baby find your breast. They may also get larger, for similar reasons.

Your nipples will slowly return to their normal color (and usually their size) after you've given birth and are done breastfeeding, if you plan to.

No Symptoms Yet

Even though symptoms are uncomfortable, a lot of moms worry when they don't have them: *Is everything with the pregnancy okay?* The absence of symptoms does not necessarily mean that something is wrong. Levels of hCG (the pregnancy hormone) can vary a lot, especially in the beginning. Your symptoms may start a bit later, or you may just be one of the (lucky) women who don't experience the usual symptoms. (About 30 percent of women won't have nausea, for example.) So try not to worry, but if you do, talk to your provider.

It would also be interesting to chat with your mom, aunts, and sisters to see what symptoms they experienced. Research finds that nausea, hyperemesis gravidarum, cholestasis, blood clots, and preeclampsia all have hereditary links.

Restless Leg Syndrome

Restless leg syndrome (RLS) can be wildly irritating. It often feels like you have bugs crawling on your legs. You may have itching and burning and want desperately to move your legs around. Many women find that moving their legs vigorously for a few minutes does help the symptom resolve.

Let your provider know that you have RLS. Research has found that increasing iron, folic acid, and magnesium can help, so your provider may want to assess your levels.

You can also try working on improving your sleep quality using the tricks listed under "Insomnia" on page 440 and "Fatigue" on page 435.

Satiety

See "Getting Full Quickly" on page 437.

Sciatic Pain

Sciatic pain is when the sciatic nerve, which runs from your lower back into your thigh, gets irritated, and it can be super-uncomfortable. You might experience pain (in your back, bottom, and leg), tingling, difficulty walking, and numbness. There are many aspects of pregnancy that can lead to sciatic pain: your growing baby and uterus putting pressure on parts of your body in new ways, the changing curvature of your spine and back, and the changes to the bones in your pelvis as it prepares for birth.

Stretching the muscles in your lower back, bottom, and legs can help. One easy stretch to try is to put your hands on a table or the back of a chair, and keeping your legs straight, bend at the waist and stick your bottom out behind you to stretch the lower back and hamstrings.

You can also sit on a chair and then cross one leg over the other so that the outside of the calf or ankle is resting on the top of the other thigh or knee. Lean forward slightly, hold for 10 seconds, and then switch sides.

Prenatal yoga and swimming are also great for loosening up tight muscles during pregnancy. You can also visit a massage therapist or chiropractor for gentle treatments.

Sensitivity to Smell

Many women find that they become extra sensitive to smells when they are pregnant. People have theorized that this is a protective evolutionary measure in that it helps prevent women from eating food that has spoiled or is otherwise dangerous. Others believe it has to do with the increased blood flow to all parts of the body—nose included. Still others say it's a hormone thing.

The research is inconclusive. Studies that support the idea that pregnant women have a better sense of smell are limited. But if I have learned anything in my day, it is to believe a pregnant lady when she says something. So, mama, if you say you can smell your co-worker's salad dressing three rooms away, I believe you.

Try to get plenty of fresh air by opening windows and taking breaks outside. If you find a smell you do like, see if you can find a transportable version to carry with you. A little bottle of peppermint essential oil can do wonders for hiding yucky odors. And don't be afraid to stick up for yourself. Asking people to tone down their perfume usage or cigarette smoke around you is more than acceptable and fair.

Shortness of Breath

Feeling short of breath can come at various moments in pregnancy. Early on, progesterone can increase your breathing rate, which makes you feel like it's harder to get air in. The increase in blood volume and related faster heartbeat can make you breathe harder—especially when exercising or walking up stairs. As your pregnancy progresses and your baby gets bigger, more pressure is applied to your diaphragm, the muscle under your lungs, which can make it harder to take a full breath. All of these things can make you pretty uncomfortable.

Getting regular exercise will help with this because it will strengthen all the muscles involved. When you feel short of breath, listen to your body. If you are hunched over or in a position where your lungs may be squished, try sitting up taller to give them more room to do their work. You can also try standing or getting on your hands and knees to give the baby more room (and give your poor diaphragm a break). Sleeping with your head and back propped on pillows can make you more comfortable at night.

You can also refer to Brooke Cates's diaphragmatic breathing practice in the "Move" section on page 119, which may help significantly.

While this symptom is common, be careful not to overlook something more serious that could be going on. If your heart is beating fast, you feel dizzy or light-headed, your chest or head hurts, you have a fever, or you are struggling to breathe, call 911.

Skin Darkening
See "Mask of Pregnancy and Skin Darkening" on page 442.

Sleep Challenges
See "Fatigue" on page 435 or "Insomnia" on page 440.

Slower Digestion
See "Getting Full Quickly" on page 437.

Snoring
During pregnancy, the tissues in your body can swell. It can happen in many places, such as your vagina, your gums, and even in your nose. This nasal swelling can lead to more mucus, and both of these factors can lead to

snoring. It's also possible that you have just always been a snorer, and that is continuing into pregnancy.

Snoring is annoying to deal with because it likely makes it harder for you (and your partner) to sleep. It can also be dangerous if it becomes sleep apnea (when you stop breathing for long periods). If you do have a bed partner, or a friend who can spend a few nights over, ask them to pay attention to how you are breathing at night. If they notice pauses or gasping, let your provider know right away. Other symptoms of sleep apnea are waking up with a dry mouth, headaches, having trouble sleeping at night, and being really tired during the day (from the lack of sleep).

A 2013 study found that women who snore are at higher risk for developing preeclampsia, having a C-section, and giving birth to a small baby, so snoring is not to be taken lightly. If you are at all concerned, speak with your provider about possible testing and solutions.

If your snoring is just snoring, you could try over-the-counter nasal strips to help your nostrils open a bit. You may also find that changing positions helps. Lie on your side or elevate your head with some pillows.

For ideas on how to deal with the constant congestion, see "Congestion" on page 433.

Spider Veins
Spider veins are tiny red and blue lines that may start to appear on your body (often on your legs) during pregnancy. They get their name because they look like spiderwebs. These tiny pregnancy "goddess webs" (it's all in the mindset, mama) are caused by the increase in blood volume in your body. This extra blood applies more pressure to your

veins, which can enlarge them, making them more visible. If you spend a lot of time on your feet, you may be more susceptible.

Spider veins are usually not anything to worry about. They may even slowly fade after you've given birth. In the meantime, here are some tricks to try:

- Exercise. Moving your body in a way that feels good can help improve circulation, which may relieve pressure on the veins. Consider a variety of types of movement, including yoga and swimming, where you can work out without spending the whole time standing.

- Put your feet up. As often as you can throughout the day, find a few minutes to sit with your legs elevated on a coffee table or chair. This will help drain some blood out of your legs.

- Try compression stockings. Compression stockings are support stockings specially designed to reduce the amount of blood that pools in your legs. These bad boys are not going to be the hottest item in your wardrobe, but goodness, do they feel good.

- Go maxi. Wear loose-fitting, drapey clothing, especially around your waist, to improve blood flow.

- Avoid crossing your legs.

- Sleep on your left side.

After the baby is born, if you still have your spider veins and are unhappy with them, you can chat with a vein specialist about options like injections and laser therapy. These procedures may not be covered by insurance.

Spotting and Vaginal Bleeding

Potential causes of spotting and vaginal bleeding might be:

- Implantation bleeding. When the embryo implants into your uterine lining, a small amount of blood can be released.

- Vaginal exam or vaginal sex. The higher-than-normal blood volume in your body can make the more sensitive parts of your body (like your gums and your cervix) bleed more easily. So, if your cervix is "bumped" during an exam or sex, it may bleed a little.

- Vaginal infection. Sometimes bacteria can irritate your cervix and make it bleed.

- Miscarriage. Vaginal bleeding is sometimes associated with miscarriage. (See chapter 4, "Miscarriage and Loss," to read more about miscarriages.)

- Complications with the pregnancy, such as placental issues. (See "Placental Issues," page 474.)

If you have spotting or vaginal bleeding, call your provider. They may suggest some blood work or an ultrasound to check on the pregnancy. If you experience heavy bleeding (filling a pad with blood in an hour or two), go to the emergency room right away.

Stretch Marks

Also known as your "mama stripes," stretch marks may form on your skin to accommodate the ways your body is changing to grow your baby. Up to 90 percent of women get stretch marks somewhere on their bellies, legs, breasts, or arms. They can be darker than your skin tone or lighter, and some are more noticeable than others.

There are usually two schools of thought on stretch marks. The first is to work hard to prevent and treat. Women try all kinds of massage, oils and lotions (store-bought and DIY), and even postpartum laser removal to correct stretch marks (which is likely expensive and not covered by most insurance plans). Stretch marks often improve on their own but do not go away completely after pregnancy. Unfortunately, we haven't found the magic solution yet, though there is research underway.

The second, and opposite, way of thinking about stretch marks is to fully embrace them. There is a movement to encourage women to wear their stripes with honor and celebrate how they represent all that their body has accomplished.

Mama, you may feel however you feel about your stretch marks. If you are proud of them, rock them. If you really wish they'd go away, that's okay, too. And if you aren't sure yet, then give yourself time. Pregnancy changes us in a thousand ways, and there is no one ideology that will work for everyone. Do what you need to do to feel good in your body.

Swelling

Swelling in pregnancy, also called edema, is incredibly common. In addition to your growing baby, your placenta, and an increased fat store, your body is hard at work making more blood and fluid to help support all of these changes and extra activity.

All this extra fluid can make you look—and feel—fairly swollen.

Your growing baby and uterus also put a lot of pressure on your circulatory and lymphatic system, which can contribute to the swelling as well.

Some women start to notice the swelling early on, but it usually develops during the second and third trimesters. Although we often have little control over it, some triggering factors include:

- Standing for a long time
- Prolonged activity
- Hot weather
- Excessive sodium chloride (salt) intake
- Low levels of potassium
- High levels of caffeine
- Dehydration

To decrease swelling, try wearing compression stockings, staying very well hydrated, and elevating your feet and legs for 10- to 20-minute periods throughout the day.

There are times where swelling can be concerning.

Until fairly recently, swelling was one of the symptoms used to diagnose preeclampsia, a condition of high blood pressure during pregnancy. It is no longer part of the diagnostic criteria, yet many women with elevated blood pressure do have swelling. (See "Preeclampsia" on page 466.)

Swelling can also be associated with a blood clot or deep vein thrombosis, or DVT (see page 459), a skin infection, or an underlying medical condition such as a heart problem.

Be sure to report any of the following symptoms:

- Pain, redness, hardness, and swelling in an area of your body
- One leg that is more swollen than the other
- Swelling in your face or hands
- Headache
- Light-headedness
- Belly pain
- Difficulty breathing
- Fever

These symptoms should serve as red flags, especially for black women, who have a higher risk of a DVT and related complications.

Vaginal Discharge

Vaginal discharge gets a bad rap, but the truth is that not only is it normal, it is the sign of a healthy vagina (and cervix). Many women find that they have more vaginal discharge during pregnancy as their bodies respond to the high levels of hormones and prepare for labor.

Normal vaginal discharge is clear or whitish, carries no unusual scent, and should not irritate your skin. If the discharge is yellow, green, bloody, or chunky or smells foul or fishy, let your provider know. If your vaginal area is itchy, burning, or painful, let them know as well.

Toward the end of pregnancy, women can experience extra discharge, and sometimes it can be hard to tell if it is normal or if your water broke. For more on water breaking, see page 239.

Varicose Veins

Varicose veins occur when your growing uterus applies pressure to your inferior vena cava, a big vein that carries blood from the lower half of your body to your heart. This results in a backflow of blood, which can put pressure on and enlarge veins. The result can

be varicose veins—veins that are enlarged and easily seen or felt through the skin.

To deal with these pests, check out the recommendations listed under "Spider Veins" on page 446.

An important note (especially for black women): It's important to be aware of the potential for a deep vein thrombosis (DVT; see page 459). If you notice a spot on your body (often one leg) that is hot, red, hard, and painful, it could be a less-concerning vein inflammation, but call your provider or go to an emergency room right away for good measure. And *don't* try to massage it.

Vivid Dreams

Dreaming is a way for our brains to process information. It makes sense that in pregnancy, when our bodies and our brains have *so* much new information swirling around (hormones, symptoms, worries, excitement), our dreams can become vivid and downright odd.

If you are still able to get rest and are not bothered by them, these vivid dreams are okay. And hey, you may have some funny stories to tell later. But if they are scary, impact your sleep, or are causing you anxiety, don't be afraid to reach out for help. Talking to a therapist may help you address an underlying cause. Some women find that recording their dreams in a journal can be therapeutic.

Vulvar Varicosities

Vulvar varicosities are varicose veins that develop on your vulva (the tissue outside of your vagina) and groin, and about 1 out of 5 women will experience them during pregnancy. We have the increased blood volume and weight of the growing uterus to thank for these gems. If you have them, you may be able to see and feel bluish veins through your skin, or you may feel pulsing or pressure or experience pain with sex. Vulvar varicosities can be alarming, as they can grow to be quite large.

Talk to your provider. Often you will just watch and wait, as they usually won't impact your pregnancy or birth, though this can change if they are very large or other complications develop.

To prevent or improve vulvar varicosities, try the recommendations listed under "Spider Veins" on page 446. If you notice a spot on your vulvar area that is hot, red, hard, or painful, this could be a sign of a more serious condition like a deep vein thrombosis (see page 459), so call your provider or go to an emergency room right away. And *don't* try to massage it.

Water Breaking

At some point, the bag of water (amniotic sac) that has been housing your baby will open, releasing the fluid. See "Water Breaking" on page 239 for more information.

Tests and Complications

The intention of this section is to provide you with the details of the tests and possible complications you may encounter throughout your pregnancy journey or that you may simply be curious about. Please use this section in the way that serves you best! Many mamas will choose to only read about items that come up for them, dipping in and out as needed. Others may want to read it from start to finish. And still others may not want to read it at all—no hard feelings, promise.

Remember, your primary source of information and guidance for your pregnancy and birth is always your health-care provider.

The content of this section is arranged by category and then alphabetically within each of those categories. Here's what you'll find:

- Prenatal Tests   452
- Fetal Testing   454
- Pregnancy Complications   458
- Sexually Transmitted Infections During Pregnancy   470
- Placental Issues   474
- Umbilical Cord Issues   476
- Birth Complications   476
- Postpartum Complications   481
- Other Issues   482

A NOTE ABOUT TESTS

There are a great many tests available today to help assess the health of a woman, her pregnancy, and the growing fetus. Before we dig into these, it's important to reflect on what you want because these tests are optional. Your provider may strongly encourage some (based on your personal health information), but ultimately, the decision is yours to make.

Some women choose to have all the available tests done, while others decline all of them. The majority of women probably fall somewhere in the middle.

To make the decision, start with questions. You can review this list of questions with your provider:

- What is the test looking for?
- What information are we hoping to gather from this test?
- How will it be done (blood draw, ultrasound, and so on)?
- What are the risks?
- What is the cost, and is it covered by my insurance? (You may need to call your insurance company for the answer to this one.)
- How will the results of this test impact me, my pregnancy, or my baby?
- Do you recommend this test for me?

With this information, you can then make your decision.

Each test presents its pros and cons, and it can be difficult to decide what to do. My general recommendation is to consider what you will do with the information you gain.

For example, perhaps you are trying to decide if you want to assess the chance that your baby may be born with a chromosomal abnormality.

If the test comes back saying your baby has a very low chance of having a chromosomal abnormality, will that help you to feel more relaxed during your pregnancy? Or would you rather not think about this knowledge one way or the other?

If the test comes back saying that your baby has a high chance of having a chromosomal abnormality, will you then choose to have an amniocentesis (more on those in a bit) to get more reliable information?

If you do choose an amniocentesis, and it reveals that your baby does indeed have a chromosomal abnormality, does that impact your decision-making moving forward? Will you, for example, appreciate knowing this information so you can begin to make special plans for caring for the baby? Will you choose to terminate the pregnancy? If the answer to both of those questions is no, perhaps you may not want to have the testing at all.

Again, it's complicated. But just like with all of pregnancy and parenting, there is no one right way to do things. The world is full of ideas and judgment, but in these moments, focus on your needs and desires and your provider's guidance.

PRENATAL TESTS

Antibody Screening (*Rh Factor*)
See "About Rhesus (Rh) Factor" on page 178.

Blood Type
This test will tell you what type of blood you have. Blood types start with letters (A, B, AB, or O) and end with either positive or negative—for example, A positive or AB negative. This is important information to have in the unlikely event of needing a blood transfusion. It is also important when considering the potential need for certain medications (see "About Rhesus (Rh) Factor" on page 178).

Carrier Screening Preconception
These saliva or blood-based tests check whether you and your partner or sperm donor "carry" a genetic mutation that could lead to an inherited disorder for your future children, such as cystic fibrosis, sickle cell disease, thalassemia, Canavan disease, Tay-Sachs disease, and more.

These disorders are recessive. This means that if your baby gets an affected gene from you but a normal one from your partner or sperm donor, they will be fine: They will be a carrier, but they won't have the disorder. But if they get an affected gene from each of you (there is a 25 percent chance of this if you are both carriers), they will develop the disorder.

If you opt to be screened for these diseases, it is ideal to do so before you try to conceive. If you find out that you and your partner share a recessive gene, you can plan for a wider range of options to address it. A genetic counselor can offer you advice about the condition and help you make informed choices about preventive assisted reproductive techniques and embryo screenings.

There are other genetic tests available, and more coming out regularly, so be sure to talk to your provider about which are best for you.

If you're already pregnant and decide you want carrier screening, you might want to do it as early as possible in your pregnancy so that you have as many options for further diagnostics as possible.

Some genetic mutations are more common for certain ethnicities, so it may be beneficial to discuss this information with your provider or genetic counselor to guide which tests may be most pertinent to you. For example, cystic fibrosis is most common in Caucasian people, Tay-Sachs disease is most common in people of Eastern European Jewish (Ashkenazi) descent, sickle cell anemia is more common among people of African, Central and South American, Middle Eastern, Asian, and Mediterranean descent.

Complete Blood Count (CBC)

This test looks at the overall health of your blood and can pick up on a number of potential concerns (for example, anemia, infections, or clotting disorders). A CBC will assess your red blood cell count, your white blood cell count, hemoglobin, hematocrit, and platelets.

Glucose Challenge Test

See "Testing for Gestational Diabetes Mellitus (GDM)" on page 161.

Hepatitis Test

See "Hepatitis B Vaccine" on page 276 and "Hepatitis" on page 472.

HIV and AIDS Tests

See "HIV" on page 473.

Pap Smears

A pap smear is a screening test that looks for abnormal cells on your cervix that could potentially be (or turn into) cervical cancer. ACOG recommends that if you are from 21 to 29 years old, you have a pap smear every 3 years, and if you are from 30 to 65, you have a pap smear and HPV testing every 5 years (more on HPV on page 471).

During a pap smear, your provider will use a speculum to get a better view of your cervix and then gently sweep your cervix with a brush (that looks like a little cotton swab). Pap smears are considered safe during pregnancy, just know that they can cause some spotting, which can feel scary when you are pregnant.

Receiving abnormal pap smear results can be stressful, especially so when you're pregnant. The good news is that abnormal cells on your cervix should not impact your pregnancy or fetus. Depending on the specific results, your provider may recommend a colposcopy, a procedure in which a small sample of cervical tissue is removed and assessed to determine if further testing should be done. More testing and potential treatments will likely be postponed until after you give birth.

Rubella Immunity

Rubella, or German measles, is a virus that can cause mild flu-like symptoms, and it can be dangerous for fetuses. If you have received an MMR vaccine, you are likely immune to rubella, which means that your baby is not at risk. Early prenatal care often involves a test to see if you are immune. Unfortunately, it is not safe to be vaccinated once you are pregnant, so if you haven't entered the TTC (trying to conceive) phase, this is a great time to get vaccinated. If you are already pregnant and not immune to rubella, take extra precautions to avoid people who may have the virus and report any concerning symptoms right away.

After your baby is born, you can receive the vaccination if you choose to.

Syphilis Test

See "Syphilis" on page 473.

Amniocentesis

An amniocentesis (amnio) is a procedure to sample the fluid that surrounds the baby. This amniotic fluid contains your baby's DNA, so it can be used to test for genetic disorders. The results show the relevant features of your baby's chromosomes. An amnio can also identify intrauterine infections and check on your baby's health if Rh factor is a concern or if there are other developmental issues. It is generally recommended for women over 35, although the need is determined by your provider. Amniocentesis is usually performed between week 15 and week 20 and does carry some risks, so it is important to be informed about them. According to the Society for Maternal-Fetal Medicine, amniocentesis is associated with a miscarriage rate of 1 in 300 to 500.

During the procedure, the doctor performs an ultrasound to determine the position of your baby and uterus. Then they insert a hollow needle through your belly into the uterus and draw out a sample of the fluid. No anesthetic is needed, but you may feel stinging and cramping as a result of the needle. Recovery is usually short and requires just a day of rest and a week of lower-than-usual activity. Results can take up to 2 weeks, depending on what is being tested.

Amniotic Fluid Index (AFI) and Maximum Vertical Pocket (MVP)

To check your amniotic fluid level, your provider may use information gathered in two types of non-invasive ultrasounds.

Amniotic fluid index (AFI)   Imagine that there are two lines that divide your uterus into four equal sections—one that goes up and down and one that goes side to side. The four sections are called pockets. The provider will measure how much fluid is in each pocket and then combine them to establish your AFI. Values between 5 and 25 centimeters are considered normal, but the average measurement is 14. It is also normal for the number to decrease as you approach the end of your pregnancy. A value of less than 5 is considered oligohydramnios (too little amniotic fluid; see "Oligohydramnios" on page 464) and may be cause for induction. On the other hand, too much fluid is a condition known as polyhydramnios (see "Polyhydramnios" on page 466).

Maximum vertical pocket (MVP)   This is the vertical dimension in centimeters of the largest pocket of amniotic fluid (that isn't also the space being occupied by the umbilical cord). A normal value is greater than 2 and less than 8. Less is considered oligohydramnios, and more is polyhydramnios.

Biophysical Profile (BPP)

A BPP combines a nonstress test (see "Nonstress Test" on page 457) with an ultrasound to get an overall assessment of the baby and pregnancy. The goal of a BPP is to detect possible problems early enough to deliver the baby before complications arise.

A BPP ultrasound looks at five things:

- Amniotic fluid level
- Baby's practice breathing movement
- Baby's movement
- Baby's tone (ability to bend and flex limbs)
- Results of the nonstress test

Each category can get a possible 2 points.

A score of 8 to 10 is considered normal, 6 is uncertain, and 4 or less is abnormal and could be a reason for induction.

Chorionic Villus Sampling (CVS)

CVS tests are one method of testing for certain disorders and chromosomal abnormalities in the fetus by looking at the chorionic villi, which are wisps of placental tissue that contain your baby's DNA. It can be done as early as 10 weeks. Placental tissue will be extracted from your uterus by a catheter inserted into your cervix or by needle into the abdomen. The tissue will be genetically analyzed for certain disorders. The procedure carries a small (0.35 percent) risk of miscarriage. It may sting and induce some cramping, but after a day of rest, you are cleared to resume normal activity.

The benefit of a CVS is that it can be done earlier in the pregnancy than an amniocentesis.

Doppler Ultrasound

This is a different type of ultrasound that presents a picture of the function of veins and arteries, which can be used to view the baby's blood flow. In a high-risk pregnancy, a Doppler ultrasound may be used in the third trimester to check how blood is flowing from the placenta to the baby or whether the baby has anemia. The results of the ultrasound may determine whether an induction is necessary or if other measures are needed to protect the baby's health.

Noninvasive Prenatal Testing (NIPT) and Multiple Marker Screening

NIPT identifies Down syndrome and a few other chromosomal conditions through a blood sample. NIPT is available starting at 10 weeks of pregnancy, and for some, it's also an

A NOTE ON 3D ULTRASOUNDS

One of the highlights of expecting a baby is daydreaming about what that baby looks like. It is no wonder that 3D ultrasounds are so popular! They can give detailed images of that adorable face you have been working so hard to bake (fair warning, though, the images are not always perfect, and the baby may have a bit of a smooshed look).

While these are so appealing and satisfy your urge to know, I should tell you that the Food and Drug Administration (FDA) and ACOG caution against the routine use of 3D ultrasounds. There are a few concerns. First, we just don't know if there are long-term effects from repeat ultrasounds, so some providers counsel that unless it is medically indicated, it is best avoided, just in case. The other concern is that sometimes these ultrasounds happen outside of medical facilities, so the staff training may be different from what you have grown used to, and they may not be able to give you medically correct information.

All this said, there may be future medical uses for these detailed looks inside, as evidence suggests that they may be able to detect structural abnormalities that 2D ultrasounds cannot.

If a 3D ultrasound is important to you, consider asking your provider to recommend a reputable service.

exciting proposition because it can reveal the baby's sex earlier than we've ever been able to know. Results take about a week.

The multiple marker screening occurs between 15 and 20 weeks and looks for the same chromosome abnormalities as well as neural tube defects. Since the multiple marker test, also known as quad screening, is not as accurate as the NIPT, you may not encounter it at all.

The results from the NIPT and the multiple marker screening don't necessarily indicate whether your baby has a chromosomal condition. They give you probabilities. Normal test results do not guarantee an absence of problems, and an abnormal result doesn't rule out a healthy baby. You'll need to get advice from your practitioner about how to interpret all the results.

To get a definitive diagnosis for something like Down syndrome, or other chromosomal disorders, you will also need to have chorionic villus sampling or amniocentesis if your NIPT indicates a high probability.

WHEN AN ULTRASOUND REVEALS A PROBLEM

An anatomy scan can identify issues ranging from a marker (a characteristic that may be indicative of a chromosomal abnormality) to a severe problem (such as a heart deformity).

Mama, I wish so badly that I could give you specific guidance here, because if this has happened, you are likely reeling. You are learning firsthand that the worry that comes from loving a child starts much earlier than birth, and it can be so stressful. So often, an ultrasound finding is just one piece of a much larger story, and without all the information, I cannot give you the answers you are craving.

What I will say is to voice your needs loudly. Your provider, who does understand your story, can help you. They are there to answer your questions and address your concerns, so please do not hesitate to lean on them. They can assess your risk factors and give you the information you need to understand how worried—if at all—you need to be and what your options are. Ask to schedule an extra appointment, so you can go over your concerns in more depth. Request to be referred to a genetic counselor who can explain the specifics and a social worker who can support your needs: Most hospitals have them, and they are often covered by insurance. You may also consider additional resources as needed, such as therapists, spiritual leaders, and support groups.

If your team diagnoses a high likelihood for a problem, do not hesitate to advocate for yourself. Ask for everything that you need, including a mental health therapist to help you cope with the profound stress that often comes with these diagnoses. Social workers will have information about support groups and local resources as well. Your provider will know the best specialists to refer you to. And you need to continue to stand in your truth, every day, and remember that taking care of yourself during this difficult time is the most important thing you can do.

You are not alone, mama.

Nonstress Tests

You may be asked to get a fetal nonstress test in the later part of your pregnancy for a variety of reasons (for example, going past your due date, the development of conditions such as gestational diabetes, or concern over decreased fetal movement). This is a simple and painless procedure focused on measuring your baby's heart rate and checking to make sure that it is responding appropriately to rest and to uterine activity.

You may be instructed to eat right before the test because that can encourage the baby to move around more. Two round monitors will be placed on your belly—one at the top of your belly to "watch" for possible contractions and one on the bottom of your belly to listen to the heartbeat. The monitoring will last for about 20 minutes (though this can run longer, so be sure to pee first!). The provider will look at the paper or electronic "strip" generated during the test to ensure everything looks normal.

Ultrasound

This technology involves transmitting short pulses of high-frequency, low-intensity sound waves through the uterus to create an image of the fetus, placenta, and surrounding organs. The first one can be performed as early as 6 weeks, and it is often called the "dating" scan, because it can reveal the age of the fetus, and show whether it is a single fetus or multiples. Ultrasounds done during the second and third trimesters can usually reveal genitalia, the baby's position, and whether there may be any developmental abnormalities.

When performed in early pregnancy, ultrasounds are done transvaginally, using a special probe inserted into the vagina. After the first trimester, they are usually performed transabdominally, with a transducer that scans the belly surface. You will lie down on a table next to the ultrasound technician, who will coat your belly with a conductive gel and then position the wand in various spots to reveal the anatomy beneath. Reading ultrasounds is not intuitive, so your technician can explain what you are seeing. A routine ultrasound will last about 30 minutes, and you may be given a picture of your baby—one to keep for the memory book!

Ultrasounds can also be used to assess your cervical length if there is concern about preterm labor.

Nuchal Translucency There is a very important fluid-filled area on the back of the baby's neck, the size of which can be indicative of the diagnosis of Down syndrome. This space will be measured and computed during the nuchal translucency ultrasound to create an individualized assessment that also factors in the mother's age. If the chance of Down syndrome is high, you may also be offered chorionic villus sampling (see "Chorionic Villus Sampling (CVS)" on page 455).

Anatomy Scan Between 18 and 20 weeks, most providers recommend having an ultrasound called an anatomy scan to check on all the body parts of your growing baby.

The technician will take photos (called sonograms) of various parts of your baby so that a doctor can look at them to make sure everything is developing normally. They'll look at the brain, heart, spine, limbs, bones, face, internal organs, and yes, the genitalia. This is the ultrasound where you may be able to find out the sex of your baby if you want to.

They will also check on the size of your baby, as well as the placenta and your uterus, ovaries, and cervix (sometimes they will need to use a vaginal probe for this part).

A 2013 study reports that ultrasounds are good, but not perfect, at identifying abnormalities. They detect 70 to 90 percent of nervous system problems, 40 to 50 percent of heart problems, 25 to 70 percent of urinary tract problems, 46 to 100 percent of abdominal and digestive problems, 20 to 50 percent of bone problems, and 7 to 55 percent of cleft lips and palates. Technology advances all the time, but it is important to keep in mind that an ultrasound is a tool, and not a flawless one.

PREGNANCY COMPLICATIONS

To be diagnosed with a pregnancy complication is rough, mama. This can leave you feeling stressed, scared, and disappointed. When you envisioned your pregnancy, this was not part of it. It is understandable and justifiable to be angry—not that you need justification. Your feelings matter, especially now.

If you can, remember that most women with pregnancy complications—and their sweet babies—are fine! Just attend all your prenatal appointments, ask tons of questions, and be very gentle on yourself.

Advanced Maternal Age

I will be honest, I hesitated to add this piece to a section entitled "Tests and Complications." Mama, your age is not a complication. More and more women are getting pregnant later in life, and most of them have perfectly fine outcomes. You may have a few factors to be aware of.

Women who will give birth when they are 35 or older are categorized as having an "advanced maternal age." Sometimes it is also called an "elderly" or "geriatric" pregnancy, to which we say, "Um, seriously?" Can we agree to change that to a "fabulous woman in her prime" pregnancy?

It is important to consider age in pregnancy because there may be some risk factors present for *fabulous women in their prime*, such as gestational diabetes (see "Gestational Diabetes Mellitus (GDM)" on page 460), placenta problems (see "Placental Issues" on page 474), and postpartum hemorrhage (see "Postpartum Hemorrhage: Warning Signs" on page 350). Your provider will help you determine what specific risks might be present for you and appropriate steps to decrease them.

Bacterial Vaginosis (BV)

Bacterial vaginosis, or BV, is the most common vaginal infection for women: About 29 percent of women have had it. BV is not a sexually transmitted infection (though women who are sexually active are more likely to experience it). BV results from an imbalance in the amounts of good and bad bacteria in the vagina. (This is one of the reasons douching is not recommended, as it disturbs this balance. See "Taking Care of Your Vagina During Pregnancy" on page 104 for a reminder on how to take care of your vagina.) BV can often have no symptoms, but if it does, they may include a fishy vaginal odor, grayish-white vaginal discharge, and vaginal itching and burning. BV can increase your risk of getting other STIs and having a preterm delivery during pregnancy. BV is diagnosed by looking at the discharge under a microscope and is treated with an antibiotic.

Bed Rest

Occasionally a prenatal complication will necessitate the modification or scaling back of certain activities and types of work (lifting heavy objects, repetitive movements, and spending prolonged periods of time on your feet or sitting). It is important to note that ACOG no longer recommends routine bed rest as effective for preventing premature birth, miscarriage, or other issues.

If you have been prescribed bed rest, despite the new guidelines, make sure you understand why your doctor has chosen this option. Some worry that bed rest can lead to psychological and physical issues, so this warrants a detailed conversation with your provider about the risks and benefits as well as ways to minimize any consequences that could come up.

Cervical Insufficiency

The cervix is normally closed and firm before and during the beginning of pregnancy. Closer to birth, it will shorten, soften, and open (that is, dilate). Cervical insufficiency is when it begins to open too soon, putting you at risk of premature birth or miscarriage. The treatment involves close monitoring. Your provider may recommend progesterone suppositories or injections, which could help prevent a preterm delivery. Or they may recommend a procedure called cerclage, which sutures the cervix closed until labor.

Cholestasis

Cholestasis, or intrahepatic cholestasis of pregnancy (ICP), is when a mother's liver decreases its ability to excrete bile acids (a substance that aids in digestion) from her body, which means that the baby can also experience a backup of bile acids. Hispanic women and women with indigenous American ancestry are at a higher risk of developing ICP.

Symptoms of cholestasis can be:

- Severe itching, often on the palms of the hands and soles of the feet
- Right upper belly pain
- Dark-colored urine
- Light-colored bowel movements
- Tiredness

Cholestasis can increase the risk of fetal complications, so it is treated very seriously. Be sure to report symptoms right away (call your provider; you don't have to wait until your next appointment). If your provider suspects cholestasis, they will do some blood tests. If those tests indicate that you have it, you may be prescribed a medication to reduce the amount of bile acids in your blood, as well as medication to help manage the unbearable itching. You will also have frequent monitoring to make sure the baby is okay, and you may be induced before your due date. Symptoms usually get better a few days after giving birth.

Deep Vein Thrombosis (DVT)

These are blood clots that can form in veins. While the risk of a DVT increases for all women during pregnancy, because your body is producing more of the component of blood responsible for clotting, this risk is especially dangerous for black women. Other symptoms of a blood clot include pain that gets worse with movement, hardness, and redness. You might also notice one leg is more swollen than the other. And while the most common site for a blood clot is in your lower legs, they can occur in other parts of the body as well.

If you think you may have a DVT, avoid massaging the area and call your provider or go to the hospital right away. And if you have chest pain or a fast heartbeat, difficulty breathing, or a bloody cough, go to the ER or call 911.

Depression During Pregnancy

Getting down and feeling hopeless can happen to anyone at any time, but because of hormonal changes (the rapid increase in estrogen and progesterone), pregnant women have a higher likelihood of experiencing depression. ACOG estimates that 14 to 23 percent of women experience depression while pregnant, though much more emphasis is placed on women who experience it postpartum.

If you are consistently feeling down and have a bleak outlook or feelings of despair, you should absolutely mention this to your health-care provider. For a complete list of symptoms of mental health concerns, see "Postpartum Mental Health" on page 343. If you are having thoughts about harming yourself or others, call 911 or go the nearest emergency room. There are many resources available to help women cope with depression, including support groups, education, therapy, and medications. Getting the help you need during pregnancy will allow you set out on the right foot once baby arrives.

Fetal Alcohol Syndrome (FAS)

Babies in utero who are exposed to alcohol can develop a syndrome characterized by certain facial features, learning disabilities, deformities, heart defects, vision and hearing difficulties, and behavioral issues. The recommendation from medical authorities is to abstain from drinking any alcohol during pregnancy because we don't know what amount can cause FAS. While the syndrome is incurable, early treatment can address many of the symptoms. If you are worried about your alcohol consumption, talk honestly and openly with your health-care provider about what you can do to protect your baby.

Flu

Getting the flu during pregnancy is potentially serious, as you are more likely than nonpregnant adults to experience complications. Most providers recommend getting a flu vaccine during flu season before and during pregnancy. And the Centers for Disease Control recommends routine flu vaccinations for all pregnant women as well. Contracting the flu puts you at risk of preterm labor and premature birth, and fevers may be linked to various birth defects and developmental problems in the baby. Furthermore, pregnant women who get the flu are at increased risk of complications, such as pneumonia. If you experience any symptoms of the flu, call your provider right away.

Gestational Diabetes Mellitus (GDM)

Occurring in 2 to 10 percent of pregnancies, GDM is when a pregnant woman develops high blood sugar, usually after the 20-week mark. If you are diagnosed with GDM, your provider will work with you to develop the best treatment plan, which can vary depending on your scenario. Dietary changes are almost always recommended and involve limiting refined carbohydrates. Exercise can help your body process blood sugar. You will be given a device to check your blood sugar at home. The bad news is that you will be pricking your fingers with a needle multiple times per day. The good news is that after they get over the initial nervousness factor, most women find that this is a generally tolerable annoyance. By tracking your blood sugar, your provider will help you determine if diet change alone is sufficient to keep your levels stable or if medications need to be added as well.

Women with GDM often have additional ultrasounds and nonstress tests (see "Nonstress Tests" on page 457) in the third trimester to monitor their babies. Sometimes, inductions are recommended at 39 weeks (see "Induction of Labor" on page 301).

GDM usually goes away after the baby is born. (*Hooray!*) It is important to note, though, that women with GDM do have a higher risk of developing type 2 diabetes later in life. Speak with both your obstetrics and primary care providers about steps to take to decrease your risk moving forward.

Mama, getting diagnosed with GDM is stressful. I know a lot of women who are really disappointed by this one. There are risks, yes, but many women go on to have a lovely and healthy pregnancy, birth, and baby. Stick to the treatment plan, take good care of yourself, and try to take some deep breaths. See "Testing for Gestational Diabetes Mellitus (GDM)" on page 161 for more information.

Group B Strep (GBS)
See "Group B Strep" on page 212.

HELLP Syndrome
This is a rare complication, thought to be related to preeclampsia, that often develops after preeclampsia has been identified.

HELLP stands for:

H Hemolysis (when red blood cells break down)
EL Elevated liver enzymes
LP Low platelet counts (the part of blood that allows for clotting)

The symptoms of HELLP can include headaches, blurry vision, upper right belly pain, nausea, high blood pressure, protein in the urine, and bleeding. If you experience any of these, call your provider immediately. The diagnosis will be made with a blood test. HELLP can cause severe problems for the mother and baby, such as placental abruption and fluid in the lungs, so it is not taken lightly.

HELLP syndrome usually occurs in the third trimester. There are medications to help with the severity of it, but ultimately the fastest way to treatment is delivery of the baby. Depending on how far along you are, your provider may advise medications to help mature the baby's lungs, followed by an induction.

Hernias
A hernia is a rare condition in which a small hole develops in the muscles of the abdomen or groin that protect and enclose your organs. When your belly grows and expands during pregnancy, pressure on this abdominal wall can enlarge existing hernias or create new ones.

A hernia can be felt as a soft lump around your navel or groin area, and it may become painful when you are active or cough or sneeze. If you notice it is becoming painful or is bulging further, it may indicate that it is becoming "strangulated," or stuck inside your abdominal wall and losing access to your blood supply. You may also experience nausea and vomiting. Contact your provider, as you may need quick treatment. Hernias can be repaired with surgery with little risk to the pregnancy, although depending on the urgency, you will likely wait until after birth.

High Blood Pressure (*Hypertension*)

Your blood pressure measures the force of your blood against the walls of your arteries. The number on top of the reading is the pressure when your heart beats (systolic), and the bottom number is the pressure in between beats (diastolic). A high reading is when either of both of these numbers is 140/90 or higher.

High blood pressure in pregnancy can come in several forms: chronic high blood pressure (if you had it before you ever became pregnant or develop it early in pregnancy), gestational hypertension or pregnancy-induced hypertension (high blood pressure that develops after week 20 of pregnancy), or preeclampsia (see "Preeclampsia" on page 466).

It is important to note that non-Hispanic black women are much more likely to be diagnosed with all forms of high blood pressure, and suffer preeclampsia disproportionately.

Speak up about any symptoms you have, including:

- Swelling
- Rapid weight gain
- Headache
- Nausea and vomiting
- Pain on the right side of your belly
- Changes in how much you pee

You do not have to (and should not) wait until your next appointment to report any of these symptoms. Call now. It's okay if it is a false alarm, but it may not be.

Elevated blood pressure in pregnancy can be incredibly stressful. And then people are telling you to be calm, so you don't raise your blood pressure, which makes you even more stressed! "Try to relax" is *not* helpful. Unfortunately though, there is some truth to it. If you've been diagnosed with any form of hypertension, see if you can view it as your mandate to lavish yourself with love and self-care.

High-Risk Pregnancies

A pregnancy is considered high risk if the risks of complications for the mother or her fetus are higher than average. You may eventually require attention from a perinatologist or maternal-fetal medicine (MFM) specialist, who coordinates specialized care with the obstetrics team. Pregnancies can begin as high risk if the mother has a preexisting condition, or they can become high risk as they progress due to developing conditions or fetal problems.

Love note time! Mama, this stinks. You are doing #allthethings and trying to be healthy, you want desperately to have a healthy baby, and yet this "high-risk" label follows you, reminding you to be nervous. I can't take that away, but what I can do is remind you that with the right attention and care, it is very possible to have a healthy baby (or two or three, if multiples are what makes you high risk). You can get through this. And think about how much stronger you will be because of it. Blowout diapers? Please, that's easy. Grocery store toddler meltdowns? Kid, you don't scare me. Everything else that motherhood will throw at you? You've got that, too.

Hyperemesis Gravidarum (*Excessive Nausea and Vomiting*)

Nausea and vomiting in pregnancy is common, and while difficult to get through, it is generally manageable and goes away around the end of the first trimester. Hyperemesis gravidarum (HG) is an entirely different beast.

HG is defined as severe nausea and vomiting in pregnancy that causes weight loss, dehydration, and electrolyte imbalances. It is fairly rare, affecting only 1 percent of pregnant women.

We don't fully know why some people get such severe nausea during pregnancy, though a recent study suggests that there is a genetic component to it. Indeed, there is a strong hereditary aspect to HG. If your mother or a sister had it, you are at a much higher risk of having it as well. And if you've had it in a previous pregnancy, there is a good chance you will have it again. Women with HG tend to experience nausea into their second trimester, and some will even have it their entire pregnancy.

It is very possible that you will require medical attention with HG in the form of medications and even hospitalization. If you go 24 hours without being able to keep food or water down, or if you feel light-headed or just really ill, call your provider or head to an emergency room.

HG can take a huge emotional toll. It can be draining to feel so rotten for that long. It can also be isolating, as it is difficult to leave the house and do all the things you normally love to do. Lastly, you may be experiencing some degree of unhelpful comments from people who don't really understand the extent to which you are suffering:

"Yeah, I threw up a few times when I was pregnant, too."

"Well, at least you know it's a baby that's causing it and not an illness."

"It's in your head. Just try to distract yourself."

Thanks, guys.

There is light, though, mama. This will get better. You will be able to e-a-t again, and life will return to normal. Until then, do not be afraid to advocate for yourself. Get the medical treatment you need and take care of your mental health as well. If you feel depressed or like hurting yourself, call a therapist or 911 right away.

For ideas on some general nausea remedies, see "Nausea and Vomiting" on page 442.

Intrauterine Growth Restriction (*IUGR*)

IUGR is when the developing fetus is growing at a slower rate than normal. It can be noticed first when a provider feels your uterus and baby through your belly, but it is diagnosed officially with an ultrasound. Causes of IUGR can be wide ranging:

- Placenta issues that prevent enough nutrients from reaching the baby
- High blood pressure
- Infections (mother or baby)
- Genetic or organ problems in baby
- Smoking during pregnancy
- Exposure to high levels of radiation
- Exposure to drugs during pregnancy
- Multiple pregnancies

IUGR can either be symmetrical (the baby's body is small all over) or asymmetrical (only the abdomen is smaller than normal).

If you are diagnosed with IUGR, you and your baby will be closely monitored. It is possible that your provider will recommend induction and early delivery if it appears that your baby will be healthier on the outside than they are on the inside. But it is also possible to carry an IUGR pregnancy to full term. It all depends on your specific scenario.

Iron-Deficiency Anemia

During pregnancy, your blood volume increases by up to 45 percent. This commonly causes a drop in your levels of iron, which is required to make hemoglobin, the protein that helps your red blood cells transport oxygen to your cells. Most cases of iron-deficiency anemia are easy to treat with nutrition and supplements. You may not even notice the telltale sign of fatigue, since that's also the hallmark of pregnancy. If you eat meat, increasing the amount you consume is the easiest way to boost your iron. Choosing more beans, chicken, fish, eggs, and fortified grains will also up your hemoglobin. See more about iron-deficiency anemia in "Pump That Iron" on page 199.

Listeriosis

Listeria is a kind of bacteria that is found in some contaminated foods like uncooked meats and vegetables, raw milk, and processed foods. This is why your provider cautioned you against eating soft cheese, deli meats, raw fish, and any food that may not have been properly handled, cooked, or refrigerated. Pregnant women are more susceptible to getting infected by listeria, which causes listeriosis. Watch for flu-like symptoms (vomiting, headaches, and nausea) and consult your provider if you experience any of these. Early antibiotic treatment can prevent complications like premature birth and infant infection.

Multiple Babies

Certain complications will be more common in a multiple pregnancy, including:

- Preterm labor, which occurs before the 37th week of gestation
- Anemia
- Gestational diabetes, which causes an increase in blood glucose levels during pregnancy
- Gestational hypertension
- Preeclampsia
- Hyperemesis gravidarum
- Polyhydramnios, which is the accumulation of too much amniotic fluid in the uterus
- Miscarriage
- Stillbirth
- Vanishing twin syndrome, when one or more babies dies in the womb, but one baby survives
- Postpartum depression
- Postpartum hemorrhage

Multiples are more likely to be born prematurely and to have neonatal health problems that require them to stay in the hospital longer than singletons. They are often born with lower birth weight, may grow more slowly, and may have a higher chance of birth defects. Yet most healthy multiples have just the same needs as single babies. It's the parents who may require more rest and support, so it will be essential for you to plan and assemble your village to help. See "Twins, Triplets, and Beyond" on page 117 for more information.

Oligohydramnios

Oligohydramnios occurs when there is too little amniotic fluid surrounding the fetus.

It is diagnosed by ultrasound and occurs in about 4 percent of pregnancies. Causes can include a slowly leaking amniotic sac, a pregnancy that has gone past its due date, intrauterine growth restriction (see page 463), a birth defect in the baby that makes it harder for them to make urine (which results in less amniotic fluid), problems with the placenta, maternal blood pressure issues, and maternal dehydration.

Too little amniotic fluid can lead to an increased risk of preterm delivery, growth restriction for the baby, and decreased amounts of oxygen getting to the baby because the umbilical cord does not have enough liquid to float around in and thus gets compressed.

Sometimes, a simple bag of IV fluid to rehydrate does the trick. It is also possible to insert fluid through amniocentesis. In labor, oligohydramnios can be managed with something called an amnioinfusion, where fluid is put into the uterus through a small tube inserted through the opening in the cervix. Depending on how far along the pregnancy is, the providers may recommend induction of labor.

Pelvic Girdle Pain

Pelvic girdle pain (PGP) is the broad term used to describe pain in the joints of the pelvis. The hormone relaxin helps to relax your pelvis so that your baby can fit through during birth: This is a good thing, but it can also lead to pain and potential injury, which can be quite unpleasant. In addition to the impact of relaxin, your pelvis is stressed by the weight of your growing uterus and baby. All of this can lead to an achy pelvis (and an unhappy mama).

There are two types of PGP:

- **Sacroiliac Joint Dysfunction (SJD)** The sacroiliac joint connects the pelvis to the spine. You may have pain in your lower back, on one or both sides, and it may travel down your leg or legs.

- **Symphysis Pubis Dysfunction (SPD)** At the front of the pelvis, two bones and ligaments are connected to a joint made of cartilage, called the symphysis pubis. With all the changes going on with the pelvis, this space usually widens a bit, and sometimes too far, in a condition called symphysis pubis dysfunction (or separated symphysis). SPD can cause back pain as well as pain in the front of your pelvis and between your legs. Movement often makes it worse.

PGP is relatively common among pregnant women, but that does not mean you just need to endure it. Let your provider know about any discomfort you're experiencing. They can refer you to a physical therapist (which may be covered by insurance) who can help treat it and prevent it from getting worse.

Other ideas to try include wearing a maternity support belt, ice packs (apply for 20 minutes at a time, up to four times per day), sleeping on your side with a pillow between your legs, and receiving care from an experienced prenatal massage therapist, chiropractor, or acupuncturist.

And don't forget to check the "Move" section in each chapter to learn how to strengthen your core and pelvic floor safely. That will help too.

Pica

If you find that you are craving foods with no nutritional value, primarily nonfood items, you might have pica. Common cravings include ice, chalk, paper, tissue, dirt, paint chips, toothpaste, coffee grounds, and soap, though this list can go on and on. As many as 1 in 4 pregnant women will experience pica.

It's suspected that pica may be caused by deficiencies in iron and other vitamins. So, if you are having these cravings, let your provider know. They can help you assess your diet and iron levels and see if adjustments are necessary. It is also important to avoid acting on the cravings as much as possible. Eating non-food materials can expose you and your baby to unhealthy toxins and bacteria. Even chewing ice can damage your teeth. This one may feel embarrassing to talk about but remember that it is common and not your fault, and there is help.

Polyhydramnios

Polyhydramnios occurs when there is too much amniotic fluid. It is diagnosed by an ultrasound, and occurs in up to 2 percent of pregnancies. Causes of polyhydramnios can include gestational diabetes, a pregnancy with multiples, a birth defect in the baby that makes it harder for them to process the amniotic fluid normally, infections, and Rh incompatibility.

Women with polyhydramnios are at a higher risk of preterm birth, prolapsed cord, the water breaking early, hemorrhage after birth, and issues with the placenta. When polyhydramnios is diagnosed, providers first try to find out the underlying cause because often when that is addressed, the fluid level normalizes. It is also possible to release some of the extra fluid through the amniocentesis procedure. Depending on how severe the polyhydramnios is, the medical team will make a recommendation about continuing with the pregnancy or inducing labor early.

Postterm Pregnancy

See chapter 15, "Beyond 40 Weeks."

Preeclampsia

Preeclampsia is a condition that only occurs in pregnancy and happens in about 3 to 5 percent of pregnancies. It usually develops after the 20-week mark. The hallmark of preeclampsia is elevated blood pressure along with protein in your urine. The protein is detected by a quick pee-in-a-cup test at your provider's office, or possibly by a 24-hour urine collection.

The normal blood pressure of a pregnant woman should be around 120/80. The severity of preeclampsia depends on the specific blood pressure numbers (abnormal blood pressures need to be present twice, at least 4 hours apart, to confirm diagnosis) and whether or not other concerning factors are present (such as other symptoms or worrisome blood tests). Your provider will make this diagnosis.

There are many theories about what causes preeclampsia; unfortunately, we're still not exactly sure of the cause. However, scientists have discovered that there is a connection to proteins made and released into the woman's bloodstream by her placenta. There are a few factors that increase the risk of developing this condition:

- History of high blood pressure prior to pregnancy
- First pregnancies
- Women with a family history of preeclampsia
- Women who have had preeclampsia in the past

- Multiple pregnancies
- Women with a BMI over 30
- Women under the age of 20 or over the age of 40
- New sperm source (that is, a new partner or sperm donor)

In many cases, women find out they have preeclampsia at a regular prenatal appointment when their blood pressure is found to be high. There are some symptoms to look out for, including:

- Headaches
- Changes in your vision
- Dizziness or light-headedness
- Tiredness
- Nausea and vomiting
- Sharp pain in your upper right belly
- Difficulty breathing (call 911 in this case)
- Decreased urine

If you have any of these symptoms, call your provider right away.

Preeclampsia can cause damage to a woman's kidneys, liver, and other organs. It can also affect the placenta, which could cause harm to the baby. In extremely rare cases, preeclampsia can evolve into eclampsia, where a woman experiences seizures. In rare instances, women can also develop HELLP syndrome (see page 461).

The only cure for preeclampsia is giving birth. Some women may be given medication to control their blood pressure, but this won't cure the condition.

Depending on how far along you are in your pregnancy, you may be given steroids to help your baby's lungs develop faster, so they're ready to be born sooner. You and your medical team may decide that it's safer for the baby to be born than to continue the pregnancy with preeclampsia. Your baby may need to spend some time in the NICU if they are born early.

In severe cases of preeclampsia, in order to prevent seizures, women are given a medication through an IV called magnesium sulfate before and during labor, as well as for the first day after. Magnesium sulfate can make you feel pretty crummy, unfortunately, but your nurses and provider will be keeping a very close eye on you to make sure you're safe.

One note: It is possible to have a totally normal pregnancy and develop postpartum preeclampsia, or extended episodes of high blood pressure after you give birth. It usually occurs within 48 hours of giving birth, though it can happen up to 6 weeks after. If you experience any of the symptoms listed above, call your provider immediately.

Preterm Prelabor Rupture of Membranes (PPROM)

PPROM is when the water breaks before the 37th week of pregnancy. Symptoms are usually the same as term rupture of membranes (see "Water Breaking" on page 239).

The concern with PPROM is the risk for infection (since the protective layer of the membranes is broken) and problems with the placenta (such as an abruption; see "Placental Abruption" on page 474). In 57 percent of the cases, the baby is born within a week of PPROM, so there is a chance for prematurity depending on the timing (see "Preterm Labor and Premature Babies" on page 242).

Treatment will depend on many factors, such as how far along you are in your pregnancy and whether there are any other complications and risk factors present. There is a chance that you will need to be hospitalized and monitored closely, and your provider may recommend medication to help the baby's lungs mature in the event that birth will occur prematurely, as well as antibiotics to prevent infection.

It is also possible (though very rare) that membranes can rupture before the pregnancy is considered viable, which is of course, incredibly difficult. If this happens to you, join us in chapter 4 for some support.

PUPPP

Otherwise known as pruritic urticarial papules and plaques of pregnancy (and sometimes called polymorphic eruption of pregnancy, or PEP), this is an incredibly itchy rash that can develop on your belly, thighs, arms, and bottom and usually starts during the third trimester. When you report intense itching to your provider, the first thing they will do is make sure that you don't have cholestasis, which is potentially dangerous. If it is "just" PUPPP, the good news is that it is harmless to you and your baby, but that doesn't mean that it is easy to deal with.

Treating PUPPP is all about minimizing your discomfort, and you may have to experiment with some options to find what works best for you. Your provider may prescribe a steroid cream. You can also try lotions; fragrance-free and mild is usually your best bet to avoid further aggravating the skin. A few to try might be coconut oil, shea butter, or aloe. Oatmeal baths can also feel soothing on irritated skin, as can placing ice packs on the irritated areas (just don't put ice directly on your skin, and apply for only about 15 to 20

minutes, or until it gets uncomfortable). Take heart: Your PUPPP should go away on its own when your little pup arrives.

Rhesus (Rh) Factor Incompatibility
See "About Rhesus (Rh) Factor" on page 178.

Toxoplasmosis
There's a potential pathogen lurking in some cat waste that can cause a rare but serious blood infection. Cat owners may develop immunity to toxoplasma, but pregnant women are more susceptible to it. It can also be transmitted through having contact with infected raw meat, gardening without gloves (see "Gardening During Pregnancy" on page 133), and eating unwashed produce. A good practice is to have someone else deal with cat litter throughout the duration of your pregnancy, keep cats off counters, and be vigilant about hygiene. Toxoplasmosis in the first and second trimesters has been linked to premature birth, low birth weight, fever, jaundice, and abnormalities of the retina and brain. Since symptoms aren't usually evident, it's important that your provider address your risk of toxoplasmosis, identify any existing infection, and treat it with a long course of antibiotics. See "Pets" on page 164 for more info on handling cats and other pets safely.

Thyroid Issues
The thyroid is a gland in the neck that controls your metabolism, the process by which your body converts food into energy. All of the changes that occur during pregnancy can make you more at risk to experience thyroid-related problems. There are two concerns: when your thyroid does not make

enough metabolism-controlling hormones, it is called hypothyroidism, and when it makes too much, it is called hyperthyroidism.

Symptoms of hypothyroidism may include:

- Feeling cold
- Fatigue
- Difficulty concentrating
- Swelling
- Dry skin
- Cramps
- Weight gain

(As you can see, these are almost all symptoms associated with pregnancy, so you may not suspect that anything is wrong.)

Symptoms of hyperthyroidism may include:

- Feeling hot
- Rapid heart rate
- Weight loss
- Trouble sleeping
- Nervousness

Thyroid issues can cause complications with your pregnancy. The good news is that they can be easily treated with medication, so definitely speak with your provider if you have any concerns.

Yeast Infections

Yeast infections, also called candidiasis, occur when the yeast that normally exists in and around the vagina begins to grow too much. Yeast infections often lead to vaginal itching or burning, painful urination and sex, and vaginal discharge that looks white and chunky, kind of like cottage cheese.

Yeast infections are generally not considered dangerous, but they are super-annoying. There are over-the-counter remedies available, but it is always a good idea to check in with your provider first to confirm that it really is a yeast infection and not something that requires a different type of treatment.

Of note, the CDC recommends that when pregnant women use antifungal medication creams and ointments, they choose the 7-day course to minimize the concentration of each dose.

There are a number of natural treatments for yeast infections that some women prefer: tea tree oil, probiotics, yogurt, and garlic, to name a few. Unfortunately, these methods are currently understudied, so it is hard to say how effective they are.

It is possible to pass a yeast infection on to your baby during birth, who might then develop thrush (see "Thrush (Candida or Yeast Infection)" on page 400).

Check out "Taking Care of Your Vagina During Pregnancy" on page 104 for pointers on how to prevent yeast infections during pregnancy.

Of note, it is also possible to get yeast infections on your skin (such as under your breasts). If you have itching or a rash, let your provider know. They can likely prescribe an antifungal cream.

Zika

Zika is a virus transmitted through mosquito bites or having sex with someone who has Zika. It can also be passed from a woman to her growing fetus. Symptoms of Zika include fever, headaches, joint pain, muscle aches, and rashes, but it is also possible to not have any symptoms. Zika itself is not usually too dangerous for adults. But if passed on to a developing fetus, it can cause miscarriage, stillbirth, birth defects, and congenital Zika syndrome. Zika has been linked to microcephaly, a rare neurological condition in which the baby is born with a smaller head and possibly a smaller brain and other developmental disorders. Unfortunately, there is no known cure for Zika at the time of writing this book.

There are areas of the world with much higher rates of Zika, so women who are pregnant or may become pregnant are encouraged not to travel to those areas—this goes for the person with the sperm as well. If you, your partner, or your sperm donor has traveled to high-risk areas, it is recommended that you wait 3 months before trying to conceive, to ensure that no one has Zika. Since these high-risk areas can change, your best bet is to check with your provider and the CDC website to see what the current recommendations are and to get more information about testing.

If you live in an area that is high risk for Zika, prevention is key. To avoid mosquito bites, wear long sleeves, long pants, socks, and hats; avoid going outside during sunset; consider sleeping under mosquito netting; and talk to your provider about the best bug repellent to use. DEET has not been found to cause problems in fetuses.

If you have been diagnosed with Zika, it is likely that you will have additional prenatal testing to monitor the fetus.

SEXUALLY TRANSMITTED INFECTIONS DURING PREGNANCY

Sexually transmitted infections (STIs) (also called sexually transmitted diseases, or STDs) are on the rise in the US—by quite a lot. Syphilis, for example, has seen a 76 percent increase since 2013. That means that we all have to take STIs seriously.

STIs are just like any other infection in the body—the presence of an unwanted bacteria or virus. The difference with STIs is that they also come along with social implications that are generally unpleasant and hard to deal with. There can be stigma or embarrassment, and in the case of a partnership, the potential that one of the members has had sex outside of that partnership. Remember that this does not necessarily mean someone cheated: An STI may have been acquired before you ever met each other. In addition, STIs in the context of pregnancy can be even tougher to deal with because they can be passed on to the baby, sometimes leading to serious consequences.

In short, STIs are their own kind of stressful.

So here is what we are going to do—together, and without judgment. Let's break down the steps and handle them one at a time:

1 Take a deep breath. I know, I know, that's annoying right now. But mama, you have to take care of your whole self right now, and the first step is to take a deep breath and send yourself some love.

2 Try not to be shy. It can feel uncomfortable to have these conversations with medical providers, but to the extent that you can, the more honest you are, the better they will be able to help you. You should be treated with respect, no matter your concern.

3 If you have not yet been diagnosed and are in the "Do I have an STI?" stage, get tested right away. It is normal to be nervous about the potential results you'll receive, but the sooner you know, the sooner you can get treated, thus reducing the risk to you and your baby. You can go to your doctor or midwife for testing or find a clinic nearby (like Planned Parenthood) that can offer same-day and low-cost appointments and testing.

4 Once you have a diagnosis, follow through with the treatment plan, which is often a one-time dose of medication.

5 If you have a partner, or people you have sex with, they need to know so that they can be tested and treated—for their sake and yours—because they can reinfect you if you have sex with them again and they are untreated. This is a tough conversation, no doubt. If you are nervous about your safety while having it, consider broaching the subject either in a public space where you feel safe or while talking in the presence of a counselor or medical provider.

6 Avoid sex again until you know that you and your partners are infection-free.

7 Depending on the infection type, there may be additional recommendations to minimize the risk for the baby.

8 Once the medical side of things is checked off, you might have more mental bandwidth to deal with the social implications (which may or may not exist, depending on your scenario). Remember that counseling is available for individuals and couples, and it may be incredibly helpful if this is a stressful time for you.

If you believe the test is not accurate, you can always request a repeat test. Mistakes can happen.

One more thing about STIs: It is important to know that they can be transmitted during all types of sex (vaginal, oral, and anal) and can be transmitted whether you have sex with women or men. Also, ejaculation does not need to occur in order to pass on an STI. Many women, pregnant and not, choose to ask their parters to use condoms to significantly decrease their risk of getting an STI.

Chlamydia

Chlamydia is a common STI, with an estimated 1.7 million cases in the US in 2017. Chlamydia is caused by a bacteria, and if left untreated, it can result in pelvic inflammatory disease (see "Pelvic Inflammatory Disease (PID)" on page 473), ectopic pregnancies (see "Ectopic Pregnancy" on page 57), and infertility in women or prostate issues in men. Chlamydia is tough to diagnose without testing because less than 30 percent of women and 10 percent of men have symptoms, so it often goes unnoticed and untreated. This is why your provider may recommend yearly screening. If you do have symptoms, they may include vaginal discharge, a cervix that bleeds easily, painful urination, and pelvic pain.

Chlamydia can be passed to a baby during birth, and the baby may be at risk for pneumonia and eye infections. Chlamydia is easily treated with antibiotics.

Genital Warts and HPV

Genital warts are painless (though sometimes itchy) white or skin-colored bumps that appear around your genital area. They are often described as looking like cauliflower. Genital warts may develop months or years after exposure to a strain of the human papillomavirus, or HPV, which is an STI that affects up to 80 percent of people. Genital warts are usually not considered dangerous, though they are contagious. They often go away on their own or can be removed using surgical, freezing, or laser techniques.

HPV is not likely dangerous for your growing baby; it is rare that it can be passed on to the baby. The concern with HPV is that some of the variations of the virus (known as strains) can cause the cells of the cervix to mutate and become cancerous. The strain that causes genital warts is not usually the strain that causes cancer in the cervix, vagina, vulva, anus, penis, throat, or mouth.

Many times, HPV resolves on its own, with no threat of cancer or other concerns.

With any history of HPV, it is important to have routine pap smears so that if the cervical cells start to become worrisome, they can be detected and treated (see "Pap Smears" on page 453 for more on abnormal pap smears during pregnancy).

There is an HPV vaccine available, though it is not recommended during pregnancy.

Gonorrhea

Gonorrhea is another common STI that occurs in adults. Men may have discharge from their penises and painful urination. Unfortunately, most women with gonorrhea do not have symptoms, which means that infection can be overlooked. Symptoms might include vaginal bleeding, vaginal discharge, and painful urination. You may also have rectal discharge, rectal bleeding, and painful bowel movements if the infection is in your rectum.

Gonorrhea during pregnancy can lead to the water breaking early, inducing early labor, and it can also infect the amniotic fluid and cause eye infections in the baby. Gonorrhea is treatable with an antibiotic, and early treatment minimizes the risk for the baby and you.

Hepatitis

While hepatitis is often a sexually transmitted infection, there are other ways it can be passed to someone that do not involve sex. Hepatitis infections consist of three strains: A, B, and C. They are all a viral infection of the liver, and are passed on through bodily secretions like semen, blood, feces, vaginal discharge, and urine.

Hepatitis B

We are concerned about all forms of hepatitis during pregnancy, but hepatitis B gets the most attention. If a mother is diagnosed with hepatitis B, she has a 90 percent chance of passing it on to her newborn unless treatment is given immediately at birth. This is why it is recommended that all pregnant women are tested for the disease. Read more about hepatitis B on page 276.

Hepatitis B vaccinations are also recommended for all newborns. If you have concerns, speak to your baby's provider about them for the best and most personalized guidance. (See "Hepatitis B Vaccine" on page 276.)

Herpes

Herpetic lesions can occur in the vagina or on the cervix, vulva, anus, and even thighs and buttocks. If a mother is infected with the herpes virus before or during the first part of pregnancy, she has a very low chance of passing it along to the baby. If a woman is infected later in pregnancy, her immune system will not have created antibodies to protect herself and her baby from the virus. Herpes in infants can be serious, so be sure that you and your sexual partners are not infected or are being treated before baby is born.

If you have herpes, your provider will likely prescribe antiviral medications to take daily starting at 36 weeks to minimize the risk of having an open lesion during your birth. If you have a lesion in an area that the baby could come into contact with, you will likely need to have a C-section so that the baby does not come into contact with the lesion on the way through the birth canal.

Herpes lesions can also appear on and around the mouth as cold sores. It is important to know that the virus can be transmitted when someone has an active cold sore, so people with one should not kiss your baby.

HIV

If a pregnant woman is HIV positive, the risk of transmitting the virus to her baby is reduced if she is able to stay healthy. However, the virus can be passed along to the baby in utero, during birth, and while breastfeeding. New medications can reduce the risk of passing the virus to just 2 percent or less. ACOG recommends that women with HIV can have vaginal births if their viral load is sufficiently low after treatment, and scheduled C-sections before the onset of labor are recommended for women with high viral loads. Newborns can also receive antiretrovirals after birth to lessen the risk of contracting HIV.

Pelvic Inflammatory Disease (PID)

If an STI goes untreated, it can sometimes lead to pelvic inflammatory disease, or PID. Essentially, the bacteria from the STI make their way farther up the reproductive tract, infecting more areas of the pelvis. Symptoms of PID may include fever, lower abdominal pain, painful sex and urination, abnormal vaginal discharge, and vaginal bleeding, though it is also possible not to have symptoms. PID can lead to infertility, ectopic pregnancies, and severe infections that require hospitalization. While uncommon in pregnancy, pregnant women with PID may be more likely to have a preterm birth or may become sicker from the infection. The good news is that PID is treatable with antibiotics, and if caught early, can resolve quickly.

Syphilis

Syphilis is an STI that occurs in phases when untreated. In the first phase, you may notice a chancre on your genital area, which is a painless, hard, little sore. The second phase can bring sores on your feet and palms, as well as fever, weight loss, hair loss, swollen lymph nodes, and fatigue. Syphilis then goes into its latent phase, in which you will have no symptoms; this can last for years. The last phase of syphilis is called the late phase, and it is serious. It can cause problems with your brain, spinal cord, heart, and eyes.

Syphilis during pregnancy can cause problems such as miscarriage and stillbirth, preterm birth, and issues with the placenta and umbilical cord, but when women get treatment before 26 weeks in pregnancy, the babies usually do well.

The very good news is that syphilis is very easily treated: Just one injection of an antibiotic usually does the trick.

Trichomoniasis

Trichomoniasis, sometimes called "trick," is an STI caused by a parasite (it can also rarely be transmitted in nonsexual ways, like from towels and clothing). Only about 30 percent of people with trichomoniasis have symptoms, which might include genital itching, burning, pain, and vaginal or penile discharge. One of the concerns with trichomoniasis is that it can make the tissue in the vagina fragile, which puts you at a higher risk for getting other STIs, such as HIV. If trichomoniasis occurs during pregnancy, there is a higher risk for preterm delivery and low-birth-weight babies. Prompt treatment is important, with a medication taken by mouth.

PLACENTAL ISSUES

Low-Lying Placenta

A low-lying placenta has an edge that is within 2 centimeters of the cervix but doesn't actually cover the cervix. Sometimes they are treated just like previas, though it may also be possible to safely have a vaginal birth with a low-lying placenta.

If you have a low-lying placenta or placenta previa, your provider may advise you not to have sex or put anything in your vagina and to avoid many types of exercise, such as running and squatting.

Placenta Attachment Problems

Rarely the placenta attaches too deeply to the uterus. There are three types of this attachment:

Placenta Accreta   The placenta normally attaches to the surface of the uterine wall, but with this condition, it grows into the wall.

Placenta Increta   The placenta grows into the uterine muscles.

Placenta Percreta   The placenta grows through the uterine wall.

These can all be dangerous complications because after the baby is born, the placenta cannot detach from the uterus normally, causing a lot of bleeding. This leads to some of the same complications as a retained placenta (see "Retained Placenta" on page 475). Cesarean section is usually recommended as the mode of delivery. Depending on the severity of the particular situation, the entire uterus may need to be removed, though your provider will certainly avoid this when at all possible.

Placenta Previa

Normally the placenta attaches to the uterus somewhere in the upper half, but occasionally it attaches much lower and covers part or all of the cervix (the opening of the uterus, which dilates). This is diagnosed with an ultrasound. An obstructed cervix is troublesome because it physically blocks the baby from passing through during birth and puts you at a higher risk for bleeding. As the lower part of the uterus and the cervix thin in labor, it can cause the placenta to bleed.

Some women are diagnosed with placenta previa during the anatomy scan ultrasound around 20 weeks, but it resolves itself in 90 percent of women. As the uterus grows, the location of the placenta moves up, and things can proceed normally. If it doesn't, Cesarean sections are necessary for giving birth. If you have placenta previa, your provider may advise you not to have sex or put anything in your vagina and to avoid many types of exercise, like running and squatting.

Placental Abruption

This is when the placenta completely or partially detaches from the uterine wall. The concern here is that the placenta cannot provide oxygen to the baby if it is not getting oxygen from the uterus. There is also a risk for heavy bleeding. Symptoms may include vaginal bleeding, frequent uterus contractions, general belly tightening, and belly or back pain. Placental abruption usually results in an emergency Cesarean section.

Placental Infarction

In a placental infarction, blood supply to one area of the placenta is cut off, causing the placental cells in that area to die. A small infarct is often nothing to worry about. A large one, or one that is in the middle of the placenta, could limit the blood supply to that area and lead to placental insufficiency (see next entry, "Placental Insufficiency"). Infarcts can occur with preeclampsia or hypertension or on their own.

Placental Insufficiency

Placental insufficiency occurs when the placenta is not able to provide the baby with all of the oxygen and nutrients they need to grow and thrive in utero. Sometimes this can be caused by a placenta that does not develop properly or by a number of pregnancy complications, such as preeclampsia, diabetes, and anemia, as well as factors such as smoking and drug use and going past your due date. If the baby is not getting what they need from the placenta, they may show slowed growth or a decrease in their movement, but it is also possible that there will be no symptoms.

If placental insufficiency is suspected, your provider may recommend additional tests to check on the baby's well-being. They may decide that induction of labor (see "Induction of Labor" on page 301) is the safest option for both of you.

Retained Placenta

Rarely, a piece or all of the placenta stays inside the uterus instead of being expelled during the third stage of labor (see chapter 20, "Third Stage of Labor: Giving Birth to the Placenta"). If the placenta has not been delivered within 30 minutes, it will be considered retained, and intervention will be required to prevent infection, hemorrhage, and other complications. Your provider may be able to manually remove the placenta with their hand. Sometimes peeing can help because a full bladder may prevent the uterus from contracting properly to release the placenta. Medication may also be used. If none of these work, a surgical procedure may be required.

Succenturiate Lobe

A succenturiate lobe is a small piece of placenta that grows apart from the main placenta; this can also be called an accessory lobe. The presence of the lobe is usually not a problem in itself, but it can increase the risk of other problems, like a vasa previa (see next entry, "Vasa Previa"). It's also possible that the lobe becomes detached during birth, so it will be important for your provider to do a detailed assessment of the placenta after birth.

Vasa Previa

In vasa previa, some of the fetus's umbilical blood vessels run across or near the cervix, without the protection of the umbilical cord. The worry with a vasa previa is that during labor, the vessels can be damaged, which would result in significant blood loss. When a vasa previa is detected during pregnancy, a C-section is recommended as the optimal mode of delivery.

Velamentous Cord Insertion

Velamentous cord insertion means that the blood vessels that are normally protected by the umbilical cord run through the membranes of the amniotic sac instead of connecting directly into the placenta via the umbilical cord. This means that the vessels are exposed and could be damaged, which would result in significant bleeding. This could happen, for example, if the amniotic sac were to break, since the vessels are within that membrane.

Velamentous cord insertions can be discovered on ultrasounds. If one is found, your provider will recommend an increase in monitoring, and depending on where the vessels are, a C-section may be necessary.

UMBILICAL CORD ISSUES

Single Umbilical Artery

Most umbilical cords contain two arteries and one vein. Occasionally, in less than 1 percent of singleton pregnancies and less than 5 percent of twin pregnancies, an ultrasound will discover that an umbilical cord has only one artery. If this is the only abnormal finding, there is a good chance that it will not impact the baby. About 20 percent of the time, a single umbilical artery can represent a genetic problem or a structural problem in the baby's renal, cardiac, nervous, or digestive systems. If a single umbilical artery is found, your provider may recommend additional testing to see if there is an underlying condition. If identified, treatment will vary depending on the diagnosis.

Umbilical Cord Cyst

This is a little sac of fluid on the umbilical cord, sometimes identified by ultrasounds. Cysts may be present in up to 3 percent of all umbilical cords. Sometimes they go away on their own, though some are related to genetic conditions in the baby. If a genetic disorder is suspected, your provider may recommend additional testing to explore underlying causes. In the case of an umbilical cord cyst, C-section may be the preferred mode of birth, as there is less of a chance of injury to the cyst, which could cause problems for the baby during birth.

Umbilical Cord Knot

Sometimes, as the fetus is flipping around in the uterus, they can tie the umbilical cord into a knot. A jellylike substance called Wharton's jelly coats the umbilical cord and makes it slippery, which means that usually the knot does not become too tight. If it does become tight, it could decrease oxygen flow to your baby. You might start to feel less movement from your baby (see "Kick Counts" on page 178). If so, head to the hospital right away. If an abnormal heart rate is detected, an emergency C-section may be recommended.

BIRTH COMPLICATIONS

This is a reminder that this book is your guide to use as you see fit. None of this is required reading, especially the following section. Take a minute to check in with yourself. Are you most relaxed when you have all of the possible information? Then, carry on, mama. But if intense medical situations make you uncomfortable, consider skipping this next bit.

Ultimately, here is what you need to know. Birth complications happen, but they are rare; many of them are exceptionally rare. Your provider and team have been trained extensively in how to manage these, and improved interventions are continually being developed. If you have specific concerns about your risk for any of these complications, speak with your provider.

Amniotic Fluid Embolism (AFE)

In this incredibly rare complication (approximately 1 out of 40,000 pregnancies in North America), amniotic fluid (or sometimes fetal hair or cells) enters the mother's bloodstream.

This triggers a severe reaction in the mother's body that can cause life-threatening cardiac and respiratory problems. Symptoms include a sudden feeling of anxiety, difficulty breathing, nausea, and changes in the fetal heart rate. We do not currently know what the exact risk factors for AFE are.

If an AFE is diagnosed, the baby will likely be delivered via emergency C-section, and

WHEN YOUR BABY NEEDS NICU CARE

Seeing your baby in the neonatal intensive care unit (NICU) may be overwhelming or shocking. They may be intubated (where a small tube is inserted through their mouth to help them breathe) and wired to machines. If your baby is premature, their skin will be translucent and thin and possibly covered with fine hair. Seeing a tiny being in such a state can trigger difficult feelings. Bring someone you can rely on to support your emotional state and comfort you.

If your infant is premature, they will likely receive all of their fluids by IV for the first bit of time, and they will probably need to remain in an incubator. When the time comes, baby will start being fed breast milk or formula through a tube, and it's something you can get involved in. Skin-to-skin contact is incredibly important, and this practice, known as kangaroo care, is becoming more and more common, especially for premature babies. Studies show that it can help babies gain weight faster and stabilize their heart rate, and ultimately, these babies go home sooner than babies who remain clothed or spend most of their time in an incubator.

There will be times when you can't hold your baby, but you may be permitted to touch them, and you can always sing or talk to them so that your voice becomes familiar and comforting. They'll take in all those good vibes.

Don't be afraid to ask questions until you understand what is going on with your baby's health and care. Medical terminology can be confusing, and doctors and nurses can be busy. You should feel empowered to get the information you need to make decisions about your baby's treatment.

It is not easy to go through the anxiety and uncertainty of a NICU stay, and the health community is finding that many parents who have NICU experiences emerge with a need for more mental health support and sometimes even post-traumatic stress interventions. If you and your family are having a tough time during or after a NICU stay, it's very important to reach out to your providers and let them know so that you can get proper support. Many hospitals offer support groups for parents of NICU babies.

medical support will be provided to the woman and baby. Distressingly, AFEs can often be fatal for the woman and the baby, though research is underway to develop better understanding of this horrible complication and to find more treatment options.

Birth Asphyxia

Birth asphyxia is a rare complication that means that the baby's brain did not receive enough oxygen at the time of birth, which can lead to a condition called hypoxic ischemic encephalopathy. It can be caused by rare complications such as meconium aspiration (see page 479), umbilical cord prolapse (see page 240), shoulder dystocia (see page 480), prematurity, or other conditions. If a baby experiences asphyxia, they will likely be born limp, quiet, and possibly blue. Your provider will take emergency measures to get the baby breathing. If you are having a home or birth center birth, your midwife has emergency equipment with her to start this process until the baby is transferred to the care of a nearby hospital.

The care depends on the baby's specific conditions and the severity of their symptoms. Some babies have minimal consequences from birth asphyxia, though serious ones are possible, including seizures, brain damage, and death.

Cephalopelvic Disproportion

Cephalopelvic disproportion, CPD, occurs when the baby's head does not fit through the mother's pelvis, either due to the size of the baby's head or the size and shape of the mother's pelvis. Though there are ways to assess the size and shape of a woman's pelvis before she is in labor, CPD is usually diagnosed during labor, when labor does not progress, or when a baby does not move down during pushing.

CPD is tricky, to put it mildly. The American College of Nurse-Midwives has reported that only 1 out of 250 pregnancies has a true CPD in the US (this may vary in different parts of the world). Yet CPD is cited as the most common reason for Cesarean sections. The reality is that many of these C-sections could be unnecessary. The problem is that we don't know whether it was truly necessary until after the baby has been born.

If I may offer a behind-the-scenes look at this: This is a stressful topic for a lot of providers. No one wants to perform an unnecessary C-section. This is a small piece of a larger conversation surrounding the high number of C-sections we see today, one without an easy answer.

In the meantime, if you are worried about or diagnosed with CPD, I would encourage thorough conversation with your provider. Different providers will feel differently about the best way to manage it, so if you have strong preferences, you can work to find someone with whom you align.

Of note, a recent study found that Asian women who have babies with white men have a higher risk of Cesarean section, even though their babies were of a similar weight as those of white women. The study authors suggest that this may be due to smaller than average pelvises among Asian women that may not be able to accommodate larger babies.

When in labor, you might try spending as much time as possible moving, and in an upright position, to encourage the baby to get into the optimal position for birth.

Chorioamnionitis (*or Intra-amniotic Infection*)

Chorioamnionitis is an infection or inflammation of the membranes that make up the bag of water (called the amnion and the chorion). The amniotic fluid, placenta, and umbilical cord can be infected as well. It most often occurs during labor and happens in up to 4 percent of pregnancies. Though it cannot always be predicted, chorioamnionitis is more likely to occur in long labors when the water has been broken for a long time, if the woman receives many vaginal exams, or if she has internal monitoring (see "Internal Monitors" on page 306).

A woman with chorioamnionitis will likely have a fever and elevated heart rate and possibly tenderness at the top of her uterus (the fundus) and foul-smelling amniotic fluid. The baby may also have an elevated heart rate. Chorioamnionitis is diagnosed based on symptoms because taking a sample of amniotic fluid and testing it for infection takes too long and may pose additional risks.

In addition to the risks of infection, chorioamnionitis can make it more likely that a woman will need a Cesarean section because the uterus may not be able to produce contractions that are as effective. For this reason, she may also have an increased risk of postpartum hemorrhage.

If you are diagnosed with chorioamnionitis, your provider will recommend IV antibiotics and close monitoring. When the baby is born, they will be watched closely for signs of infection, though when chorioamnionitis is diagnosed and treated, outcomes tend to be good.

Malposition

See "Baby Positions" on page 198.

Meconium Aspiration

Meconium is the name of a baby's first poop. It resembles tar: black or dark green, sticky, and thick. Sometimes babies will poop before they are born or just as they are being born. This occurs in about 8 percent of full-term births. Oftentimes there is nothing to worry about. My mother loves to tell the story about how green and covered with meconium I was when I was born (sorry, Mom).

If the baby breathes in this meconium, it is called meconium aspiration, which is rare, occurring in less than 0.1 percent of births. If the baby does breathe in the meconium, they can experience difficulty getting enough oxygen and develop an infection. Your baby may require close monitoring in a hospital (either in the nursery or the NICU), where pediatricians will recommend treatments as necessary. Babies with meconium aspiration tend to do well long term.

Precipitous Labor and How to Deliver a Baby

A precipitous birth is a birth that happens very quickly, within 3 hours of the start of regular contractions. They are not common, especially for women having their first babies.

The likelihood of not making it to your birthing place, or your provider not making it to you, is very low. This said, as you'll soon learn from parenthood, it's always good to be prepared.

In the name of preparedness, have your birth partner read the following section too, for good measure.

I know the idea of delivering a baby sounds wild. I still remember how hard I had to focus on keeping my hands from shaking during those first births. But try to stay calm and focused. Mom's body and the baby will do much of the work on their own. Your job is to guide the baby out, so they don't fall. They are a little slippery, but you will be okay.

In the unlikely event that a precipitous birth happens, here is what to do:

1 Call 911 (unless you are planning a home birth, and your provider will arrive shortly). They may arrive after the baby is out but can assist should a complication arise and can escort mom and baby to a medical facility for evaluation.

2 Ensure safety. Pull over if you are driving, for example.

3 Wash your hands if you have time or use hand sanitizer.

4 Take a deep breath.

5 As the baby's head emerges, allow it to come into your hands. Do not pull on the head. You are catching.

6 The baby's shoulders will follow, and the baby's body will likely just come into your hands and forearms. Grasp the baby by the shoulders or upper arms after both shoulders are born and gently guide the baby out.

7 Place the baby on mom's belly and cover them with a dry towel (or shirt or anything cleanish that you can find).

8 Do not cut the umbilical cord.

9 Do not pull on the umbilical cord. The placenta will deliver itself.

Remember, this is for emergencies only. I do not recommend planned unassisted births.

Shoulder Dystocia

Shoulder dystocia is a relatively rare birth complication that occurs in about 1 out of 150 births. Normally, after the head is delivered, the shoulders slip out of the birth canal easily. In a shoulder dystocia, the baby's shoulders get "stuck" on the mother's pelvic bones, and then baby cannot come out right away. The concern with this is that the umbilical cord may be compressed during the time of the dystocia, which means that the baby may get decreased amounts of oxygen.

Another possible complication, which occurs in a small number of dystocias, is a brachial plexus injury, in which nerves in the baby's arm and shoulder are damaged. This usually resolves over time, although permanent injury is possible. Physical therapy can improve outcomes. It is also possible that a baby's arm or collarbone can be broken as the provider works to deliver the baby. I know this sounds scary, mama, but this isn't common, and broken bones usually heal quickly—especially in these little ones.

Shoulder dystocias are obstetric emergencies. A series of maneuvers will be used to move the baby so that the shoulders can pass through. If this happens to you, try to stay as focused as you can on what your provider is saying, as they may ask you to move in specific ways.

When the baby is born, they will likely be immediately evaluated by the provider and may require NICU care.

There are some risk factors for shoulder dystocias: big babies, gestational diabetes, and maternal BMI greater than 30, but more often than not, it is unpredictable.

Umbilical Cord Prolapse

See "Umbilical Cord Prolapse" on page 240.

Umbilical Cord Wrapped Around the Neck (*Nuchal Cord*)

See "Nuchal Cord" on page 262.

Uterine Inversion

An inverted uterus is one that is turned partially or completely inside-out by the placenta as it goes through the cervix. A crude analogy is to think of a pulling a sock inside-out. It is incredibly rare, affecting 2.9 out of 10,000 deliveries. If a uterus inverts, the immediate course of action is for the provider to use their hand to manually return the uterus to its correct position and shape and then administer medications to help the uterus contract. Occasionally, surgery is required to fix it. Again, mama, this is rare.

Uterine Rupture

Uterine rupture is a rare complication in which part of the uterus tears, usually late in pregnancy or during labor. The tear can be very small (sometimes called a window) or large enough that the fetus can actually pass through it into the woman's abdomen. When a uterine rupture occurs, the woman might experience severe pain, vaginal bleeding, and a sudden decrease in contractions, and the monitor will likely show a drop in the baby's heart rate. An emergency C-section will be ordered to deliver the baby and examine the extent of damage to the uterus. In some cases, the uterus must be removed.

Vaginal and Perineal Lacerations (*Tearing*)

Sometimes as a baby is being born, the tissue in a woman's vagina or perineum (the area between the vagina and the anus) tears. For more info on managing the worry of this, see "Tearing" on page 261.

There are four degrees of tearing (first degree and second degree are much more common than third and fourth):

- First degree: The skin of the perineum tears.
- Second degree: The muscle of the perineum tears.
- Third degree: The muscles of the perineum and the muscle around the anus, called the anal sphincter, tear.
- Fourth degree: The tear goes through the anal sphincter and into the rectum. These tears are rare.

POSTPARTUM COMPLICATIONS

Plugged or Clogged Duct

See "Plugged or Clogged Duct" on page 400.

Postoperative Ileus

After any type of abdominal surgery (such as a Cesarean section), there is a small risk for a postoperative ileus, a complication in which the intestines stop moving food along, which could lead to a blockage. Symptoms of an ileus include pain, constipation, inability to pass gas, and nausea and vomiting.

Your medical team will monitor you closely for signs of an ileus; this is why you are not allowed to eat right away following a Cesarean birth. If you do develop an ileus, treatment options include anything from wait and see to surgery. For more about this, see "Cesarean Section Healing" on page 352.

Postpartum Hemorrhage

See "Postpartum Hemorrhage: Warning Signs" on page 350.

Postpartum Infections

Postpartum women have a lowered immune response, which means that infections that go untreated are potentially more serious. If you notice any of the symptoms below, you should contact your provider as soon as possible.

Cellulitis and Wound Infection   It is possible for a C-section incision site to become infected. If this happens, you might have a fever and chills, excessive pain, redness, oozing and pus, or an opening of the wound. Report any of these symptoms right away. Treatment is usually very effective. For more on C-section incisions and infection prevention, see "Cesarean Section Healing" on page 352.

Endometritis   Endometritis is an infection in the uterus. It can bring on fever, chills, or an overall feeling of discomfort. Other symptoms include pain in the lower abdomen or lochia (vaginal discharge) that smells particularly bad.

Mastitis   One breast with a red, painful, hard area along with fever, chills, muscle aches, headache, and fatigue could be signs of mastitis, a breast infection (see "Mastitis" on page 399).

Urinary Tract Infection   Difficult or painful urination, or a feeling of urgency with very little coming out, could be signs of a urinary tract infection (see "Urinary Tract Infections" on page 354).

Spinal Headache

In rare cases, spinal fluid can leak out of the tiny insertion site of spinal or epidural anesthesia (see the diagram "Injection into the Epidural Space" on page 294). This changes the fluid balance and pressure, which can cause very significant headaches. To treat a spinal headache, an anesthesiologist can do a procedure called a blood patch, where they use a small amount of your blood to "patch" the leak, which allows your body to rebalance.

OTHER ISSUES

Chromosomal or Other Congenital Abnormality

If your baby has been diagnosed with a chromosomal or other congenital abnormality, there are a million possible ways you might feel right now—likely a combination of all of them. Worries and thoughts of what comes next may consume you. Visit us at mother.ly /becomingmama for specific articles dealing with these topics.

Stillbirth

If you are reading this section, perhaps you have received unbelievably devastating news.

When a baby dies after the 20th week of pregnancy, before birth, it is called an intrauterine fetal demise (IUFD), or stillbirth. Having helped women who have had IUFDs give birth, I can only begin to imagine what you are going through, and my heart is aching for your loss.

Babies die before birth for a variety of reasons. Some have anomalies that are incompatible with life, such as a chromosomal abnormality. Some are the victims of something that has gone wrong with the pregnancy, such as a tight knot in the umbilical cord. Many times, there are no obvious indications that point to the cause of the death. An autopsy can sometimes point to a reason.

Stillbirth occurs in about 1 percent of pregnancies in the US. Many problems that led to stillbirths in the past are now recognized earlier in pregnancy, and measures are taken to greatly minimize the risk. If you have received news that your baby has died, your provider will discuss options with you, which often includes inducing your labor as soon as possible. Your provider will also discuss with you how you want to handle the actual birth. Do you want to hold the baby for as long as possible? Who do you want in the room with you when you give birth? Do you want an autopsy?

There are often support groups available to help you with your grief, and professional counseling is always available. If you plan to get pregnant again, you will likely be offered testing either before you get pregnant or during the pregnancy to help ensure a healthy outcome.

Termination

The termination of a pregnancy, otherwise called an abortion, reaches into every category of our lives: medical, emotional, psychological, social, familial, financial, spiritual, religious, logistical, and political. All of these factors are intertwined into a complicated and deeply personal story that only you know. Your reasons for being here right now are more complex than can possibly be addressed within these pages, perhaps more complex than any of us can understand in a lifetime. In that complexity can come isolation.

It is so important that no matter where you find yourself on this spectrum of possibilities, you know that you are not alone.

Consider for a few moments what type of support you need right now. Do you need guidance making a decision, or do you need support around a decision that you have made?

Think about what that support needs to feel like; this will be different for everyone. What type of energy do you need to be around? It is okay to seek out people who provide that energy, while distancing yourself from people who tend to reinforce unhealthy response patterns.

Next, decide which types of professionals will be helpful to you. This may include your doctor or midwife, geneticist, social workers, mental health therapist, termination doula, or spiritual guides. Lean on these professionals. Ask for what you need. It is their job and honor to be with you. Seeking out a support group of people who have had similar experiences, whether you choose to terminate or not, can also be incredibly powerful.

Keep in mind that humans are opinionated and often eager to share their opinions. To the extent that you can, remember that only you know the full story and understand the complicated landscape of emotions within you. Don't be afraid to tell people exactly what you need:

"I have decided to terminate the pregnancy. I need you to come with me to my appointments."

"I have made the decision not to terminate the pregnancy, and I need you to support me after I give birth."

If people respond in ways that are unhelpful, unkind, or unsupportive, it is likely a reflection of their own experiences and beliefs, not yours. It is okay to protect yourself emotionally while you feel vulnerable.

Through it all, take care of yourself. You can do this, whatever *this* is.

Writer's Acknowledgments

Rarely at a loss for words, I find myself struggling to find a way to adequately acknowledge all the people who helped bring *Becoming Mama* into the world. It took—and I swear this is true and completely unplanned—exactly 280 days to write this book (which you now know is 40 weeks, the length of a full-term pregnancy). This is wildly appropriate, as gestating and giving birth to this book has been one of the most meaningful experiences of my life. And through it all, I have been surrounded by a "birth team" for whom I will be forever grateful.

To begin, this book—and all the wonder that is Motherly—started because two women had an idea. From the inspiration, tireless work, and loving guidance of founders Jill Koziol and Liz Tenety, Motherly was born. Motherly is more than a brand; it is a way of life, and I am deeply honored to have been on this journey with them and the fantastic team they have assembled. In addition to making the magic of Motherly happen daily, the fiercely talented and dedicated group at #TeamMotherly contributed their ideas, support, and time to make this book a reality.

The shining star from #TeamMotherly on this book-creating adventure has been Anne-Marie Gambelin, without whom I would have been completely lost. Her intelligence, creativity, work ethic, passion, and warmth buoyed this entire process from day one, and I am eternally grateful for her efforts and presence in my life.

And to Anne Hill, Motherly's Art Director, I am forever in awe of your talent and vision, and so incredibly grateful that you unleashed those superpowers on *Becoming Mama*.

I am not sure how I got lucky enough to be under the wing of such a rock-star publishing group composed of Jaime Schwalb and the entire Sounds True team and my fabulous editors, Jessica Carew Kraft and Rachel Lehmann-Haupt, but I will take it. I can never thank them enough for all they have done.

Thank you to Andrea Barzvi for all her invaluable guidance in helping us to ensure that this book reaches as many women as possible and positively impacts their motherhood journeys.

When I found out that Stepha Lawson agreed to illustrate *Becoming Mama*, I cried. Her art is magic, and it has elevated the entire experience of this book.

I am truly humbled when I look at the list of experts who have contributed their knowledge, time, and art to this book. Thank you for joining me on this mission to redefine pregnancy and empower women.

To the Motherly community, please know that you are behind everything we do. You inspire us every day with your bravery, compassion, energy, and vulnerability, and we cannot thank you enough for welcoming us into your lives. To all who contributed insight, quotes, and ideas to the creation of this book, your efforts mean more than you know.

Erica Green and Caroline Pincus, thank you for sharing your time and insights and helping us create a resource that is meaningful for all mamas. To Sarah Bjorkman, MD, Motherly's Medical Advisor, you have been a guiding light of knowledge since the very beginning of Motherly. Your dedication to Motherly, this book, and to women is profound, and we feel so lucky to have you on our team. And heartfelt gratitude to Miriam Mahler, CNM, for devoting countless hours to this project and for never failing to come into my room in the middle of the night to tell me how many babies you delivered that day.

Thank you to Seth Bardo for making me fall in love with writing and to Julia Lange Kessler, CM, DNP, FACNM; Jeanne Murphy, PhD, CNM, FACNM; Richard Jennings, CNM; Maura Larkin, CNM; and all the midwives at Bellevue Hospital in New York City for transforming me into a midwife and making me love birth.

To my family and friends, who have forever been my backbone, I could not have done this without you. Finally, and perhaps most difficult to articulate in words, is my gratitude for my husband and children. You four are my entire world. Thank you for your patience. Thank you for your encouragement. Thank you for choosing me. Saya, Asher, and Wilder, thank you for making me a mama.

Notes

CHAPTER 1
Deciding to Have a Baby and Preparing to Get Pregnant

In fact, studies have been done...
Kate Sweeny et al., "Waiting for a Baby: Navigating Uncertainty in Recollections of Trying to Conceive," *Social Science & Medicine* 141 (September 2015): 123–132, doi.org/10.1016/j.socscimed.2015.07.031.

Women may struggle with the unpredictability...
Sweeny et al., "Waiting for a Baby," 123–132

However, it is possible that high levels of stress...
Germaine M. Buck Louis et al., "Stress Reduces Conception Probabilities Across the Fertile Window: Evidence in Support of Relaxation," *Fertility & Sterility* 95, no. 7 (June 2011): 2184–2189, doi.org/10.1016/j.fcrtnstert.2010.06.078.

Researchers are finding more...
Elmaric Botha, Teri Gwin, and Christina Purpora, "The Effectiveness of Mindfulness Based Programs in Reducing Stress Experienced by Nurses in Adult Hospital Settings: A Systematic Review of Quantitative Evidence Protocol," *JBI Database of Systematic Reviews and Implementation Reports* 13, no. 10 (October 2015): 21–29, doi.org/10.11124/jbisrir-2015-2380.

...stress reduction, less anxiety and depression...
Françoise Roy Malis, Thorsten Meyer, and Mechthild M. Gross, "Effects of an Antenatal Mindfulness-Based Childbirth and Parenting Programme on the Postpartum Experiences of Mothers: A Qualitative Interview Study," *BMC Pregnancy and Childbirth* 17, no. 1 (February 2017): 57, doi.org/10.101650140-6736(18)30311-8.

In fact, research has found...
Judith Stephenson et al., "Before the Beginning: Nutrition and Lifestyle in the Preconception Period and Its Importance for Future Health," *Lancet* 391, no. 10132 (May 2018): 1830–1841, doi.org/10.1186/s12884-017-1240 9.

The appointment itself will likely...
Ines Kersten et al., "Chronic Diseases in Pregnant Women: Prevalence and Birth Outcomes Based on the SNiP-study," *BMC Pregnancy and Childbirth* 14 (February 2014): 75, doi.org/10.1186/1471-2393-14-75.

Of note, the Centers for Disease Control...
"Pregnant Women & Influenza (Flu)," National Center for Immunization and Respiratory Diseases (NCIRD), Centers for Disease Control and Prevention, last modified February 12, 2019, cdc.gov/flu/protect/vaccine/pregnant.htm.

Your male partner or sperm donor...
Anthony Paul O'Brien et al., "Men's Preconception Health: A Primary Health-Care Viewpoint," *American Journal of Men's Health* 12, no. 5 (September 2018): 1575–1581, doi.org/10.1177/1557988318776513.

Here are just a few of the ways that a healthy mouth...
Kim A. Boggess and Burton L. Edelstein, "Oral Health in Women During Preconception and Pregnancy: Implications for Birth Outcomes and Infant Oral Health," *Maternal and Child Health Journal* 10, supplement 1 (September 2006): 169–174, doi.org/10.1007/s10995-006-0095-x.

A healthy mouth can also decrease...
Kim A. Boggess, "Maternal Oral Health in Pregnancy," *Obstetrics & Gynecology* 111, no. 4 (April 2008): 976–986, doi.org/10.1097/AOG.0b013e31816a49d3.

...and cancer...
K. S. Rajesh et al., "Poor Periodontal Health: A Cancer Risk?" *Journal of Indian Society of Periodontology* 17, no. 6 (November–December 2013): 706–710, doi.org/10.4103/0972-124X.124470.

If you do not have health insurance...
Healthcare.gov, US Centers for Medicare & Medicaid Services, accessed January 10, 2019, healthcare.gov.

Almost all dental procedures are considered safe...
Oral Health Care During Pregnancy Steering Committee, *Oral Health Care During Pregnancy: Practice Guidance for Maryland's Prenatal and Dental Providers* (Baltimore: Maryland Department of Health, 2018), acog.org/-/media/Sections/MD/Public/MDOralHealthPregnancyGuide.pdf?dmc=1&ts=20181121T2152076401.

The findings from a 2018 review...
Tadele Girum and Abebaw Wasie, "Return of Fertility After Discontinuation of Contraception: A Systematic Review and Meta-Analysis," *Contraception and Reproductive Medicine* 3 (July 2018): 9, doi.org/10.1186/s40834-018-0064-y.

Condoms tend to be less effective . . .
James Trussell, "Contraceptive Failure in the United
    States," *Contraception* 83, no. 5 (May 2011): 397–404,
    doi.org/10.1016/j.contraception.2011.01.021.

CHART: ACOG Prenatal Nutrition Guidelines . . .
"Nutrition During Pregnancy," American College of
    Obstetricians and Gynecologists, February 2018,
    acog.org/-/media/Womens-Health/nutrition-in
    -pregnancy.pdf.

These can be found on the FDA website . . .
"Survey Data on Lead in Women's and Children's
    Vitamins," US Food & Drug Administration,
    January 12, 2018, fda.gov/food/metals/survey
    -data-lead-womens-and-childrens-vitamins.

Registered dietician and nutritionist. . .
"Folic Acid: The Vitamin That Helps Prevent
    Birth Defects," New York State Department of
    Health, last modified April 2007, health.ny.gov/
    publications/1335/.

In fact, 40 to 50 percent of women develop . . .
Noran M. Abu-Ouf and Mohammed M. Jan, "The
    Impact of Maternal Iron Deficiency and Iron
    Deficiency Anemia on Child's Health," *Saudi
    Medical Journal* 36, no. 2 (February 2015): 146–149,
    ncbi.nlm.nih.gov/pmc/articles/PMC4375689/.

Vitamin C helps iron get absorbed . . .
"Iron: Fact Sheet for Health Professionals," National
    Institutes of Health, US Department of Health and
    Human Services, updated August 22, 2019, ods
    .od.nih.gov/factsheets/Iron-HealthProfessional/.

Eating 1 tablespoon of blackstrap molasses . . .
"Anemia," Milton S. Hershey Medical Center, Penn
    State Hershey, updated December 19, 2015,
    pennstatehershey.adam.com/content
    .aspx?productId=107&pid=33&gid=000009.

Research is showing that people in developed countries . . .
Elaine Patterson et al., "Health Implications of High
    Dietary Omega-6 Polyunsaturated Fatty Acids,"
    Journal of Nutrition and Metabolism 2012 (April
    2012): 539426, doi.org/10.1155/2012/539426.

Research has also shown that DHA supplementation . . .
Danielle Swanson, Robert Block, and Shaker A.
    Mousa,"Omega-3 Fatty Acids EPA and DHA: Health
    Benefits Throughout Life," *Advances in Nutrition* 3,
    no. 1 (January 2012): 1–7, doi.org/10.3945
    /an.111.000893.

And continued supplementation . . .
Connye N. Kuratko et al., "The Relationship of
    Docosahexaenoic Acid (DHA) with Learning and
    Behavior in Healthy Children: A Review," *Nutrients*
    5, no. 7 (July 2013): 2777–2810, doi.org/10.3390
    /nu5072777.

A nonjudgmental note for smokers . . .
Patrick Drake, Anne K. Driscoll, and T. J. Mathews,
    "Cigarette Smoking During Pregnancy: United
    States, 2016," National Center for Health Statistics
    Data Brief, no. 305, February 2018, cdc.gov/nchs
    /data/databriefs/db305.pdf.

Substances in cigarettes can make . . .
Clotilde Dechanet et al., "Effects of Cigarette Smoking
    on Embryo Implantation and Placentation and
    Analysis of Factors Interfering with Cigarette
    Smoke Effects (Part II)," *Gynecology, Obstetrics &
    Fertility* 39, no.10 (October 2011): 567–574,
    doi.org/10.1016/j.gyobfe.2011.07.023.

Cigarettes can lead to serious pregnancy complications . . .
Joseph R. DiFranza, C. Andrew Aligne, and Michael
    Weitzman, "Prenatal and Postnatal Environmental
    Tobacco Smoke Exposure and Children's Health,"
    Pediatrics 113, Supplement 3 (April 2004), 10071115,
    doi.org/10.1542/peds.2010-2850.

And children who were exposed to cigarettes . . .
Anders Bjerg et al., "A Strong Synergism of Low Birth
    Weight and Prenatal Smoking on Asthma in
    Schoolchildren," *Pediatrics* 127, no. 4 (April 2011):
    1007–1115, pediatrics.aappublications.org/content
    /127/4; Toshihiro Ino, "Maternal Smoking During
    Pregnancy and Offspring Obesity: Meta-Analysis,"
    Pediatrics International 52, no. 1 (February 2010):
    94–99, doi.org/10.1111/j.1442-200X.2009.02883.x.

Lastly, research indicates . . .
Jason R. Kovac, Abhinav Khanna, and Larry I.
    Lipshultz, "The Effects of Cigarette Smoking on
    Male Fertility," *Postgraduate Medicine* 127, no. 3
    (April 2015): 338–341, doi.org/10.1080/00325481.20
    15.1015928.

Some studies have said it's just fine . . .
Cristina Lopez-del Burgo et al., "Alcohol and Difficulty
    Conceiving in the SUN Cohort: A Nested Case-
    Control Study," *Nutrients* 7, no. 8 (July 2015):
    6167–6178, doi.org/10.3390/nu7085278.

A 2017 review of nineteen studies . . .
Dazhi Fan et al., "Female Alcohol Consumption and
    Fecundability: A Systematic Review and Dose-
    Response Meta-Analysis," *Scientific Reports*
    7, no. 1 (October 2017): 13815, doi.org/10.1038
    /s41598-017-14261-8.

Also of note, despite the possible impact of alcohol . . .
Audrey J. Gaskins et al., "Prepregnancy Low to Moderate Alcohol Intake Is Not Associated with Risk of Spontaneous Abortion or Stillbirth," *Journal of Nutrition* 146, no. 4 (April 2016): 799–805, doi.org/10.3945/jn.115.226423.

While some studies have found that caffeine . . .
Amelia K. Wesselink et al., "Caffeine and Caffeinated Beverage Consumption and Fecundability in a Preconception Cohort," *Reproductive Toxicology* 62 (July 2016): 39–45, doi.org/10.1016/j.reprotox.2016.04.022.

A 2018 study led by Boston University . . .
Lauren A. Wise et al., "Marijuana Use and Fecundability in a North American Preconception Cohort Study," *Journal of Epidemiology and Community Health*, 72, no. 3 (December 2017): 208–215. doi.org/10.1136/jech-2017-209755.

ACOG, however, states . . .
"Marijuana Use During Pregnancy and Lactation," Committee Opinion No. 722, American College of Obstetricians and Gynecologists, *Obstetrics and Gynecology* 130 (2017): e205–e209, acog.org/clinical-guidance-and-publications/committee-opinions/committee-on-obstetric-practice/marijuana-use-during-pregnancy-and-lactation.

Though research is always evolving here . . .
TD Metz et al., "Medical Marijuana Use, Adverse, Pregnancy Outcomes, and Neonatal Morbidity," *Am J Obstet* Gynecol 217, no. 4 (October 2017): e1-8, doi.org/10.1016%2Fj.ajog.2017.05.050.

Researchers found that women who get . . .
Jacqueline D. Kloss et al., "Sleep, Sleep Disturbance, and Fertility in Women," *Sleep Medicine Reviews* 22 (August 2015): 78–87, doi.org/10.1016/j.smrv.2014.10.005.

You can also consider seeking treatment . . .
Kloss et al., "Sleep, Sleep Disturbance, and Fertility," 78–87.

And this goes for men too . . .
Lauren Anne Wise et al., "Male Sleep Duration and Fecundability in a North American Preconception Cohort Study," *Fertility and Sterility* 109, no. 3 (March 2018): 453–459, doi.org/10.1016/j.fertnstert.2017.11.037.

There are chemicals in our air . . .
"Picture of America: Reproductive Outcomes," Centers for Disease Control and Prevention, National Center for Environmental Health, last modified April 6, 2017, cdc.gov/pictureofamerica/pdfs/Picture_of_America_Reproductive_Outcomes.pdf.

A major medical organization . . .
"Reproductive and Developmental Environmental Health," FIGO International Federation of Gynecology and Obstetrics, figo.org/working-group-reproductive-and-developmental-environmental-health.

The Environmental Working Group puts out . . .
Sonya Lunder, "EWG's 2019 Shopper's Guide to Pesticides in Produce™," Environmental Working Group, March 20, 2019, ewg.org/foodnews/summary.php.

Scientists have found that it takes women . . .
Erica Silvestris et al., "Obesity as Disruptor of the Female Fertility," *Reproductive Biology and Endocrinology* 16, no. 1 (March 2018): 22, doi.org/10.1186/s12958-018-0336-z.

A BMI over 25 may . . .
Damian Best, Alison Avenell, and Siladitya Bhattacharya, "How Effective Are Weight-Loss Interventions for Improving Fertility in Women and Men Who Are Overweight or Obese? A Systematic Review and Meta-Analysis of the Evidence," *Human Reproduction Update* 23, no. 6 (November 2017): 681–705, doi.org/10.1093/humupd/dmx027.

One explanation for this . . .
Christopher J. Brewer and Adam H. Balen, "The Adverse Effects of Obesity on Conception and Implantation," *Reproduction* 140, no. 3 (September 2010): 347–364, doi.org/10.1530/REP-09-0568.

The good news: A woman with a BMI over 25 . . .
Best et al., "How Effective Are Weight-Loss Interventions?" 681–705.

Women who exercise more . . .
Osnat Hakimi and Luiz-Claudio Cameron, "Effect of Exercise on Ovulation: A Systematic Review," *Sports Medicine* 47, no. 8 (August 2017): 1555–1567, doi.org/10.1007/s40279-016-0669-8.

This goes for males as well . . .
Amy C. Roberts et al., "Overtraining Affects Male Reproductive Status," *Fertility and Sterility* 60, no. 4 (October 1993): 686–692, doi.org/10.1016/S0015-0282(16)56223-2.

Of course, this is a very personal matter . . .
Kate Sweeny et al., "Waiting for a Baby: Navigating Uncertainty in Recollections of Trying to Conceive," *Social Science & Medicine* 141 (September 2015): 123–132, doi.org/10.1016/j.socscimed.2015.07.031.

Sometimes fertility issues can be hereditary . . .
"Genetic Causes of Female Infertility," Reproductive Science Center of New Jersey, January 2019, fertilitynj.com/infertility/female-infertility/genetic-causes/.

If your mother went through menopause . . .
Kelly Fitzgerald, "Daughter's Fertility Predicted by Mother's Age at Menopause," Medical News Today, November 7, 2012, medicalnewstoday.com/articles/252465.php.

In fact, in 2015, for the first time . . .
"General Fertility Rates," National Center for Health Statistics, Centers for Disease Control and Prevention, October 16, 2018, cdc.gov/nchs/nvss/vsrr/natality-dashboard.htm.

If you will be a single parent . . .
"The Majority of Children Live with Two Parents, Census Bureau Reports," Release Number CB16-192, US Census Bureau, November 17, 2016, census.gov/newsroom/press-releases/2016/cb16-192.html.

If you encounter these issues in your workplace . . .
"Filing a Charge of Discrimination," US Equal Employment Opportunity Commission, February 2019, eeoc.gov/employees/charge.cfm.

CHAPTER 2
The Extraordinary Anatomy of Pregnancy and Birth

Historically, Western obstetrical medicine . . .
Steph Yin, "Why Textbooks May Need to Update What They Say About Birth Canals," *New York Times*, October 27, 2018, nytimes.com/2018/10/27/health/birth-canals-evolution.html.

There are several hormones . . .
Sunil K. Kota et al., "Endocrinology of Parturition," *Indian Journal of Endocrinology and Metabolism* 17, no. 1. (January–February 2013): 50–59, doi.org/10.4103/2230-8210.107841.

A groundbreaking 2018 study . . .
Lia Betti and Andrea Manica, "Human Variation in the Shape of the Birth Canal Is Significant and Geographically Structured," *Proceedings of the Royal Society B: Biological Sciences* 285, no. 1889 (October 24, 2018), doi.org/10.1098/rspb.2018.1807.

It is estimated that 513,000 girls . . .
Howard Goldberg et al., "Female Genital Mutilation/Cutting in the United States: Updated Estimates of Women and Girls at Risk, 2012," *Public Health Reports* 131 (March–April 2016): 1–8, uscis.gov/sites/default/files/USCIS/Humanitarian/Special%20Situations/fgmutilation.pdf.

CHAPTER 3
How to Conceive

Tracking your ovulation, otherwise known as charting . . .
Marlies Manders et al., "Timed Intercourse for Couples Trying to Conceive," Cochrane Database of Systematic Reviews 2015, no. 3 (March 2015): CD011345, doi.org/10.1002/14651858.CD011345.pub2.

Research has found that apps . . .
Sarah Johnson, Lorrae Marriott, and Michael Zinaman, "Can Apps and Calendar Methods Predict Ovulation with Accuracy?" *Current Medical Research and Opinion* 34, no.9 (September 2018): 1587–1594, doi.org/10.1080/03007995.2018.1475348.

There are wearable devices that can help . . .
Mohaned Shilaih et al., "Modern Fertility Awareness Methods: Wrist Wearables Capture the Changes in Temperature Associated with the Menstrual Cycle," *Bioscience Reports* 38, no. 6 (November 2018), doi.org/10.1042/BSR20171279.

. . . and the research on their efficacy is promising . . .
Mohaned Shilaih et al., "Pulse Rate Measurement During Sleep Using Wearable Sensors, and Its Correlation with the Menstrual Cycle Phases: A Prospective Observational Study," *Scientific Reports* 7 (May 2017): 1294, doi.org/10.1038/s41598-017-01433-9.

There is also variation in how the urine-based tests . . .
Sonya Godbert et al., "Comparison Between the Different Methods Developed for Determining the Onset of the LH Surge in Urine During the Human Menstrual Cycle," *Archives of Gynecology and Obstetrics* 292, no.5 (November 2015): 1153–1116, doi.org/10.1007/s00404-015-3732-z.

It does seem that accuracy picks up . . .
Antonio Rene Leiva et al., "Urinary Luteinizing Hormone Tests: Which Concentration Threshold Best Predicts Ovulation?" *Frontiers in Public Health* 5 (November 2017): 320, doi.org/10.3389/fpubh.2017.00320.

Stay horizontal for about 15 to 30 minutes after sex . . .
Inge M. Custers et al., "Immobilisation Versus Immediate Mobilisation After Intrauterine Insemination: Randomised Controlled Trial," *BMJ* 339 (October 2009): b4080, doi.org/10.1136/bmj.b4080.

A 2018 study found that reducing the number . . .
Jessica A. Grieger et al., "Pre-Pregnancy Fast Food and Fruit Intake Is Associated with Time to Pregnancy," *Human Reproduction* 33, no. 6 (June 2018): 1063–1070, doi.org/10.1093/humrep/dey079.

Drinking one or more sugar-sweetened drinks . . .
Elizabeth E. Hatch et al., "Intake of Sugar-Sweetened
Beverages and Fecundability in a North American
Preconception Cohort," *Epidemiology* 29, no. 3
(May 2018): 369–378, doi.org/10.1097/EDE
.0000000000000812.

The same study on fast food found . . .
Grieger et al., "Pre-Pregnancy Fast Food," 1063–1070.

But after examining . . .
Marinus J. C. Eijkemans et al., "Too Old to Have
Children? Lessons from Natural Fertility
Populations," *Human Reproduction* 29, no. 6 (June
2014): 1304–1312, doi.10.1093/humrep/deu056.

Research finds that receiving support . . .
Arthur L. Greil, Kathleen Slauson-Blevins, and Julia
McQuillan, "The Experience of Infertility: A Review
of Recent Literature," *Sociology of Health & Illness* 32,
no.1 (January 2010): 140–162, doi.org/10.1111/j.1467
-9566.2009.01213.x.

About 1 out of every 9 women . . .
"How Common Is Infertility?" National Institute of
Health, US Department of Health and Human
Services, last modified February 8, 2018, nichd
.nih.gov/health/topics/infertility/conditioninfo
/common.

This is the cause of infertility in 25 to 30 percent . . .
Su Jen Chua, Valentine A. Akande, and Ben Willem J.
Mol, "Surgery for Tubal Infertility," Cochrane
Database of Systematic Reviews 2017, Intervention,
no. 1 (January 2017)): CD006415, doi.org/10.1002
/14651858.CD006415.pub3.

The field of epigenetics . . .
Magdalena Janecka et al., "Advanced Paternal Age
Effects in Neurodevelopmental Disorders: Review
of Potential Underlying Mechanisms," *Translational
Psychiatry* 7, no. 1 (January 2017): e1019,
doi.org/10.1038/tp.2016.294.

CHAPTER 4
Miscarriage and Loss

In these heartbreaking moments . . .
Ajahn Chah, "It's Like This: 108 Dhamma Similes," trans.
Thanissaro Bhikkhu, 2013, buddhismnow.files
.wordpress.com/2014/02/itslikethis-ajahn-chah.pdf.

From 11 to 22 percent of clinically recognized pregnancies . . .
Lyndsay Ammon Avalos, Claudia C. Galindo, and
De-Kun Li, "A Systematic Review to Calculate
Background Miscarriage Rates Using Life Table
Analysis," *Birth Defects Research* 94, no. 6 (June
2012): 417–423, doi.org/10.1002/bdra.23014.

Spotting is fairly common . . .
Christopher Everett, "Incidence and Outcome of
Bleeding Before the 20th Week of Pregnancy:
Prospective Study from General Practice," *BMJ* 315,
no.799 (July 1997): 32–34, doi.org/10.1136/bmj.315
.7099.32.

It occurs in about 25 percent of pregnancies . . .
Mark Deutchman, Amy Tanner Tubay, and David K.
Turok, "First Trimester Bleeding," *American Family
Physician* 79, no. 11 (June 2009): 985–994, aafp.org
/afp/2009/0601/p985.html.

Although tissue sampling is usually recommended . . .
"Early Pregnancy Loss," ACOG Practice Bulletin 200,
American College of Obstetricians and
Gynecologists, *Obstetrics & Gynecology* 132 (August
29, 2018): e197–e207, acog.org/clinical
-guidance-and-publications/practice-bulletins
/committee-on-practice-bulletins-gynecology
/early-pregnancy-loss.

*From 60 to 85 percent of miscarriages require no
interventions*
Clarissa Kripke, "Expectant Management vs. Surgical
Treatment for Miscarriage," *American Family
Physician* 74, no. 7 (October 2006): 1125–1126, aafp.
org/afp/2006/1001/p1125.html.

About 71 percent of women will have completed miscarriage . . .
"Early Pregnancy Loss," ACOG Practice Bulletin 200,
e197-207.

The risk that not all the tissue would be removed . . .
"Early Pregnancy Loss," ACOG Practice Bulletin 200,
e197-207.

An ectopic pregnancy is a rare complication . . .
Norah M. van Mello et al., "Ectopic Pregnancy: How
the Diagnostic and Therapeutic Management Has
Changed," *Fertility & Sterility* 98, no. 5 (November
2012): 1066–1073, doi.org/10.1016/j.fertnstert.2012
.09.040.

Also called a hydatidiform mole or gestational trophoblastic . . .
"Molar Pregnancy," Mayo Clinic, updated December 14,
2017, mayoclinic.org/diseases-conditions
/molar-pregnancy/symptoms-causes/syc-20375175.

However, more current research is showing . . .
Adam J. Wolfberg et al., "Low Risk of Relapse After
Achieving Undetectable hCG Levels in Women
with Complete Molar Pregnancy," *Obstetrics &
Gynecology* 104, no. 3 (September 2004): 551–554,
doi.org/10.1097/01.aog.0000136099.21216.45.

Miscarriage after an induced...
"Induced Abortion," Frequently Asked Questions, American College of Obstetricians and Gynecologists, May 2015, acog.org/Patients/FAQs /Induced-Abortion.

Put a head of cabbage in your refrigerator...
Avinesh Rona Disha et al., "Effect of Chilled Cabbage Leaves vs. Hot Compression on Breast Engorgement Among Post Natal Mothers Admitted in a Tertiary Care Hospital," *Nursing and Midwifery Research Journal* 11, no. 1 (January 2015): 24–32, medind.nic.in/nad/t15/i1/nadt15i1p24.pdf.

Research has shown that when partners...
Kristen M. Swanson et al., "Miscarriage Effects on Couples' Interpersonal and Sexual Relationships During the First Year After Loss: Women's Perceptions," *Psychosomatic Medicine* 65, no. 5 (September/October 2003): 902–910, doi.org/10.1097/01.psy.0000079381.58810.84.

Some providers do not recommend red raspberry leaf tea...
Lone Holst, Svein Haavik, and Hedvig Nordeng, "Raspberry Leaf: Should It Be Recommended to Pregnant Women?" *Complementary Therapies in Clinical Practice* 15, no. 4 (November 2009): 204–208, doi.org/10.1016/j.ctcp.2009.05.003.

In 2016, researchers looked into the impact...
Clemence Due, Stephanie Chiarolli, and Damien W. Riggs, "The Impact of Pregnancy Loss on Men's Health and Wellbeing: A Systematic Review," *BMC Pregnancy and Childbirth* 17 (November 2017): 380, doi.org/10.1186/s12884-017-1560-9.

...and perhaps for a shorter period of time than women...
G. W. S. Kong et al., "Gender Comparison of Psychological Reaction After Miscarriage: A 1-Year Longitudinal Study," *BJOG* 117, no. 10 (September 2010): 1211–1219, doi.org/10.1111/j.1471-0528.2010 .02653.x.

For same-sex partners of women who have miscarried...
Petra Boynton, "Miscarriage: You Don't Have to Be Strong for Me," *Lancet* 385 (January 2015): 222–223, thelancet.com/pdfs/journals/lancet/PIIS0140 -6736(15)60047-2.pdf.

One of the keys to going through a miscarriage...
Annsofie Adolfsson et al., "Guilt and Emptiness: Women's Experiences of Miscarriage," *Health Care for Women International* 25, no. 6 (June/July 2004): 543–560, doi.org/10.1080/07399330490444821.

The couples who can find harmony...
Adolfsson et al., "Guilt and Emptiness," 543–560.

The medical community has routinely encouraged...
"Early Pregnancy Loss," ACOG Practice Bulletin 200, e197–207.

If you are part of a spiritual or religious community...
Maryam Allahdadian and Alireza Irajpour, "The Role of Religious Beliefs in Pregnancy Loss," *Journal of Education and Health Promotion* 4 (December 2015): 99, doi.org/10.4103/2277-9531.171813.

In 2007, Danuta Wojnar conducted...
Danuta Wojnar, "Miscarriage Experiences of Lesbian Couples," *Journal of Midwifery & Women's Health* 52, no. 5 (September–October 2007): 479–485, doi.org/10.1016/j.jmwh.2007.03.015.

Recurrent miscarriage is rare...
"Repeated Miscarriage," Frequently Asked Questions, American College of Obstetricians and Gynecologists, May 2016, acog.org/patients/faqs /repeated-miscarriages.

After three miscarriages, providers will...
"Repeated Miscarriage."

Recurrent miscarriages can be caused by...
"Repeated Miscarriage."

ACOG states that while the general recommendation...
"Early Pregnancy Loss," ACOG Practice Bulletin 200, e197–207

Of note, a 2010 study of over thirty thousand women...
Eleanor Love, et al., "Effect of Interpregnancy Interval on Outcomes of Pregnancy After Miscarriage: Retrospective Analysis of Hospital Episode Statistics in Scotland," *BMJ* 341 (August 2010): c3967, doi.org/10.1136/bmj.c3967.

CHAPTER 5
Finding Out You Are Pregnant and Your First Weeks of Pregnancy

Psst: Close to 50 percent of our Motherly community...
"2018 State of Motherhood Survey," Motherly, May 7, 2018, motherly.s3.amazonaws.com/motherly%20 state%20of%20motherhood%20survey%20results _cleaned%20and%20weighted.pdf.

In Southeast Asia, the word for placenta...
Anne Fadiman, *The Spirit Catches You and You Fall Down* (New York: Farrar, Straus and Giroux, 1997), 5.

hCG values by weeks since LMP...
"Human Chorionic Gonadotropin (hCG): The Pregnancy Hormone," American Pregnancy Association, americanpregnancy.org/while -pregnant/hcg-levels/.

ACOG states that there are no known long-term dangers...
"Ultrasound Exams," Frequently Asked Questions, American College of Obstetricians and Gynecologists, updated June 2017, acog.org/patients/faqs/ultrasound-exams.

Research has found that incorporating relaxation...
Gian Mauro Manzoni et al., "Relaxation Training for Anxiety: A Ten-Years Systematic Review with Meta-Analysis," *BMC Psychiatry* 8 (June 2008): 41, doi.org/10.1186/1471-244X-8-41.

Almost 50 percent of pregnancies in the US...
"Unintended Pregnancy in the United States," Guttmacher Institute, updated January 2019, guttmacher.org/fact-sheet/unintended -pregnancy-united-states.

...and 40 percent of pregnancies in the world...
Gilda Sedgh, Susheela Singh, and Rubina Hussain, "Intended and Unintended Pregnancies Worldwide in 2012 and Recent Trends," *Studies in Family Planning* 45, no. 3 (September 2014): 301–314, doi.org/10.1111/j.1728-4465.2014.00393.x.

Many medical professionals agree on the "all or none phenomenon"...
Margaret P. Adam, "The All-or-None Phenomenon Revisited," *Birth Defects Research Part A: Clinical and Molecular Teratology* 94, no. 8 (August 2012): 664–669, doi.org/10.1002/bdra.23029.

Women who have unplanned pregnancies...
Katherine Barton et al., "Unplanned Pregnancy and Subsequent Psychological Distress in Partnered Women: A Cross-Sectional Study of the Role of Relationship Quality and Wider Social Support," *BMC Pregnancy and Childbirth* 17, no. 1 (January 2017): 44, doi.org/10.1186/s12884-017-1223-x.

About 1 out of every 475 women will not know they are pregnant...
Marco Del Giudice, "The Evolutionary Biology of Cryptic Pregnancy: A Re-Appraisal of the 'Denied Pregnancy' Phenomenon," *Medical Hypotheses* 68, no. 2 (September 2006): 250–258, doi.org/10.1016 /j.mehy.2006.05.066.

Survivors often report that in the context of prenatal care...
Lauren Sobel et al., "Pregnancy and Childbirth After Sexual Trauma: Patient Perspectives and Care Preferences," *Obstetrics & Gynecology* 132, no. 6 (December 2018): 1461–1468, doi.org/10.1097 /aog.0000000000002956.

CHAPTER 6
Choosing a Birthplace and Provider

Research shows that choosing a birthing place...
Anke B. Witteveen et al., "Pregnancy Related Anxiety and General Anxious or Depressed Mood and the Choice for Birth Setting: A Secondary Data-Analysis of the DELIVER Study," *BMC Pregnancy and Childbirth* 16 (November 2016): 363, doi.org/10.1186 /S12884-016-1158-7.

If your family is LGBTQ+ or you are concerned...
Erin Wingo, Natalie Ingraham, and Sarah C. M. Roberts, "Reproductive Health Care Priorities and Barriers to Effective Care for LGBTQ People Assigned Female at Birth: A Qualitative Study," *Women's Health Issues* 28, no. 4 (July–August 2018): 350–357, doi.org/10.1016/j.whi.2018.03.002.

Most women in the US (about 98 percent)...
Marian F. MacDorman, Tom J. Matthews, and Eugene R. Declercq, "Trends in Out-of-Hospital Births in the United States, 1990–2012," NCHS Data Brief 144 (Hyattsville, MD: National Center for Health Statistics, 2014), 1–8, cdc.gov/nchs/data/databriefs /db144.pdf.

For example, over 50 percent of women giving birth in hospitals...
"Epidural Anesthesia," American Pregnancy Association, updated July 15, 2019, american pregnancy.org/labor-and-birth/epidural/.

About 7 percent of babies spend some time in the NICU...
Beth Skwarecki, "NICU Admission Rates Rising for Infants of All Weights," Medscape Medical News, July 28, 2015, medscape.com/viewarticle/848722.

Research has found that birth centers are a safe option...
Susan Rutledge Stapleton, Cara Osborne, and Jessica Illuzzi, "Outcomes of Care in Birth Centers: Demonstration of a Durable Model," *Journal of Midwifery and Women's Health* 58, no. 1 (January/ February 2013): 3–14, doi.org/10.1111/jmwh.12003.

In 1938, 50 percent of babies...
Ruth Zielinski, Kelly Ackerson, and Lisa Kane Low, "Planned Home Birth: Benefits, Risks, and Opportunities," *International Journal of Women's Health* 7 (April 2015): 361–377, doi.org/10.2147/IJWH .S55561.

For example, up to 20 percent of women in the Netherlands...
Zielinski et al., "Planned Home Birth," 361–377.

In general, home births involve fewer interventions...
Ole Olsen and Jette A. Clausen, "Planned Hospital Birth Versus Planned Home Birth," Cochrane Database of Systematic Reviews 2012, no. 9 (September 2012), CD000352, doi.org/10.1002 /14651858.cd000352.pub2.

According to ACOG, "High-quality evidence..."
"Planned Home Birth," ACOG Committee Opinion No. 697, American College of Obstetricians and Gynecologists," *Obstetrics and Gynecology* 129 (April 2017; Reaffirmed 2018): e117–122, acog.org /clinical-guidance-and-publications/committee -opinions/committee-on-obstetric-practice /planned-home-birth.

For example, the American College of Nurse-Midwives . . .
American College of Nurse-Midwives "Midwifery
    Provision of Home Birth Services," clinical bulletin
    no. 14, *J Midwifery Women's Health* 61, no. 1 (2015):
    127-133, doi.org/10.1111/jmwh.12431.

*The American Academy of Pediatrics (AAP) agrees with
ACOG . . .*
American Academy of Pediatrics, "Planned Home
    Birth," *Pediatrics* 131, no. 5 (May 2013), pediatrics.
    aappublications.org/content/131/5/1016.

The ACNM states that "Internnational . . .
"Home Birth," Position Statement, American College of
    Nurse-Midwives, May 2011, midwife.org/acnm/files
    /acnmlibrarydata/uploadfilename/000000000251
    /home%20birth%20aug%202011.pdf.

The Midwives Alliance of North America (MANA) . . .
"Homebirth Study One-Page Fact Sheet," Midwives
    Alliance of North America, mana.org
    /healthcare-policy/homebirth-study-fact-sheet.

Of note, ACOG estimates that one-fourth of home births . . .
"Planned Home Birth," e117-122.

The infant mortality and preterm delivery rates . . .
Lisa Rosenthal and Marci Lobel, "Explaining Racial
    Disparities in Adverse Birth Outcomes: Unique
    Sources of Stress for Black American Women,"
    Social Science & Medicine 72, no. 6 (March 2011):
    977–983, doi.org/10.1016/j.socscimed.2011.01.013.

. . . and there is a higher risk for pregnancy-related illnesses . . .
Lindsay K. Admon et al., "Racial and Ethnic Disparities
    in the Incidence of Severe Maternal Morbidity
    in the United States, 2012–2015," *Obstetrics &
    Gynecology* 132, no. 5 (November 2018): 1158–1166,
    doi.org/10.1097/aog.0000000000002937.

New York Times reporter Erica Green . . .
Erica Green, in a phone interview with the author,
    December 14, 2018.

About 6 percent of women in the US . . .
Katy B. Kozhimannil et al., "Potential Benefits
    of Increased Access to Doula Support During
    Childbirth," *American Journal of Managed Care* 20,
    no. 8 (August 2014): e340–e352, ncbi.nlm.nih.gov
    /pubmed/25295797.

A large review of research found that doulas . . .
Ellen D. Hodnett et al., "Continuous Support for
    Women During Childbirth," Cochrane Database
    of Systematic Reviews 2011, no. 2 (February 2011):
    CO003766, doi.org/10.1002/14651858.cd003766.pub5.

A 2017 study in Iran . . .
Mozhgan Firouzbakht et al., "The Effect of Perinatal
    Education on Iranian Mothers' Stress and Labor
    Pain," *Global Journal of Health Science* 6, no. 1 (2014):
    61–68, doi.org/10.5539/gjhs.v6n1p61.

A 2008 study published in the journal Birth *. . .*
Susan K. McGrath and John H. Kennell, "A
    Randomized Controlled Trial of Continuous Labor
    Support for Middle-Class Couples: Effect on
    Cesarean Delivery Rates," *Birth* 35, no. 2 (June
    2008): 92–97, doi.org/10.1111/j.1523-536x.2008.00221.x.

Chiropractors use hands-on techniques . . .
Kent Jason Stuber, Shari Wynd, and Carol Ann Weis,
    "Adverse Events from Spinal Manipulation in the
    Pregnant and Postpartum Periods: A Critical
    Review of the Literature," *Chiropractic & Manual
    Therapies* 20, (March 2012): 8,
    doi.org/10.1186/2045-709x-20-8.

Some women also report that routine chiropractic . . .
Joel Alcantara et al., "The Use of the Patient Reported
    Outcomes Measurement Information System
    and the RAND VSQ9 to Measure the Quality of
    Life and Visit-Specific Satisfaction of Pregnant
    Patients Under Chiropractic Care Utilizing the
    Webster Technique," *Journal of Alternative and
    Complementary Medicine* 24, no. 1 (January 2018):
    90–98, doi.org/10.1089/acm.2017.0162.

People seek acupuncture care for a vast number . . .
Lars G. Westergaard et al., "Acupuncture on the
    Day of Embryo Transfer Significantly Improves
    the Reproductive Outcome in Infertile Women:
    A Prospective, Randomized Trial," *Fertility and
    Sterility* 85, no. 5 (May 2006): 1341–1346,
    doi.org/10.1016/j.fertnstert.2005.08.070.

Research has found that when done . . .
Jimin Park et al., "The Safety of Acupuncture During
    Pregnancy: A Systematic Review," *Acupuncture
    in Medicine* 32, no. 3 (June 2014): 257–266, doi.
    org/10.1136/acupmed-2013-010480; Caroline
    Smith, C. Crowther, and Justin Beilby, "Pregnancy
    Outcome Following Women's Participation in a
    Randomised Controlled Trial of Acupuncture to
    Treat Nausea and Vomiting in Early Pregnancy,"
    Complementary Therapies in Medicine 10, no. 2 (June
    2002): 78–83, doi.org/10.1054/ctim.2002.0523.

But women report wonderful results . . .
Thaís Romera Bergamo et al., "Findings and
    Methodological Quality of Systematic Reviews
    Focusing on Acupuncture for Pregnancy-Related
    Acute Conditions," *Acupuncture in Medicine* 36,
    no. 3 (June 2018): 146–152, doi.org/10.1136/acupmed
    -2017-011436.

... including decreased pelvic and back pain ...
Elizabeth Soliday and Debra Betts, "Treating Pain in Pregnancy with Acupuncture: Observational Study Results from a Free Clinic in New Zealand," *Journal of Acupuncture and Meridian Studies* 11, no. 1 (February 2018): 25–30, doi.org/10.1016/j.jams.2017.11.005.

... decreased depressive symptoms ...
Rachel Manber et al., "Acupuncture for Depression During Pregnancy: A Randomized Controlled Trial," *Obstetrics & Gynecology* 115, no. 3 (March 2010): 511–520, doi.org/10.1097/aog.0b013e3181cc0816.

In addition, a form of acupuncture called moxibustion ...
Isabella Neri et al., "Acupuncture Plus Moxibustion to Resolve Breech Presentation: A Randomized Controlled Study," *Journal of Maternal-Fetal and Neonatal Medicine* 15, no. 4 (May 2004): 247–252, doi.org/10.1080/14767050410001668644.

The benefits can be quite remarkable ...
Tiffany Field, "Pregnancy and Labor Massage," *Expert Review of Obstetrics & Gynecology* 5, no. 2 (March 2010): 177–181, doi.org/10.1586/eog.10.12.

CHAPTER 7
Month 2, Weeks 5–8

From 11 to 22 percent of clinically recognized pregnancies ...
Lyndsay Ammon Avalos, Claudia C. Galindo, and De-Kun Li, "A Systematic Review to Calculate Background Miscarriage Rates Using Life Table Analysis," *Birth Defects Research* 94, no. 6 (June 2012): 417–423, doi.org/10.1002/bdra.23014.

Almost 25 percent of women in the US ...
"Intimate Partner Violence During Pregnancy," Information Sheet, World Health Organization, 2011, apps.who.int/iris/bitstream/handle/10665/70764/who_rhr_11.35_eng.pdf?sequence=1.

In addition to the immediate consequences ...
Hafrún Finnbogadóttir and Anna-Karin Dykes, "Increasing Prevalence and Incidence of Domestic Violence During the Pregnancy and One and a Half Year Postpartum, as Well as Risk Factors: A Longitudinal Cohort Study in Southern Sweden," *BMC Pregnancy and Childbirth* 16 (October 2016): 327, doi.org/10.1186/s12884-016-1122-6.

Seven ways hydration can help ...
Barry M. Popkin, Kristen E. D'Anci, and Irwin H. Rosenberg, "Water, Hydration and Health," *Nutrition Reviews* 68, no. 8 (August 2010): 439–458, doi.org/10.1111/j.1753-4887.2010.00304.x.

Did you know that learning to use your core ...
Cynthia M. Chiarello et al., "The Effects of an Exercise Program on Diastasis Recti Abdominis in Pregnant Women," *Journal of Women's Health Physical Therapy* 29, no.1 (April 2005): 11–16, doi.org/10.1097/01274882-200529010-00003.

As you get closer to giving birth, your areolas ...
Vincenzo Zanardo et al., "Maternal Areola pH: A Chemical Basis for Mother-Infant Recognition," *Early Human Development* 121 (June 2018): 33–36, doi.org/10.1016/j.earlhumdev.2018.05.001.

CHAPTER 8
Month 3, Weeks 9–12

Researchers have found that during a first pregnancy ...
Neil A. Segal et al., "Pregnancy Leads to Lasting Changes in Foot Structure," *American Journal of Physical Medicine and Rehabilitation* 92, no. 3 (March 2013): 232–240, doi.org/10.1097/phm.0b013e31827443a9.

By the time your baby is born, your brain ...
Catherine Caruso, "Pregnancy Causes Lasting Changes in a Woman's Brain," *Scientific American*, December 19, 2016, scientificamerican.com/article/pregnancy-causes-lasting-changes-in-a-womans-brain/.

In early pregnancy, women who know ...
Aytul Corbacioglu et al., "The Role of Pregnancy Awareness on Female Sexual Function in Early Gestation," *Journal of Sexual Medicine* 9, no.7. (July 2012): 1897–1903, doi.org/10.1111/j.1743-6109.2012.02740.x.

If you are having oral sex ...
Giovanni Sisti, Sorbi Flavia, and Fambrini Massimiliano, "Inherent Dangers in Orogenital Sex During Pregnancy," *Journal of Basic and Clinical Reproductive Sciences* 2, no.1 (January–June 2013), doi.org/10.4103/2278-960X.112570.

If you are feeling helpless ...
Sigrid Elsenbruch et al., "Social Support During Pregnancy: Effects on Maternal Depressive Symptoms, Smoking and Pregnancy Outcome," *Human Reproduction* 22, no. 3 (March 2007): 869–877, doi.org/10.1093/humrep/del432.

You are more at risk ...
Mitali Mahapatra, "A Clinical Study on Symptomatic Urinary Tract Infection During Pregnancy," *The Antiseptic*, March 2016, 31, theantiseptic.in/uploads/medicine/a%20clinical%20study%20on%20symptomatic%20urinary%20tract%20infection%20during%20pregnancy.pdf.

Psst: Sometimes decreased libido . . .
Margaret A. De Judicibus and Marita P. McCabe, "Psychological Factors and the Sexuality of Pregnant and Postpartum Women," *Journal of Sex Research* 39, no. 2 (May 2002): 94–103, doi.org/10.1080/0022449 0209552128.

CHAPTER 9
Month 4, Weeks 13–17

This program has become a tradition . . .
Ying Lau, "Traditional Chinese Pregnancy Restrictions, Health-Related Quality of Life and Perceived Stress Among Pregnant Women in Macao, China," *Asian Nursing Research* 6, no. 1 (March 2012): 27–34, doi.org/10.1016/j.anr.2012.02.005.

Because you are stimulating their inner ear's . . .
Gianluca Esposito et al., "Infant Calming Responses During Maternal Carrying in Humans and Mice," *Current Biology* 23, no. 9 (May 2013): 739–745, doi.org/10.1016/j.cub.2013.03.041.

To keep yourself safe, always wear gloves . . .
"Reducing Risks of Birth Defects," Frequently Asked Questions, American College of Obstetricians and Gynecologists, February 2018, acog.org/patients/faqs/reducing-risks-of-birth-defects.

Your breasts are starting to make colostrum . . .
Melissa Cole, "Lactation After Perinatal, Neonatal, or Infant Loss," *Clinical Lactation* 3, no. 3 (2012): 94–100, lunalactation.com/final_clinical_lactation.pdf.

Did you know that more than 10 percent of soon-to-be fathers . . .
Anthony P. O'Brien et al., "New Fathers' Perinatal Depression and Anxiety Treatment Options: An Integrative Review," *American Journal of Men's Health* 11, no. 4 (July 2017): 863–876, doi.org/10.1177/1557988316669047.

This may be higher if mama is also depressed . . .
James F. Paulson and Sharnail D. Bazemore, "Prenatal and Postpartum Depression in Fathers and Its Association with Maternal Depression: A Meta-Analysis," *JAMA* 303, no. 19 (May 2010): 1961–1969, doi.org/10.1001/jama.2010.605.

There is also some research into female partners' . . .
Lori E.Ross, Leah Steele, and Beth Sapiro, "Factors for Perinatal Depression in Same-Sex Parents," *Journal of Midwifery & Women's Health* 50, no. 6 (November–December 2005): e65–e70, doi.org/10.1016/j.jmwh.2005.08.002.

And third, new parents with depression . . .
Sylia Wilson and C. Emily Durbin, "Effects of Paternal Depression on Fathers' Parenting Behaviors: A Meta-Analytic Review," *Clinical Psychology Review* 30, no. 2 (March 2010): 167–180, doi.org/10.1016/j.cpr.2009.10.007.

It's confidential, and whether you begin . . .
"What Is Depression?" American Psychiatric Association, psychiatry.org/patients-families/depression/what-is-depression.

About 56 percent of pregnant women are employed . . .
"Employment Considerations During Pregnancy and the Postpartum Period," ACOG Committee Opinion No. 733, American College of Obstetricians and Gynecologists, *Obstetrics and Gynecology* 131, no. 4 (April 2018): e115–e123, doi.org/10.1097/aog.0000000000002589.

Maternity Leave Around the World
Katie Warren, "Here's What Maternity Leave Looks Like Around the World," *Insider*, May 15, 2018, insider.com/maternity-leave-around-the-world-2018-5; Matt Turner, "Here's How Much Paid Leave New Mothers and Fathers Get in 11 Different Countries," *Business Insider*, September 7, 2017, businessinsider.com/maternity-leave-worldwide-2017-8.

Getting Parental Leave as an LGBTQ+ Parent . . .
Sabia Prescott, "Queer Families Still Struggle to Access Leave," *Slate*, February 7, 2018, slate.com/human-interest/2018/02/even-after-gay-marriage-many-queer-families-cant-access-leave.html.

CHAPTER 10
Month 5, Weeks 18–22

Some studies have found that the soy protein isolates . . .
Mark Messina and Geoffrey Redmond, "Effects of Soy Protein and Soybean Isoflavones on Thyroid Function in Healthy Adults and Hypothyroid Patients: A Review of the Relevant Literature," *Thyroid* 16, no. 3 (March 2006): 249–258, doi.org/10.1089/thy.2006.16.249.

When you have high blood protein levels . . .
"Edema, What Is It?" Harvard Health Publishing, Harvard Medical School, December 2018, health.harvard.edu/a_to_z/edema-a-to-z.

A note on salt: While we often hear . . .
Kei Asayama and Yutaka Imai, "The Impact of Salt Intake During and After Pregnancy," *Hypertension Research* 41, no. 1 (January 2018): 1–5, doi.org/10.1038/hr.2017.90.

Mediterranean Chickpea Salad
Crystal Karges, "3 Easy Mason Jar Salad Recipes for Kids (and Busy Mamas, Too!)," Crystal Karges Nutrition, June 8, 2018, crystalkarges.com/blog/simple-summer-salads-kids-will-like-to-eat?rq=salad%20jar.

Pregnancy can pose unique challenges . . .
Erica P. Gunderson, "Childbearing and Obesity in Women: Weight Before, During, and After Pregnancy," *Obstetrics and Gynecology Clinics of North America* 36, no. 2 (June 2009): 317–332, doi.org/10.1016/j.ogc.2009.04.001.

Researchers have now found that what you eat . . .
Jessica L. Saben et al., "Maternal Metabolic Syndrome Programs Mitochondrial Dysfunction via Germline Changes Across Three Generations," *Cell Reports* 16, no.1 (June 2016): 1–8, doi.org/10.1016/j.celrep.2016.05.065.

Recent research has called the long-standing belief . . .
"Do Ovaries Continue to Produce Eggs During Adulthood?" Public Library of Science, Science Daily, July 26, 2012, sciencedaily.com/releases/2012/07/120726180259.htm.

You may also be eligible to apply . . .
"2019 Open Enrollment Is Over. Still Need Health Insurance?" US Centers for Medicare & Medicaid Services, January 2019, healthcare.gov.

The American Academy of Pediatrics recommends . . .
"Used Car Seats," American Academy of Pediatrics, aap.org/en-us/about-the-aap/aap-press-room/aap-press-room-media-center/pages/used-car-seats.aspx.

CHAPTER 11
Month 6, Weeks 23–27

Your body and brain physically change . . .
Elseline Hoekzema et al., "Pregnancy Leads to Long-Lasting Changes in Human Brain Structure," *Nature: Neuroscience* 20, no. 2 (February 2017): 287–296, doi.org/10.1038/nn.4458.

Your DNA changes . . .
Nancy Shute, "Beyond Birth: A Child's Cells May Help or Harm the Mother Long After Delivery," *Scientific American*, April 30, 2010, scientificamerican.com/article/fetal-cells-microchimerism/.

While we learn in science classes that we are unique . . .
Hilary S. Gammill et al., "Pregnancy, Microchimerism, and the Maternal Grandmother," *PLOS One* 6, no. 8 (August 2011): e24101, doi.org/10.1371/journal.pone.0024101.

By looking at developing twins . . .
Janelle Weaver, "Social Before Birth: Twins First Interact with Each Other as Fetuses," *Scientific American: Mind*, January 1, 2011, scientificamerican.com/article/social-before-birth/.

Even at this early stage, it appears . . .
Weaver, "Social Before Birth."

The American Diabetes Association recommends . . .
"Classification and Diagnosis of Diabetes: Standards of Medical Care in Diabetes—2018," *Diabetes Care* 41, supplement 1 (January 2018): S13–S27, doi.org/10.2337/dc18-S002.

From 2 to 10 percent of pregnant women will develop . . .
Brindles Lee Macon and Winnie Yu, "Gestational Diabetes," Healthline, June 25, 2018, healthline.com/health/gestational-diabetes.

GDM may run in families . . .
Nael Shaat and Leif Groop, "Genetics of Gestational Diabetes Mellitus," *Current Medicinal Chemistry* 14, no. 5 (2007): 569–583, doi.org/10.2174/092986707780059643

Of note, women who have immigrated to the US . . .
Lili Yuen and Vincent W. Wong, "Gestational Diabetes Mellitus: Challenges for Different Ethnic Groups," *World Journal of Diabetes* 6, no. 8 (July 2015): 1024–1032, doi.org/10.4239/wjd.v6.i8.1024.

Expecting a Baby in Finland
Helena Lee, "Why Finnish Babies Sleep in Cardboard Boxes," *BBC News Magazine*, June 4, 2013, bbc.com/news/magazine-22751415.

For example, it is possible that having 28 jelly beans . . .
Michael E. Lamar et al., "Jelly Beans as an Alternative to a Fifty-Gram Glucose Beverage for Gestational Diabetes Screening," *American Journal of Obstetrics and Gynecology* 181, no. 5 (November 1999): 1154–1157, doi.org/10.1016/s0002-9378(99)70099-2.

. . . or 10 Twizzlers . . .
Diana A. Racusin et al., "Twizzlers as a Cost-Effective and Equivalent Alternative to the Glucola Beverage in Diabetes Screening," *Diabetes Care* 36, no. 10 (October 2013): e169–e170, doi.org/10.2337/dc13-1130.

This is not yet a well-proven alternative . . .
Diane Farrar et al., "Different Strategies for Diagnosing Gestational Diabetes to Improve Maternal and Infant Health," Cochrane Database of Systematic Reviews 2017, no. 8 (August 2017), doi.org/10.1002/14651858.CD007122.pub4.

Ensure that your travel destination does not . . .
"Vaccines. Medicines. Advice," Centers for Disease Control and Prevention, cdc.gov/travel.

If you are planning to take a flight . . .
Morteza Izadi et al., "Do Pregnant Women Have a Higher Risk for Venous Thromboembolism Following Air Travel?" *Advanced Biomedical Research* 4 (February 2015): 60, doi.org/10.4103 /2277-9175.151879.

The American Society for Blood and Marrow Transplantation . . .
William T. Shearer et al., "Cord Blood Banking for Potential Future Transplantation," American Academy of Pediatrics, *Pediatrics* 140, no. 5 (November 2017), pediatrics.aappublications.org /content/140/5/e20172695.

Private cord blood banking can be expensive . . .
Shearer et al., "Cord Blood Banking."

For these reasons, the American Academy of Pediatrics . . .
Shearer et al., "Cord Blood Banking."

Unfortunately, many experts recommend . . .
Aaron M. Milstone, Allison George Agwu, and Frederick J. Angulo, "Alerting Pregnant Women to the Risk of Reptile-Associated Salmonellosis," *Obstetrics & Gynecology* 107, no. 2 (February 2006): 516–518, doi.org/10.1097/01.aog.0000187950 .37065.87.

. . . and children younger than 5 . . .
"Advice for Pet Reptile Owners," Centers for Disease Control and Prevention, last updated August 20, 2014, cdc.gov/salmonella/cotham-04-14/advice-pet -owners.html.

Good news: Research finds that when babies . . .
Tove Fall et al., "Early Exposure to Dogs and Farm Animals and the Risk of Childhood Asthma," *JAMA Pediatrics* 169, no. 11 (November 2015): e153219, doi. org/10.1001/jamapediatrics.2015.3219.

Babies who live with cats . . .
Eija Bergroth et al., "Respiratory Tract Illnesses During the First Year of Life: Effect of Dog and Cat Contacts," *Pediatrics* 130, no.2 (August 2012): 211–220, doi.org/10.1542/peds.2011-2825.

You probably have some inkling that your placenta . . .
Graham J. Burton and Eric Jauniaux, "What Is the Placenta?" *American Journal of Obstetrics and Gynecology* 213, no. 4 (October 2015): S6.e1–S6.e4, doi.org/10.1016/j.ajog.2015.07.050.

Studies find that when women have positive . . .
Laura M. Schwab-Reese, Ellen J. Schafer, and Sato Ashida, "Associations of Social Support and Stress with Postpartum Maternal Mental Health Symptoms: Main Effects, Moderation, and Mediation," *Women & Health* 57, no. 6 (July 2017): 723–740, doi.org/10.1080/03630242.2016.1181140.

Researchers have found that stay-at-home mothers . . .
Maricar Santos, "When You Factor in Family Duties, the Average Working Mom Works 98 Hours a Week," Working Mother, updated May 9, 2018, workingmother.com/when-you-factor-in-family -duties-average-working-mom-works-98-hours -week?src=soc&dom=fb.

. . . their workload would garner a salary . . .
"Moms: We Know You're Worth It. But How Much Is 'It' Really Worth?" Salary.com, updated December 2017, salary.com/articles/stay-at-home-mom/.

In Motherly's 2018 State of Motherhood Survey . . .
"2018 State of Motherhood Survey," Motherly, motherly.s3.amazonaws.com/Motherly%20 state%20of%20motherhood%20survey%20results _cleaned%20and%20weighted.pdf.

Women are more educated . . .
Richard Fry, Ruth Igielnik, and Eileen Patten, "How Millennials Today Compare with Their Grandparents 50 Years Ago," Fact Tank, Pew Research Center, March 16, 2018, pewresearch.org /fact-tank/2018/03/16/how-millennials-compare -with-their-grandparents/.

Increasingly, women are running their own businesses . . .
"Women Business Owners Statistics," National Association of Women Business Owners, updated, December, 2017, nawbo.org/resources /women-business-owner-statistics.

According to the Bureau of Labor Statistics Consumer Price Index . . .
"CPI Inflation Calculator," Official Data Foundation, Alioth LLC, January 11, 2019,officialdata.org/1988 -dollars-in-2018.

That means that $10 in 2018 had the purchasing power . . .
"Median and Average Sales Prices of New Homes Sold in United States," US Census Bureau, updated December 2018, census.gov/construction/nrs /pdf/uspricemon.pdf.

When you factor in that just from 2000 to 2015 . . .
"Median and Average Sales Prices of New Homes Sold in United States."

In heterosexual relationships between 2010 and 2014 . . .
Cassie Rushing and Misti Sparks, "The Mother's Perspective: Factors Considered When Choosing to Enter a Stay-at-Home Father and Working Mother Relationship," *American Journal of Men's Health* 1, no. 4 (July 2017): 1260–1268, doi.org/10.1177/1557988317693347.

Plus, about a quarter of all moms . . .
"The Majority of Children Live with Two Parents, Census Bureau Reports," United States Census Bureau, November 17, 2016, census.gov/newsroom/press-releases/2016/cb16-192.html.

In a study on how American culture views . . .
Elizabeth Paré and Heather Dillaway, "'Staying at Home' Versus 'Working': A Call for Broader Conceptualizations of Parenthood and Paid Work," *Michigan Family Review* 10, no. 1 (2005): 66–85, doi.org/10.3998/mfr.4919087.0010.105.

Motherly mamas agree: About 78 percent . . .
Heather Marcoux, "Motherhood Survey: Millennial Mothers Demand More Support from Government and Society," Motherly, May 13, 2018, mother.ly/news/2018-state-of-motherhood-survey-millennial-mothers-need-more-support.

CHAPTER 12
Month 7, Weeks 28–31

Of note, on rare occasions babies let us know . . .
Jason H. Collins, "Umbilical Cord Accidents," *Biomed Central Pregnancy and Childbirth* 12, supplement 1 (August 2012): A7, doi.org/10.1186/1471-2393-12-S1-A7.

They are derived from blood products . . .
"Frequently Asked Questions," RhoGAM, Kedrion Biopharma, Inc., last modified June 2018, rhogam.com/faq/.

ACOG recommends that all pregnant women receive . . .
"Frequently Asked Questions for Pregnant Women Concerning Tdap Vaccination," American College of Obstetricians and Gynecologists, 2015, acog.org/-/media/departments/immunization/tdap-vaccine-mailing/tear-pad-faqtdap.pdf.

Women who report significant sleep difficulty . . .
Lianne M. Tomfohr et al., "Trajectories of Sleep Quality and Associations with Mood During the Perinatal Period," *Sleep* 38, no. 8 (August 2015): 1237–1245, doi.org/10.5665/sleep.4900.

In parts of India, starting in the seventh month . . .
Abdul Rashid Gatrad, Manabendra Ray, and Aziz Sheikh, "Hindu Birth Customs," *Archives of Disease in Childhood* 89, no. 12 (December 2004): 1094–1097, doi.org/10.1136/adc.2004.050591.

In fact, 60 percent of grandparents take . . .
Ye Luo et al., "Grandparents Providing Care to Grandchildren: A Population-Based Study of Continuity and Change," *Journal of Family Issues* 33, no. 9 (September 2012): 1143–1167, doi.org/10.1177/0192513x12438685.

If support from family members . . .
Jacqueline Howard, "The Costs of Child Care Around the World," CNN, updated April 25, 2018, cnn.com/2018/04/25/health/child-care-parenting-explainer-intl/index.html.

. . . couples spend an average of 25.6 percent of their income . . .
Willem Adema, Chris Clarke, and Olivier Thévenon, "Who Uses Childcare? Background Brief on Inequalities in the Use of Formal Early Childhood Education and Care (ECEC) Among Very Young Children," Social Policy Division, OECD Directorate of Employment, Labor and Social Affairs, updated June 2016, oecd.org/els/family/who_uses_childcare-backgrounder_inequalities_formal_ecec.pdf.

In Denmark, for example, couples spend . . .
Howard, "The Costs of Child Care."

Well, researchers have found there is a significant . . .
Janet A. DiPietro et al., "What Does Fetal Movement Predict About Behavior During the First Two Years of Life?" *Developmental Psychobiology* 40, no. 4 (May 2002): 358–371, doi.org/10.1002/dev.10025.

Eventually, they build up their immunity . . .
Saskia Hullegie et al., "First-Year Daycare and Incidence of Acute Gastroenteritis," *Pediatrics* 137, no. 5 (May 2016): e20153356, doi.org/10.1542/peds.2015-3356.

The normal window for birth . . .
Gordon C. S. Smith, "Use of Time to Event Analysis to Estimate the Normal Duration of Human Pregnancy," *Human Reproduction* 16, no. 7 (July 2001): 1497–1500, doi.org/10.1093/humrep/16.7.1497.

CHAPTER 13
Month 8, Weeks 32–35

Researcher Judith A. Lothian wrote in a study . . .
Judith A. Lothian, "Do Not Disturb: The Importance of Privacy in Labor," *Journal of Perinatal Education* 13, no.3 (Summer 2004): 4–6, doi.org/10.1624/105812404x1707.

You don't need a research study to tell you . . .
Colleen Fisher, Yvonne Hauck, and Jenny Fenwick, "How Social Context Impacts on Women's Fears of Childbirth: A Western Australian Example," *Social Science and Medicine* 63, no. 1 (July 2006): 64–75, doi.org/10.1016/j.socscimed.2005.11.065.

There is a scientifically demonstrated phenomenon . . .
Giuseppe Mancia et al., "Diagnosis and Management of Patients with White-Coat and Masked Hypertension," *Nature Reviews Cardiology* 8, no. 12 (August 2011): 686–693, doi.org/10.1038/nrcardio.2011.115; Elsa Lena Ryding et al., "An Evaluation of Midwives' Counseling of Pregnant Women in Fear of Childbirth," *Acta Obstetricia et Gynecologica Scandinavica* 82, no.1 (January 2003): 10–17, doi.org/10.1080/j.1600-0412.2003.820102.x.

Studies have found that almost 80 percent of women . . .
Ryding et al., "An Evaluation of Midwives' Counseling of Pregnant Women," 10–17.

I want to convey to you, warrior mama . . .
Kathrin Stol and Wendy Hall, "Vicarious Birth Experiences and Childbirth Fear: Does It Matter How Young Canadian Women Learn About Birth?" *Journal of Perinatal Education* 22, no. 4 (Fall 2013): 226–233, doi.org/10.1891/1058-1243.22.4.226.

Getting therapy . . .
Elisabet Rondung, Johanna Thomtén, and Örjan Sundin, "Psychological Perspectives on Fear of Childbirth," *Journal of Anxiety Disorders* 44 (December 2016): 80–91, doi.org/10.1016/j.janxdis.2016.10.007.

Research shows that at least 85 to 90 percent . . .
Martin E. P. Seligman, "The Effectiveness of Psychotherapy: The Consumer Reports Study," *American Psychologist* 50, no. 12 (December 1995): 965–974, doi.org/10.1037/0003-066x.50.12.965.

Project LETS (Let's Erase the Stigma) . . .
"Emergency Action for Panic Attacks," Project LETS, accessed May 10, 2019, letserasethestigma.com/emergency-action-for-panic-attacks.

Starting around week 25 . . .
Jessica Timmons, "When Can a Fetus Hear?" Healthline, January 5, 2018, healthline.com/health/pregnancy/when-can-a-fetus-hear#1.

Their heart rate goes up . . .
Gabriella A. Ferrari et al., "Ultrasonographic Investigation of Human Fetus Responses to Maternal Communicative and Non-Communicative Stimuli," *Frontiers in Psychology* 7 (March 2016): 354, doi.org/10.3389/fpsyg.2016.00354.

What's more, recent studies have also found . . .
Christine Moon, Hugo Lagercrantz, and Patricia K. Kuhl, "Language Experienced in Utero Affects Vowel Perception After Birth: A Two-Country Study," *Acta Paediatrica* 102, no. 2 (February 2013): 156–160, doi.org/10.1111/apa.12098.

And even in the womb, little ones respond . . .
Viola Marx and Emese Nagy, "Fetal Behavioural Responses to Maternal Voice and Touch," *PLOS One* 10, no. 6 (June 2015): e0129118, doi.org/10.1371/journal.pone.0129118.

Research also shows that music . . .
T. Christina Zhao and Patricia K. Kuhl, "Musical Intervention Enhances Infants' Neural Processing of Temporal Structure in Music and Speech," *Proceedings of the National Academy of Sciences* 113, no. 19 (May 2016): 5212–5217, doi.org/10.1073/pnas.1603984113.

Psst: A 2018 study found that pregnant women who took naps . . .
Lulu Song et al., "Afternoon Napping During Pregnancy and Low Birth Weight: The Healthy Baby Cohort Study," *Sleep Medicine* 48 (August 2018): 35–41, doi.org/10.1016/j.sleep.2018.03.029.

Your provider may recommend a repeat HIV screening . . .
"An Opt-Out Approach to HIV Screening," Centers for Disease Control and Prevention, updated September 9, 2019, cdc.gov/hiv/group/gender/pregnantwomen/opt-out.html.

Research finds that more than half . . .
Carola Eriksson, Göran Westman, and Katarina Hamberg, "Experiential Factors Associated with Childbirth-Related Fear in Swedish Women and Men: A Population Based Study," *Journal of Psychosomatic Obstetrics & Gynecology* 26, no.1 (March 2005): 63–72, doi.org/10.1080/01674820400023275; Suzanne Hanson et al., "Paternal Fears of Childbirth: A Literature Review," *Journal of Perinatal Education* 18, no. 4 (2009): 12–20, doi.org/10.1624/105812409x474672.

Children who grow up with a strong sense of connection . . .
Patrice Marie Miller and Michael Lamport Commons, "The Benefits of Attachment Parenting for Infants and Children: A Behavioral Developmental View," *Behavioral Development Bulletin* 16, no. 1 (2010): 1–14, doi.org/10.1037/h0100514.

Attachment Parenting International has laid out . . .
"API's Eight Principles of Parenting," Attachment
Parenting International, updated December 2018,
attachmentparenting.org/principles/api. © 1994,
2007, 2009, 2014, 2017, 2018, 2019 Attachment
Parenting International. "API's Eight Principles
of Parenting" define the parenting approach
commonly referred to as Attachment Parenting.
They were created by Attachment Parenting
International to reflect parenting choices that
promote a child's secure attachment. "API's Eight
Principles of Parenting" can be found in its entirety
at attachmentparenting.org/principles/api.

But is it any wonder that a whopping 59 percent of car seats . . .
"Child Passenger Safety: Get the Facts," Centers
for Disease Control and Prevention, updated
September 13, 2019, cdc.gov/motorvehiclesafety
/child_passenger_safety/cps-factsheet.html.

CHAPTER 14
Month 9, Weeks 36–40

Research has found that doing the test on yourself . . .
Hillary Mount, F. Chris Vincent, and Lara Handler,
"Self-Administered GBS Testing in Pregnant
Women," *American Family Physician* 90, no. 10
(November 2014): 729–730, aafp.org/afp/2014/1115
/p729.html.

Between 1 and 2 percent of babies . . .
"Group B Strep Infection," March of Dimes, updated
November 2013, marchofdimes.org/complications
/group-b-strep-infection.aspx.

DNA-based tests that can give results . . .
Maria Isabel S. Gouvea et al., "Accuracy of a Rapid
Real-Time Polymerase Chain Reaction Assay for
Diagnosis of Group B *Streptococcus* Colonization
in a Cohort of HIV-Infected Pregnant Women,"
Journal of Maternal-Fetal and Neonatal Medicine 30,
no. 9 (2017): 1096–1101, doi.org/10.1080/14767058
.2016.1205021.

A macrosomic baby, or big baby . . .
Jacques S. Abramowicz and Jennifer T. Ahn, "Fetal
Macrosomia," UpToDate, last updated July 31, 2019,
uptodate.com/contents/fetal-macrosomia.

Macrosomia is not that common . . .
Mahin Najafian and Maria Cheraghi, "Occurrence
of Fetal Macrosomia Rate and Its Maternal and
Neonatal Complications: A 5-Year Cohort Study,"
ISRN Obstetrics and Gynecology 2012 (2012): 353791,
doi.org/10.5402/2012/353791.

There are some factors that can make you more at risk . . .
Najafian and Cheraghi, "Occurrence of Fetal
Macrosomia," 353791.

However, this is no longer the case as rates have dropped . . .
"Prevention of Early-Onset Group B Streptococcal
Disease in Newborns," Committee Opinion
No. 782, American College of Obstetricians and
Gynecologists, *Obstetrics and Gynecology* 134 (2019):
e19-40, acog.org/clinical-guidance-and
-publications/committee-opinions/committee-on
-obstetric-practice/prevention-of-early-onset-group
-b-streptococcal-disease-in-newborns.

*Providers may use this information to make
recommendations . . .*
Suneet P. Chauhan et al., "Suspicion and Treatment of
the Macrosomic Fetus: A Review," *American Journal
of Obstetrics and Gynecology* 193, no. 2, (August
2005): 332–346, doi.org/10.1016/j.ajog.2004.12.020.

In fact, overestimation of fetal weight . . .
Kelly B. Zafman, Eric Bergh, and Nathan S. Fox,
"Accuracy of Sonographic Estimated Fetal Weight
in Suspected Macrosomia: The Likelihood of
Overestimating and Underestimating the True
Birthweight," *The Journal of Maternal-Fetal and
Neonatal Medicine* 1, no. 6 (September 2018): 201,
doi.org/10.1080/14767058.2018.1511697.

Another important point to consider . . .
Lauren Jansen et al., "First Do No Harm:
Interventions During Childbirth," *Journal of
Perinatal Education* 22, no. 2 (Spring 2013): 83–92,
doi.org/10.1891/1058-1243.22.2.83.

Many providers recommend additional testing . . .
"STDs During Pregnancy: CDC Fact Sheet (Detailed),"
Centers for Disease Control and Prevention,
updated February 11, 2016, cdc.gov/std/pregnancy
/stdfact-pregnancy-detailed.htm.

Easy Baked Pesto Chicken
Crystal Karges, "Easy Basil Pesto Chicken Bake
Recipe," Crystal Karges Nutrition, March 17, 2019,
crystalkarges.com/blog/easy-basil-pesto-chicken
-bake-recipe.

In India, women might observe . . .
Catherine Gigante-Brown, "Postpartum Practices
Worldwide: How the World Takes Care of Moms
and Babies," Ravishly, August 18, 2015, ravishly.
com/2015/08/18/postpartum-practices-worldwide
-how-world-takes-care-moms-and-babies.

In Japan, women may practice ansei . . .
Gigante-Brown, "Postpartum Practices Worldwide."

Multiples are more likely to come early . . .
Roshni R. Patel et al., "Does Gestation Vary by Ethnic Group? A London-Based Study of over 122,000 Pregnancies with Spontaneous Onset of Labour," *International Journal of Epidemiology* 33, no. 1 (February 2004): 107–113, doi.org/10.1093/ije /dyg238.

CHAPTER 15
Beyond 40 Weeks

"Now is the time to appreciate the magic . . .
Colleen Temple, "To the Mama About to Give Birth—There's Magic in the Waiting," Motherly, January 2019, mother.ly/life/to-the-mama-about-to-give -birth-theres-magic-in-the-waiting.

We believe that, in addition to a number of maternal factors . . .
Jossimara Polettini et al., "Telomere Fragment Induced Amnion Cell Senescence: A Contributor to Parturition?" *PLOS One* 10, no. 9 (September 2015): e0137188, doi.org/10.1371/journal.pone.0137188.

ACOG states that testing should start . . .
"When Pregnancy Goes Past Your Due Date," Frequently Asked Questions, American College of Obstetricians and Gynecologists, updated June 2017, acog.org/patients/faqs/when-pregnancy -goes-past-your-due-date#postterm.

Some people may choose . . .
"Ask the Expert: Baby Showers. Is It Against the Rules, or Just a Superstition?" My Jewish Learning, January 2019, myjewishlearning.com/article/ask -the-expert-baby-showers/.

The research jury is still out . . .
Josephine Kavanagh, Anthony J. Kelly, and Jane Thomas, "Sexual Intercourse for Cervical Ripening and Induction of Labour," Cochrane Database of Systematic Reviews 2001, no. 2 (April 2008): CD003093, doi.org/10.1002/14651858.cd003093.

Gently massaging your nipples can release . . .
Kaori Takahata et al., "Effects of Breast Stimulation for Spontaneous Onset of Labor on Salivary Oxytocin Levels in Low-Risk Pregnant Women: A Feasibility Study," *PLOS One* 13, no. 2 (February 2018): e0192757, doi.org/10.1371/journal.pone .0192757.

It therefore may effectively start labor . . .
Gulbahtiyar Demirel and Handan Guler, "The Effect of Uterine and Nipple Stimulation on Induction with Oxytocin and the Labor Process," *Worldviews on Evidence-Based Nursing* 12, no. 5 (October 2015): 273–280, sigmapubs.onlinelibrary.wiley.com/doi /abs/10.1111/wvn.12116.

One small study found that it actually increased . . .
Nilanchali Singh et al., "Breast Stimulation in Low-Risk Primigravidas at Term: Does It Aid in Spontaneous Onset of Labour and Vaginal Delivery?" *Biomed Research International* 2014 (November 2014): 695037, doi.org/10.1155/2014 /695037.

It's important to note that since the studies have . . .
Deepa Maheswari Narasimhulu and Ling Zhu, "Uterine Tachysystole with Prolonged Deceleration Following Nipple Stimulation for Labor Augmentation," *Kathmandu University Medical Journal* 13, no. 51 (July–September 2015): 268–270, doi.org/10.3126/kumj.v13i3.16820.

Evening primrose oil . . .
Mahnaz Kalati et al., "Evening Primrose Oil and Labour, Is It Effective? A Randomised Clinical Trial," *Journal of Obstetrics and Gynaecology* 38, no. 4 (May 2018): 488–492, doi.org/10.1080/01443615.2017.1386165.

Red raspberry leaf tea . . .
Michele Simpson et al., "Raspberry Leaf in Pregnancy: Its Safety and Efficacy in Labor," *Journal of Midwifery and Women's Health* 46, no. 2 (March–April 2001): 51–59, doi.org/10.1016/S1526-9523 (01)00095-2.

Blue and black cohosh . . .
Aviva Romm, "Blue Cohosh: History, Science, Safety, and Midwife Prescribing of a Potentially Fetotoxic Herb," *Yale Medicine Thesis Digital Library* 88 (September 2009), elischolar.library.yale.edu /ymtdl/88; Matthew J. Blitz, Michelle Smith-Levitin, and Burton Rochelson, "Severe Hyponatremia Associated with Use of Black Cohosh During Prolonged Labor and Unsuccessful Home Birth," *American Journal of Perinatology Reports* 6, no. 1 (March 2016): e121–124, doi.org/10.1055/s-0036- 1579537.

Comfrey root . . .
Cynthia Belew, "Herbs and the Childbearing Woman: Guidelines for Midwives," *Journal of Nurse-Midwifery* 44, no. 3 (May–June 1999): 231–252, doi.org/10.1016/S0091-2182(99)00043-9.

A small study found that there is an increased chance ...
Sedighe Azhari et al., "Evaluation of the Effect of Castor Oil on Initiating Labor in Term Pregnancy," *Saudi Medical Journal* 27, no. 7 (July 2006): 1011–1014, ncbi.nlm.nih.gov/pubmed/16830021.

... we don't have strong enough research ...
Anthony J. Kelly, Josephine Kavanagh, and Jane Thomas, "Castor Oil, Bath and/or Enema for Cervical Priming and Induction of Labour," Cochrane Database of Systematic Reviews 2013, no. 7 (July 2013: CD003099, doi.org/10.1002/14651858 .cd003099.pub2.

Studies have found that acupuncture ...
Caroline A. Smith, Caroline A. Crowther, and Suzanne J. Grant, "Acupuncture for Induction of Labour," Cochrane Database of Systematic Reviews 2013, no. 8 (August 2013): CD002962, doi.org/10 .1002/14651858.CD002962.pub3; Judith M. Schlaeger et al., "Acupuncture and Acupressure in Labor," *Journal of Midwifery and Women's Health* 62, no. 1 (January/February 2017): 12–28, doi.org/10.1111 /jmwh.12545.

CHAPTER 16
When Pregnancy Is Hard

Pregnant women who have completed mindfulness
Cassandra Dunn, Emma Hanieh, Rachel Roberts, and Roselind Powrie, "Mindful Pregnancy and Childbirth: Effects of a Mindfulness-Based Intervention on Women's Psychological Distress and Well-Being in the Perinatal Period," *Archives of Women's Mental Health* 15, no. 2 (April 2012): 139–143, doi.org/10.1007/s00737-012-0264-4.

CHAPTER 17
Going into Labor

However, there are some other milestones ...
Catherine Y. Spong, "Defining 'Term' Pregnancy: Recommendations from the Defining 'Term' Pregnancy Workgroup," *JAMA* 309, no. 23 (June 2013): 2445–2446, doi.org/10.1001/jama.2013.6235.

Only 4 percent of women have their babies ...
Andrew P. MacKenzie, Courtney D. Stephenson, and Edmund F. Funai, "Prenatal Assessment of Gestational Age, Date of Delivery, and Fetal Weight," UpToDate, last updated July 8, 2019, uptodate.com/ contents/prenatal-assessment-of-gestational-age -date-of-delivery-and-fetal-weight.

If this is your second time giving birth ...
Ka Ying Bonnie Ng and Philip J. Steer, "Prediction of an Estimated Delivery Date Should Take into Account Both the Length of a Previous Pregnancy and the Interpregnancy Interval," *European Journal of Obstetrics & Gynecology and Reproductive Biology* 201 (June 2016): 101–107, doi.org/10.1016/j .ejogrb.2016.03.045.

In fact, studies have found that 40 weeks and 3 days ...
Anna S. Oberg et al., "Maternal and Fetal Genetic Contributions to Postterm Birth: Familial Clustering in a Population-Based Sample of 475,429 Swedish Births," *American Journal of Epidemiology* 177, no. 6 (March 2013): 531–537, doi.org/10.1093/aje /kws244.

... or 40 weeks and 5 days ...
Anne Marie Jukic et al., "Length of Human Pregnancy and Contributors to Its Natural Variation," *Human Reproduction* 28, no. 10 (October 2013): 2848–2855, doi.org/10.1093/humrep/det297.

You may be more likely to go past your due date if ...
Oberg et al., "Maternal and Fetal Genetic Contributions," 531-537.

A study found that as due dates approached ...
Marla V. Anderson and M. D. Rutherford, "Evidence of a Nesting Psychology During Human Pregnancy," *Evolution and Human Behavior* 34, no. 6 (November 2013): 390–397, doi.org/10.1016/j.evolhumbehav .2013.07.002.

For about 10 percent of women ...
"Premature Rupture of Membranes (PROM)/Preterm Premature Rupture of Membranes (PPROM)," Children's Hospital of Philadelphia, May 2019, chop.edu/conditions-diseases/premature-rupture -membranes-prompreterm-premature-rupture -membranes-pprom.

Of note, over 75 percent of women with PROM ...
Armando Pintucci et al., "Premature Rupture of Membranes at Term in Low Risk Women: How Long Should We Wait in the 'Latent Phase'?" *Journal of Perinatal Medicine* 42, no 2 (March 2014): 189–196, doi.org/10.1515/jpm-2013-0017.

Of the 90 percent of women who don't ...
"Premature Rupture of Membranes."

Their babies win cool-entry awards ...
"Caul, or Face Veil, Occasionally Present at Birth," Medical College of Wisconsin, HealthLink, updated January 24, 2005, healthlink.mcw.edu/article /901311432.html.

Very rarely (in about 0.16 to 0.18 percent of pregnancies) . . .
Tetsuya Kawakita, Chun-Chih Huang, and Helain J.
  Landy, "Risk Factors for Umbilical Cord Prolapse
  at the Time of Artificial Rupture of Membranes,"
  American Journal of Perinatology Reports 8, no. 2
  (April 2018): e89–e94, doi.org/10.1055/s-0038
  -1649486.

While you wait for the paramedics . . .
Waleed Ali Sayed Ahmed and Mostafa Ahmed Hamdy,
  "Optimal Management of Umbilical
  Cord Prolapse," *International Journal of Women's
  Health* 10 (August 2018): 459–465, doi.org/10.2147
  /ijwh.s130879.

You will likely be more comfortable . . .
"New Professional Recommendations to Limit Labor
  and Birth Interventions: What Pregnant Women
  Need to Know," Childbirth Connection, March 2017,
  nationalpartnership.org/our-work/resources/health
  -care/maternity/professional-recommendations-to
  -limit-labor-and-birth-interventions.pdf.

About 1 in 10 babies is born prematurely . . .
"Premature Birth," National Center for Chronic Disease
  Prevention and Health Promotion, Centers for
  Disease Control and Prevention, updated June 13,
  2019, cdc.gov/features/prematurebirth/index.html.

. . . but the vast majority of these are born after . . .
Pierre-Yves Ancel, François Goffinet, and the
  EPIPAGE-2 Writing Group, "Survival and Morbidity
  of Preterm Children Born at 22 Through 34 Weeks'
  Gestation in France in 2011: Results of the
  EPIPAGE-2 Cohort Study," *JAMA Pediatrics* 169, no.
  3 (2015): 230–238, doi.org/10.1001/jamapediatrics
  .2014.3351.

For babies born as early as 26 weeks . . .
Hannah C. Glass et al., "Outcomes for Extremely
  Premature Infants," *Anesthesia and Analgesia* 120,
  no. 6 (June 2015): 1337–1351, doi.org/10.1213
  /ane.0000000000000705.

Studies have shown that non-Hispanic black babies . . .
Heather H. Burris, James W. Collins, Jr., and Robert O.
  Wright, "Racial/Ethnic Disparities in Preterm Birth:
  Clues from Environmental Exposures," *Current
  Opinion in Pediatrics* 23, no. 2 (April 2011): 227–232,
  ncbi.nlm.nih.gov/pmc/articles/pmc3753013/.

Lesbian and bisexual women have a significantly higher risk . . .
Bethany G. Everett et al., "Sexual Orientation
  Disparities in Pregnancy and Infant Outcomes,"
  Maternal and Child Health Journal 23, no. 1 (January
  2019): 72–81, doi.org/10.1007/s10995-018-2595-x.

. . . likely stemming from prejudicial treatment . . .
"Guiding Principles to Achieving Equity in Preterm
  Birth," March of Dimes Prematurity Collaborative,
  February 2017, marchofdimes.org/materials/pc18
  -02%20prematuritycollaborative2018summitreport
  _final.pdf.

CHAPTER 18
First Stage of Labor: Dilating and Effacing

It decreases with increasing maternal age . . .
Mary N. Zaki, Judith U. Hibbard, and Michelle A.
  Kominiarek, "Contemporary Labor Patterns and
  Maternal Age," *American Journal of Obstetrics &
  Gynecology* 122, no. 5 (November 2013): 1018–1024,
  ncbi.nlm.nih.gov/pmc/articles/pmc3894623/.

For example, a study found that black women . . .
Mara B. Greenberg et al., "Are There Ethnic
  Differences in the Length of Labor?" *Obstetrics &
  Gynecology* 195, no. 3 (September 2006): 743–748,
  doi.org/10.1016/j.ajog.2006.06.016.

Women with a higher body mass index . . .
Sara Carlhäll, Karin Källén, and Marie Blomberg,
  "Maternal Body Mass Index and Duration of Labor,"
  *European Journal of Obstetrics and Gynecology and
  Reproductive Biology* 171, no. 1 (November 2013):
  49–53, doi.org/10.1016/j.ejogrb.2013.08.021.

This curve shows that women having their first babies . . .
Jeremy L. Neal et al., "'Active Labor' Duration and
  Dilation Rates Among Low-Risk, Nulliparous
  Women with Spontaneous Labor Onset: A
  Systematic Review," *Journal of Midwifery and
  Women's Health* 55, no. 4 (July–August 2010):
  308–318, doi.org/10.1016/j.jmwh.2009.08.004.

The problem: His study included . . .
Rebecca Dekker, "Friedman's Curve and Failure
  to Progress: A Leading Cause of Unplanned
  Cesareans," Evidence Based Birth, updated April 26,
  2017, evidencebasedbirth.com/friedmans-curve
  -and-failure-to-progress-a-leading-cause-of
  -unplanned-c-sections/.

Recent research suggests that for low-risk . . .
Neal et al. "'Active Labor' Duration."

In 2010, Zhang and colleagues . . .
Jun Zhang et al., "Contemporary Patterns of
  Spontaneous Labor with Normal Neonatal
  Outcomes," *Obstet Gynecol* 116, no. 6 (December
  2010): 1281-12-87, doi.org/ 10.1097/AOG.0b013e
  3181fdef6e.

It can last roughly from 8 to 12 hours . . .
"Stages of Childbirth: Stage I," American
  Pregnancy Association, updated July 16, 2019,
  americanpregnancy.org/labor-and-birth/first
  -stage-of-labor/.

You'll have a lot of adrenaline pumping . . .
Siw Alehagen et al., "Catecholamine and Cortisol
  Reaction to Childbirth," *International Journal of
  Behavioral Medicine* 8, no. 1 (March 2001): 50–65,
  doi.org/10.1207/s15327558ijbm0801_04.

Walking during early labor . . .
Michele Ondeck, "Healthy Birth Practice #2:
  Walk, Move Around, and Change Positions
  Throughout Labor," *Journal of Perinatal Education*
  23, no. 4 (Fall 2014): 188–193, doi.org/10.1891/1058
  -1243.23.4.188.

Even if you can only drift off . . .
Catherine E. Milner and Kimberly A. Cote, "Benefits of
  Napping in Healthy Adults: Impact of Nap Length,
  Time of Day, Age, and Experience with Napping,"
  Journal of Sleep Research 18, no. 2 (June 2009): 272–
  281, doi.org/10.1111/j.1365-2869.2008.00718.x.

Active labor lasts an average of 7.7 hours . . .
Leah L. Albers, "The Duration of Labor in Healthy
  Women," *Journal of Perinatology* 19, no. 2 (March
  1999): 114–119, doi.org/10.1038/sj.jp.7200100.

It is usually the shortest phase of the first stage . . .
"Stages of Childbirth," American Pregnancy
  Association.

Research finds that when women have . . .
Meghan A. Bohren et al., "Continuous Support for
  Women During Childbirth," Cochrane Database
  of Systematic Reviews 2017, no. 7 (July 2017):
  CD003766, doi.org/10.1002/14651858.cd003766.pub6.

CHAPTER 19
Second Stage of Labor: Pushing

First-time moms push for an average of . . .
Vivienne Souter et al., "364: Length of the Second
  Stage of Labor in Nulliparas in a Contemporary US
  Hospital Population," *American Journal of Obstetrics
  and Gynecology* 218, no. 1 (January 2018): S225–S226,
  doi.org/10.1016/j.ajog.2017.10.300.

Of note, recent research shows that immediate pushing . . .
Alison G. Cahill et al., "Effect of Immediate vs. Delayed
  Pushing on Rates of Spontaneous Vaginal Delivery
  Among Nulliparous Women Receiving Neuaxial
  Analgesia," *JAMA* 320, no. 14 (2018): 1444-1454,
  doi.org/ 10.1001/jama.2018.13986.

Pushing in an upright position . . .
Janesh K. Gupta et al., "Position in the Second Stage of
  Labour for Women Without Epidural Anaesthesia,"
  Cochrane Database of Systematic Reviews 2017, no.
  5 (May 2017): CD002006, doi.org/10.1002/14651858
  .cd002006.pub4.

Therefore, women should push in the positions . . .
Gupta et al., "Position in the Second Stage."

This is the most commonly used position . . .
Joyce T. DiFranco and Marilyn Curl, "Healthy Birth
  Practice #5: Avoid Giving Birth on Your Back
  and Follow Your Body's Urge to Push," *Journal of
  Perinatal Education* 23, no. 4 (Fall 2014): 207–210,
  doi.org/10.1891/1058-1243.23.4.207.

Squatting can allow gravity to help . . .
"Positions for Labour and Birth," Spiritual Birth, April 12,
  2011, spiritualbirth.net/positions-for-labour-and-birth.

Based on drawings and sculptures . . .
Lauren Dundes, "The Evolution of Maternal Birthing
  Position," *American Journal of Public Health* 77, no. 5
  (May 1987): 638–641, ajph.aphapublications.org/doi
  /pdf/10.2105/ajph.77.5.636.

Perineal massage during pregnancy . . .
Michael M. Beckmann and Owen M. Stock, "Antenatal
  Perineal Massage for Reducing Perineal Trauma,"
  Cochrane Database of Systematic Reviews 2013, no.
  4 (April 2013): CD005123, doi.org/10.1002/14651858
  .cd005123.pub3.

By lying on your left side . . .
Bruno Carbonne et al., "Maternal Position During
  Labor: Effects on Fetal Oxygen Saturation
  Measured by Pulse Oximetry," *Obstetrics &
  Gynecology* 88, no. 5 (November 1996): 797–800,
  doi.org/10.1016/0029-7844(96)00298-0.

In 2015, 9 percent of women in the United Kingdom . . .
Henry Taylor et al., "Neonatal Outcomes of
  Waterbirth: A Systematic Review and Meta-
  Analysis," *BMJ Archives of Disease in Childhood—
  Fetal and Neonatal Edition* 101, no. 4 (July 2016):
  F357–F365, doi.org/10.1136/archdischild
  -2015-309600.

At this point, studies have shown that water birth . . .
Rowena Davies et al., "The Effect of Waterbirth on
  Neonatal Mortality and Morbidity: A Systematic
  Review and Meta-Analysis," *JBI Database of
  Systematic Reviews and Implementation Reports* 13, no.
  10 (October 2015): 180–231, doi.org/10.11124
  /jbisrir-2015-2105; Jennifer Vanderlaan, Priscilla J.
  Hall, and MaryJane Lewitt, "Neonatal Outcomes
  with Water Birth: A Systematic Review and Meta-
  Analysis," *Midwifery* 59 (April 2018): 27–38,
  doi.org/10.1016/j.midw.2017.12.023.

The American Association of Birth Centers . . .
"Water Birth," ACNM Position Statement:
    Hydrotherapy During Labor and Birth, November
    2016, midwife.org/water-birth.

*However, the American College of Obstetricians and
Gynecologists . . .*
"Immersion in Water During Labor and Delivery," ACOG
    Committee Opinion Number 679, American College
    of Obstetricians and Gynecologists, *Obstetrics and
    Gynecology* 128 (2016): e231–e236, acog.org/clinical
    -guidance-and-publications/committee-opinions
    /committee-on-obstetric-practice/immersion-in
    -water-during-labor-and-delivery.

Prevention of tearing may be possible . . .
Vigdis Aasheim et al., "Perineal Techniques During
    the Second Stage of Labour for Reducing Perineal
    Trauma," Cochrane Database of Systematic
    Reviews 2017, no. 6 (June 2017): CD006672,
    doi.org/10.1002/14651858.CD006672.pub3.

Some midwives and doctors will apply warm . . .
Aasheim et al., "Perineal Techniques."

Your provider may also massage . . .
Carmen Imma Aquino et al., "Perineal Massage During
    Labor: a Systematic Review and Meta-Analysis
    of Randomized Controlled Trials," *The Journal of
    Maternal-Fetal and Neonatal Medicine* (September
    2018): 1–13, doi.org/10.1080/14767058.2018.1512574.

Birth Tradition in Islam
"Muslim Birth Rites," BBC, August 18, 2008, bbc.co.uk
    /religion/religions/islam/ritesrituals/birth.shtml.

Another way to reduce tearing . . .
Zohre Ahmadi et al., "Effect of Breathing Technique of
    Blowing on the Extent of Damage to the Perineum
    at the Moment of Delivery: A Randomized Clinical
    Trial," *Iranian Journal of Nursing and Midwifery
    Research* 22, no. 1 (January–February 2017): 62–66,
    doi.org/10.4103/1735-9066.202071.

Tears are often smaller than episiotomies . . .
Roberto L. Lede, José M. Belizán, and Guillermo
    Carroli, "Is Routine Use of Episiotomy Justified?"
    American Journal of Obstetrics and Gynecology 174, no.
    5 (May 1996): 1399–1402, doi.org/10.1016/S0002
    -9378(96)70579-3.

The very good news is that . . .
Hong Jiang et al., "Selective Versus Routine Use of
    Episiotomy for Vaginal Birth," Cochrane Database
    of Systematic Reviews 2017, no. 2 (February 2017):
    CD000081, doi.org/10.1002/14651858.cd000081.pub3.

Did you know that about 25 percent of babies . . .
Morarji Peesay, "Nuchal Cord and Its Implications,"
    Maternal Health, Neonatology and Perinatology 3,
    no. 28 (December 2017), doi.org/10.1186/s40748-017
    -0068-7.

CHAPTER 20
Third Stage of Labor: Giving Birth to the Placenta

Postpartum hemorrhage occurs in 2 to 5 percent . . .
" Practice Bulletin No. 183: Postpartum Hemorrhage,"
    American College of Obstetricians and
    Gynecologists, *Obstetrics & Gynecology* 130, no. 4
    (October 2017): e168–e186, clinicalinnovations
    .com/wp-content/uploads/2017/10/acog_practice
    _bulletin_no_183_postpartum-hemorrhage-2017.
    pdf; Fiona Urner, Roland Zimmermann, and
    Alexander Krafft, "Manual Removal of the Placenta
    After Vaginal Delivery: An Unsolved Problem in
    Obstetrics," *Journal of Pregnancy* 2014 (April 2014):
    274651, doi.org/10.1155/2014/274651.

Retained placenta occurs in 0.6 to 3 percent . . .
Andrew D. Weeks, "The Retained Placenta," *African
    Health Science* 1, no. 1 (August 2001): 36–41, ncbi
    .nlm.nih.gov/pmc/articles/pmc2704447/; Urner,
    Zimmermann, and Krafft, "Manual Removal of the
    Placenta After Vaginal Delivery," 274651.

Uterine inversion occurs in 0.002 to 0.033 percent . . .
Rui Filipe Monteiro Leal et al., "Total and Acute
    Uterine Inversion After Delivery: A Case Report,"
    Journal of Medical Case Reports 8, no. 347 (October
    2014), doi.org/10.1186/1752-1947-8-347.

ACOG recommends delaying cord clamping . . .
"Delayed Umbilical Cord Clamping After Birth,"
    Committee Opinion No. 684, American College
    of Obstetricians and Gynecologists, *Obstetrics and
    Gynecology* 129 (2017): e5–e10, acog.org/clinical
    -guidance-and-publications/committee-opinions
    /committee-on-obstetric-practice/delayed
    -umbilical-cord-clamping-after-birth.

Expectant management means that your provider . . .
Cecily M. Begley et al., "Active Versus Expectant
    Management for Women in the Third Stage of
    Labour," Cochrane Database of Systematic Reviews
    2015, no. 3 (February 2019): CD007412, doi.org/10
    .1002/14651858.cd007412.pub4.

More research is needed in this area . . .
Begley et al., "Active Versus Expectant Management,"
    CD007412.

... but does not have obvious benefits ...
"Active Management of the Third Stage of Labor,"
Position Statement, The American College of Nurse-Midwives (ACNM), updated September 2017,
midwife.org/acnm/files/acnmlibrarydata/
uploadfilename/000000000310/amtsl-ps-final-10-10-17.pdf.

As of 2017, the World Health Organization ...
"Postpartum Hemorrhage," American College
of Obstetricians and Gynecologists, *WHO
Recommendations for the Prevention and Treatment
of Postpartum Haemorrhage* (Geneva: World Health
Organization, 2012), midwife.org
/acnm/files/cclibraryfiles/filename
/000000003875/who-2012-recommendations
-prevention-pph.pdf.

CHAPTER 21
Fourth Stage of Labor:
The First Hours of Motherhood

In addition to the sheer loveliness of skin-to-skin ...
World Health Organization, *Kangaroo Mother Care: A
Practical Guide*, Department of Reproductive Health
and Research (Geneva: World Health Organization,
2003), apps.who.int/iris/bitstream/handle/10665
/42587/9241590351.pdf;jsessionid=d17a5f6f41c1eb
2f66c1f617dc1648ce?sequence=1; Ellen O. Boundy
et al., "Kangaroo Mother Care and Neonatal
Outcomes: A Meta-Analysis," *Pediatrics* 137, no. 1
(January 2016), doi.org/10.1542/peds.2015-2238;
Elizabeth R. Moore et al., "Early Skin-to-Skin
Contact for Mothers and Their Healthy Newborn
Infants," *Cochrane Database of Systematic Reviews*
2012, no. 5 (May 2012): CD003519, doi.org/10.1002
/14651858.cd003519.pub3.

There is a ton to be gained (by everyone involved) ...
Kerstin Hedberg Nyqvist et al., "Towards Universal
Kangaroo Mother Care: Recommendations and
Report from the First European Conference and
Seventh International Workshop on Kangaroo
Mother Care," *Acta Paedatricia* 99, no. 6 (June 2010):
820–826, doi.org/10.1111/j.1651-2227.2010.01787.x.

As many as 15 percent of newborns will have ...
"Infant and Child Hip Dysplasia," International Hip
Dysplasia Institute, hipdysplasia.org
/developmental-dysplasia-of-the-hip/faq/.

The vast majority of pediatricians recommend ...
David L. Hill, "Erythromycin Ointment," Healthy
Children, American Academy of Pediatrics, updated
May 11, 2012, healthychildren.org/english/ages
-stages/prenatal/delivery-beyond/pages/
erythromycin-ointment.aspx.

The CDC therefore recommends that a newborn's ...
"Hepatitis B VIS," Centers for Disease Control and
Prevention, updated August 15, 2019, cdc.gov
/vaccines/hcp/vis/vis-statements/hep-b.html.

Without preventive measures, 0.25 to 1.7 percent ...
"Controversies Concerning Vitamin K and the
Newborn," Committee on Fetus and Newborn
Pediatrics, American Academy of Pediatrics,
Pediatrics 112, no.1 (July 2003): 191–192, doi.org/10
.1542/peds.112.1.191.

The AAP recommends routine administration of vitamin K ...
"Controversies Concerning Vitamin K," 191-192.

Jaundice is quite common: about 50 percent of full-term ...
Anthony Kwaku Akobeng, "Neonatal Jaundice,"
American Family Physician 71, no. 5 (March 2005):
947–948, aafp.org/afp/2005/0301/p947.html.

Jaundice can be treated by placing the baby ...
Fadhil M. Salih, "Can Sunlight Replace Phototherapy
Units in the Treatment of Neonatal Jaundice? An In
Vitro Study," *Photodermatology, Photoimmunology
and Photomedicine* 17, no. 6 (December 2001):
272–277, doi.org/10.1111/j.1600-0781.2001.170605.x.

Studies have looked at the rate the bilirubin ...
Academy of Breastfeeding Medicine Protocol
Committee, "ABM Clinical Protocol #22:
Guidelines for Management of Jaundice in the
Breastfeeding Infant Equal to or Greater Than 35
Weeks' Gestation," *Breastfeeding Medicine* 5, no. 2
(April 2010), 87–93, doi.org/10.1089/bfm.2010.9994.

The March of Dimes lists a number of conditions ...
"Newborn Screening Tests for Your Baby," March of
Dimes, updated February 2016, marchofdimes.
org/baby/newborn-screening-tests-for-your-baby.
aspx?gclid=eaiaiqobchmizpxisvw13giv2ywzch
obogodeaayasaaegjcipd_bwe.

CHAPTER 22
Pain and Coping Techniques

When your skin or tissues experience the pain ...
Eric L. Garland, "Pain Processing in the Human
Nervous System: A Selective Review of Nociceptive
and Biobehavioral Pathways," *Primary Care: Clinics
in Office Practice* 39, no.3 (September 2012): 561–571,
doi.org/10.1016/j.pop.2012.06.013.

Pain can also stimulate fear ...
Emma E. Biggs, Ann Meulders, and Johan W. S.
Vlaeyen, "Chapter 7: The Neuroscience of Pain and
Fear," in *Neuroscience of Pain, Stress, and Emotion:
Psychological and Clinical Implications*, ed. Mustafa
al'Absi and Magne Arue Flaten (Cambridge, MA:
Academic Press, 2016): 133–157, doi.org/10.1016
/B978-0-12-800538-5.00007-8.

The obstetrical dilemma, a theory . . .
Colin Barras, "The Real Reasons Why Childbirth Is So Dangerous and Painful," BBC: Earth, December 22, 2016, bbc.com/earth/story/20161221-the-real -reasons-why-childbirth-is-so-painful-and-dangerous.

When some of our ancestors started to rely . . .
Barras, "The Real Reasons."

People have different tolerance levels of pain . . .
Laura Y. Whitburn et al., "The Meaning of Labour Pain: How the Social Environment and Other Contextual Factors Shape Women's Experiences," *BMC Pregnancy and Childbirth* 17, no. 1 (May 2017): 157, doi.org/10.1186/s12884-017-1343-3.

One study found that when women interpret pain . . .
Whitburn et al., "The Meaning of Labour Pain."

Wendy Christiaens and colleagues . . .
Wendy Christiaens, Mieke Verhaeghe, and Piet Bracke, "Pain Acceptance and Personal Control in Pain Relief in Two Maternity Care Models: A Cross-National Comparison of Belgium and the Netherlands," *BMC Health Services Research* 10, no. 1 (September 2010): 268, doi.org/10.1186/1472-6963-10-268.

As Brooke Cates has taught throughout . . .
Gretchen Cuda, "Just Breathe: Body Has a Built-In Stress Reliever," National Public Radio, December 6, 2010, npr.org/2010/12/06/131734718/just-breathe -body-has-a-built-in-stress-reliever.

And studies have found that deep breathing . . .
Mahin Kamalifard et al., "The Efficacy of Massage Therapy and Breathing Techniques on Pain Intensity and Physiological Responses to Labor Pain," *Journal of Caring Sciences* 1, no. 2 (May 2012): 73–78, doi.org/10.5681/jcs.2012.011.

A small study found that women who spent 20 minutes . . .
Shu-Ling Lee et al., "Efficacy of Warm Showers on Labor Pain and Birth Experiences During the First Labor Stage," *Journal of Obstetric, Gynecologic, and Neonatal Nursing* 42, no. 1 (January–February 2013): 19–28, doi.org/10.1111/j.1552-6909.2012.01424.x.

Similar outcomes have been found . . .
Elizabeth R. Cluett et al., "Immersion in Water During Labour and Birth," *Cochrane Database of Systematic Reviews* 2018, no. 5 (May 2018): CD000111, doi. org/10.1002/14651858.CD000111.pub4.

In one study, women who sat on a birth ball . . .
Meei-Ling Gau et al., "Effects of Birth Ball Exercise on Pain and Self-Efficacy During Childbirth: A Randomised Controlled Trial in Taiwan," *Midwifery* 27, no. 6 (December 2011): e293–e300, doi.org/10 .1016/j.midw.2011.02.004.

Most women up to 5 foot 8 inches tall . . .
"Using a Birthing Ball," BabyCentre, updated April 2019, babycentre.co.uk/a1048463/using-a-birthing-ball.

A small study in 2015 found that women with epidurals . . .
Christina Marie Tussey et al., "Reducing Length of Labor and Cesarean Surgery Rate Using a Peanut Ball for Women Laboring with an Epidural," *Journal of Perinatal Education* 24, no. 1 (January 2015): 16–24, doi.org/10.1891/1058-1243.24.1.16.

A small study in Australia found that hypnobirthing . . .
Julie Phillips-Moore, "Birthing Outcomes from an Australian HypnoBirthing Programme," *British Journal of Midwifery* 20, no. 8 (August 2012): 558–564, doi.org/10.12968/bjom.2012.20.8.558.

Another study found that while hypnobirthing . . .
Soo Downe et al., "Self-Hypnosis for Intrapartum Pain Management in Pregnant Nulliparous Women: A Randomized-Controlled Trial of Clinical Effectiveness," *Obstetric Anesthesia Digest* 36, no. 2 (June 2016): 102, doi.org/10.1097/01.aoa.00004826 39.34055.36.

Several small studies have found that aromatherapy . . .
Rajavadi Tanvisut, Kuntharee Traisrisilp, and Theera Tongsong, "Efficacy of Aromatherapy for Reducing Pain During Labor: A Randomized Controlled Trial," *Archives of Gynecology and Obstetrics* 297, no. 5 (May 2018): 1145–1150, doi.org/10.1007/s00404-018-4700 -1; Mansoreh Yazdkhasti and Arezoo Pirak, "The Effect of Aromatherapy with Lavender Essence on Severity of Labor Pain and Duration of Labor in Primiparous Women," *Complementary Therapies in Clinical Practice* 25 (November 2016): 81–86, doi.org/10.1016/j.ctcp.2016.08.008; Sepideh Hamdamian et al., "Effects of Aromatherapy with *Rosa damascena* on Nulliparous Women's Pain and Anxiety of Labor During First Stage of Labor," *Journal of Integrative Medicine* 16, no. 2 (March 2018): 120–125, doi.org/10.1016/j.joim.2018.02.005.

To learn more about essential oils . . .
"Find an Aromatherapist," National Association for Holistic Aromatherapy, January 2019, naha.org/find -an-aromatherapist.

Studies have found that vocalizing . . .
Bali Yogitha et al., "Complimentary Effect of Yogic Sound Resonance Relaxation Technique in Patients with Common Neck Pain," *International Journal of Yoga* 3, no. 1 (January–June 2010): 18–25, doi.org /10.4103/0973-6131.66774.

And laboring women often later report...
Jan Marie Barbieri, "Addressing Perceived Pain in Childbirth: A Music Therapy Voicework Intervention Design" (master's thesis, Concordia University, 2015), spectrum.library.concordia.ca/979869/.

Massage during labor can be...
Caroline A. Smith et al., "Massage, Reflexology and Other Manual Methods for Pain Management in Labour," Cochrane Database of Systematic Reviews 2018, no. 3 (March 2018): CD009290, doi.org/10.1002/14651858.cd009290.pub3.

A study found that women who had pressure...
Fatemeh Dabiri and Arefeh Shahi, "The Effect of LI4 Acupressure on Labor Pain Intensity and Duration of Labor: A Randomized Controlled Trial," *Oman Medical Journal* 29, no. 6 (November 2014): 425–429, doi.org/10.5001/omj.2014.113.

Similarly, the Sanyinjiao point...
Reginaldo Roque Mafetoni and Antonieta Keiko Kakuda Shimo, "The Effects of Acupressure on Labor Pains During Child Birth: Randomized Clinical Trial," *Revista Latino-Americana de Enfermagem* 24 (August 2016): e2738, doi.org/10.1590/1518-8345.0739.2738.

A small study found that when women held hands...
Pavel Goldstein, Irit Weissman-Fogel, and Simone G. Shamay-Tsoory, "The Role of Touch in Regulating Inter-Partner Physiological Coupling During Empathy for Pain," *Scientific Reports* 7, (June 2017): 3252, nature.com/articles/s41598-017-03627-7.

Some studies have found sterile water injections...
"Approaches to Limit Intervention During Labor and Birth," ACOG Committee Opinion No. 766, American College of Obstetricians and Gynecologists, *Obstetrics and Gynecology* 133, no. 2 (February 2019): e164–e173, acog.org/clinical-guidance-and-publications/committee-opinions/committee-on-obstetric-practice/-/media/committee-opinions/committee-on-obstetric-practice/co766.pdf.

The drugs may pass to the baby...
"Medications for Pain Relief During Labor and Delivery," Frequently Asked Questions, American College of Obstetricians and Gynecologists, updated May 2017, acog.org/patients/faqs/medications-for-pain-relief-during-labor-and-delivery.

Also note that these drugs do not increase...
"WHO Recommendation on Opioid Analgesia for Pain Relief During Labour," World Health Organization, updated February 17, 2018, extranet.who.int/rhl/topics/preconception-pregnancy-childbirth-and-postpartum-care/care-during-childbirth/care-during-labour-1st-stage/who-recommendation-opioid-analgesia-pain-relief-during-labour.

Research has found nitrous oxide to be safe...
Judith P. Rooks, "Safety and Risks of Nitrous Oxide Labor Analgesia: A Review," *Journal of Midwifery and Women's Health* 56, no. 6 (November–December 2011): 557–565, doi.org/10.1111/j.1542-2011.2011.00122.x.

It is also shown to be the pain relief method...
Millicent Anim-Somuah et al., "Epidural Versus Non-Epidural or No Analgesia for Pain Management in Labour," Cochrane Database of Systematic Reviews 2018, no. 5. (May 2018): CD000331, doi.org/10.1002/14651858.cd000331.pub4.

An epidural is different from a spinal...
"Cesarean Sections, Pregnancy and Birth: What Are the Pros and Cons of Regional and General Anesthetics?" Informed Health Online, updated March 22, 2018, ncbi.nlm.nih.gov/books/nbk279566/.

A large study in 2019 found that women...
Naama Srebnik et al., "The Impact of Epidural Analgesia on the Mode of Delivery in Nulliparous Women That Attain the Second Stage of Labor," *Journal of Maternal-Fetal & Neonatal Medicine* (January 2019), doi.org/10.1080/14767058.2018.1554045.

And a 2018 study of 11,000 women...
Millicent Anim-Somuah et al., "Epidural Versus Non-Epidural or No Analgesia for Pain Management in Labour," Cochrane Database of Systematic Reviews, May 21, 2018, doi.org/10.1002/14651858.CD000331.pub4.

A recent large review of more than 15,000 women...
Ban Leong Sng et al., "Early Versus Late Initiation of Epidural Analgesia for Labour," Cochrane Database of Systematic Reviews, October 9, 2014, doi.org/10.1002/14651858.CD007238.pub2.

If you're worried about the effect...
Anim-Somuah et al., "Epidural Versus Non-epidural."

The risks of general anesthesia...
"Cesarian Sections, Pregnancy, and Birth."

In most cases, the exposure time . . .
"FDA Drug Safety Communication: FDA Review Results in New Warnings About Using General Anesthetics and Sedation Drugs in Young Children and Pregnant Women," US Food and Drug Administration, December 14, 2016, fda.gov/drugs /drug-safety-and-availability/fda-drug-safety -communication-fda-review-results-new-warnings -about-using-general-anesthetics-and.

CHAPTER 23
Interventions

Past research has indicated that inductions . . .
Lauren Jansen et al., "First Do No Harm: Interventions During Childbirth," *Journal of Perinatal Education* 22, no.2 (Spring 2013): 83–92, doi.org/10.1891/1058-1243.22.2.83.

There appears to be a higher risk of stillbirth . . .
Kate F. Walker et al., "Randomized Trial of Labor Induction in Women 35 Years of Age or Older," *New England Journal of Medicine* 374, no. 9 (March 2016): 813–822, doi.org/10.1056/NEJMoa1509117.

In 2018, a large, randomized study . . .
William Grobman, "LB01: A Randomized Trial of Elective Induction of Labor at 39 Weeks Compared with Expectant Management of Low-Risk Nulliparous Women," *American Journal of Obstetrics and Gynecology* 218, no. 1 (January 2018): S601, doi.org/10.1016/j.ajog.2017.12.016.

Welcoming a child into the world . . .
Heather Marcoux, "Getting Induced May Not Increase Your Risk for C-Sections, Says New Study," Motherly, August 20, 2018, mother.ly/news/getting -induced-doesnt-increase-risk-c-section.

While providers may use AROM . . .
Rebecca M. D. Smyth, S. Kate Alldred, and Carolyn Markham, "Amniotomy for Shortening Spontaneous Labour," Cochrane Database of Systematic Reviews 2013, no. 6 (January 2013): CD006167, doi. org/10.1002/14651858.cd006167.pub4.

Induced and augmented labors . . .
Shuqin Wei et al., "Early Amniotomy and Early Oxytocin for Prevention Of, or Therapy For, Delay in First Stage Spontaneous Labour Compared with Routine Care," Cochran Database of Systematic Reviews, August 7, 2013, doi.org/10.1002/14651858 .CD006794.pub4.

However, current research suggests . . .
Andrea Ciardulli et al., "Less-Restrictive Food Intake During Labor in Low-Risk Singleton Pregnancies: A Systematic Review and Meta-Analysis," *Obstetrics and Gynecology* 129, no. 3 (March 2017): 473–480, doi.org/10.1097/aog.0000000000001898.

ACOG even states that . . .
"Oral Intake During Labor," ACOG Committee Opinion No. 441, American College of Obstetricians and Gynecologists, *Obstetrics and Gynecology* 114 (2009): 714, acog.org/clinical-guidance-and -publications/committee-opinions/committee-on -obstetric-practice/oral-intake-during-labor.

What's more, EFM has been found to increase . . .
Zarko Alfirevic et al., "Continuous Cardiotocography (CTG) as a Form of Electronic Fetal Monitoring (EFM) for Fetal Assessment During Labour," Cochrane Database of Systematic Reviews 2017, no. 2. (February 2017): CD006066, doi.org/10 .1002/14651858.cd006066.pub3.

ACOG states that intermittent auscultation . . .
"Intrapartum Fetal Heart Rate Monitoring: Nomenclature, Interpretation, and General Management Principles," Practice Bulletin Number 106, *Obstetrics and Gynecology* 114, no. 4 (July 2009): 192-202, acog.org/clinical-guidance-and -publications/practice-guidelines-and-reports- search?keyword=%20intermittent%20auscultation.

. . . and ACNM goes further to say that it is . . .
"Intermittent Auscultation for Intrapartum Fetal Heart Rate Surveillance," Clinical Bulletin, American College of Nurse-Midwives, *Journal of Midwifery and Women's Health* 60, no. 5 (September–October 2015): 626-632, doi.org/10.1111/jmwh.12372.

They involve tools (the vacuum or the forceps) . . .
Joyce A. Martin et al., "Births: Final Data for 2017," *National Vital Statistics Reports* 67, no. 8 (November 2018): 1-49, cdc.gov/nchs/data/nvsr/nvsr67 /nvsr67_08-508.pdf.

Vacuums tend to be more common . . .
Fidelma O'Mahony, G. Justus Hofmeyr, and Vijay Menon, "Choice of Instruments for Assisted Vaginal Delivery," Cochrane Database of Systematic Reviews 2010, no. 11 (November 2010): CD005455, doi.org/10.1002/14651858.cd005455.pub2.

Various scalp, head, and eye injuries . . .
Ali and Norwitz, "Vacuum-Assisted Vaginal Delivery," 5-17.

The short-term maternal risks from operative deliveries . . .
O'Mahony, Hofmeyr, and Menon, "Choice of Instruments," CD005455.

CHAPTER 24
Cesarean Births

As I have shared on Motherly . . .
Diana Spalding, "10 C-Section Myths We'd Like to
Clear Up Right Now," Motherly, March 2019,
mother.ly/life/6-c-section-myths-wed-like-to-clear
-up-right-now.

High HIV viral load . . .
Brenna Hughes and Susan Cu-Uvin, "Patient
Education: HIV and Pregnancy (Beyond the
Basics)," UpToDate, June 8, 2018, uptodate.com
/contents/hiv-and-pregnancy-beyond-the-basics.

Shaving pubic hair is not usually done . . .
Vittorio Basevi and Tina Lavender, "Routine Perineal
Shaving on Admission in Labour," Cochrane
Database of Systematic Reviews 2014, no. 11
(November 2014): CD001236, doi.org/10.1002
/14651858.cd001236.pub2.

Studies have found that routine urinary catheters . . .
Divya Pandey et al., "Indwelling Catheterization in
Caesarean Section: Time to Retire It!" *Journal of
Clinical & Diagnostic Research* 9, no. 9 (September
2015): QC01–QC04, doi.org/10.7860/jcdr/2015/13495
.6415; Azza Mohamed Nasr et al., "Evaluation of the
Use vs. Nonuse of Urinary Catheterization During
Cesarean Delivery: A Prospective, Multicenter,
Randomized Controlled Trial," *Journal of
Perinatology* 29, no. 6 (June 2009): 416–421, doi.org
/10.1038/jp.2009.4.

The outermost skin layer will be closed . . .
A. Dhanya Mackeen et al., "Suture Compared with
Staple Skin Closure After Cesarean Delivery: A
Randomized Controlled Trial," *Obstetrics and
Gynecology* 123, no. 6 (June 2014): 1169–1175, doi.org
/10.1097/aog.0000000000000227.

At this point, we do not have enough research . . .
"Vaginal Seeding," ACOG Committee Opinion
No. 725, American College of Obstetricians and
Gynecologists, *Obstetrics and Gynecology* 130, no. 5
(November 2017): e274–e278, doi.org/10.1097
/aog.0000000000002402.

But a large review of studies . . .
Jeanne-Marie Guise et al., "Systematic Review of the
Incidence and Consequences of Uterine Rupture in
Women with Previous Caesarean Section," *BMJ* 329,
no. 7456 (July 2004): 19–25, doi.org/10.1136/bmj.329
.7456.19.

About 60 to 80 percent of women who try . . .
"Vaginal Birth After Cesarean Delivery," ACOG
Practice Bulletin Number 184, *Obstetrics and
Gynecology* 130, no. 5 (November 2017): e217-233,
ncbi.nlm.nih.gov/pubmed/29064970.

ACOG's guidelines state that in consultation . . .
"Vaginal Birth After Cesarean Delivery," e217-233.

*Know the facts. The American College of Obstetricians and
Gynecologists . . .*
"Vaginal Birth After Cesarean (VBAC): Resource
Overview," American College of Obstetricians and
Gynecologists, February 2019, acog.org/Womens
-Health/Vaginal-Birth-After-Cesarean-VBAC;
"Vaginal Birth After Cesarean Delivery," Position
Statement, American College of Nurse-Midwives,
December 2011, midwife.org/acnm/files/acnm
librarydata/uploadfilename/000000000090
/vbac%20dec%202011.pdf.

Some women who have Cesarean sections . . .
"What Is Bengkung Belly Binding?" CAPPA, August 22,
2018, cappa.net/what-is-bengkung-belly-binding.

CHAPTER 25
Birth Plans

Many cultures around the world . . .
Zainab Reza, "Placenta Traditions from Around the
World: Different Cultures, Different Beliefs,"
Babygaga, March 9, 2015, babygaga.com/placenta
-traditions-from-around-the-world-different
-cultures-different-beliefs/.

It is important to note that there are no big studies . . .
Emily Hart Hayes, "Consumption of the Placenta in the
Postpartum Period," *Journal of Obstetrics, Gynecology
& Neonatal Nursing* 45, no. 1 (January-February 2016):
78–89, doi.org/10.1016/j.jogn.2015.10.008; Sarah
Hollister, "Health Implications to Consider with
Placenta for Consumption," January 2019, static1
.squarespace.com/static/537fb379e4b0fe1778d0f178
/t/59b9b176a803bb401f2d9889/1505341814834
/health+implications+to+consider+with+placenta
+for+consumption%2c+researched_update.pdf.

In a lotus birth, the umbilical cord is not cut . . .
Laura A. Zinsser, "Lotus Birth: A Holistic Approach on
Physiological Cord Clamping," *Women and Birth* 31,
no. 2 (April 2018): e73–e76, doi.org/10.1016/j.wombi
.2017.08.127.

CHAPTER 26
Self-Nurturing and the Fourth Trimester

Research has found that even little catnaps . . .
Catherine E. Milner and Kimberly A. Cote, "Benefits of
  Napping in Healthy Adults: Impact of Nap Length,
  Time of Day, Age, and Experience with Napping,"
  Journal of Sleep Research 18, no. 2 (June 2009):
  272–281, doi.org/10.1111/j.1365-2869.2008.00718.x.

P.S. Etiquette expert Emily Post . . .
"Top Baby Shower Etiquette Questions," Emily Post
  Institute, January 2019, emilypost.com/advice/top
  -baby-shower-etiquette-questions/.

Postpartum Tradition in Brazil
Rebeca Duran, "Gift-giving Culture in Brazil," The
  Brazil Business, June 21, 2013, thebrazilbusiness
  .com/article/gift-giving-culture-in-brazil.

In fact, an investigation done by the nonprofit . . .
Sharon Lerner, "The Real War on Families: Why the U.S.
  Needs Paid Leave Now," *In These Times*, August 18,
  2015, inthesetimes.com/article/18151/the-real-war
  -on-families.

Not only does nourishment allow your body to heal . . .
Thalia M. Sparling et al., "Nutrients and Perinatal
  Depression: A Systematic Review," *Journal of
  Nutritional Science* 6 (December 2017): e61, doi.org
  /10.1017/jns.2017.58.

There is so much pressure on new moms . . .
Meghan E. Lovering et al., "Exploring the Tripartite
  Influence Model of Body Dissatisfaction in
  Postpartum Women," *Body Image* 24 (March 2018):
  44–54, doi.org/10.1016/j.bodyim.2017.12.001.

Studies have linked dieting . . .
Rachel F. Rodgers et al., "A Biopsychosocial Model of
  Body Image, Disordered Eating, and Breastfeeding
  Among Postpartum Women," *Appetite* 126 (July
  2018): 163–168, doi.org/10.1016/j.appet.2018.04.007.

Overnight Oats
Crystal Karges, "Basic Overnight Oat Recipe for
  Breastfeeding Moms," Crystal Karges Nutrition,
  February 13, 2018, crystalkarges.com/blog/basic
  -overnight-oat-recipe-for-breastfeeding-mamas.

*Up to 25 percent of women experience postpartum
depression . . .*
"Depression and Postpartum Depression: Resource
  Overview," American College of Obstetricians and
  Gynecologists, March 2019, acog.org/womens
  -health/depression-and-postpartum-depression.

*But did you know that the brain undergoes massive
changes . . .*
Paula J. Brunton and John A. Russell, "The Expectant
  Brain: Adapting for Motherhood," *Nature Reviews
  Neuroscience* 9, no. 1 (January 2008): 11–25, nature
  .com/articles/nrn2280.

Neuroscientist Jodi L. Pawluski and colleagues . . .
Jodi L. Pawluski, Kelly G. Lambert, and Craig H. Kinsley,
  "Neuroplasticity in the Maternal Hippocampus:
  Relation to Cognition and Effects of
  Repeated Stress," *Hormones and Behavior* 77 (January
  2016): 86–97, doi.org/10.1016/j.yhbeh.2015.06.004.

During pregnancy, our brains lose grey matter . . .
Pawluski, Lambert, and Kinsley, "Neuroplasticity in
  the Maternal Hippocampus," 86-97.

One theory is that the loss . . .
Elseline Hoekzema et al., "Pregnancy Leads to Long-
  Lasting Changes in Human Brain Structure," *Nature
  Neuroscience* 20, no. 2 (February 2017): 287–296,
  doi.org/10.1038/nn.4458.

So on that premise, researchers studied mothers . . .
Alexandra Tornek et al.; "Music Effects on EEG in
  Intrusive and Withdrawn Mothers with Depressive
  Symptoms," *Psychiatry Interpersonal & Biological
  Processes* 66, no. 3 (Fall 2003): 234–243, doi.org/10
  .1521/psyc.66.3.234.25157.

To the Mama Who Had a Traumatic Birth . . .
Diana Spalding, "When I Tell You About My Difficult
  Birth, Here's What I Need You to Do," Motherly,
  February 2019, mother.ly/life/when-i-tell-you
  -about-my-difficult-birth-heres-what-i-need-you-to-do.

Trauma is defined as . . .
Oxford English Dictionary, s.v. "trauma," accessed
  January 2019, en.oxforddictionaries.com
  /definition/trauma.

CHAPTER 27
Postpartum Physical Recovery

It takes about 6 weeks . . .
Elizabeth R. Cluett, Jo Alexander, and Ruth M.
  Pickering, "What Is the Normal Pattern of Uterine
  Involution? An Investigation of Postpartum Uterine
  Involution Measured by the Distance Between the
  Symphysis Pubis and the Uterine Fundus Using a
  Paper Tape Measure," *Midwifery* 13, no. 1 (March
  1997): 9–16, doi.org/10.1016/S0266-6138(97
)90027-9.

Native American women may be at an increased risk . . .
Salam E. Chalouhi et al., "Risk of Postpartum Hemorrhage Among Native American Women," *Obstetrics and Gynecology* 131, no. 3 (December 2015): 269–272, doi.org/10.1016/j.ijgo.2015.05.037.

And black women who have postpartum hemorrhages . . .
C. Gyamfi-Bannerman et al., "Postpartum Hemorrhage Outcomes and Race," *American Journal of Obstetrics and Gynecology* 219, no. 2 (August 2018): 185.e1-185.e10, doi.org/10.1016/j.ajog. 2018.04.052.

With either type of delivery, tampons . . .
Ramesh Venkataraman and Sat Sharma, "Toxic Shock Syndrome," Medscape, updated May 7, 2018, emedicine.medscape.com/article/169177-overview.

With a huge caveat, the standard answer . . .
Alison J. Macarthur and Colin Macarthur, "Incidence, Severity, and Determinants of Perineal Pain After Vaginal Delivery: A Prospective Cohort Study," *American Journal of Obstetrics and Gynecology* 191, no. 4 (October 2004): 1199–1204, ajog.org/article/s0002-9378(04)00227-3/fulltext.

Yes, most women (95 percent, in fact) . . .
Macarthur and Macarthur, "Incidence, Severity, and Determinants," 1199-1206.

A study found that Reiki resulted in . . .
Tulay Sagkal Midilli and İsmet Eşer, "Effects of Reiki on Post-Cesarean Delivery Pain, Anxiety, and Hemodynamic Parameters: A Randomized, Controlled Clinical Trial," *Pain Management Nursing* 16, no. 3 (June 2015): 388–399, doi.org/10.1016/j.pmn.2014.09.005.

Studies have found that chewing sugar-free gum . . .
Farideh Mohsenzadeh Ledari et al., "Chewing Sugar-Free Gum Reduces Ileus After Cesarean Section in Nulliparous Women: A Randomized Clinical Trial," *Iranian Red Crescent Medical Journal* 15, no. 4 (April 2013): 330–334, doi.org/10.5812/ircmj.6458.

UTIs can be more common during pregnancy . . .
John E. Delzell Jr. and Michael L. Lefevre, "Urinary Tract Infections During Pregnancy," *American Family Physician* 61, no. 3 (February 2000): 713–720, mcgill.ca/familymed/files/familymed/urinary_tract_infections_during_pregnancy_-_american_family_physician.pdf.

Researchers have not yet found concrete evidence . . .
Jennifer L. Hallock and Victoria L. Handa, "The Epidemiology of Pelvic Floor Disorders and Childbirth: An Update," *Obstetrics and Gynecology Clinics of North America* 43, no. 1 (March 2016): 1–13, doi.org/10.1016/j.ogc.2015.10.008.

Your GI tract also slows down . . .
Joseph S. Davison, Mary C. Davison, and David M. Hay, "Gastric Emptying Time in Late Pregnancy and Labour," *BJOG* 77, no. 1 (January 1970): 37–41, doi.org/10.1111/j.1471-0528.1970.tb03405.x.

Some women like to get their squat on . . .
Shigetsugu Takano and Dana R. Sands, "Influence of Body Posture on Defecation: A Prospective Study of 'The Thinker' Position," *Techniques in Coloproctology* 20, no. 2 (February 2016): 117–121, doi.org/10.1007/s10151-015-1402-6.

New moms there don't suffer as much from incontinence . . .
Siv Mørkved and Kari Bø, "Effect of Postpartum Pelvic Floor Muscle Training in Prevention and Treatment of Urinary Incontinence: A One-Year Follow Up," *BJOG* 107, no. 8 (August 2000): 1022–1028, doi.org/10.1111/j.1471-0528.2000.tb10407.x.

It doesn't seem quite fair that . . .
K. Lauren Barnes, Theodore A. Stern, and Lori R. Berkowtiz, "Postpartum Fecal and Flatal Incontinence: Silence, Stigma, and Psychological Interventions," *Primary Care Companion for CNS Disorders* 19, no. 5 (October 2017): 17602164, doi.org/10.4088/pcc.17f02164.

Postpartum night sweats can be quite annoying . . .
Rebecca C. Thurston et al., "Prospective Evaluation of Hot Flashes During Pregnancy and Postpartum," *Fertility and Sterility* 100, no.6 (December 2013): 1667–1672, doi.org/10.1016/j.fertnstert.2013.08.020.

They tend to start to go away around week 2 . . .
Thurston et al., "Prospective Evaluation of Hot Flashes," 1667-1672.

Following is a guide . . .
"Birth Control," Options for Sexual Health, updated March 2018, optionsforsexualhealth.org/birth-control-pregnancy/birth-control-options/effectiveness.

Research estimates that anywhere from 30 to 100 percent . . .
Nina Kimmich et al., "Rektusdiastase und Schwangerschaft" [Diastasis Recti Abdominis and Pregnancy], *Praxis* 2015, no. 104 (July 2015): 803–806, doi.org/10.1024/1661-8157/a002075; Patrícia Gonçalves Fernandes da Mota et al., "Prevalence and Risk Factors of Diastasis Recti Abdominis from Late Pregnancy to 6 Months Postpartum, and Relationship with Lumbo-Pelvic Pain," *Manual Therapy* 20, no. 1 (February 2015): 200–205, doi.org/10.1016/j.math.2014.09.002.

If you are not breastfeeding, you can expect . . .
Andrew M. Kaunitz, Courtney A. Schreiber, and
Kristen Eckler, "Postpartum Contraception:
Initiation and Methods," UpToDate, updated
October 24, 2018, uptodate.com/contents/
postpartum-contraception-initiation-and-methods.

CHART: Birth Control Methods . . .
"Birth Control Method Comparison Chart," American
Sexual Health Association, updated 2013,
ashasexualhealth.org/pdfs/ContraceptiveOptions.pdf.

CHART: Birth Control Methods (Skyla) . . .
"About Skyla," Bayer, March 2019, skyla-us.com/what
-is-skyla.php.

CHART: Birth Control Methods (Plan B) . . .
"What's the Plan B Morning-After Pill?"Planned
Parenthood, March 2019, plannedparenthood.org
/learn/morning-after-pill-emergency-contraception
/whats-plan-b-morning-after-pill.

CHAPTER 28
Your Baby and Bonding

The official statement by the AAP . . .
"Newborn Male Circumcision," American Academy of
Pediatrics, August 27, 2012, aap.org/en-us/about
-the-aap/aap-press-room/pages/newborn-male
-circumcision.aspx.

A report from 2016 . . .
Brian J. Morris et al., "Estimation of Country-Specific
and Global Prevalence of Male Circumcision,"
Population Health Metrics 14, no. 4 (April 2016): 11,
doi.org/10.1186/s12963-016-0073-5.

It ranges from almost none . . .
Morris, et al., "Estimation of Country-Specific,"11.

Prevention of urinary tract infections . . .
"Male Circumcision," Task Force on Circumcision,
American Academy of Pediatrics, *Pediatrics* 130, no.
3 (September 2012), doi.org/10.1542/peds.2012-1990.

Circumcision Care . . .
"Newborn Male Circumcision," Frequently Asked
Questions, American College of Obstetricians and
Gynecologists, updated June 2017, acog.org
/patients/faqs/newborn-male-circumcision.

Your baby will go through nearly four thousand diapers . . .
Elizabeth Vargas, Howie Masters, and Michael
Mendelsohn, "Diapers and Showers and Sodas, Oh
My!" *ABC News*, April 10, 2008, abcnews
.go.com/2020/story?id=4618854&page=1.

When this happens, it is recommended . . .
Peter Liaw et al., "Infant Deaths in Sitting Devices,"
Pediatrics 144, no. 1 (July 2019): e20182576,
doi.org/10.1542/peds.2018-2576.

I encourage parents to use Dr. Harvey Karp's Five S's . . .
Harvey Karp, *The Happiest Baby on the Block: The New
Way to Calm Crying and Help Your Newborn Baby
Sleep Better*, 2nd ed. (New York: Bantam, 2015).

Studies have shown that an emotionally secure child . . .
Wendy M. Troxel et al., "Negative Emotionality
Moderates Associations Among Attachment,
Toddler Sleep, and Later Problem Behaviors,"
Journal of Family Psychology 27, no. 1 (February 2013):
127–136, doi.org//10.1037/a0031149.

SUID is extremely rare . . .
"Sudden Unexpected Infant Death and Sudden Infant
Death Syndrome," Centers for Disease Control and
Prevention, updated September 13, 2019, cdc.gov
/sids/data.htm.

Babies who receive breast milk during the first 2 months . . .
"Breastfeeding for Two Months Halves Risk of SIDS:
Researchers Determine Duration Needed for
Protective Benefit for Baby," ScienceDaily, October
30, 2017, sciencedaily.com/releases/2017/10
/171030123401.htm.

AAP's position is that parents should . . .
"American Academy of Pediatrics Announces New Safe
Sleep Recommendations to Protect Against SIDS,
Sleep-Related Infant Deaths," American Academy of
Pediatrics, October 24, 2016, aap.org/en-us
/about-the-aap/aap-press-room/pages/american
-academy-of-pediatrics-announces-new-safe-sleep
-recommendations-to-protect-against-sids.aspx.

Wedges and positioners can actually lead . . .
"Do Not Use Infant Sleep Positioners Due to the Risk of
Suffocation," US Food & Drug Administration, April
18, 2018, fda.gov/forconsumers/consumerupdates
/do-not-use-infant-sleep-positions-due-to-risk
-suffocation.

The AAP recommends that the safest place . . .
"American Academy of Pediatrics Announces."

One study found that 25 percent of mothers . . .
Kathleen Kendall-Tackett, Zhen Cong, and Thomas
W. Hale, "Mother-Infant Sleep Locations and
Nighttime Feeding Behavior," *Clinical Lactation* 1
(Fall 2010): 27–30, babiesincommon.com/docs
/mother-infant-sleep-locations-2.pdf.

Other recommendations for safe bed sharing...
"Safe Cosleeping Guidelines: Guidelines to Sleeping Safe with Infants," Mother-Baby Behavioral Sleep Laboratory, University of Notre Dame, February 2019, cosleeping.nd.edu/safe-co-sleeping -guidelines/.

For more, visit dontshake.org...
"What Is the Period of PURPLE Crying Program?" National Center on Shaken Baby Syndrome, March 2019, dontshake.org/purplecrying.

A study was done where mothers who spoke...
Elise A. Piazza, Marius Cătălin Iordan, and Casey Lew-Williams, "Mothers Consistently Alter Their Unique Vocal Fingerprints When Communicating with Infants," *Current Biology* 27 no. 20 (October 2017): P3162–3167.E3, doi.org/10.1016/j.cub.2017 .08.074.

In fact, evidence suggests that babies who are read to...
"Reading with Children Starting in Infancy Gives Lasting Literacy Boost: Shared Book-Reading That Begins Soon After Birth May Translate into Higher Language and Vocabulary Skills Before Elementary School," ScienceDaily, May 4, 2017, sciencedaily .com/releases/2017/05/170504083146.htm.

Giving your baby a very light massage...
Sónia Vicente, Manuela Veríssimo, and Eva Diniz, "Infant Massage Improves Attitudes Toward Childbearing, Maternal Satisfaction and Pleasure in Parenting," *Infant Behavior and Development* 49 (November 2017): 114–119, sciencedirect.com/ science/article/pii/s0163638316302375?via%3dihub.

Newborn Care in Nigeria
"11 Unique Birthing Traditions Around the World," *Huffington Post*, updated December 7, 2017, huffpost. com/entry/world-birthing-traditions_n_7033790.

One of the most important things to do is to mount...
"Product Instability or Tip-Over Injuries and Fatalities Associated with Televisions, Furniture and Appliances, 2017 Report," US Consumer Product Safety Commission, October 2017, cpsc.gov/s3fs -public/product-instability-or-tip-over-report-oct- 2017_stamped.pdf?6zpgeccrrlwpm51kopcsrk8r2 jsbpokd.

According to anchorit.gov...
Anchor It, Consumer Product Safety Commission, February 2019, anchorit.gov.

The International Hip Dysplasia Institute provides...
"Baby Carriers & Other Equipment," IHDI Educational Statement, February 2019, hipdysplasia.org/ developmental-dysplasia-of-the-hip/prevention /baby-carriers-seats-and-other-equipment/.

CHAPTER 29
Breastfeeding

Exclusively breastfeeding an infant...
"Optimizing Support for Breastfeeding as Part of Obstetric Practice," ACOG Committee Opinion No. 756, American College of Obstetricians and Gynecologists, *Obstetrics and Gynecology* 132 (2018): e187–e196, acog.org/clinical-guidance-and -publications/committee-opinions/committee -on-obstetric-practice/optimizing-support-for -breastfeeding-as-part-of-obstetric-practice.

If breastfeeding is causing so much pain...
Olivia Scobie, "Postpartum Depression and Intensive Mothering: How Western Cultural Expectations of Motherhood Shape Maternal Mental Health in New Parents," *Canadian Social Work* 19, no 1. (Autumn 2017): 39–50.

As we'll discuss, organizations like the AAP...
"Optimizing Support for Breastfeeding," e187–196.

As an example, a 2017 study...
John M. D. Thompson et al., "Duration of Breastfeeding and Risk of SIDS: An Individual Participant Data Meta-Analysis," *Pediatrics* 140, no. 5 (November 2017), doi.org/10.1542/peds.2017-1324.

In fact, the Affordable Care Act now requires...
"Understanding Health Care Coverage," American College of Obstetricians and Gynecologists, March 2019, acog.org/about-acog/acog-departments /breastfeeding/understanding-health-care-coverage.

But as the writer Zuzana Boehmová said...
Zuzana Boehmová, "Stop Saying Breast Milk Is Free," *Slate*, February 13, 2018, slate.com/human-interest /2018/02/breast-milk-isnt-free.html.

Positive effects of breastfeeding for baby...
"Breastfeeding and the Use of Human Milk," Policy Statement, *American Academy of Pediatrics* 129, no. 3 (March 2012), pediatrics.aappublications.org /content/129/3/e827.full#content-block.

The American Academy of Pediatrics (AAP) recommends...
"Breastfeeding and the Use of Human Milk."

Women who have experienced trauma...
Lauren Sobel et al., "Pregnancy and Childbirth After Sexual Trauma: Patient Perspectives and Care Preferences," *Obstetrics and Gynecology* 132, no. 6 (December 2018): 1461–1468, doi.org/10.1097 /aog.0000000000002956.

This has no bearing on your ability to make milk...
"Colostrum: Prenatal/Antenatal Expression," La Leche League International, January 2019, llli.org /breastfeeding-info/colostrum-prenatal-antenatal -expression/.

In most women, the right breast produces more milk . . .
Janet L. Engstrom et al., "Comparison of Milk Output from the Right and Left Breasts During Simultaneous Pumping in Mothers of Very Low Birthweight Infants," *Breastfeeding Medicine* 2, no. 2 (June 2007): 83–91, doi.org/10.1089/bfm.2006.0019.

Mothers of boys tend to produce more milk . . .
Marissa Fessenden, "Boys and Girls May Get Different Breast Milk," *Scientific American*, December 1, 2012, scientificamerican.com/article/boys-and-girls-may -get-different-breast-milk/.

A mother's age and number of past babies . . .
"Milk Volume," chap. 6 in *Nutrition During Lactation* (Washington, DC: National Academies Press, 1991), 80–112, nap.edu/read/1577/chapter/6.

For this reason, most breastfeeding support people . . .
Jacqueline C. Kent et al., "Volume and Frequency of Breastfeedings and Fat Content of Breast Milk Throughout the Day," *Pediatrics* 117, no. 3 (March 2006): e387-395, pediatrics.aappublications.org /content/117/3/e387.short.

Lactation Cookie Bites
Crystal Karges, "Easy No Bake Lactation Bites Recipe for the Busy Breastfeeding Mom," Crystal Karges Nutrition, July 14, 2019, crystalkarges.com/blog /easy-no-bake-lactation-bites-recipe-for-the-busy -breastfeeding-mom.

Studies have found, though, that nipple confusion . . .
Emily Zimmerman and Kelsey Thompson, "Clarifying Nipple Confusion," *Journal of Perinatology* 35, no. 11 (November 2015): 895–899, researchgate.net /publication/280091118_clarifying_nipple_confusion.

It is actually quite common (about 1 out of 7 babies) . . .
Nagate Raghavendra Reddy et al., "Clipping the (Tongue) Tie," *Journal of Indian Society of Periodontology* 18, no. 3 (May–June 2014): 395–398, doi.org/10.4103/0972-124x.134590.

A study also found that stress and lack of sleep . . .
Betsy Foxman et al., "Lactation Mastitis: Occurrence and Medical Management Among 946 Breastfeeding Women in the United States," *American Journal of Epidemiology* 155, no. 2 (January 2002): 103–114, doi.org/10.1093/aje/155.2.103.

Historically, gentian violet (a blue dye) . . .
"Gentian Violet," Drugs and Lactation Database (LactMed), National Library of Medicine (US), updated December 3, 2018, ncbi.nlm.nih.gov/books /NBK501869/.

It is legal to breastfeed in public . . .
"Breastfeeding State Laws," Maternal and Child Health Bureau, National Conference of State Legislators (NCSL), updated April 30, 2019, ncsl.org/research/ health/breastfeeding-state-laws.aspx.

Studies have found that sugar in the barley . . .
Berthold V. Koletzko and Frauke Lehner, "Beer and Breastfeeding," in *Short and Long Term Effects of Breast Feeding on Child Health, Advances in Experimental Medicine and Biology*, vol. 478 (Boston: Springer, 2002): 23–28, link.springer.com/chapter /10.1007%2F0-306-46830-1_2.

However, in general, research has found that alcohol . . .
Julie Mennella, "Alcohol's Effect on Lactation," *Alcohol Research and Health: The Journal of the National Institute on Alcohol Abuse and Alcoholism* 25 no. 3 (February 2001): 230–234, researchgate.net /publication/11548375_alcohols_effect_on_lactation.

And alcohol may also temporarily change . . .
Julie A. Mennella and Gary K. Beauchamp, "The Transfer of Alcohol to Human Milk: Effects on Flavor and the Infant's Behavior," *New England Journal of Medicine* 325, no. 14 (October 1991): 981– 985, doi.org/10.1056/nejm199110033251401.

The alcohol amount in your breast milk . . .
"Drinking Alcohol and Breastfeeding," La Leche League International, January 2019, llli.org/breastfeeding -info/alcohol/.

If you want to drink while breastfeeding . . .
"Drinking Alcohol and Breastfeeding."

To get highly specific, the American Academy of Pediatrics . . .
"Breastfeeding and the Use of Human Milk," Policy Statement, Section on Breastfeeding, American Academy of Pediatrics, *Pediatrics* 129, no. 3 (March 2012), pediatrics.aappublications.org/content/129 /3/e827.full.

Get a team feeding plan . . .
Chantal Lau, "Breastfeeding Challenges and the Preterm Mother-Infant Dyad: A Conceptual Model," *Breastfeeding Medicine* 13, no. 1 (January 2018): 8–17, doi.org/10.1089/bfm.2016.0206.

CHAPTER 30
Pumping and Bottle-Feeding

If your pumped milk will spend more than 4 hours . . .
"Proper Storage and Preparation of Breast Milk," Centers for Disease Control and Prevention, updated August 6, 2019, cdc.gov/breastfeeding /recommendations/handling_breastmilk.htm.

The other factor to consider is where . . .
"Break Time for Nursing Mothers Provision,"
Section 7(r) of the Fair Labor Standards Act, US
Department of Labor, March 23, 2010, dol.gov/whd
/nursingmothers/sec7rflsa_btnm.htm.

Section 7 of the Fair Labor Standards Act . . .
"Break Time for Nursing Mothers Provision."

When you're done pumping . . .
"How to Keep Your Breast Pump Kit Clean: The
Essentials," Centers for Disease Control and
Prevention, updated May 20, 2019, cdc.gov
/healthywater/hygiene/healthychildcare
/infantfeeding/breastpump.html.

If you are pumping once per day . . .
Jacqueline C. Kent et al., "Volume and Frequency of
Breastfeedings and Fat Content of Breast Milk
Throughout the Day," *Pediatrics* 117, no. 3 (March
2006): e387–395, doi.org/10.1542/peds.2005-1417.

Earlier than 4 weeks can cause nipple confusion . . .
Emily Zimmerman and Kelsey Thompson, "Clarifying
Nipple Confusion," *Journal of Perinatology* 35, no. 11
(November 2015): 895–899, doi.org/10.1038/jp.2015.83.

. . . which may make them prefer a bottle . . .
Marianne Neifert, Ruth Lawrence, and Joy Seacat,
"Nipple Confusion: Toward a Formal Definition,"
Journal of Pediatrics 126, no. 6 (June 1995): S125–S129,
doi.org/10.1016/S0022-3476(95)90252-x.

To locate a milk bank . . .
"Find a Milk Bank," Human Milk Banking Association
of North America, hmbana.org/find-a-milk-bank
/overview.html.

Studies have found that unofficial donations . . .
Maude St-Onge, Shahnaz Chaudhry, and Gideon
Koren, "Donated Breast Milk Stored in Banks
Versus Breast Milk Purchased Online," *Canadian
Family Physician* 61, no. 2 (February 2015): 143–146,
ncbi.nlm.nih.gov/pubmed/25676644.

. . . and AAP cautions against them . . .
"New American Academy of Pediatrics
Recommendations Aim to Ensure Safe Donor
Human Milk Available for High Risk Infants Who
Need It," American Academy of Pediatrics,
December 10, 2016, aap.org/en-us/about-the-aap
/aap-press-room/pages/new-american-academy-of
-pediatrics-recommendations-aim-to-ensure-safe
-donor-human-milk-available-for-high-risk-infants
-who.aspx.

CHAPTER 31
**Postpartum Love and Village
and Returning to Work**

Research has found that within 3 years . . .
Marc S. Schulz, Carolyn Pape Cowan, and Philip A.
Cowan, "Promoting Healthy Beginnings:
A Randomized Controlled Trial of a Preventive
Intervention to Preserve Marital Quality During the
Transition to Parenthood," *Journal of Consulting and
Clinical Psychology* 74, no. 1 (February 2006): 20–31,
doi.org/10.1037/0022-006x.74.1.20.

*Just as every individual could benefit from seeing a
therapist . . .*
Kurt Hahlweg and Howard J. Markman, "Effectiveness
of Behavioral Marital Therapy: Empirical Status of
Behavioral Techniques in Preventing and
Alleviating Marital Distress," *Journal of Consulting
and Clinical Psychology* 56, no. 3 (June 1988): 440–447,
doi.org/10.1037/0022-006x.56.3.440.

New research shows that it is optimal for women to wait . . .
Laura Schummers et al., "Association of Short
Interpregnancy Interval with Pregnancy Outcomes
According to Maternal Age," *JAMA Internal Medicine*
178, no.12 (December 2018): 1661–1670, doi.org/10
.1001/jamainternmed.2018.4696.

*One thing to keep in mind is that persistent lack of sexual
desire . . .*
Margaret A. De Judicibus and Marita P. McCabe,
"Psychological Factors and the Sexuality of Pregnant
and Postpartum Women," *Journal of Sex Research* 39,
no. 2 (May 2002): 94–103, doi.org/10.1080/002244
90209552128.

With over 70 percent of mothers employed . . .
"Employment Characteristics of Families, 2018," News
Release, Bureau of Labor Statistics, US Department
of Labor, April 18, 2019, bls.gov/news.release/pdf
/famee.pdf.

Symptom Checker

After 28 weeks, if your baby has hiccups . . .
Jason H. Collins, "Umbilical Cord Accidents," *BMC
Pregnancy and Childbirth* 12, no. 1 (August 2012): A7,
doi.org/10.1186/1471-2393-12-s1-a7.

Hormonal changes cause your body to respond . . .
Shailesh M. Gondivkar, Amol Gadbail, and Revant
Chole, "Oral Pregnancy Tumor," *Contemporary
Clinical Dentistry* 1, no. 3 (July–September 2010):
190–192, doi.org/10.4103/0976-237x.72792.

Ensure that you are getting enough vitamin D...
Thomas Dietrich et al., "Association Between Serum Concentrations of 25-hydroxyvitamin D and Gingival Inflammation," *American Journal of Clinical Nutrition* 82, no. 3 (September 2005): 575–580, doi.org/10.1093/ajcn/82.3.575.

...and vitamin C...
Pirkko J. Pussinen et al., "Periodontitis Is Associated with a Low Concentration of Vitamin C in Plasma," *Clinical and Diagnostic Lab Immunology* 10, no. 5 (September 2003): 897–902, doi.org/10.1128/cdli.10.5.897-902.2003.

Probiotics can help too...
Anirban Chatterjee, Hirak Bhattacharya, and Abhishek Kandwal, "Probiotics in Periodontal Health and Disease," *Journal of Indian Society of Periodontology* 15, no. 1 (January–March 2011): 23–28, doi.org/10.4103/0972-124x.82260.

Carpal tunnel (wrist pain) is super-common...
Robert H. Ablove and Tova Ablove, "Prevalence of Carpal Tunnel Syndrome in Pregnant Women," *WMJ: Official Publication of the State Medical Society of Wisconsin* 108, no. 4 (July 2009): 194–196, ncbi.nlm.nih.gov/pubmed/19753825.

Probiotics, like those found in kefir...
İlker Turan et al., "Effects of a Kefir Supplement on Symptoms, Colonic Transit, and Bowel Satisfaction Score in Patients with Chronic Constipation: A Pilot Study," *Turkish Journal of Gastroenterology* 25, no. 6 (December 2014): 650–656, doi.org/10.5152/tjg.2014.6990.

Daily exercise has been linked to improved bowel...
Sherri A. Longo et al., "Gastrointestinal Conditions During Pregnancy," *Clinics in Colon and Rectal Surgery* 23, no. 2 (June 2010): 80–89, doi.org/10.1055/s-0030-1254294.

I have been there, as have so many others...
Katherine Sapra et al., "Signs and Symptoms Associated with Early Pregnancy Loss: Findings from a Population-Based Preconception Cohort," *Human Reproduction* 31, no. 4 (April 2016): 887–896, doi.org/10.1093/humrep/dew010.

In their 2016 study, researcher Katherine Sapra...
Sapra et al., "Signs and Symptoms," 887-896.

There are lots of little tricks to try...
Vazquez, "Heartburn in Pregnancy," 1411.

Pregnant women need to add 1 to 2 hours...
"How Much Sleep Do I Need?" National Institutes of Health, US Department of Health and Human Services, updated April 29, 2019, nichd.nih.gov/health/topics/sleep/conditioninfo/how-much#3.

The hormone progesterone causes...
Juan C. Vazquez, "Heartburn in Pregnancy," *BMJ Clinical Evidence* 2015 (September 2015): 1411, researchgate.net/publication/281621281_heartburn_in_pregnancy.

Skipping breakfast and irregular eating...
Marie-Pierre St-Onge, Anja Mikic, and Cara E. Pietrolungo, "Effects of Diet on Sleep Quality," *Advances in Nutrition* 7, no. 5 (September 2016): 938–949, doi.org/10.3945/an.116.012336.

Unfortunately, insomnia can be connected...
Michele L. Okun and Louise M. O'Brien, "Concurrent Insomnia and Habitual Snoring Are Associated with Adverse Pregnancy Outcomes," *Sleep Medicine* 46 (June 2018): 12–19, doi.org/10.1016/j.sleep.2018.03.004.

Mask of Pregnancy and Skin Darkening...
Ivan Bolanča et al., "Chloasma: The Mask of Pregnancy," *Collegium Antropologicum* 32, no. 2 (October 2008): 139–141, ncbi.nlm.nih.gov/pubmed/19140277.

About 70 percent of women experience at least...
Guannan Bai et al., "Associations Between Nausea, Vomiting, Fatigue and Health-Related Quality of Life of Women in Early Pregnancy: The Generation R Study," *PLOS One* 11, no. 11 (November 2016): e0166133, doi.org/10.1371/journal.pone.0166133.

Anthropologist Kari Moca writes that morning sickness...
Kari Moca, "Morning Sickness," Reproductive Biology and Disease, Center for Academic Research and Training in Anthropogeny, January 2019, carta.anthropogeny.org/moca/topics/morning-sickness.

While they are marketed for decreasing seasickness...
Nancy M. Steele et al., "Effect of Acupressure by Sea-Bands on Nausea and Vomiting of Pregnancy," *Journal of Obstetric, Gynecologic and Neonatal Nursing* 30, no. 1 (January–February 2001): 61–70, doi.org/10.1111/j.1552-6909.2001.tb01522.x.

Ginger comes in many forms and can help...
Anne Matthews et al., "Interventions for Nausea and Vomiting in Early Pregnancy," Cochrane Database of Systematic Reviews 2010, no. 9 (September 2010): CD007575, doi.org/10.1002/14651858.cd007575.pub2.

Vitamin B6 (pyridoxine)...
Matthews et.al., "Interventions for Nausea and Vomiting," CD007575.

About 30 percent of women won't have nausea...
Mario Festin, "Nausea and Vomiting in Early Pregnancy," *BMJ Clinical Evidence* 2014 (March 2014): 1405, ncbi.nlm.nih.gov/pmc/articles/PMC3959188/.

Research finds that nausea, hyperemesis gravidarum . . .
Yafeng Zhang et al., "Familial Aggregation of Hyperemesis Gravidarum," *American Journal of Obstetrics and Gynecology* 204, no. 3 (March 2011): 230.e1–230.e7, doi.org/10.1016/j.ajog.2010.09.018.

. . . cholestasis . . .
"Intrahepatic Cholestasis of Pregnancy," US National Library of Medicine, September 10, 2019, ghr.nlm.nih.gov/condition/intrahepatic-cholestasis-of-pregnancy.

. . . blood clots . . .
Paola Devis and M. Grace Knuttinen, "Deep Venous Thrombosis in Pregnancy: Incidence, Pathogenesis and Endovascular Management," *Cardiovascular Diagnosis and Therapy* 7, no. 3 (December 2017): S309–S319, doi.org/10.21037/cdt.2017.10.08.

. . . preeclampsia . . .
"Preeclampsia," US National Library of Medicine, September 10, 2019, ghr.nlm.nih.gov/condition/preeclampsia#inheritance.

Research has found that increasing iron . . .
L. R. Patrick, "Restless Legs Syndrome: Pathophysiology and the Role of Iron and Folate," *Alternative Medicine Review* 12, no. 2 (June 2007): 101–102, ncbi.nlm.nih.gov/pubmed/17604457.

Studies that support the idea that pregnant women . . .
Š. Podzimek et al., "The Evolution of Taste and Perinatal Programming of Taste Preferences," *Physiological Research* 67, no. 3 (November 2018): S421–S429, ncbi.nlm.nih.gov/pubmed/30484669.

A 2013 study found that women who snore . . .
"Pregnant Women Who Snore at Higher Risk for C-Sections, Delivering Smaller Babies," Science Daily, October 31, 2013, sciencedaily.com/releases/2013/10/131031153457.htm.

Up to 90 percent of women get stretch marks . . .
Benjamin Farahnik et al., "Striae Gravidarum: Risk Factors, Prevention, and Management," *International Journal of Women's Dermatology* 3, no. 2 (June 2017): 77–85, doi.org/10.1016/j.ijwd.2016.11.001.

Vulvar varicosities are varicose veins that develop . . .
Nicholas Fassiadis, "Treatment for Pelvic Congestion Syndrome Causing Pelvic and Vulvar Varices," *International Angiology* 25, no. 1 (March 2006): 1–3, researchgate.net/publication/7256858_treatment_for_pelvic_congestion_syndrome_causing_pelvic_and_vulvar_varices.

Tests and Complications

Carrier Screening Preconception . . .
"Carrier Screening," Frequently Asked Questions: Pregnancy, American College of Obstetricians and Gynecologists, December 2018, acog.org/-/media/for-patients/faq179.pdf.

For example, cystic fibrosis is most common . . .
"Cystic Fibrosis," Genetics Home Reference, National Institutes for Health, updated September 10 2019, ghr.nlm.nih.gov/condition/cystic-fibrosis#statistics.

. . . Tay-Sachs disease is most common in . . .
"Tay-Sachs Disease," National Tay-Sachs and Allied Diseases Association of Delaware Valley, February 2019, tay-sachs.org/taysachs_disease.php.

. . . sickle cell anemia is more common among . . .
"Sickle Cell Disease," American Society of Hematology, February 2019, hematology.org/patients/anemia/sickle-cell.aspx.

According to the Society for Maternal-Fetal Medicine, amniocentesis . . .
"Risks of Chorionic Villus Sampling and Amniocentesis," Society for Maternal-Fetal Medicine, accessed May 28, 2019, smfm.org/publications/156-risks-of-chorionic-villus-sampling-and-amniocentesis.

It is also normal for the number to decrease . . .
Shripad Hebbar et al., "Reference Ranges of Amniotic Fluid Index in Late Third Trimester of Pregnancy: What Should the Optimal Interval Between Two Ultrasound Examinations Be?" *Journal of Pregnancy* 2015 (January 2015): 319204, doi.org/10.1155/2015/319204.

A BPP combines a nonstress test . . .
Frank A. Manning et al., "Fetal Assessment Based on Fetal Biophysical Profile Scoring: In 19,221 Referred High-Risk Pregnancies," *American Journal of Obstetrics and Gynecology* 157, no. 4 (October 1987): 880–884, doi.org/10.1016/S0002-9378(87)80077-7.

The procedure carries a small (0.35 percent) risk . . .
Jaroslaw Beta et al., "Risk of Miscarriage Following Amniocentesis and Chorionic Villus Sampling: A Systematic Review of the Literature," *Minerva Ginecologica* 70, no. 2 (April 2018): 215–219, smfm.org/publications/156-risks-of-chorionic-villus-sampling-and-amniocentesis.

A 2013 study reports that ultrasounds are good . . .
Maria Daniela Renna et al., "Sonographic Markers for Early Diagnosis of Fetal Malformations," *World Journal of Radiology* 5, no. 10 (October 2013): 356–371, doi.org/10.4329/wjr.v5.i10.356.

It is important to consider age in pregnancy . . .
Matthew C. Jolly, et al., "The Risks Associated with Pregnancy in Women Aged 35 Years or Older," *Human Reproduction* 15, no. 11 (November 2000): 2433–2437, ncbi.nlm.nih.gov/pubmed/11056148.

Bacterial vaginosis, or BV, is the most common . . .
Emilia H. Koumans et al., "The Prevalence of Bacterial
Vaginosis in the United States, 2001–2004:
Associations with Symptoms, Sexual Behaviors, and
Reproductive Health," *Sexually Transmitted Diseases*
34, no. 11, (November 2007): 864–869, doi.org/10.1097
/olq.0b013e318074e565.

This is one of the reasons douching is not . . .
Roberta B. Ness et al., "Douching in Relation to
Bacterial Vaginosis, Lactobacilli, and Facultative
Bacteria in the Vagina," *Obstetrics and Gynecology*
100, no. 4 (October 2002): 765–772, doi.org/10.1016
/S0029-7844(02)02184-1.

It is important to note that ACOG no longer . . .
"Management of Preterm Labor," Practice Bulletin
No. 127, Committee on Practice Bulletins—
Obstetrics, American College of Obstetricians and
Gynecologists, *Obstetrics and Gynecology* 119, no. 6
(June 2012): 1308–1317, doi.org/10.1097/aog.0b013e3
1825af2f0.

All this said, there may be future medical uses . . .
Eberhard Merz and Sonila Pashaj, "Advantages of 3D
Ultrasound in the Assessment of Fetal Abnormalities,"
Journal of Perinatal Medicine 45, no. 6 (August 2017):
643–650, doi.org/10.1515/jpm-2016-0379.

Hispanic women and women with indigenous . . .
Laura N. Bull et al., "Intrahepatic Cholestasis of
Pregnancy (ICP) in US Latinas and Chileans:
Clinical Features, Ancestry Analysis, and Admixture
Mapping," *PLOS One* 10, no. 6 (June 2015): e0131211,
doi.org/10.1371/journal.pone.0131211.

And while the most common site for a blood clot . . .
"Deep Vein Thrombosis (DVT) in Pregnancy," Your
Pregnancy and Baby Guide, National Health Service
(UK), last reviewed March 27, 2018, nhs.uk/conditions
/pregnancy-and-baby/dvt-blood-clot-pregnant/.

ACOG estimates that 14 to 23 percent of women . . .
"Depression and Postpartum Depression: Resource
Overview," Women's Health Care Physicians,
American College of Obstetricians and Gynecologists,
January 2019, acog.org/womens-health
/depression-and-postpartum-depression.

And the Centers for Disease Control recommends . . .
"What Vaccines Are Recommended for You," Centers
for Disease Control and Prevention, October
2, 2018, cdc.gov/vaccines/adults/rec-vac/index.
html; Pranita D. Tamma et al., "Safety of Influenza
Vaccination During Pregnancy," *American Journal
of Obstetrics and Gynecology* 201, no. 6 (December
2009): 547–552, doi.org/10.1016/j.ajog.2009.09.034.

Occurring in 2 to 10 percent of pregnancies, GDM . . .
Brindles Lee Macon and Winnie Yu, "Gestational
Diabetes," Healthline, June 25, 2018, healthline.com
/health/gestational-diabetes.

It is fairly rare, affecting only 1 percent . . .
Caitlin Dean et al., "Recurrence Rates of Hyperemesis
Gravidarum in Pregnancy: A Systematic Review
Protocol," *JBI Database of Systematic Reviews and
Implementation Reports* 15, no. 11 (November 2017):
2659–2665, doi.org/10.11124/jbisrir-2016-003271.

We don't fully know why some people . . .
Emily Glover, "For Mothers with Extreme Morning
Sickness, Study Offers New Hope," Motherly, April
5, 2018, mother.ly/news/for-mothers-with-extreme
-morning-sickness-study-offers-new-hope.

Indeed, there is a strong hereditary aspect . . .
Marlena S. Fejzo et al., "High Prevalence of Severe
Nausea and Vomiting of Pregnancy and Hyperemesis
Gravidarum Among Relatives of Affected Individuals,"
*European Journal of Obstetrics, Gynecology, and
Reproductive Biology* 141, no. 1 (November 2008):
13–17, doi.org/10.1016/j.ejogrb.2008.07.003.

And if you've had it in a previous pregnancy . . .
Dean et al., "Recurrence Rates of Hyperemesis
Gravidarum," 2659–2665.

Smoking during pregnancy . . .
Claire Infante-Rivard et al., "Absence of Association of
Thrombophilia Polymorphisms with Intrauterine
Growth Restriction," *New England Journal of
Medicine* 347 (July 2002): 19–25, doi.org/10.1056
/nejm200207043470105.

Exposure to high levels of radiation . . .
Pamela M. Williams and Stacy Fletcher, "Health
Effects of Prenatal Radiation Exposure," *American
Family Physician* 82, no. 5 (September 2010):
488–493, researchgate.net/publication/46168816
_health_effects_of_prenatal_radiation_exposure.

But it is also possible to carry an IUGR pregnancy . . .
Lesley M. McCowan, Francesc Figueras, and Ngaire
H. Anderson, "Evidence-Based National Guidelines
for the Management of Suspected Fetal Growth
Restriction: Comparison, Consensus, and
Controversy," *American Journal of Obstetrics and
Gynecology* 219, no. 2 (February 2018): S855–S868,
doi.org/10.1016/j.ajog.2017.12.004.

It is diagnosed by ultrasound . . .
Perry Friedman and Dotun Ogunyemi,
"Oligohydramnios," in *Obstetric Imaging: Fetal
Diagnosis and Care*, 2nd ed., ed. Joshua A. Copel et al.
(Philadelphia: Elsevier, 2018), 511–515.

Causes can include . . . intrauterine growth restriction . . .
Shripad Hebbar et al., "Reference Ranges of Amniotic Fluid Index in Late Third Trimester of Pregnancy: What Should the Optimal Interval Between Two Ultrasound Examinations Be?" *Journal of Pregnancy* 2015 (January 2015): 319204, ncbi.nlm.nih.gov/pmc/articles/pmc4312643/.

As many as 1 in 4 women will experience . . .
Emily J. Fawcett, Jonathan M. Fawcett, and Dwight Mazmanian, "A Meta-Analysis of the Worldwide Prevalence of Pica During Pregnancy and the Postpartum Period," *International Journal of Gynecology and Obstetrics* 133, no. 3 (June 2016): 277–283, doi.org/10.1016/j.ijgo.2015.10.012.

Polyhydramnios occurs when there is too much . . .
Hebbar et al., "Reference Ranges of Amniotic Fluid Index," 319204.

It is diagnosed by an ultrasound . . .
Amr Hamza et al., "Polyhydramnios: Causes, Diagnosis and Therapy," *Geburtshilfe und Frauenheilkunde* 73, no. 12 (December 2013): 1241–1246, doi.org/10.1055/s-0033-1360163.

Preeclampsia is a condition that only occurs . . .
Cande V. Ananth, Katherine M. Keyes, and Ronald J. Wapner, "Preeclampsia Rates in the United States, 1980-2010: Age-Period-Cohort Analysis," *BMJ* 347 (November 2013): f6564, doi.org/10.1136/bmj.f6564.

In 57 percent of the cases . . .
Tanya M. Medina and D. Ashley Hill, "Preterm Premature Rupture of Membranes: Diagnosis and Management," *American Family Physician* 73, no. 4 (February 2006): 659–664, aafp.org/afp/2006/0215/p659.html.

Of note, the CDC recommends . . .
"Vulvovaginal Candidiasis," 2015 Sexually Transmitted Diseases Treatment Guidelines, Centers for Disease Control and Prevention, June 4, 2015, cdc.gov/std/tg2015/candidiasis.htm; Lauren B. Angotti, Lara C. Lambert, and David E. Soper, "Vaginitis: Making Sense of Over-the-Counter Treatment Options," *Infectious Diseases in Obstetrics and Gynecology* 2007 (August 2007): 97424, doi.org/10.1155/2007/97424.

DEET has not been found to cause problems . . .
Rose McGready et al., "Safety of the Insect Repellent N,N-diethyl-M-toluamide (DEET) in Pregnancy," *American Journal of Tropical Medicine and Hygiene* 65, no. 4 (October 2001): 285–289, doi.org/10.4269/ajtmh.2001.65.285.

Syphilis, for example, has seen a 76 percent increase . . .
"Sexually Transmitted Disease Surveillance 2017," Centers for Disease Control and Prevention, October 15, 2018, cdc.gov/std/stats17/default.htm.

Chlamydia is a common STI . . .
"Chlamydia: CDC Fact Sheet (Detailed)," Centers for Disease Control and Prevention, October 4, 2016, cdc.gov/std/chlamydia/stdfact-chlamydia-detailed.htm.

If you have herpes, your provider will likely prescribe . . .
"ACOG Releases Guidelines on Managing Herpes in Pregnancy," Practice Guideline, *American Family Physician* 77, no. 3 (February 2008): 369–370, aafp.org/afp/2008/0201/p369.html.

ACOG recommends that women with HIV . . .
"Labor and Delivery Management of Women with Human Immunodeficiency Virus Infection," ACOG Committee Opinion No. 751, American College of Obstetricians and Gynecologists, *Obstetrics and Gynecology* 132 (2018): e131–e137, acog.org/clinical-guidance-and-publications/committee-opinions/committee-on-obstetric-practice/labor-and-delivery-management-of-women-with-human-immunodeficiency-virus-infection.

Sometimes they are treated just like previas . . .
Atsuko Taga et al., "Planned Vaginal Delivery Versus Planned Cesarean Delivery in Cases of Low-Lying Placenta," *Journal of Maternal-Fetal and Neonatal Medicine* 30, no. 5 (March 2017): 618–622, doi.org/10.1080/14767058.2016.1181168.

Some women are diagnosed with placenta previa . . .
"Placenta Previa," Mayo Clinic, March 6, 2018, mayoclinic.org/diseases-conditions/placenta-previa/symptoms-causes/syc-20352768.

Velamentous cord insertion means that the blood vessels . . .
Monica Mihaela Cîrstoiu et al., "Velamentous Cord Insertion: An Important Obstetrical Risk Factor," *Gineco.edu* 12, no. 3 (2016): 124-134, doi.org/10.18643/gieu.2016.129.

Occasionally, in less than 1 percent of singleton pregnancies . . .
"MFM Consult: Single Umbilical Artery: What You Need to Know," Contemporary OB/GYN, October 1, 2010, contemporaryobgyn.net/modern-medicine-now/mfm-consult-single-umbilical-artery-what-you-need-know.

About 20 percent of the time . . .
"Umbilical Cord Conditions," March of Dimes, last reviewed June 2016, marchofdimes.org/complications/umbilical-cord-conditions.aspx.

Cysts may be present in up to 3 percent . . .
Leyre Ruiz Campo et al., "Prenatal Diagnosis of
    Umbilical Cord Cyst: Clinical Significance and
    Prognosis," *Taiwanese Journal of Obstetrics and
    Gynecology* 56, no. 5 (October 2017): 622–627,
    doi.org/10.1016/j.tjog.2017.08.008.

In this incredibly rare complication . . .
"What Is Amniotic Fluid Embolism?" AFE Foundation,
    March 2019, afesupport.org/what-is-amniotic
    -fluid-embolism.

We do not currently know what the exact risk factors . . .
"What Is Amniotic Fluid Embolism?"

The American College of Nurse-Midwives has reported . . .
"Cephalopelvic Disproportion (CPD)," Labor and Birth,
    American Pregnancy Association, updated August
    2015, americanpregnancy.org/labor-and-birth
    /cephalopelvic-disproportion/.

Yet CPD is cited as the most common reason . . .
James M. Nicholson and Lisa C. Kellar, "The Active
    Management of Impending Cephalopelvic
    Disproportion in Nulliparous Women at Term: A
    Case Series," *Journal of Pregnancy* 2010 (July 2010):
    708615, doi.org/10.1155/2010/708615.

Of note, a recent study found that Asian women . . .
Michelle Brandt, "Asian-White Couples Face Distinct
    Pregnancy Risks, Stanford/Packard Study Finds,"
    Stanford Medicine News Center, October 1, 2008,
    med.stanford.edu/news/all-news/2008/10/asian
    -white-couples-face-distinct-pregnancy-risks
    -stanfordpackard-study-finds.html.

Chorioamnionitis is an infection or inflammation . . .
Alan Thevenet N. Tita, "Intra-amniotic Infection
    (Clinical Chorioamnionitis or Triple I)," UpToDate,
    updated September 3, 2019, uptodate.com
    /contents/intra-amniotic-infection-clinical
    -chorioamnionitis-or-triple-i.

It most often occurs during labor . . .
Alan Thevenet N. Tita and William W. Andrews,
    "Diagnosis and Management of Clinical
    Chorioamnionitis," *Clinics in Perinatology* 37,
    no. 2 (June 2010): 339–354, doi.org/10.1016/j.clp
    .2010.02.003.

This occurs in about 8 percent of full-term . . .
Cyril Fischer et al., "A Population-Based Study of
    Meconium Aspiration Syndrome in Neonates Born
    Between 37 and 43 Weeks of Gestation,"
    International Journal of Pediatrics 2012, no. 2
    (January 2012): 321545, doi.org/10.1155/2012/321545.

Shoulder dystocia is a relatively rare . . .
"Shoulder Dystocia," Royal College of Obstetricians and
    Gynaecologists, March 2013, rcog.org.uk
    /globalassets/documents/patients/patient
    -information-leaflets/pregnancy/pi-shoulder
    -dystocia.pdf.

It is incredibly rare, affecting 2.9 out of . . .
Sarah L. Coad, Leanne S. Dahlgren, and Jennifer A.
    Hutcheon, "Risks and Consequences of Puerperal
    Uterine Inversion in the United States, 2004
    through 2013," *American Journal of Obstetrics and
    Gynecology* 217, no. 3 (September 2017): 377.e1–377.
    e6, doi.org/10.1016/j.ajog.2017.05.018.

Stillbirth occurs in about 1 percent of pregnancies . . .
"What Is Stillbirth?" Centers for Disease Control and
    Prevention, May 9, 2019, cdc.gov/ncbddd/stillbirth
    /facts.html.

Illustration Credits

Index

Note: Bold page numbers denote figures.

blood sugar (*continued*)
  gestational diabetes and, 161–62,
    460–61
  glucose challenge test, 161
  stabilizing with diet, 165
  sweet potatoes and, 132
blood type, 452
blood work, 103
body
  anatomy, 21–33
  changes in pregnancy, 115–16
  pregnant body, **28**
  trusting your body, 209, 211
  See also anatomy; growth of baby
    and uterus; symptoms in
    pregnancy
body mass index (BMI), 14–15, 150
  BMI categories, 15
  gestational diabetes and, 150
  stigma and, 150
body weight. *See* weight; weight gain
bonding
  anatomy scan of baby and,
    143–45, 146
  attuning to baby, 116
  endorphins and, 31
  imagining relationship with baby,
    116, 177–78
  letter to your baby, 211–12
  in month 2, 99
  in month 3, 116
  in month 4, 130
  in month 5, 143–45
  in month 6, 160
  in month 7, 177–78
  in month 8, 196
  in month 9, 211–12
  oxytocin and, 30
  postpartum, 363–85
bone broth, 180
bottle-feeding, 410
  jaundice and, 277–78
boundaries, establishing, 336
bowel movement, in postnatal
  period, 354–56
brain of baby
  development in pregnancy, 110,
    171, 180
  eating fat and protein for, 171
brain of mother, changes in
  pregnancy, 116, 343
bras, 400–401, 432

nursing, 400–401
Braxton-Hicks contractions, 178,
  196, 212, 241, 432
breakouts (pimples), 432
breast milk, 393
  colostrum, 135, 393, 403
  "coming in" of milk, 393, 401
  oversupply of, 398
  storage of, 409–10, **409**
breast soreness/tenderness, 99,
  116, 432
breastfeeding, 387–403
  alcohol consumption and, 402–3
  areolas and, 112, 146, 391–92
  benefits for baby, 390, 393
  benefits for mama, 390
  breast anatomy and, 391–92, **391**
  breastfeeding pillows, 401
  "breastfeeding shouldn't hurt"
    phrase, 398–99
  clogged ducts, 400
  cluster feeding, 393
  combination feeding, 410
  diaper rash and, 369
  dysphoric milk ejection reflex
    (D-MER), 400
  engorged breasts, 393, 398
  estrogen levels and, 392
  feeding tube systems and, 401
  feeding your baby, 394–400
  food restrictions, 342
  fun facts about, 392
  gear for, 400–401
  handwashing before, 400
  how to know if baby is done
    feeding, 394
  how to know if baby is getting
    enough milk, 393, 394–95
  hunger cues, 394
  lactation consultants, 339, 397, 403
  lactation cookie bites, 395
  latching, 395, 398–99
  laws on public breastfeeding, 402
  lip and tongue ties (baby's), 399
  mastitis and, 399–400
  in NICU, 403
  nipple confusion and, 397, 410
  nursing bras, 400–401
  nutrition for, 340, 394, 398
  on-demand feeding, 392–93
  oxytocin and, 350, 392
  positions for, 395–97, **396**
  positions for, after C-section, 353
  postpartum doulas and, 339

prolactin and, 31, 392
in public, 402
pumping and dumping, 402–3
reflux by baby and, 398
resumption of period delayed
  by, 360
sadness and, 400
starting in first hours after birth,
  270, 272–73
starting, tips for, 397
sucking by baby, 204, 392
as supply and demand system, 392
support groups, 397
thrush and, 400
time frame for continuing (in
  months), 390–91
time involved in, 390, 393, 396–97
trauma history and, 391
troubleshooting, 397–400
uterine contractions and, 350
vitamin D supplements during, 390
work protections for, 408
See also pumping and
  bottle-feeding
breastmilk pumping. *See* pumping
  and bottle-feeding
breasts
  anatomy, 391–92, **391**
  bras and, 400–401, 432
  breast soreness/tenderness, 99,
    116, 432
  changes in pregnancy, 112, 115, 116
  colostrum and, 135, 393
  engorged, 393, 398
  infection of: mastitis, 399–400, 482
  infection of: thrush, 400
  nipple and areola darkening, 112,
    116, 146, 444
  nipples, 391, **391**, 392
  prenatal breast assessment, 397
  sensitivity, sex and, 124
breathing
  diaphragmatic breathing, 119–22
  in labor, 288
  and postpartum bowel
    movement, 355–56
  rate, for newborns, 277
  shortness of breath, 119, 178, 196,
    212, 445–46
breathing of baby
  after birth, 275
  amniotic fluid and, 140
  breaths per minute, 202
  placenta, gas exchange in, 166

breathing of baby (*continued*)
    surfactant and, 183
    in week 17, 139–40
    in week 29, 183
    in week 33, 202

breech babies, **197**, 198

Cesarean section and, 311
    moxibustion (acupuncture
        technique) for, 94
    turning, tricks for, 93, 198–99
    vaginal birth of, 198
    Webster technique for, 93

C-section. *See* Cesarean birth

caffeine, 11, 439

calcium, 9

candida or yeast infection, 400, 469
    thrush, 378

cannabidiol (CBD), 12

car seats, 152
    installation of, 206

carbohydrates, 165, 340

carpal tunnel, 432–33

castor oil, 227

Cates, Brooke, 25, 31

catheter, urinary, 296, 312, 352

cats, 164, 468
    toxoplasmosis and, 133, 468

CBD (cannabidiol), 12

cellulitis, 482

cephalopelvic disproportion
    (CPD), 478

cervical insufficiency, 459

cervical mucus, 39
    mucus plus, 122

Cervidil, 303

cervix, 27–28, 246
    anatomy of, **26**, 27–28, **27**
    dilation of, 28, **29**, 246–47
    during labor, 27–28, **29**, 246–47
    effacing of, 27–28, **29**
    fully dilated (10 cm), 28, **29**
    mucus plus, 122
    normal length of, 29
    obstructed (placenta previa), 474
    position during cycle, 40
    softening of, 27, 207, 246

Cesarean births (C-section), 309–20
    birth of placenta during, 313
    clothing and items after, 318

descriptions by mothers, 315–16
elective, 311
emergency unplanned, 312, 314–15
epidurals and, 295, 312
general anesthesia for, 314–15
gentle Cesareans, 311–12, 314
healing and recovery after, 352–53
incision, and stitching of, 313–14
induction of labor and C-section
    rates, 302
meditation for, 318–19
nonemergency unplanned, 311–12
number of C-sections
    recommended, 316
partners during, 312–13, 316
planned, 311, 314
previous C-sections and, 311, 316
procedures during, 312–14
reasons for, 311, 312
spinal block for, 295, 312
timing for birth by, 313
trial of labor after Cesarean
    (TOLAC), 316–17
types of, 311–13
vaginal birth after Cesarean
    (VBAC), 316–17
vaginal bleeding after, 351
vaginal seeding and, 314
wound infection postpartum, 482

charting your cycle, 12

chemical pregnancy, 53, 57

chemicals, toxic and endocrine-
    disrupting, 12–14

child, inviting to witness the birth, 185

childcare, 196–99, 419–20
    au pair, 188–89
    babysitter/nanny, 188
    co-ops, 187–88
    daycare/preschool, 189
    factors in, 186–87
    family members or friends, 186, 187
    finding, 196–99
    nanny shares, 188
    parent helpers, 189

China, postpartum recovery in, 129

chiropractors, 93, 429
    stimulation of labor by, 227

chlamydia, 471

cholestasis, 459
    induction of labor for, 301
    itching and, 441, 459

chorioamnionitis (intra-amniotic
    infection), 479

chorionic villus sampling (CVS),
    117, 455

chromosomal abnormalities, 53,
    65, 482
    Down syndrome (trisomy 21),
        117, 130
    Edwards syndrome (trisomy
        18), 117
    Patau syndrome (trisomy 13), 117
    screening for, 117, 130, 456

cigarette smoking, quitting, 10–11

circumcision, 365–66

clary sage oil, 227

cleaner, household, 13

clitoris, **24**, 29, **30**
    nerve endings in, 29

Clomid, 48

cluster feeding, 393

coconut water, 108

colic, 375

collagen, consuming in diet, 180–81

colostrum, 135, 393, 403

comfrey root, 227

complementary medicine, 49

complete blood count (CBC), 103, 453

complex carbohydrates, 165

complications. *See* birth
    complications; pregnancy
    complications

compression stockings, 161, 447, 448

conception, 35–49
    active lifetime of sperm and eggs,
        40–41
    age and, 44, 47
    basal temperature and, 39–40
    cervical mucus and, 39
    cervical position and, 40
    fertile period, 40–41
    fertility chart (downloadable), 38
    fertility treatments and, 45–49
    fertilization, 37, 40–41
    food recommendations for, 42
    how often to have sex, 41
    if you don't get pregnant, 43–45
    infertility and, 45
    keeping sex fun, 41, 42
    menstrual cycle and, 37–38
    monitoring/tracking your
        ovulation, 38–40, 42
    months needed to achieve, 41
    ovulation and, 37–41

gestational diabetes mellitus
(GDM) (*continued*)
induction of labor and, 301
risk factors, 161, 162
testing for, 161–62
getting full quickly, 16, 178, 212,
437–38
getting pregnant, 1–94
anatomy and, 21–33
choosing a birthplace and
provider, 83–94
conception, 35–49
decision to become pregnant, 3–19
finding out you are pregnant,
71–81
miscarriage and loss, 51–69
ginger, 119, 443
giving birth. *See* labor
glucose challenge test (GCT), 161, 162
glucose tolerance test (GTT), 162
glycine, 180–81
gonorrhea, 472
grief, 66–67
for arrival of period, 45
over miscarriage, 55, 60, 62, 66–67
groin pain, 130, 145, 161, 178, 196,
212, 438
round ligament pain, 438
group B strep (GBS), 212–14, 240
controversy over, 213–14
growing baby terminology, 75
growth of baby and uterus
baby at month 2 (weeks 5-8), **106**
baby at month 3 (weeks 9-12), **121**
baby at month 4 (weeks 13-17), **134**
baby at month 5 (weeks 18-22), **149**
baby at month 6 (weeks 23-27), **169**
baby at month 7 (weeks 28-31), **182**
baby at month 8 (weeks 32-35), **200**
baby at month 9 (weeks 36-40), **217**
fundal height, 145–46, **146**, 178, 197
growth spurt (third trimester), 180
halfway milestone, 145
palpation of abdomen to
determine, 130
quickening, 131
ultrasound anatomy scan for
baby, 143–45, 457–58
using tape measure to assess
growth, 145–46
guilt feelings, 58, 67, 77, 206
letting go of, 111

hair
baby's (lanugo), 148–50, 189–90,
216
hair growth during pregnancy, 438
loss, postpartum, 356–57
pubic, 104
The Happiest Baby on the Block
(Karp), 372
hCG. *See* human chorionic
gonadotropin
head
cephalopelvic disproportion
(CPD), 478
of newborn, **274**, 275
headaches, 130, 145, 438–39
causes of, 438
hydration and, 107
migraines, 439
spinal headache, 482
health disparities, 90
health insurance, 7, 152–53
Affordable Care Act and, 7, 153
for baby/newborn, 380
community resources for, 79
determining your coverage, 153
Medicaid, 153
option to make changes in, 152–53
health visits/appointments. *See*
prenatal provider visits
hearing, baby's sense of, 148, 155, 196
hearing test for newborns, 278
music for baby, 196
talking and reading to baby, 148, 196
heart
mother's, in pregnancy, 116
of newborn, 274, 275
of newborn, ductus arteriosus
in, 275
pumping in early embryo, 111
heart rate of baby
in early embryo, 108
in month 9, 214
monitoring during labor, 205–6
emergency C-section and, 312
newborn's, 277
heart rate of mother, increase in,
178, 439
heartbeat of baby
first detection of, 75
first sounds on ultrasound, 117, 125
first visible on ultrasound, 108
heart rate, 108, 117

listening to at provider visit, 130,
145, 161, 178, 197
heartburn, 439–40
as symptom in pregnancy, 130, 145,
161, 178, 196, 199, 212
HELLP syndrome, 461
help
asking for, 338–39
partner, 16
providers, choosing, 78, 89–94
hemolysis (HELLP syndrome), 461
hemorrhoids, 439–40
during pregnancy, 130, 145, 161,
178, 196, 212, 439–40
postpartum, 356
hepatitis, 472
hepatitis B, 472
hepatitis B vaccine, 276, 472
testing for, 103, 276, 472
hernias, 461–62
herpes, 472–73
C-section and, 311, 473
hiccups, baby's, 131, 161, 178, 429
high blood pressure (hypertension),
462
high risk pregnancies, 462
hip squeeze, 290, **290**
hips of baby, 275
babywearing and, 275, 383
hip dysplasia, 275, 383
HIV, 473
testing, 103, 197, 473
viral load, C-section and, 311
home birth, 88–89
APGAR scors and, 88
professional attendants for, 88, 89
safety of, 88, 89
transfer to hospital, 307
hormones, 30–31
adrenaline and noradrenaline, 31
anti-Mullerian hormone (AMH),
45–46
from corpus luteum, 37
cortisol, 30–31
endorphins, 31
estrogen, 30
fertility screening tests, 46–47
follicle-stimulating hormone
(FSH), 37, 47
human chorionic gonadotropin
(hCG), 38, 73–75

hormones (*continued*)
oxytocin, 30
progesterone, 30
prolactin, 31, 291
prostaglandin, 31
relaxin, 31, 207
hospitals, 85–87
"Baby Friendly", 272, 273
epidurals and, 86
NICU in, 87, 243, 477
operating room and resources of, 85–86
professionals allowed to attend births in, 86
recommended for these situations, 86
"rooming in" at, 272
hot flashes, 178, 196, 212, 440
household duties, sharing, 416
HPV, 471–72
Hugo point (acupressure), 292, **292**
human chorionic gonadotropin (hCG), 38
amount detected by pregnancy tests, 74
functions of, 73
levels after miscarriage, 59
levels throughout pregnancy, 73, 74
pregnancy tests and, 38, 73, 74–75
human papilloma virus (HPV), 471–72
humidifier, 431
hydration. *See* water (hydration)
hyperactivity, umbilical cord and, 178
hyperemesis gravidarum (HG), 444, 463
hypertension, 462
hypnobirthing, 290–91
hysterosalpingogram, 47

ibuprofen, not to be taken during pregnancy, 434, 439
iliacus muscle, **23**, 24
implantation, 37
bleeding and, 447
cramping and, 434
in vitro fertilization (IVF), 46, 48
incomplete miscarriage, 59
incontinence, 307, 354
fecal, 356

India
postpartum nurturing in, 218
pregnancy tradition in, 181
induction of labor, 301–4
artificial rupture of membranes (AROM), 303
augmentations, 304
elective inductions, 302
Foley bulb, 303
home methods for inducing, 226–28, 302
hormones and, 303–4
Pitocin and, 304
practitioner methods for, 302–4
prostaglandin medications, 303
reasons for, 301–2
subsequent C-section and, 302
sweeping or stripping the membranes, 302–3
worry about, 301
See also interventions
infant mortality
home birth and risk of, 88
stillbirth, 482–83
women and babies of color, 90
infection
bacterial vaginosis, 458
chorioamnionitis (intra-amniotic infection), 479
herpes, 311, 472
HIV, 311
mastitis, 399–400, 482
postpartum, 482
and preterm prelabor rupture of membranes (PPROM), 467
risk after water breaks, 240, 303
thrush, 400
urinary tract infections (UTIs), 123
uterine, 350
of uterus (endometritis), 482
wound infection (after C-section), 482
yeast (candidiasis), 469
infertility, 45
and mood/anxiety disorders, 77
inner core muscles. *See* core muscles
inner thigh squeezes, 181–83, 218
insomnia, 440–41
insurance, 152–53
health insurance, 7, 152–53, 380
life insurance, 153
intermittent fetal heart rate monitoring, 306

interventions, 299–307
beyond due date, 301
fetal monitoring, 305–6
forceps delivery, 306–7
induction of labor, 301–4
internal monitors, 306
intrauterine pressure catheter (IUPC), 306
intravenous (IV) therapy, 305
operative vaginal deliveries, 306–7
personal preferences, stating, 325
reasons for, 301–2
transfer from to hospital, 307
vacuum delivery, 306
worry about, 301
See also Cesarean births; induction of labor
intra-amniotic infection (chorioamnionitis), 479
intracervical insemination (ICI), 48
intrahepatic cholestasis of pregnancy (ICP), 459
intrauterine growth restriction (IUGR), 463–64
induction of labor for, 301
intrauterine insemination (IUI), 48
intrauterine pressure catheter (IUPC), 306
intravaginal insemination (IVI), 48
intravenous (IV) therapy, 305
iron, 9–10, 147
iron-deficiency anemia, 201, 464
iron-rich foods, 201, 340–41
paired with vitamin C, 199
restless leg syndrome and, 444
itching, 161, 178, 196, 212, 441
PUPPP and, 441
items for baby, 173–74

Japan, postpartum nurturing in, 218
jaundice, in newborns, 277–78
Judaism, pregnancy tradition in, 226

Keating, Catherine, 68–69
Kegel exercises, 32
kick counts, 178

labia majora, 29, **30**
labia minora, 29, **30**

pain and coping techniques
    (*continued*)
    contractions, characteristics of,
        284, 285
    coping skills, usefulness of, 287
    culture and pain, 286
    difference of labor pain (vs. other
        pain), 284
    epidurals, 295–97
    experience of pain, 285–87
    first-hand descriptions of labor
        pain, 284–85
    general anesthesia, 297
    hip squeeze, 290, **290**
    holding hands, 293
    however you feel is OK, 285–86
    hypnobirthing, 290–91
    intense pain as sign of
        complications, 286
    listing in birth plan, 324–25
    massage, 292
    medical coping methods, 293–97
    medications for pain, how they
        work, 293–94
    middle-school dance, 288
    music, 293
    nitrous oxide (laughing gas), 294
    nonmedical coping methods,
        287–93
    opioids, 293–94
    pain tolerance levels, 286
    peanut balls, 289–90
    pudendal block, 295
    purpose of pain, 283
    reasons for pain in birthing, 283–85
    rebozos, 290
    spinal block, 295, 312
    sterile water injections, 293
    twilight sleep, 247
    vocalization, 291–92
    water therapy, 288–89
palpation of abdomen, 130
Pap smear, 103, 453
parenting, 177, 202–4, 415–16
    Eight Principles of, 202–3
    parent helpers, 189
    single parenthood, 419
    See also childcare
partner, 16
    active labor, role in, 249
    Cesarean birth and, 312–13, 316
    couples counseling, 79
    couples therapy, 415
    cutting the cord, 266

delivery, assisting with, 262, 479–80
depression and, 136
fear, experience of, 202
household duties, sharing, 416
joining in meditation, 194–96
making time as a couple, 417
medical history of, 101
newborn care and parenting, 415–16
postpartum transitions, 338
preconception health visit for, 7
pushing during labor, support for,
    255, 258
questions for, 17
sex after the birth, 417–19
skin-to-skin and, 271
staying in communication, 44
staying in the zone, 184
support after miscarriage, 60
support for pregnancy
    symptoms, 123
transition (in labor), role in, 250
water therapy, bringing a bathing
    suit for, 287
Patau syndrome, 117
peanut balls, 289–90
pediatricians, 203
pelvic exams, 7, 102–4
    at first prenatal visit, 102–4
    reasons for, 103
    speculum and, 102–3
    tricks for making easier, 102–3
pelvic floor, 24–25, **24**
    belly pump exercise and, 132–35, 183
    physical therapy (postpartum), 355
pelvic girdle, 23–24, **23**
    pelvic girdle pain (PGP), 465
    sacroiliac joint dysfunction, 465
    symphysis pubis dysfunction
        (SPD), 465
pelvic inflammatory disease (PID), 473
pelvic pain, 465
    exercises for, 181–83
pelvis, 23–24, **23**
    changes in pregnancy, 115
    expansion and contraction of, 23–24
    ligaments of, 23
    pelvic floor, 24–25, **24**
    pelvic girdle (bones), 23–24, **23**
    pelvic muscles, **23**, 24
    relaxin hormone and, 207
    variations in anatomy of, 31
peppermint tea, 119

perinatal mood and anxiety
    disorders (PMADs), 77
perineal massage, 260
perineal pain, remedies for, 351–52
    burning sensation when peeing, 353
    padsicles, 351–52
    sitz bath, 351
perineum, 28–29, **28**, **30**
    episiotomies, 262
    ring of fire, 261
    tearing (during labor), 261–62, 481
perineum bottle, 354
pesticides, 133
pets, 164, 468
physical exam (first prenatal
    visit), 102–5
physical recovery, postpartum, 347–61
    birth control and, 357, **358–59**
    bleeding, 349–51
    constipation, 356
    diastasis recti, 357–60, **357**
    exercise, 360–61
    fecal incontinence, 356
    getting your period, 360
    hair loss, 356–57
    healing after C-section, 352–53
    hemorrhoids, 356
    incontinence, 354
    night sweats, 356
    passing gas, 352
    peeing, 353–54
    pelvic floor physical therapy, 355
    pooping, 354–56
    urinary tract infections, 354
    uterus, healing of, 349–51
    vaginal healing, 351–52
pica (nonfood cravings), 436, 465–66
pimples, 432
pineapple, 228
Pitocin, 266, 304
placenta, 166, **166**
    cells crossing, 160
    functions of, 166
    gas exchange and, 166
    giving birth to, 166, 265–67, 313
    human chorionic gonadotropin
        made by, 38, 73
    looking at, after birth, 166, 267
    for multiple fetuses, 166
    placentophagy (ingesting the
        placenta), 326–27
    retained placenta, 266, 475

sciatic pain, 445

seat belt, wearing while pregnant, 132

seaweed, 181

second trimester (weeks 13-27), 100, 128, 129

self-care
  on finding out you are pregnant, 77–78
  making time for, 111
  mama ritual, 205–7
  postpartum, 333–46
  while trying to conceive, 43, 45
  See also self-nurturing, postpartum

self-massage, 94

self-nurturing, postpartum, 333–46, 416–17
  birth story, writing down, 335
  bonding and taking care of newborn, 363–85
  boundaries, establishing, 336
  eating and dieting, 337, 340
  getting help, 338–39
  golden rules for, 336–39
  maternity/family leave time, 338
  nutrition, 337, 339–43
  postpartum doulas, 93, 339
  postpartum mental health, 343–45
  rules for visitors, 339
  sleep, 336
  thank-you notes, time for, 337
  trusting yourself, 337–38
  See also newborn; newborn care

semen analysis, 47

senses of baby
  hearing, 148, 155, 196
  sight, 180
  taste, 136
  touch, 160

septic miscarriage, 59

serosa (perimetrium), **26**, 27

sex
  after giving birth, 417–19
  during pregnancy, 122–24
  having to induce labor, 226
  how often to have for conception, 41
  keeping sex fun, 41, 42
  lubricants for, 122
  oral sex, 123
  orgasms and, 122–23
  oxytocin and, 226
  positions for, 122, 124

return to, after miscarriage/loss, 62
safety of, during pregnancy, 122–23
sex drive, 123–24, 419
staying horizontal after, 42
timing for insemination, 41–42
urinary tract infections (UTIs) and, 123

sex of baby
  genitals visible on ultrasound, 146
  noninvasive prenatal testing and (month 3), 117, 456
  ultrasound anatomy scan and, 144, 457

sexually transmitted infections (STIs), 470–74
  chlamydia, 471
  genital warts and HPV, 471–72
  gonorrhea, 472
  hepatitis, 472
  herpes, 472–73
  HIV, 473
  pelvic inflammatory disease (PID) and, 473
  syphilis, 473
  testing for, 103, 470
  trichomoniasis, 473–74

shaken baby syndrome, 375–76

sharing
  about miscarriage, 62–64
  about pregnancy, 109
  about trying to conceive (TTC), 17–18
  hiding the news about pregnancy, 109–10
  when to share about pregnancy, 109

shaving of pubic hair, 104

shiitake mushrooms, 181

Short-Term Disability (STD) program, 138

shortness of breath, 119, 178, 196, 212, 445–46

shoulder dystocia, 480

SIDS (sudden infant death syndrome), 372–75

sight, baby's sense of, 180

single parent, village (resources) for, 18

single parenthood, 419

sitz bath, 351, 356, 440

size of baby
  estimating with ultrasound, 214, 225–26

macrosomic (big) (9 pounds, 15 ounces), 213
  See also growth of baby

skin darkening, 99, 442

skin of baby, 163–65

skin-to-skin contact, 271–72, 477

skull of newborn, **274**, 275
  soft spots (fontanels), 274, 275

sleep hygiene, 440–41

sleep, of baby
  co-sleeping and bed sharing, 373–74
  newborns, 369–75
  safe sleep for newborn, 372–75
  SIDS prevention, 372–75
  sleep habits to establish, 370–72
  sleeping on the back, 373
  in womb, 207

sleep, of mother, 440–41
  back pain and, 429
  challenges in pregnancy, 178, 181, 196, 212
  insomnia, 440–41
  naps (for mother), 196, 248, 370, 435
  postpartum needs for, 336
  prenatal needs for, 12, 435
  sleep hygiene, 440–41
  vivid dreams, 196, 212, 449

smells, sensitivity to, 99, 116, 445

smoking, quitting, 10–11

snacks, 165, 215–16, 438, 443
  early labor snacks, 216

snoring, 161, 178, 196, 212, 446

social connections, 168–70

social interaction (of baby), 160

social media, 170

Social Security card for baby, 382

soft spots (fontanels), 274, 275

Sokunbi, Bola, 153, 154, 172

sonograms, 457–58

soothing methods for newborns (5 S's), 372

sounds
  baby's first sounds (in utero), 117
  glass bangles worn in India, 181
  heartbeat of baby, 117, 125
  music, 196
  See also hearing

soy protein, 147

work (*continued*)
Family and Medical Leave Act
(FMLA), 137, 138, 139
financial considerations, 171–72
giving 30 days' notice, 137
hiring protections, 138
how to tell workplace about your
pregnancy, 137–39
LGBTQ+ parents, 139
maternity/family leave, 137, 138,
139, 338
maternity leave around the
world, 140
month 3 issues (survival mode),
124–25
month 9 issues, 220
mother as breadwinner in
family, 172
numbers of women working
during pregnancy, 136–37
Pregnancy Discrimination Act
(PDA), 138
prepregnancy issues and
questions, 18–19
returning to, 419–21
Short-Term Disability (STD)
program, 138
survey on work and motherhood,
171–72
taking leave from, 137
workplace discrimination, 18–19
world traditions for pregnancy and
postpartum period
Brazil, 337
China, 129
Europe, 254, 259
Finland, 162
India, 181, 218
Japan, 218
Mexico, 218
Navajo, 258
Nigeria, 380
Southeast Asia, 73
wrist pain (carpal tunnel), 432–33

yeast infections, 469
yoga, prenatal, 429

Zika, 161, 469–70
zone, staying in, 184
zygote, 75

Contributors

Kymberlie Berrien is a massage therapist who bridges the health-care gap for her clients who suffer with chronic pain or disease. She partners with the medical community and assists her clients to advocate for their own health care. Using techniques that address scar tissue, trigger points, inflammation, and muscle tension, Kymberlie uses a mind-body approach that addresses the cause of pain to heal the hurt, providing lasting relief for clients who have tried many other methods without success.

She enjoys working with women; especially women who have chronic pelvic or abdominal pain or suffer with an autoimmune disorder. Kymberlie is also trained to work with pregnant women and women who are dealing with infertility and seeking a natural complement to other modalities.

Kymberlie obtained her massage training and certification through the Pennsylvania School of Muscle Therapy, graduating in 2001. She also possesses specialized training in pain management and women's health as well as being a DONA-trained birth and postpartum doula.

You can find Kymberlie at berrihealthy.net.

Sarah Bjorkman, MD, is an ob-gyn who has a passion for helping modern mamas on their journey to motherhood through evidenced-based strategies for active and healthy pregnancies. Her favorite parts of her job are getting to hand babies to her pediatrician husband and coming up with creative ways to make their two-physician life a little less wild. After completing their training at Yale, Sarah and her husband moved back to the Midwest with their golden retriever, where Sarah is pursuing her fellowship in reproductive endocrinology and infertility.

You can find Sarah at mother.ly/u/dr-sarah-bjorkman.

Brooke Cates is a certified personal trainer, pre- and postnatal corrective exercise specialist, diastasis recti and core rehabilitation specialist, and pre- and postnatal holistic health coach. She is the founder and CEO of The Bloom Method, a pre- and postnatal fitness method that is redefining exercise for the modern mom.

Brooke created The Bloom Method with a desire to empower women through movement before, during, and after their pregnancies. Recognizing gaps in both the mainstream and pregnancy fitness worlds, she created a fitness method that consists of diastasis recti rehabilitation and prevention exercises, labor training, functional exercise movements, and innovative core techniques that are designed to keep women strong and thriving through pregnancy and motherhood.

In 2018, Brooke launched the first-ever pre- and postnatal virtual fitness studio, making the education, tools, and innovative fitness classes of The Bloom Method accessible to women everywhere.

You can find Brooke at thebloommethod.com.

Tiffany Dufu is founder and CEO of The Cru, a peer-coaching service for women looking to accelerate their professional and personal growth, and the author of the bestselling book *Drop the Ball: Achieving More by Doing Less*. According to foreword contributor Gloria Steinem, *Drop the Ball* is "important, path-breaking, intimate, and brave."

Named to Fast Company's League of Extraordinary Women, Tiffany has raised nearly $20 million for the cause of women and girls. She was a launch team member for Lean In and was chief leadership officer at Levo, one of the fastest-growing millennial professional networks. Prior to that, Tiffany served as president of The White House Project, as a major gifts officer at Simmons University, and as associate director of development at Seattle Girls' School.

Tiffany is a member of Women's Forum New York and Delta Sigma Theta Sorority, Inc., and is a Lifetime Girl Scout. She serves on the board of Girls Who Code and Simmons University. She lives in New York City with her husband and two children.

You can find Tiffany at findyourcru.com.

Aimee Eyvazzadeh, MD, is a board-certified ob-gyn, specializing in reproductive endocrinology and infertility. Based in the San Francisco Bay area, and host of *The Egg Whisperer Show*, she has heard story after story from people from all over the world about their struggles trying to conceive. She has gone on a mission to promote "fertility awareness." She hopes to empower women, making them more aware of their fertility levels and allowing them to be better educated about their options.

In 2014, she launched her mission by hosting "egg freezing parties." These parties offer women a chance to learn more about their fertility and ask their questions in a comfortable, safe environment with like-minded women.

Aimee is a graduate of the UCLA School of Medicine. After completing her residency in obstetrics and gynecology at Beth Israel Deaconess Medical Center and Harvard Medical School, she completed a fellowship in reproductive endocrinology and infertility at the University of Michigan. She also completed a master's degree in public health in health management and policy at the University of Michigan.

In her off time, Aimee is a mom to four rambunctious young kids.

You can find Aimee at draimee.org.

Rachel Gorton is a Certified Infant and Toddler Sleep Consultant and Motherly's Business Development Director and resident sleep expert. She lives outside of Boston with her husband, and together they have five children. She is passionate about helping parents and children get better sleep, so they can enjoy the magical moments of parenting!

You can find Rachel at mysweetsleeper.com.

Tiffany Han's standard elevator-pitch bio would tell you that she is a writer, speaker, teacher, and life coach whose work focuses on teaching smart, driven women how to embrace a new framework of success and productivity to bring their best selves to the forefront of their lives.

But really, she teaches ambitious and capable women how to raise their hands and say yes to the lives they want for themselves—and all the things they want to do, be, and say—instead of overperforming for the sake of the life that somebody else dictates for them.

As the founder of Say Yes Creative LLC, and with a degree in psychology from the University of North Carolina at Chapel Hill and a CPCC certification from the Coaches Training Institute combined with over a decade of experience in nonprofit fundraising, marketing, and sales, she brings an abundant array of academic, professional, and personal experiences to her work.

Her job is to disrupt your status quo and help you get as uncomfortable as possible because you know as well as she does that the thing you're most afraid of is precisely what you need to move forward.

You can find Tiffany at tiffanyhan.com.

Crystal Karges, MS, RDN, IBCLC, is a maternal health specialist, child-feeding expert, and food and body image coach for mothers. Crystal is passionate about helping mamas build a peaceful relationship with food and their bodies, so they can confidently nourish themselves and their kids and bring joy back to eating. Crystal is committed to providing holistic, compassionate, and evidenced-based nutrition care to mothers and families worldwide through her online blog and virtual nutrition coaching practice.

Find more motherhood and mealtime inspiration at crystalkarges.com.

Catherine Keating is the author of *There Was Supposed to Be a Baby: A Guide to Healing After Pregnancy Loss.* Her mission is to help grieving mothers navigate through their personal healing journeys. She facilitates workshops and retreats designed to support women in tending to mind, body, and spirit to rediscover their inner wisdom and wellness. Catherine is also passionate about supporting mothers who identify as a "highly sensitive person" in finding wellness in these same spaces—mind, body, spirit. She guides women in practices to nourish themselves so that they can nourish others. Catherine lives in Seattle with her husband, two children, and sweet old pup. She spends any extra time she finds reminding women to be gentle with themselves and searching for beauty in every nook and cranny. You can find her at therewassupposedtobe .com and at catherinekeating.com.

Stepha Lawson is the artist behind the illustrations in this book. She is a birth and postpartum doula, artist, counselor, mama, and plant geek in Bellingham, Washington. She is the owner of The Language of Birth, a platform dedicated to exploring how we talk about birth today and how birth talks to us. The nuanced lens through which she approaches the field of communication with birth is reflected in her illustrations—the spirited intersection of the plant and human world, which holds timeless the cycles that seek to seed, to be born, to sprout, to grow, to wither, to die away, and then to come back again. It's a language of survival and of magic.

When she is not talking or drawing or attending births, Stepha often finds herself leading packs of kids on long adventures, hiking and singing with her sister-friends, listening to self-development books on Audible, tending to becoming a better ally, and marveling in long conversations with the world around her.

You can find Stepha at languageofbirth.com.

Sharen Medrano, IBCLC, is an International Board Certified Lactation Consultant and wellness coach living in New York with her husband and two children. She works as an IBCLC in private practice and is helping the

Rockland County Department of Health in New York create "Baby Cafés," where moms can drop in for free breastfeeding help, in order to increase breastfeeding rates in the county and reduce racial disparities.

You can find Sharen at mother.ly/u /sharen-medrano.

Claire Nicogossian, LMFT, is a licensed clinical psychologist, author, writer, and mama to four daughters and resides in Rhode Island. She has a master's degree in counseling from Marymount University and a doctorate in clinical psychology from the American School of Professional Psychology at Argosy University and has over 20 years of clinical experience providing therapy to clients with a variety of presenting issues and concerns. Claire is passionate about supporting mamas throughout all phases of motherhood, encouraging self-care practices to maintain health and well-being. Her writing and work can be found on her websites, momswellbeing.com and drclaire nicogossian.com as well as through media outlets such as Motherly, Scary Mommy, Dr. Oz, *Huffington Post*, Women's Health, WebMD, Thrive Global, The Mighty, and *Essence*. She has a podcast, *In-Session with Dr. Claire*, in which she focuses on mental health and well-being in parenthood.

Chrissy Powers, LMFT, is wife to a surfer who builds houses and mother to Waylon, Zeke, and Ruby. She is a licensed marriage and family therapist, creative career coach, and host of the *Sure, Babe Podcast*. She writes with honesty about motherhood, relationships, travel, style, and life in Southern California.

You can find Chrissy at chrissypowers.com.

Niki (Amita) Saxena, MD, has been a pediatrician since 1996. She received her undergraduate degree in biochemistry from the University of California, Berkeley, in 1986, her master's of arts in cell biology from San Francisco State University in 1989, and her master's degree in business administration from Santa Clara University in 2018. In 1993 she graduated from St. Louis University School of Medicine and then completed her internship and residency at Stanford Hospital. She is a member of the American Academy of Pediatrics, American Association for Physician Leadership, San Mateo County Medical Association (serving as president 2013–2014), Sequoia Quality Care Network Board of Directors (serving as chairperson in 2013), and the Physician Strategy and Advisory Board for Dignity Health. She also served on the Advisory Board for the Sequoia Physician's Network Independent Practice Association.

She enjoys spending time with her family (both furry and human), swimming, hiking, theater, traveling, cooking and baking, dancing, and reading.

You can find Niki at pediatricwellness group.com.

Bola Sokunbi, CFEI, is a certified financial education instructor, finance expert, influencer, and founder of Clever Girl Finance, a platform that empowers and educates women to make the best financial decisions and to pursue their dreams of financial independence, so they can live life on their own terms. Her site (clevergirlfinance.com) has been voted one of the top personal finance websites for women.

Carolyn Wagner, MA, LPC, PMH-C, is a psychotherapist in private practice in the Chicago area, specializing in perinatal mental health and trauma. She is passionate about supporting moms from preconception through empty nesting. When not working, Carolyn enjoys writing, eating, traveling, and navigating life with three young, spirited kids.

You can find Carolyn at wilmettecounseling .com.

About the Writer

Diana Spalding, MSN, CNM, is a midwife, registered pediatric nurse, mother of three, and in love with everything to do with pregnancy and birth. She attended Phillips Academy Andover and then earned a bachelor of arts in anthropology at Emory University and a bachelor of science in nursing at New York University. She worked as a pediatric oncology nurse in the Bronx and then returned to NYU, where she received her master's degree in midwifery.

Diana then had the honor of attending births at Bellevue Hospital in New York City. Her role as educator evolved as a nursing school professor at Cedar Crest College and a midwifery school advisor at Georgetown University. Diana has spent time conducting public health research in Costa Rica and served as a chairperson for the American College of Nurse-Midwives Division of Global Health.

Diana is the Digital Education Editor at Motherly and is the founder of Gathered Birth, a motherhood wellness center in Media, Pennsylvania.

Her most treasured roles are as the mother of three young children and partner to her husband, all of whom amaze, surprise, and inspire her every day.

About the Authors

Jill Koziol is the cofounder and CEO of Motherly. She resides in Silicon Valley with her husband and two daughters.

Liz Tenety is the cofounder and Chief Digital Officer of Motherly. She resides with her husband and four children in New Jersey.

About Motherly

Motherly is a modern lifestyle brand redefining motherhood. We exist to change the world on behalf of a new generation of mothers, engaging an audience of over thirty million each month as the only expert-driven, woman-centered, nonjudgmental, and empowering parenting brand. Blurring digital and physical boundaries, *The Motherly Podcast* and Motherly's book series, consumer product line, and signature events create community intimacy through offline connections. Motherly was founded in 2015 by Jill Koziol, consultant and repeat entrepreneur, and Liz Tenety, an award-winning *Washington Post* editor and digital strategist. To learn more, please visit Mother.ly or follow us on Facebook @motherlymedia and Instagram @mother.ly.

M MOTHERLY

About Sounds True

Sounds True is a multimedia publisher whose mission is to inspire and support personal transformation and spiritual awakening. Founded in 1985 and located in Boulder, Colorado, we work with many of the leading spiritual teachers, thinkers, healers, and visionary artists of our time. We strive with every title to preserve the essential "living wisdom" of the author or artist. It is our goal to create products that not only provide information to a reader or listener but also embody the quality of a wisdom transmission.

For those seeking genuine transformation, Sounds True is your trusted partner. At SoundsTrue.com you will find a wealth of free resources to support your journey, including exclusive weekly audio interviews, free downloads, interactive learning tools, and other special savings on all our titles.

To learn more, please visit SoundsTrue.com.

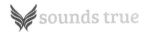 sounds true